# CORE CURRICULUM FOR PERIANESTHESIA NURSING PRACTICE

American Society of PeriAnesthesia Nurses

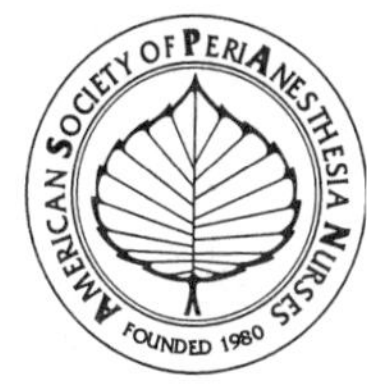


# CORE CURRICULUM FOR PERIANESTHESIA NURSING PRACTICE

## Fourth Edition

**Kim Litwack**, PhD, RN, FAAN, CFNP, CPAN, CAPA

Associate Professor
College of Nursing
University of New Mexico
Albuquerque, New Mexico

W.B. SAUNDERS COMPANY
A *Harcourt Health Sciences Company*

Philadelphia London New York St. Louis Sydney Toronto

W. B. SAUNDERS COMPANY
*A Harcourt Health Sciences Company*
The Curtis Center
Independence Square West
Philadelphia, PA 19106

**Library of Congress Cataloging-in-Publication Data**

Core curriculum for perianesthesia nursing / American Society of PeriAnesthesia Nurses : [edited by] Kim Litwack. — 4th ed.
p. cm.
Rev. ed. of: Core curriculum for post anesthesia nursing practice / [edited by] Kim Litwack. 3rd ed. c1995.
Includes bibliographical references and index.
ISBN 0-7216-7896-3
1. Post anesthesia nursing. I. Litwack, Kim. II. American Society of PeriAnesthesia Nurses. III. Core curriculum for post anesthesia nursing practice.
[DNLM: 1. Anesthesia—nursing outlines. 2. Postanesthesia Nursing outlines. 3. Perioperative Nursing outlines. WY 18.2C7972 1999]
RD51.3.C67 1999
610.73'677—dc21
DNLM/DLC

98-28129

## NOTICE

Nursing is an ever-changing field. Standard safety precautions must be followed, but as new research and clinical experience broaden our knowledge, changes in treatment and drug therapy become necessary or appropriate. Readers are advised to check the product information currently provided by the manufacturer of each drug to be administered to verify the recommended dose, the method and duration of administration, and contraindications. It is the responsibility of the treating physician relying on experience and knowledge of the patient to determine dosages and the best treatment for the patient. Neither the Publisher nor the editor assumes any responsibility for any injury and/or damage to persons or property.

THE PUBLISHER

CORE CURRICULUM FOR PERIANESTHESIA NURSING PRACTICE ISBN 0-7216-7896-3



Printed in the United States of America

Last digit is the print number: 9 8 7 6 5 4 3 2

# *Contributors*

**Deborah Brown Atsberger, MSN, RN, CPAN**

Clinical Nurse Specialist, Surgical Services, Cleveland Clinic Foundation, Cleveland, Ohio
*Interpretation of Acid-Base Balance*

**Linda M. Bernard, MS, RN**

Assistant Professor, West Suburban College of Nursing, Oak Park, Illinois
*The Pulmonary Surgical Patient*

**Tracy Britton, BSN, RN, CRNO**

Operating Room Staff Nurse, Swagel-Wootton Eye Center, Mesa, Arizona
*The Ophthalmic Surgical Patient*

**Jennifer Ruth Consla, MSN, RN, CNS, CPAN**

Perianesthesia Clinical Nurse Specialist, St. Joseph Healthcare, Albuquerque, New Mexico
*Pain Assessment and Management*

**Margaret DeFranco, MS, CRNA**

Certified Registered Nurse Anesthetist, Highland Hospital, Rochester, New York
*Fluid and Electrolyte Balance*

**Sue Dill-Calloway, JD, MSN, RN**

Director of Risk Management, Ohio Hospital Association, Columbus, Ohio
*Legal Issues in Perianesthesia Care Nursing*

**Cecil B. Drain, PhD, RN, CRNA, FAAN**

Dean, School of Allied Health Professions, Medical College of Virginia, Virginia Commonwealth University, Richmond, Virginia
*Pain Assessment and Management*

**D. George Dresden, MSN, RN, CCRN**

Staff Registered Nurse, Post Anesthesia Care Unit, St. Joseph Northeast Heights Hospital, Albuquerque, New Mexico
*Basic and Advanced Cardiac Life Support; Hemodynamic Monitoring*

**Diane E. Fritsch, MSN, RN, CCRN, CS**

Clinical Faculty, Frances Payne Bolton School of Nursing, Case Western Reserve University; Clinical Nurse Specialist, Trauma Critical Care Nursing, MetroHealth Medical Center, Cleveland, Ohio
*The Plastic Surgery and Burn Patient*

**Barbara A. Gervasio, BSN, RN, CNOR**

Surgical Service Nursing Director, Indian River Memorial Hospital, Vero Beach, Florida
*The Endocrine Surgical Patient*

**Ronald E. Harbut, PhD, MD**

Director of Anesthesia Services, Page Hospital, Page, Arizona; Samaritan Health System, Phoenix, Arizona
*Anesthetic Agents and Adjuncts*

**Frank D. Hicks, PhD, RN, CCRN**

Assistant Professor, Medical-Surgical Nursing, Niehoff School of Nursing, Loyola University Chicago, Chicago, Illinois
*The Cardiac Surgical Patient*

**William M. Kiefner, RN**

Urology Clinician, St. Joseph Medical Center, Albuquerque, New Mexico
*The Urologic Surgical Patient*

**Michael Kost, MSN, CRNA**

Program Director, Montgomery Hospital School of Anesthesia, Norristown, Pennsylvania; Adjunct Faculty, Saint Joseph's University, Philadelphia, Pennsylvania
*Conscious Sedation*

**Abigail M. Kristt, MS, RN, CCRN**

Critical Care Cardiothoracic Nursing Instructor, New York Hospital, Cornell Medical Center, New York, New York
*The Peripheral Vascular Surgical Patient*

**Kim Litwack, PhD, RN, FAAN, CFNP, CPAN, CAPA**

Associate Professor, College of Nursing, University of New Mexico, Albuquerque, New Mexico
*The Elderly Patient; Postanesthesia Complications: Respiratory, Cardiac, and Neurologic*

**Lawrence Litwack, EdD**

Professor of Counseling Psychology, Rehabilitation, and Special Education, Northeastern University, Boston, Massachusetts
*Test-Taking Techniques*

**Kathleen S. Maes, BSN, RN, CRNO**

Postanesthesia Care Unit Staff Nurse, St. Joseph Eye Surgery Center, Albuquerque, New Mexico
*The Ophthalmic Surgical Patient*

**Patricia A. Muller-Smith, EdD, RN**

Faculty, University of Tulsa, University of Oklahoma, and Northeastern Oklahoma University; Director of Education, Saint Francis Health System, Tulsa, Oklahoma
*PACU Management*

**Gratia M. Nagle, BA, CRNFA, CURN**

Surgical and Clinical Urology, Office of James R. Bollinger, MD, FACS, PC, Paoli, Pennsylvania
*The Urologic Surgical Patient*

**Gwen Lynn Nelson, MSN, RN, CNOR**

Perioperative Faculty, Delaware County Community College, Media, Pennsylvania; Clinical Educator, Valleylab, Incorporated, Boulder, Colorado
*The Gynecologic Surgical Patient*

**Debby Niehaus, BS, RN, CPAN**

Clinical Nurse III, Bethesda North Ambulatory Surgery Center, Cincinnati, Ohio
*The Surgical Patient in the Ambulatory or Short-Stay Setting*

**Denise O'Brien, BSN, RN, CPAN, CAPA**

Clinical Nurse III, Ambulatory Surgery Unit, Department of Operating Rooms/PACU, University of Michigan Health System, Ann Arbor, Michigan
*The Gastrointestinal Surgical Patient*

**Jan Odom, MS, RN, CPAN**

Clinical Nurse Specialist, Forrest General Hospital, Hattiesburg, Mississippi
*Evolution of Perianesthesia Care*

**Nancy S. Okula, BSN, RN**

Clinical Manager, PACU Anesthesiology, Egleston–Scottish Rite Children's Health Care System, Atlanta, Georgia
*The Pediatric Patient*

**Judith H. Poole, MN, RNC, FACCE**

Perinatal Outreach Education Coordinator, Department of Obstetrics and Gynecology, Carolinas Medical Center, Charlotte, North Carolina
*The Obstetric Surgical Patient*

**Laura Kull Quigley, MS, RN, ONC**

Assistant Professor, College of Nursing, Rush University; Research Assistant, Joint Replacement, Department of Orthopedic Surgery, Rush-Presbyterian–St. Luke's Medical Center, Chicago, Illinois
*The Orthopedic Surgical Patient*

**Charlene Cash Roberts, MS, RN**

Administrative Director, Ambulatory Quality, Egleston–Scottish Rite Children's Health Care System, Atlanta, Georgia
*The Pediatric Patient*

**Henry Rosenberg, MD**

Professor of Anesthesiology, Jefferson Medical College of Thomas Jefferson University; Anesthesiologist Residency Program Director, Thomas Jefferson University Hospital, Philadelphia, Pennsylvania
*Malignant Hyperthermia and Related Disorders*

**Donald Sauer, BS, RRT, RPFT**

Pulmonary Services Supervisor, Presbyterian Hospital, Albuquerque, New Mexico
*Postanesthesia Respiratory Care*

**Deborah Wright Shpritz, PhD, RN, CCRN**

Assistant Professor, University of Maryland School of Nursing, Department of Adult Health, Baltimore, Maryland
*The Neurosurgical Patient*

**Sue Silcox, AD, RN, CORLN**

Knifley, Kentucky
*The Otorhinolaryngologic and Head and Neck Surgical Patient*

**Janice Silinsky, MSA, RN, MT(ASCP)**

Director of Surgical Services, Temple University Health System, Lower Bucks Hospital, Bristol, Pennsylvania
*The Hematologic System*

**Gwen Singleton, BSN, RN, CNOR, CORLN**

Staff Nurse Level II, Neurosensory Center, The Methodist Hospital, Houston, Texas
*The Otorhinolaryngologic and Head and Neck Surgical Patient*

**Sharon L. Summers, PhD, ARNP**

Associate Professor, School of Nursing, and Family Nurse Practitioner, Family Medicine Clinic, University of Kansas Medical Center, Kansas City, Kansas
*Nursing Research*

**Mary E. Watson, MSCP, EdD, RRT**

Chair and Associate Professor of Cardiopulmonary Sciences, Northeastern University, Boston, Massachusetts
*A Systems Approach to Education of the Surgical Patient*

**Denise White, MSN, RNC**

Director, Obstetrical and Neonatal Services, University Hospital, Carolinas Healthcare System, Charlotte, North Carolina
*The Obstetric Surgical Patient*

**Maria T. Zickuhr, MSN, RN, CPAN**

Johns Hopkins Health System, Baltimore, Maryland
*Nursing Practice, Nursing Standards, and Nursing Process*

# *Reviewers*

**Barbara A. Struthers, RN, CPAN**

Commerce Township, Michigan

**Pamela E. Windle, MS, RN, CNA, CPAN, CAPA**

St. Luke's Episcopal Hospital, Houston, Texas

# *Foreword*

The practice of perianesthesia nursing continues to evolve. Advances in science, technology, surgery, anesthesia, and nursing research compel the perianesthesia nurse to update and expand his or her knowledge base. Changes in the delivery of health care include new practice settings—acute outpatient settings, office-based anesthesia delivery, and mobile surgery units. As the acuity of patients is increasing, length of stay is decreasing! Patients require educated, expert perianesthesia nurses to provide vigilant care in the critically vulnerable anesthesia recovery period. Cost-effective quality care, delivered by highly skilled, caring, intelligent nurses is the challenge for today's perianesthesia units.

The *Core Curriculum* serves as an excellent resource for perianesthesia nurses, from the beginner to the expert practitioner. It is an informative guide for students, teachers, and clinicians in this critical specialty and serves as an excellent study guide for preparing for the national perianesthesia nursing certification examinations. Revisions from the third edition reflect current concepts in perianesthesia nursing and patient care delivery. It is my hope that as you study this text, practice issues will be answered and new questions will arise that give you a deeper knowledge and understanding of perianesthesia nursing care.

**Maureen V. Iacono, BSN, RN, CPAN**
*President, American Society of PeriAnesthesia Nurses*

# Preface

The perianesthesia care nurse cares for pediatric, adult, and elderly patients. This care follows ambulatory surgical procedures and more invasive, extensive surgeries requiring inpatient hospitalization and, at times, includes intensive care. The perianesthesia care nurse cares for surgical patients with preexisting medical problems and integrates knowledge of physiology, pathophysiology, pharmacology, and nursing process in caring for patients. The perianesthesia care nurse uses principles of education in patient and family teaching and of management and administration in coordinating the delivery of patient care. The perianesthesia care nurse considers legal and ethical issues when delivering care. The content of this *Core Curriculum* is designed to reflect the scope of knowledge on which perianesthesia nursing practice is based.

This review text is designed to be a resource for perianesthesia nurses, regardless of practice setting. This text is also designed to assist the perianesthesia care nurse in preparing for the certification examination. The text is not designed as a sole reference, and the review questions are not mirror images of the certification examination. The text is designed to guide study. Each individual practitioner should assess his or her own level of experience and knowledge in developing a personal study plan.

Continuing with the successful features of the third edition of the *Core Curriculum,* this edition includes the following:

- Chapter objectives
- Chapter review questions
- Chapter-specific reference lists
- Integration of the nursing process
- Identification of nursing diagnoses

With 34 chapters, the fourth edition has added two new chapters, one on patient education and the other on intravenous conscious sedation. Every chapter continuing from the third edition was reviewed, updated, and in some cases, completely rewritten. Chapter content and review questions were reviewed for accuracy, timeliness, and clarity.

Most authors who participated in the third edition also contributed to the fourth edition. These authors, with several new contributors, were selected to provide the most current, accurate content possible. All authors are experts in their respective fields. Many are prepared at the graduate level; many are certified in their specialties.

The development of this *Core Curriculum* was sponsored and supported by the American Society of PeriAnesthesia Nurses (ASPAN).

**Kim Litwack, PhD, RN, FAAN, CFNP, CPAN, CAPA**
*Editor*

# *Acknowledgments*

The development of this *Core Curriculum* has been the work of many. I wish to thank and commend the authors who contributed chapters, responded to feedback, and, for the most part, met deadlines. This text reflects all of their expertise. I also wish to acknowledge the production work coordinated by Mary Espenschied, who was efficient, organized, and a pleasure to work with. Victoria Legnini at W.B. Saunders kept us on schedule and made sure I's were dotted and all T's were crossed. I welcome the opportunity to work with both Mary and Victoria again.

Lastly, I wish to acknowledge and thank my husband Daniel, son Jordan, and daughter Jamie for being the *Core Curriculum* of my life.

# Contents

PART ONE

# The Profession of Perianesthesia Care Nursing

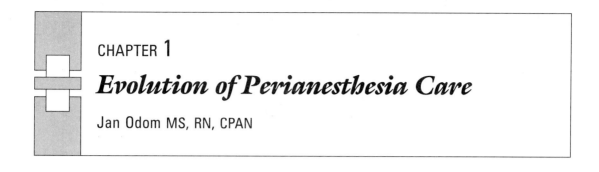

CHAPTER 1

# Evolution of Perianesthesia Care

Jan Odom MS, RN, CPAN

## OBJECTIVES

**Study of the information represented by this outline will enable the learner to:**

1. Describe three of the earliest recovery rooms.
2. Name the decade when recovery rooms became commonplace.
3. Name the one historical event that contributed most to the advent of recovery rooms.
4. Name two factors that led to the decline of recovery rooms.
5. Describe the development of the American Society of PeriAnesthesia Nurses (ASPAN).
6. List and describe three benefits brought to perianesthesia nursing by ASPAN.

Knowledge of our collective history and the evolution of postanesthesia nursing have equipped us with the tools needed to define our specialty. This knowledge is essential to developing a certification program and also guides us in resolving issues and setting goals and priorities for the specialty.

## IDENTIFICATION OF NEED FOR RECOVERY ROOM

I. **Separate Care for Postsurgical Patients**
   A. Nineteenth century
      1. New Castle Infirmary, New Castle, England (1751): rooms reserved for dangerously ill or major surgery patients
      2. Florence Nightingale, London, England (1863): separate rooms for patients to recover from immediate effects of anesthesia
   B. Twentieth century
      1. 1920s–1930s: complexity of surgeries increased
      2. 1923: Johns Hopkins Hospital, Baltimore, Maryland: three-bed neurosurgical recovery unit opened by Dandy and Firor
      3. World War II: recovery units created to provide adequate level of nursing care during nursing shortage
      4. 1942: Mayo Clinic, Rochester, Minnesota
      5. 1944: New York Hospital
      6. 1945: Ochsner Clinic, New Orleans, Louisiana

II. **Value of Recovery Room Demonstrated in Improving Surgical Care**
   A. Anesthesia Study Commission of the Philadelphia County Medical Society report (1947): one third of preventable postsurgical deaths during an 11-year period could have been prevented by improved postoperative nursing care
   B. Operating Room Committee for New York Hospital (1949): stated that adequate recovery room service was necessary for any hospital that provided surgical services

## ACCEPTANCE AND DECLINE OF RECOVERY ROOMS

**I. Impact of Changing Technology on Patient Care**
- A. 1950s: more knowledge of common postanesthesia complications
- B. 1950s–1960s: growth of surgical intensive care and postoperative respiratory support
- C. Expanding complex surgical procedures
- D. Change in anesthesia techniques and medications
- E. 1970s: recovery rooms managed routine postanesthesia patients as well as critically ill postanesthesia patients receiving respiratory and circulatory support

**II. Recovery Rooms Lose Visibility and Identity**
- A. Staffing: shortage of skilled personnel
- B. No organized body of knowledge pertinent to postanesthesia
  1. Staff performance evaluated on the basis of trial and error
  2. No territorial restrictions: in some places considered to be extension of operating room (OR)
  3. No established standards of care

## EMERGENCE OF ORGANIZED RECOVERY ROOM GROUPS

**I. Need to Identify a Special Body of Knowledge and Skills Required for Practice**
- A. Groups form to develop educational opportunities
  1. Nineteen groups organized in United States
  2. Florida Society of Anesthesiologists (FSA) initiated yearly seminar in 1969
     - a. Attended by nurses from United States and Canada
     - b. Dr. Frank McKechnie: very supportive of recovery room nurses
- B. Series of seminars sponsored by American Society of Anesthesiologists (ASA)–1970s
  1. Supported by solid attendance and strong interest
  2. Interest shown in development of recovery room nursing organization

**II. Local and State Organizations Form National Group**
- A. Regional nursing representatives met with ASA Care Team to organize national postanesthesia nurses' association
- B. Goals established
  1. Education for postanesthesia nurses
  2. Recognition of postanesthesia nursing as a specialty
- C. Steering committee formed: 1979
  1. Selection of name: American Society of Post Anesthesia Nurses (ASPAN)
  2. Preparation of bylaws
  3. Incorporation
  4. First ASPAN president: Ina Pipkin, RN, from Seattle, Washington
- D. First meeting of board of directors held October, 1980, in Orlando, Florida
- E. Charter for Component Status Granted to Alabama and Florida April 1982

## FIRST YEARS (OCTOBER 1980–APRIL 1982)

**I. Financial Development**
- A. ASA grant for legal expenses
- B. Membership dues

**II. Internal Organization Developed**
- A. Committees appointed
- B. Newsletter, *Breathline*, begun: 1981

C. Membership increased
   1. First national conference planned
   2. Regional educational meetings held

## ASPAN DEVELOPMENTS

**I. Publications**

A. 1983—*Guidelines for Standards of Care*
B. 1986—*Standards of Nursing Practice*
C. 1986—*Journal of Post Anesthesia Nursing*
D. 1986—*Post Anesthesia Nursing Review for Certification*
E. 1990—*Fifty Years of Progress in Post Anesthesia Nursing 1940–1990*
F. 1991—*Standards of Post Anesthesia Nursing Practice*
G. 1991—*Core Curriculum for Post Anesthesia Nursing Practice,* 2nd ed
H. 1992—*Standards of Post Anesthesia Nursing Practice*
I. 1992—*ASPAN Resource Manual*
J. 1993—*Postanesthesia and Ambulatory Surgery Nursing Update*—1993 (WB Saunders, publisher)
K. 1994—Pediatrics added to *Redi-Ref*
L. 1994—*ASPAN Resource Manual* published in collaboration with ABPANC
M. 1994—*Ambulatory Post Anesthesia Nursing Outline: Content for Certification*
N. 1995—*Core Curriculum for Post Anesthesia Nursing Practice,* 3rd ed
O. 1995—*Standards of Perianesthesia Nursing Practice*
P. 1996—*Certification Review for Perianesthesia Nursing* (WB Saunders, publisher)
Q. 1996—*Research Primer*
R. 1997—Competency-based orientation credentialing program
S. 1998—*Revised Redi-Ref* available
T. 1998—*Standards of Perianesthesia Nursing Practice 1998.* New additions include:
   1. Guidelines for preadmission phase
      a. Preadmission
      b. Day of surgery/procedure
   2. Guidelines for phase III (addresses ongoing care for those patients requiring extended observations/interventions after transfer/discharge from phase I or phase II)
   3. New position statements
      a. Minimum staffing in phase I PACU
      b. Registered nurse use of unlicensed assistive personnel (UAP)
      c. ICU overflow patients
U. 1999—*Core Curriculum for Ambulatory Perianesthesia Nursing Practice* (WB Saunders, publisher)
V. 1999—*Core Curriculum for Perianesthesia Nursing Practice,* 4th ed. (WB Saunders, publisher)

**II. Certification**

A. 1985: American Board of Post Anesthesia Nursing Certification (ABPANC) established
B. Certification examination developed to recognize knowledge and skill of practitioners
C. November 1986: certification examination first administered
D. Annual certified postanesthesia nurse recognition day at national conference
E. 1991: certification examination expanded to include ambulatory surgery nurses who work in preoperative and phase II areas
F. 1993–1994: separate certification examinations under development for phase I postanesthesia care unit (PACU) nurses and ambulatory postanesthesia nurses: certified postanesthesia nurse (CPAN) and certified ambulatory postanesthesia (nurse) (CAPA) designations
G. November 1994: CAPA examination first administered

H. 1996: Name changed to American Board of PeriAnesthesia Nursing Certification
I. 1998: 4191 CPANs, 1183 CAPAs, and 100 CPAN-CAPA

**III. Education**

A. National conference and annual educational program
B. Regional core curriculum workshops (2-day program available)
C. Regional ambulatory surgery workshops
D. Regional interpersonal and leadership skills workshops
E. ASPAN videotapes: overviews of postanesthesia nursing
F. National ASPAN Lecture Series established 1993
G. Joint ASPAN/AORN (Association of Operating Room Nurses) Ambulatory Surgery Symposium: 1993
H. Cosponsored Governmental Affairs Workshop with American Association of Nurse Anesthetists, the Association of Operating Room Nurses, and the American Veterans Association of Nurse Anesthetists, 1994
I. Sponsored Volunteer Leadership Institute (VLI) in Richmond, VA, September 1994
J. Participated and endorsed two AORN/Mosby seminars: Management Institute and Surgical Symposium—1995
K. Patient education videos on general anesthesia, conscious sedation, and regional anesthesia developed—1997

**IV. Specialty Representation**

A. Member of National Federation for Specialty Nursing Organizations (NFSNO) since June 1983
B. Member of National Organization Liaison Forum (NOLF)
C. Established official liaison with ASA
D. Official liaisons with following organizations
   1. Society of Gastroenterology Nurses and Associates (SGNA)
   2. Society of Critical Care Medicine (SCCM)
   3. Federated Ambulatory Surgery Association (FASA)
E. Increased networking with the following
   1. American Association of Nurse Anesthetists (AANA)
   2. Association of Operating Room Nurses (AORN)
   3. American Association of Critical Care Nurses (AACN)
F. Organizational affiliate of American Nurses' Association (ANA): 1992
G. ASPAN elected to NFSNO Executive Board 1994–1996
H. ASPAN elected to NOLF Board 1994
I. ASPAN represented at AORN Perioperative World Conference in Adelaide, Australia 1994
J. Nursing Summit held in Chicago—a coalition of all nursing leadership to discuss Nursing's Agenda for Healthcare Reform

**V. Other Highlights**

A. 1983: members encouraged to change name of workplace from recovery room to postanesthesia care unit (PACU)
B. 1989: postanesthesia nurse awareness week (PANAW) established
C. 1989: definition of immediate postanesthesia nursing expanded to include preoperative and phase II areas to incorporate ambulatory nurses working only in those areas
D. 1989: presidential award established
E. 1989: AACN formally recognized postanesthesia nursing as a critical care specialty
F. 1991: clinical excellence and outstanding achievement awards established
G. 1991: ASPAN becomes an ANA approver and provider of continuing education
H. 1992–1993: research committee offers grants and conducts Delphi study to establish postanesthesia and ambulatory surgery nursing priorities
I. 1993: American Society of Post Anesthesia Nursing Foundation established with first board of trustees

J. 1993: Organizational task force appointed to look at size and structure of ASPAN Board, dues structure, and membership voting
K. 1994: Approved concept of specialty practice groups (SPGs)
L. 1994: Ontario, Canada, becomes ASPAN's first affiliate member
M. 1994: Organizational task force conducts first planning meeting
N. 1994: Online communication by means of internet between officers and national office
O. 1995: ASPAN name change to American Society of PeriAnesthesia Nurses approved. Change took effect July 1, 1996
P. 1995: Funds for first scholarship awards donated by the ASPAN Foundation
Q. 1996: One dues structure initiated (One payment includes membership in state and national organization)
R. 1996: ASPAN website created *(http://www.aspan.org)*
S. 1996: JOPAN name changed to *Journal of PeriAnesthesia Nursing*
T. 1996: Preadmission testing SPG formed by ASPAN members
U. 1997: Newly structured board of directors met for first time April 10 in Denver, CO, after the ASPAN conference
V. 1997: ASPAN Foundation receives seat and ASPAN member attends AANA Foundation Research Scholars Program
W. 1998: First meeting of the Representative Assembly on April 21 at National Conference
X. 1998: ASPAN and the ASPAN Foundation hosted the Perioperative Temperature Consensus Conference in Bethesda, MD
Y. 1998: ASPAN membership is more than 10,000 with 40 components
Z. Management SPG formed by ASPAN members

## BIBLIOGRAPHY

American Board of PeriAnesthesia Nursing Certification: Unpublished data, 1998.

American Society of PeriAnesthesia Nurses: Personal communication. Unpublished data, 1998.

American Society of Post Anesthesia Nurses: *ASPAN Resource Manual.* Richmond, Va, The Society, 1992.

American Society of Post Anesthesia Nurses: *Fifty Years of Progress in Post Anesthesia Nursing 1940–1990.* Richmond, Va, The Society, 1990.

Bendixen H, Kinney J: History of intensive care: American College of Surgeons. In Kinney JM, Bendixen HH, Powers SR Jr (eds): *Manual of Surgical Intensive Care.* Philadelphia, WB Saunders, 1977.

Burden N: PACU nursing: Our today, our tomorrows. *J Post Anesth Nurs* 3(4):222–228, 1988.

Dunn F, Shupp M: The recovery room: A wartime economy. *Am J Nurs* 43(3):279–281, 1943.

Feeley T: The recovery room. In Miller R (ed): *Anesthesia,* vol 3, 2nd Ed. New York, Churchill Livingstone, 1986.

Fetzer SJ: Practice characteristics of the dual certificant—CPAN/CAPA. *J Perianesth Nurs* 12(4):240–244, 1997.

Frost E (ed): *Post Anesthesia Care Unit: Current Practices,* 2nd Ed. St Louis, Mosby, 1990.

Litwack K: *Post Anesthesia Care Nursing,* 2nd Ed. St Louis, Mosby–Year Book, 1995.

Luczun ME: Postanesthesia nursing: Past, present, and future. *J Post Anesth Nurs* 5(4):282–285, 1990.

Ruth H, Haugen F, Grove DD: Anesthesia study commission. *JAMA* 135(14):881–884, 1945.

Schneider M: Trends in postanesthesia nursing. *J Post Anesth Nurs* 2(3):183–188, 1987.

## REVIEW QUESTIONS

**1. The first recovery room reserved for major surgery patients was during which period?**

A. 1990s
B. 1950s
C. 1700s
D. 1800s

**2. When did recovery rooms evolve in large metropolitan hospitals?**

A. 1913–1940
B. 1875–1920
C. 1943–1970
D. 1900–1927

**3. The Anesthesia Study Commission of the Philadelphia County Medical Society found that a large percentage of postsurgical deaths could be prevented by:**

A. Better delivery of anesthesia
B. Improved postoperative nursing care
C. A decrease in rates of infection
D. More family involvement in care

**4. Recovery rooms lost identity because of what factor?**

A. No specialized equipment
B. No established standards of care
C. Too many nurses
D. Territorial restrictions

**5. Which group initiated yearly seminars?**

A. American Society of Post Anesthesia Nurses
B. American Society of Anesthesiologists
C. Florida Society of Anesthesiologists
D. American Nurses' Association

**6. What goals were established by ASPAN?**

A. Certification, publication
B. Education, recognition
C. Staffing, salary
D. Specialized equipment, seminars

**7. The first publication concerning postanesthesia nursing was:**

A. *Vital Signs*
B. *Journal of Post Anesthesia Nursing*
C. *Anesthesia Nursing*
D. *Breathline*

**8. Standards of nursing practice for postanesthesia nursing were established in what year?**

A. 1986
B. 1982
C. 1985
D. 1981

**9. The first certification examination for postanesthesia nursing was held in November 1986.**

A. True
B. False

**10. The designation for a perianesthesia nurse who receives a certification in ambulatory nursing is:**

A. Certified Associate in Perianesthesia Nursing (CAPN)
B. Certified Outpatient Surgery Nurse (COSN)
C. Certified Ambulatory PeriAnesthesia Nurse (CAPA)
D. Certified Post Anesthesia Nurse (CPAN)

**ANSWERS:** 1. D, 2. A, 3. B, 4. B, 5. C, 6. B, 7. D, 8. A, 9. A, 10. C

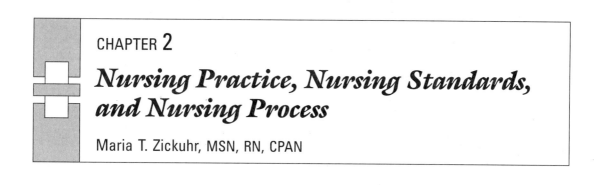

CHAPTER 2

# Nursing Practice, Nursing Standards, and Nursing Process

Maria T. Zickuhr, MSN, RN, CPAN

## OBJECTIVES

**Study of the information represented by this outline will enable the learner to:**

1. Describe the components of the nursing process.
2. Give examples of nursing diagnoses from a patient assessment.
3. Use patient assessment findings to plan and implement nursing care.
4. Describe the Nursing Interventions Classification/Nursing Outcomes Classification (NIC/NOC) System for clinical practice of choosing interventions and evaluating outcomes.
5. Give examples of process, outcome, and structure using perianesthesia nursing standards.

Standards are the foundation from which the nurse develops and expands an individual level of service. Standards not only help delineate the scope of practice but also become a tool for the nurse to facilitate each step of the nursing process. Professional nursing practice is composed of delegated, interdependent, and independent service to patients (process standards), standards of care (outcome standards), and structure standards. These standards provide the common ground for basic practice accountability.

The nursing process is the basis for all nursing action and is the essence of professional perianesthesia nursing practice. The ASPAN standard of nursing practice supports the nursing process and generic American Nurses Association (ANA) standards of nursing practice (Table 2–1). The nursing process is a problem-solving method to provide comprehensive, planned care. The process is cyclic, and the components are interrelated. During the perioperative period, it provides continuity of care among phases: preanesthesia phase, postanesthesia care in phase I, and postanesthesia care in phase II.

## NURSING PRACTICE

**I. Three Categories of Nursing Care Delivery in Perianesthesia Nursing Practice**

A. Delegated category: services nurses deliver in response to physicians' orders
   *Focus:* medical diagnosis or physicians' postoperative orders

B. Interdependent category: services nurses provide because patient has a particular health problem, medical diagnosis, or treatment plan
   *Focus:* judgments related to the task

C. Independent category: services nurses provide because patient has a particular human response or nursing diagnosis
   *Focus:* nursing diagnosis

**II. Types of Nursing Practice**

A. Institutional nursing: dependent, task-dominated practice wherein nursing service is dictated only by physicians' orders, hospital policies, and procedures

**TABLE 2–1** Relationship of *ANA Standards of Nursing Practice* (1973) and *ASPAN Standards of Nursing Practice* (1998) to Nursing Process

| NURSING PROCESS | ASSESSMENT/ DATA COLLECTION | DIAGNOSIS | PLANNING | | IMPLEMENTATION | | EVALUATION | |
|---|---|---|---|---|---|---|---|---|
| *ANA Standards of Nursing Practice* | I<br>Assessment and data collection are systematic and continuous; data accessibly communicated and recorded | II<br>Nursing diagnoses derived from health status data | III<br>Plan includes goals derived from nursing diagnoses | IV<br>Plan includes priorities and approaches to achieve goals derived from nursing diagnoses | V<br>Nursing action—provide for client participation and health promotion, maintenance | VI<br>Nursing action—assist client to maximize health capabilities | VII<br>Progress toward goal achievement is determined by patient and nurse | VIII<br>Client's progress directs new goal setting and plan revision |
| *ASPAN Standards of Nursing Practice* | VII<br>**Assessment**<br>Post anesthesia nursing practice includes systematic, continuous assessment of patient's condition; nurse ensures data are collected, documented, and communicated; professional nurse analyzes data to determine appropriate nursing interventions | | VIII<br>**Planning and Implementation**<br>Professional nurse designs and coordinates implementation of plan of care to achieve patient outcomes | | | | IX<br>**Evaluation**<br>Professional nurse continuously measures patient's progress toward designated outcomes and revises plan of care and interventions as necessary | |

B. Professional nursing: practice that includes all three categories of nursing service: delegated, interdependent, and independent

## NURSING STANDARDS

**I. Three Types of Nursing Standards**

A. Structure standards: statements describing valued attributes of the setting that directly or indirectly influence care; for example:

1. Equipment, physical plant requirements, education, annual cardiopulmonary resuscitation (CPR) recertification, staff mix, staff/patient ratios, specific policies and procedures, and teaching resources

B. Process standards: statements or standards of nursing practice delineate nursing activities or interventions to meet expected patient outcome; for example:

1. The nurse will assess patient's learning needs (preanesthesia).
2. The nurse will assess patient's level of pain (postanesthesia, phase I).
3. The nurse will provide home care instruction (postanesthesia, phase II).

C. Outcome standards: statements or standards of care that delineate expected outcomes on the basis of patient problems or nursing diagnosis; for example:

1. The patient's anxiety will be reduced to a mild level (preanesthesia)
2. The patient's pain will be reduced to a mild level (postanesthesia, phase I)
3. The patient will understand the actions and side effects of prescribed take-home medication (postanesthesia, phase II)

**II. Standards Define the Substance of Professional Nursing Practice by Delineating Scope and Content of Nursing Care**

Structure standards provide support and directly or indirectly influence that care. Both process and outcome standards are needed to define nursing care for a given nursing diagnosis or patient problem.

## COMPONENTS OF NURSING PROCESS

**I. Identification of Components** (Fig. 2–1)

A. Assessment
B. Nursing diagnosis
C. Planning

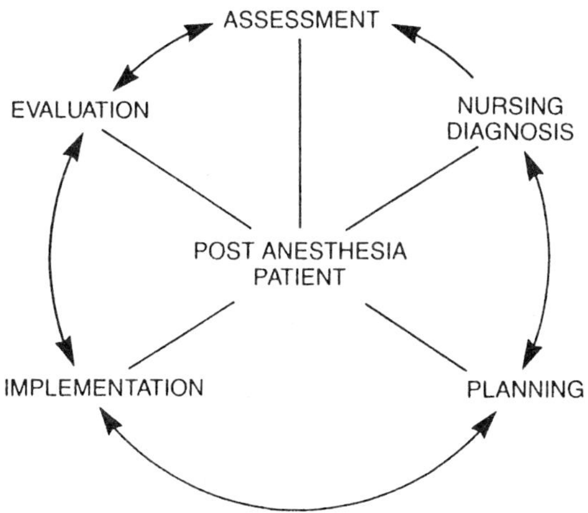


**FIGURE 2–1** Components of the nursing process.

D. Implementation
E. Evaluation/reassessment

**II. Utilization of Components**

A. Assessment
1. Critical base on which to build other components
a. Health status data (history)
(1) Physical
(2) Psychosocial: emotional, developmental, social, intellectual, and spiritual
b. Physical assessment
2. Sources for data collection
a. Preoperative teaching and interview of patient
b. Report from anesthesia care provider
c. Review of records
d. Patient's history up to point of admission
e. Initial physical assessment
f. Frequent reassessment to maintain current database

B. Nursing diagnosis*
1. Statement of potential or actual altered health status of patient (derived from assessment)
2. Requires intervention appropriate to the domain of nursing practice
3. Consists of three elements
a. Problem statement (P)
*Example:* anxiety, severe
b. Etiology or related factors (E)
*Example:* related to fear of surgical procedure
c. Defining cluster of signs and symptoms (S)
*Example:* increased pulse, increased blood pressure
4. Nursing diagnoses relevant to preanesthesia patient, postanesthesia phase-I patient, and postanesthesia phase-II patient include but are not limited to:
a. Activity intolerance
b. Airway clearance, ineffective
c. Anxiety
d. Aspiration, risk for
e. Body image disturbance
f. Body temperature, risk for altered
g. Breathing pattern, ineffective
h. Cardiac output, decreased
i. Communication, impaired verbal
j. Confusion, acute
k. Fear
l. Fluid volume deficit
m. Fluid volume excess
n. Gas exchange impaired
o. Grieving
p. Hyperthermia
q. Hypothermia
r. Individual coping, ineffective
s. Infection, risk for
t. Injury, risk for

---

*For complete listing and definitions of nursing diagnoses, see North American Nursing Diagnosis Association: *NANDA Nursing Diagnoses: Definition and Classification 1995–1996*. Philadelphia, The Association, 1994.

u. Knowledge deficit (specify)
v. Noncompliance (specify)
w. Pain
x. Peripheral neurovascular dysfunction, risk for
y. Physical mobility, impaired
z. Skin integrity, impaired
aa. Tissue perfusion, altered (specify)
bb. Urinary elimination, altered
cc. Urinary retention
dd. Ventilation, inability to sustain spontaneous
ee. Ventilation weaning response, dysfunction

5. North American Nursing Diagnosis Association (NANDA)
   a. Group of nurses and nurse educators whose task is to identify and define nursing diagnoses
   b. Publishes updated classification annually
      North American Nursing Diagnosis Association
      1211 Locust St.
      Philadelphia, PA 19107-5409
      1-800-647-9002
      www.nanda.org

C. Planning
   1. Systematic method of achieving outcomes established for each patient and done in each phase of the perioperative period
      a. Prioritize nursing diagnoses
      b. Formulate patient goals (expected outcomes)
      c. Plan alternative interventions
      d. Select nursing actions
   2. Preanesthesia goal: adequately prepare patient for surgery
      a. Physically
      b. Emotionally
      c. Psychologically
   3. Postanesthesia care, phase-I goal: smooth emergence from anesthesia
      a. Return patient to safe physiologic level
      b. Avoid complications of anesthesia
   4. Postanesthesia care, phase-II goal: assist patient in returning to safe functional level
      a. Meet written discharge criteria
      b. Provide appropriate knowledge base for home care
   5. Plan includes family
      a. Short-term expected outcomes set and discussed
      b. Outcomes must be met before discharge

D. Implementation
   1. Initiate plan or nursing interventions
   2. Each identified problem or nursing diagnosis has implications for intervention
   3. Alter plan to meet changing needs throughout perioperative period

E. Evaluation
   1. Continually evaluate responses to interventions
   2. Determine whether expected outcomes have been achieved
   3. Alter plan and nursing diagnosis as appropriate to meet changing needs
   4. Document effectiveness of intervention on patient care record
   5. Discharge summary documents evaluation of plan of care
      a. Reflects nursing process
      b. Includes:
         (1) Short-term expected outcomes that were met
         (2) Patient's current status

(3) Evaluation of patient's response to care
(4) Any special needs identified that must be included in next phase of care
6. Summary and report are transmitted to nurse responsible for next phase

## NIC/NOC SYSTEM LINKED TO NURSING DIAGNOSES

**I. Nursing Interventions Classification (NIC), Iowa Intervention Project**

A. Standardized classification of nursing interventions
1. Comprehensive (433)
2. Research-based
3. Developed deductively on the basis of practice
4. Funded by grants: National Institute of Health, National Institute of Nursing Research, Rockefeller Foundation
5. Recognized by the American Nurses Association (ANA)
6. May be linked to NANDA nursing diagnoses and NOC outcomes

B. Purpose
1. Standardize documentation
2. Provide choice of nursing interventions for a particular patient by using clinical decision making
3. Communicate treatment to other providers in a standard way
4. Provide clinical data elements for automated patient record
5. Determine cost of services provided by nurses.
6. Provide a unified nursing database to be used in the Nursing Minimum Data Set

**II. Nursing Outcomes Classification (NOC), Iowa Outcome Project**

A. Standardized classification describing patient outcomes that are responsive to nursing interventions
1. Comprehensive (190)
2. Research-based
3. Developed inductively and deductively
4. Funded by grants from the National Institute of Health, National Institute of Nursing Research, Sigma Theta Tau
5. Recognized by ANA as a classification in development
6. May be linked to NANDA nursing diagnoses (Table 2–2) and NIC interventions

B. Purpose
1. Standardize documentation
2. Provide a measure of quality on a continuum using a 5-point Likert scale rather than as discrete goals met or not met
3. Used for individual patients or groups of patients in critical paths
4. Communicates outcomes to other providers in a standard way
5. Provides clinical data elements for the Nursing Minimum Data Set to be used in automated patient records

**III. Linkage between NANDA Nursing Diagnoses, NIC, and NOC**

A. Purpose for the linkage
1. Nursing diagnoses linked to nursing interventions will provide identification of specific nursing interventions or treatments that nurses may choose to implement to resolve a specific nursing diagnosis
2. Nursing diagnoses linked to nursing outcomes will provide identification of specific outcomes that nurses may choose to monitor in patients with a specific nursing diagnosis

B. Uses of the three linked classifications
1. Individual patient plans of care
2. Grouping of patients by care paths or critical paths
3. Computer-based orientation program

**TABLE 2–2** Process of Assessing NOC Outcomes

| NURSING DIAGNOSIS | NOC OUTCOME* | NOC RATING SCALE | | | | |
|---|---|---|---|---|---|---|
| | | 1 | 2 | 3 | 4 | 5 |
| 1. Activity intolerance | Self-care—activities of daily living (ADL) | Never | Rarely | Sometimes | Often | Consistently demonstrates |
| 2. Airway clearance ineffective | Respiratory status; ventilation | Extremely | Substantially | Moderately | Mildly | Not compromised |
| 3. Anxiety | Anxiety control | Never | Rarely | Sometimes | Often | Demonstrates consistently |
| 4. Aspiration, risk for | Neurologic status | Extremely | Substantially | Moderately | Mildly | Not compromised |
| 5. Body image disturbance | Body image (adjust to change in physical appearance) | Never | Rarely | Sometimes | Often | Consistently positive |
| 6. Body temperature, risk for altered | Infection status | Severe | Substantially | Moderately | Slight | None |
| 7. Breathing pattern, ineffective | Muscle function | Extremely | Substantially | Moderately | Mildly | Not compromised |
| 8. Cardia output, decreased | Vital signs status | Extremely | Substantially | Moderately | Mildly | No deviation from expected range |
| 9. Communication, improved verbal | Cognitive orientation (identify person, place, time) | Never | Rarely | Sometimes | Often | Demonstrates consistently |
| 10. Confusion, acute | Neurologic status; consciousness | Extremely | Substantially | Moderately | Mildly | Not compromised |
| 11. Fear | Fear control | Never | Rarely | Sometimes | Often | Consistently demonstrates |
| 12. Fluid volume deficit | Hydration | Extremely | Substantially | Moderately | Mildly | Not compromised |
| 13. Fluid volume excess | Fluid balance | Extremely | Substantially | Moderately | Mildly | Not compromised |
| 14. Gas exchange, impaired | Respiratory status: gas exchange | Extremely | Substantially | Moderately | Mildly | Not compromised |
| 15. Grieving | Grief resolution | Not at all | To a slight extent | To a moderate extent | To a great extent | To a very great extent |
| 16. Hyperthermia | Thermoregulation | Extremely | Substantially | Moderately | Mildly | Not compromised |
| 17. Hypothermia | Thermoregulation | Extremely | Substantially | Moderately | Mildly | Not compromised |
| 18. Individual coping, ineffective | Coping | Never | Rarely | Sometimes | Often | Consistently demonstrates |
| 19. Infection, risk for | Fever | Severe | Substantially | Moderately | Slight | None |
| 20. Injury, risk for | Safety status; physical injury | Severe | Substantially | Moderately | Slight | None |
| 21. Knowledge deficit (specify) | Knowledge: prescribed activity, medication | None | Limited | Moderately | Substantial | Extensive |
| 22. Noncompliance (specify) | Compliance behavior | Never | Rarely | Sometimes | Often | Consistently demonstrates |
| 23. Pain | Pain level | Severe | Substantially | Moderately | Slight | None |
| 24. Peripheral neurovascular dysfunction, risk for | Tissue perfusion: peripheral | Extremely | Substantially | Moderately | Mildly | Not compromised |
| 25. Physical mobility, impaired | Mobility level | Dependent does not participate | Requires assistive person & device | Requires assistive person | Independent with assistive person | Completes independently |
| 26. Skin integrity, impaired | Tissue integrity: skin & mucous membrane | Extremely | Substantially | Moderately | Mildly | Not compromised |
| 27. Tissue perfusion altered (specify) | Tissue integrity: peripheral | Extremely | Substantially | Moderately | Mildly | Not compromised |
| 28. Urinary elimination, altered | Urinary elimination | Extremely | Substantially | Moderately | Mildly | Not compromised |
| 29. Urinary retention | Urinary elimination | Extremely | Substantially | Moderately | Mildly | Not compromised |
| 30. Ventilation, inability to sustain spontaneous | Muscle functions | Extremely | Substantially | Moderately | Mildly | Not compromised |
| 31. Ventilatory weaning response, dysfunction | Respiratory status; ventilation | Extremely | Substantially | Moderately | Mildly | Not compromised |

*This table provides an example of one possible outcome with each diagnosis and demonstrates how the outcome would be assessed using the outcome scale. Many outcomes are possible with each diagnosis.

4. Outcome measurement
5. Research

C. The classification systems: NIC, NOC, ND, and what they are not
1. The classification systems are not prescriptive
2. The outcome classification does not evaluate organizational performance
3. The outcome classification system is not specific for a particular nursing diagnosis or nursing intervention because the nurse must choose on the basis of clinical judgment
4. The outcomes are not nursing diagnoses, although they assess the same patient status
5. Patient goals are not "met or not met" but are assessed on a 5-point measurement scale
6. The outcome system is not subjective because the nurse evaluates whether the outcome is met on the basis of specific indicators for each outcome

**IV. Process to Implement into Clinical Practice*†**

A. Assess patient
B. Choose NANDA nursing diagnosis on the basis of the problem, etiology, and symptoms
C. Choose the expected outcome from the NOC outcomes before specifying the NIC intervention because the expected nursing outcome serves as the criteria from which to judge the success of a nursing intervention
D. Choose from the specific indicators listed for each outcome
E. After selecting the NOC outcome and indicators, the nurse determines the point on the outcome scale (1–5) that is the desired outcome for this individual patient. This is done for each outcome and indicator
F. The nurse then chooses the NIC interventions on the basis of clinical judgment
G. The nurse obtains a baseline rating of the patient's condition with the 1–5 outcome scale and then implements the plan of care, interventions, and treatments
H. The patient is reevaluated at specified intervals and at the time of discharge by using the outcome scale

***Summary of NIC/NOC System for Clinical Practice***

| | |
|---|---|
| **Assess** | Assess patient |
| **Plan** | Choose nursing diagnosis |
| | Choose outcome, indicators, and desired ratings |
| | Choose nursing interventions |
| | Obtain baseline ratings |
| **Implement** | Implement nursing interventions |
| **Evaluation** | Rate at intervals and at discharge |

## SUMMARY OF NURSING PROCESS IN PREANESTHESIA PHASE, POSTANESTHESIA PHASE I, AND POSTANESTHESIA PHASE II

**I. Assessment**

A. Collection of data
1. Preoperative patient interview
2. Preoperative chart review
3. Preanesthesia evaluation
4. Anesthesiologist's postanesthesia report

---

*For complete listing and definitions of standard NIC interventions see McCloskey J, Bulechek G (eds): *Iowa Intervention Project: Nursing Intervention Classification (NIC),* 2nd Ed. St Louis, Mosby, 1996.

†For complete listing, definitions, and ratings of standard NOC outcomes see Johnson M, Maas M (eds): *Iowa Outcomes Project: Nursing Outcomes Project: Nursing Outcomes Classification (NOC).* St Louis, Mosby, 1997.

5. Operating room (OR) nurse's report
6. Postanesthesia nurse's chart review
7. Postanesthesia nurse's physical assessment
   a. Phase I
   b. Phase II

B. Analysis of data
1. Implications of physical, psychologic, and sociologic status of patient
2. Relate implications to operative procedure to be performed

**II. Nursing Diagnosis**

A. Nurse-patient identification of problems amenable to nursing interventions
B. Nursing diagnosis statement
1. Problem statement
2. Etiology or related factors
3. Signs and symptoms

**III. Planning**

A. Identification of nursing actions to treat problems amenable to nursing interventions
B. Short-term goals: expected outcomes
C. Long-term goals: expected outcomes

**IV. Implementation: Nursing Actions According to Plan of Care**

**V. Evaluation: Patient's Response to Nursing Actions**

**VI. Reassessment: Preanesthesia and Postanesthesia Nurses' Continuing Assessments**

## BIBLIOGRAPHY

American Association of Critical Care Nurses: *Outcome Standards for Nursing Care of the Critically Ill.* Laguna Niguel, Calif, The Association, 1990.

American Society of PeriAnesthesia Nurses: *Standards of Perianesthesia Nursing Practice.* Richmond, Va, The Society, 1998.

Bellack J, Edlund B: *Nursing Assessment and Diagnosis,* 2nd Ed. Boston, Jones and Bartlett, 1992.

Bulechek GM et al: Report on the NIC Project: Nursing interventions used in practice. *Am J Nurs* 49(10): 59–66, 1994.

Bulechek GM, McCloskey JC (eds): *Symposium on Nursing Interventions (Nurs Clin North Am).* Philadelphia, Saunders, 1992.

Bulechek GM, McCloskey JC (eds): *Nursing Interventions: Essential Nursing Treatments,* 2nd Ed. Philadelphia, Saunders, 1992.

Bulechek GM, McCloskey JC, Donahue W: Nursing Interventions Classification (NIC): A language to describe nursing treatments. In Lang NM, (ed): *Nursing Data Systems: The Emerging Framework* (pp 115–131). Washington, DC, American Nurses Association, 1995.

Johnson M, Maas M (eds): *Iowa Outcomes Project: Nursing Outcomes Classification (NOC).* St Louis, Mosby, 1997.

Carlson JH et al: *Nursing Diagnosis: A Case Study Approach.* Philadelphia, Saunders, 1991.

Carpenito LJ: *Nursing Diagnosis: Application to Clinical Practice,* 4th Ed. Philadelphia, JB Lippincott, 1992.

Doenges M, Moorhouse M: *Application of Nursing Process and Nursing Diagnosis: An Interactive Text.* Philadelphia, FA Davis, 1992.

Doyer B, Macker N, Radovich H: Functional health patterns: The post anesthesia care unit's approach to identification. *J Post Anesth Nurs* 5(3):157–162, 1990.

Gay CR: The development of a post anesthesia record incorporating the nursing process. *J Post Anesth Nurs* 5(2):85–90, 1990.

Gettrust K, Brabec P: *Nursing Diagnosis in Clinical Practice: Guides for Care Planning.* New York, Delmar, 1992.

Griffith-Kenney J, Christensen P: *Nursing Process Application of Theories, Frameworks, and Models,* 2nd Ed. St Louis, Mosby, 1986.

Kim M, McFarland G, McLane A: *Pocket Guide to Nursing Diagnoses,* 4th Ed. St Louis, Mosby, 1991.

Ledrer J et al: *Care Planning Pocket Guide,* 4th Ed. Redwood City, Calif, Addison-Wesley Nursing, 1991.

Lewis JM, Beaulieu J: Application of nursing diagnosis to the PAR scoring system, *J Post Anesth Nurs* 2(4): 237–243, 1987.

McCloskey J, Bulechek G (eds): *Iowa Intervention Project: Nursing Interventions Classification (NIC),* 2nd Ed. St Louis, Mosby, 1996.

McCloskey JC, Bulechek GM: Defining and classifying nursing interventions. In Moritz P (ed): *Patient Outcomes Research: Examining the Effectiveness of Practice: Proceedings of the State of the Science Conference* (NIH Pub No 93-3411; pp 63–69). Washington, DC, National Institute of Nursing Research, 1993.

McCloskey JC, Bulechek GM: *Classification of Nursing Diagnoses: Proceedings of the Tenth Conference* (pp. 113–125). Philadelphia, JB Lippincott, 1994.

McFarland GK, McFarlane EA: *Nursing Diagnoses and Intervention: Planning for Patient Care,* 2nd Ed. St Louis, Mosby, 1993.

North American Nursing Diagnosis Association: *NANDA Nursing Diagnoses: Definition and Classification 1995–1996.* Philadelphia, The Association, 1994.

Pinkley CL: Exploring NANDA's definition of nursing diagnosis: Linking diagnostic judgements with the selection of outcomes and interventions. *Nursing Diagn* 2(1):26–32, 1991.

Pritchard V, Eckard JM: Standards of nursing care in the post anesthesia unit. *J Post Anesth Nurs* 5(3):P163–167, 1990.

Steelman V, Bulechek GM, McCloskey JC: Toward a standardized language to describe perioperative nursing. *Am Operating Room Nurses J* 60:786–795, 1994.

Summers S: Using nursing diagnosis to document care in the post anesthesia unit. *J Post Anesth Nurs* 4(5): 306 311, 1989.

Titler MG: Research for practice: Using NIC in nursing practice. *MEDSURG Nurs* 3(4):300–302, 1994.

Titler MG, Bulechek GM, McCloskey JC: Use of the nursing interventions classification by critical care nurses. *Crit Care Nurse,* 16(4):38–40, 45–54, Aug. 1996.

Werley HH, Lang NM (eds): *Identification of the Nursing Minimum Data Set.* New York, Springer, 1988.

Wesorick B: *Standards of nursing care: A model for Clinical Practice.* Philadelphia, JB Lippincott, 1990.

Wong DL: *Whaley and Wong's Essentials of Pediatric Nursing,* 4th Ed. St Louis, Mosby, 1993.

Zickuhr M: American Society of Post Anesthesia Nursing. In *Classification of Nursing Diagnoses, Proceedings of the Ninth Conference, NANDA.* Philadelphia, JB Lippincott, 1991.

## REVIEW QUESTIONS

**1. Which of the following is not a component of the nursing process?**

A. Implementation
B. Nursing diagnosis
C. Documentation
D. Assessment

**2. From what sources should assessment data be collected?**

A. Medical records
B. Physical assessment
C. Anesthesia report
D. All of the above
E. None of the above

**3. Nursing diagnosis:**

A. Consists of two elements, symptoms related to a cause
B. Requires intervention appropriate to the domain of nursing practice
C. Uses interdependent interventions to achieve the goal
D. Allows nurses to diagnose and treat patients

**4. What two elements are part of the planning stage of the nursing process?**

A. Standardized outcomes and interventions
B. Set of interventions and predefined evaluations
C. Plan of care and individually set goals
D. Lists of problems and goals

**5. The evaluation stage is:**

A. Continual assessment of patient responses to nursing interventions
B. Documentation of unmet goals
C. Documentation of medical orders carried out
D. None of the above

**6. Which is a correct statement about standards?**

A. Standards of nursing practice focus on patient outcomes
B. Outcome standards delineate nursing activities or interventions
C. Structure standards describe the setting that influences care
D. Process standards are standards of care

**7. Which statement is an outcome standard?**

A. The patient will receive a nursing assessment on admission to postanesthesia care unit (PACU)
B. The patient's airways are clear bilaterally
C. The patient's plan of care is evaluated before discharge
D. The patient's anxiety level is assessed on admission and discharge

**8. When assessing outcomes using the NIC/NOC System**

A. The nurse obtains a baseline rating of the outcome before implementing interventions
B. The nurse specifies nursing interventions from the Nursing Intervention Classification on the basis of clinical judgment
C. The patient is reevaluated at intervals and at discharge by use of the outcome scale
D. The nurse chooses specific indicators with each chosen outcome
E. All of the above

**ANSWERS:** 1. C, 2. D, 3. B, 4. C, 5. A, 6. C, 7. B, 8. E

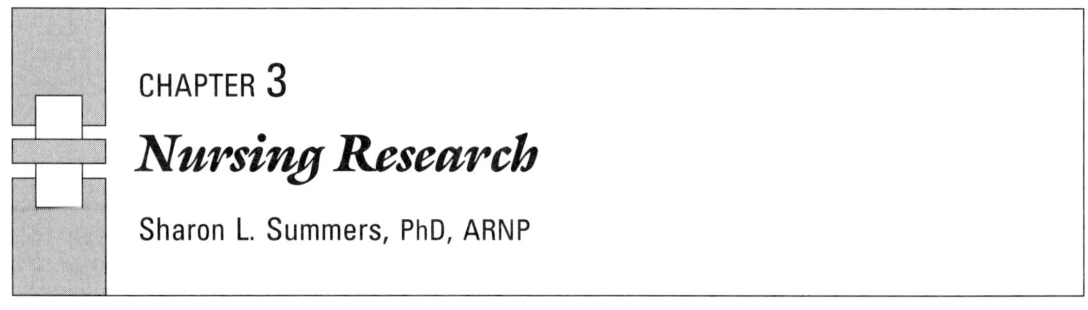

CHAPTER 3

# *Nursing Research*

Sharon L. Summers, PhD, ARNP

## OBJECTIVES

**Study of the information in this outline will enable the learner to:**

1. Define nursing research.
2. Describe the purposes of nursing research.
3. Explore why research is important for perianesthesia care unit (PACU) nurses.
4. Describe the steps in the research proposal and process.

## I. Definition of Nursing Research

A. Scientific method: controlled, systematic process for conducting studies in which data are collected under constant conditions to decrease error so that all data are collected in the same manner

B. Research: process of applying the scientific method to answer questions

C. Nursing research: process of applying the scientific method to answer questions about nursing education, nursing practice, and nursing administration

D. Subsets of these categories: studies about nurses and what nurses do in multisite multiunit care

## II. Purposes of Nursing Research

A. To apply the steps of the scientific method to answer questions or solve problems relevant to nurses and nursing practice

B. To replace trial-and-error method of data collection

C. To build nursing knowledge so that other professions do not dictate nursing practice methods that have not been validated with studies

D. For PACU nurse: studies that make an impact on the nurse and the delivery of nursing care to PACU patients

E. Therefore, to validate nursing practice to determine that what nurses do affects patient recovery

1. For example, many nursing procedures have been handed down from medicine with little or no research support
    a. Irrigating heparin locks with saline and heparin was handed down to nursing when the locks were used exclusively to inject heparin
    b. When heparin locks were used for "keep open" purposes, the saline or heparin procedure continued to be ordered
    c. Nurses' research concluded that no significant difference was found between irrigating the heparin lock with saline or heparin, and changes in institutional practices resulted

## III. Importance of Research for PACU Nurses

A. Needed to validate PACU nursing practice and to provide scientific explanations for nursing actions

1. PACU procedures handed down from anesthesia and surgery need to be validated; e.g., cough, turn, and deep breathe (CTBD)
   a. Dripps and Waters (1941) published the "stir-up" procedure to be used by nurses; article was subjective and did not cite research on which to base the need for this nursing procedure
   b. Thoren (1953) supplied research data to indicate that postcholecystectomy patients who had instructions in deep breathing, turning, and coughing with postural drainage before and after surgery had a significantly lower incidence of pulmonary complications and lower temperatures and required fewer antibiotics than patients who did not have instructions or the procedures performed
   c. Lindeman and Van Aernam (1971) validated effectiveness of this procedure in a nursing study
   d. Breslin (1981) determined that coughing was detrimental to patients without preexisting pulmonary congestion and suggested screening for patients at high risk of pulmonary complications, restricting CTDB to these patients
   e. Procedure needs to be studied by nurses to validate CTDB procedure and to explore use of techniques and technology developed since these older studies were conducted

## IV. The Research Proposal Development

A. Must precede a study for three reasons:
   1. Assists researcher to think through all steps in study so nothing is missed and to make changes before investing time and money into methods that may not yield answers to research questions or hypotheses
   2. Encourages researcher to plan study with such clarity that it can be replicated
   3. Provides an opportunity for peer review: constructive criticism from others who are knowledgeable about topic and research process for purpose of strengthening study
B. Human subjects committee or institutional review board (IRB) review is concerned with protection of human subjects; although these committees also provide peer review, they are primarily interested in ethical concerns, including:
   1. Protection of subjects from physical and psychologic harm
   2. Methods to maintain subject's anonymity and confidentiality
   3. Methods by which subjects are fully informed, including consent forms that require subject's signature
   4. Methods by which subjects can withdraw from a study without prejudice to their care
   5. Where the researcher can be contacted for further information
C. Research proposal contains steps from problem to data analysis as listed below; research report contains all steps listed below; published articles usually contain all steps in abbreviated form

## V. Steps in Research Process

A. Introduction and problem
   1. Introduction defines problem and provides background information so reader can understand why study needs to be conducted
      a. For example, an introduction could consist of one or two paragraphs that discuss PACU standards of care and staffing; it could then conclude with a problem statement describing whether a critically ill surgical patient should recover in PACU or ICU and what happens when either unit is short staffed or it is the midnight shift
B. Purpose
   1. Broad discussion given in introduction; problem then narrowed to describe purpose of study
      a. In the example above, the purpose of the study might be written as: the purpose of this study is to determine whether the quality of perianesthesia care delivered in the PACU differs from the perianesthesia care delivered in the ICU

C. Research question or hypothesis
   1. Purpose of study narrowed further to formulate research question or hypothesis
   2. Research questions are stated as questions and used when little is known about topic
      a. For the example above, the research question might be stated as: what is the difference between PACU nursing care and ICU nursing care of critically ill perianesthesia patients?
   3. Hypothesis (or hypotheses) is a specific sentence that may be stated as null (no significant difference) or directional (*X* significantly greater than *Y*); used when researcher has sufficient information about a topic to write a statement of expected outcomes or directions of outcomes
      a. For example, a null hypothesis might be stated: there is no significant difference in quality of care delivered by PACU nurses and ICU nurses when caring for critically ill perianesthesia patients
      b. Directional hypothesis may be stated: PACU nurses will provide significantly higher quality of care than ICU nurses when caring for critically ill perianesthesia patients

D. Variables
   1. Research question or hypothesis contains concepts to be studied
   2. Concept in preceding example is quality nursing care
   3. Concepts that can be measured are known as variables
      a. For example, quality nursing care can be measured with a questionnaire in which items are based on PACU nursing standards; quality of nursing care (a concept) becomes a variable because it is measurable
      b. Variables then refer to anything measured in a study, including demographic variables such as age, sex, and marital status or quality of nursing care
   4. Two other types of variables also used in research studies
      a. Independent and dependent variables are labels used in experimental and quasi-experimental designed studies when researcher introduces an intervention or does something to a subject; the intervention is the independent variable, and the outcome is the dependent variable
         (1) For example, a patient rewarming device could be considered an independent variable (intervention), and patient thermal comfort scores could be considered a dependent variable (outcome)

E. Theory, conceptual framework, or model
   1. Guides research studies
   2. Provides method where knowledge derived from a study can be incorporated or added to a body of previously existing knowledge; important so that conclusions do not stand as facts isolated from any existing body of knowledge
   3. Theory: consists of concepts, construct, and propositions tested over time so there is sufficient evidence that similar outcomes occur on repeated testing; describes, explains, predicts, and controls phenomena
      a. As stated above, concepts are words to describe events such as blood pressure
      b. Constructs: consist of several concepts and are words that represent complex events
         (1) For example, Spielberger's state-trait anxiety (construct) theory indicates that people respond to anxious events at moment of occurrence (state, which is a concept), and response is based on personality characteristics (trait, which is a concept)
      c. Propositions: statements that suggest how concepts and constructs are related
         (1) For example, research studies have confirmed that trait anxiety has a direct impact on state anxiety response (proposition)
   4. Conceptual framework: consists of concepts and constructs believed to be related; however, little research evidence suggests that events occur in any predictable pattern
      a. For example, a conceptual framework could describe how quality nursing care is related to certification (constructs); however, it would take many studies to develop this into a theory

5. Model: "picture" used to demonstrate how researcher believes concepts and constructs are related; can be used to image a theory or conceptual framework or can be used to draw an image when researcher does not know how concepts or constructs are related

F. Assumptions and limitations
 1. Discussed in studies because it is impossible to control for all errors in research
  a. Assumptions: statements assumed to be truths
   (1) For example, "it is assumed that all patients will answer questions honestly" is a frequently stated assumption
  b. Limitations: statements that describe any problems when conducting a study or drawing conclusions from study findings
   (1) For example, "a limitation of the study may be that when the nurses began a pain study on inpatient cholecystectomy patients, the procedure was changed to laser laparoscopy and 23-hour stay, which limits the results of the study"

G. Review of literature
 1. Purpose: to analyze what has been previously written or studied on proposed topic
 2. As problems are uncovered in practice, it is important to first review the literature to determine whether solutions are available before planning a study
 3. Literature cited should be published within past 5 years unless of historical relevance
 4. Should consist of both theoretic and research-based publications
  a. Theoretic literature: usually subjective, consisting of opinions, hunches, or practical experience articles found in nursing and nonnursing journals
  b. Research-based literature: studies that followed steps of scientific method, including qualitative studies (phenomenology, ethnography, grounded theory, historical studies) in which unit of analysis is words and quantitative studies (exploratory, descriptive, correlational, quasi-experimental, experimental studies) in which unit of analysis is numeric
  c. Research-based studies are also found in nursing and nonnursing journals

H. Methods
 1. Discussions regarding research design, sample and setting, ethical concerns and institutional approval, instrument(s), reliability and validity of instruments, and data analysis methods
  a. Research design: "blueprint" or plan of how study will be conducted
  b. Designs commonly used are those listed above under qualitative and quantitative definitions
  c. Designs commonly seen in quantitative studies:
   (1) Exploratory: to describe events when little is known about topic
   (2) Descriptive: to describe such variables as patient/family/nurse experiences
   (3) Correlational: to measure relationships among variables
   (4) Quasi-experimental: to measure effect of treatment or intervention on subjects, but there may or may not be a control group or randomization of subjects to treatment groups
   (5) Experimental: to measure effect of treatment or intervention; random selection or assignment of subjects into at least one experimental and one control group
  d. Designs commonly seen in qualitative studies
   (1) Phenomenological: describe phenomenon or the lived experience, i.e., the lived surgical experience of a mastectomy patient
   (2) Ethnographic: describe cultures in which the researcher becomes a part of the culture and analyzes the culture's attributes
   (3) Grounded theory: describe events in a natural setting that may contribute to theory building, i.e., caring practices of PACU nurses
   (4) Historical: systematically examine documents or interview persons for the purpose of describing events, i.e., historical development of PACUs

I. Sample and setting
   1. Sample: used to describe portion of population to be studied; after data are collected on the sample, they are referred to as subjects
      a. Types of samples
         (1) Simple random sample: random selection of study subjects from population of interest
            (a) For example, sample could be randomly selected from the population of thyroidectomy patients because it would be difficult and costly to study all patients in this category
            (b) One method: flip of a coin, which indicates that a 50:50 chance is possible for a subject to be placed in one of two groups; should more than two groups be needed, a random numbers table must be used
         (2) Stratified random samples: dividing subjects into layers or strata on the basis of specific attributes
            (a) For example, if PACU nurse wishes to study PACU standards of practice, hospitals could be stratified by geographic location and bed size
            (b) Hospitals could be randomly selected from a directory, using a random numbers table as discussed above; stratification could include east, west, north, and south locations and bed sizes of 100, 200, 300, and 400
            (c) Data could be analyzed by location and bed size for standards of practice
         (3) Systematic random sampling: random selection of sample from a list or membership roster
            (a) For example, the American Society of PeriAnesthesia Nurses (ASPAN) membership roster (population of PACU nurses) could be used to obtain a sample of PACU nurses for a study on attitudes toward research
         (4) Cluster sample: selection of a cluster of institutions in a geographic area
            (a) For example, instead of sampling PACU nurses from one hospital, a sample could be selected from several PACUs from several hospitals in a metropolitan area
         (5) Convenience or accidental sample: obtaining subjects within readily available location or handy population
            (a) For example, PACU nurse may wish to study effect of music therapy on pain in perianesthesia patients; convenience sample could be selected as patients are admitted to PACU and divided into two groups; nurse could test all patients' pain level, provide cassette players and headphones for one group of patients to listen to music, and measure amount of pain medication received by both groups
            (b) Problem with convenience samples: patients studied may not be representative of all patients admitted to all PACUs in all states
         (6) Purposive sample: selected intentionally on the basis of a particular attribute and frequently used in instrument development
            (a) For example, PACU nurse who wanted to test a new instrument to measure attitudes of ambulatory surgical patients' families regarding family visits in PACU would purposefully ask surgical patients' family members to participate in study
            (b) Problem: families studied may not be representative of all ambulatory surgical patients' families
   2. Setting description needed to describe conditions under which data were collected

J. Ethical concerns
   1. Ethical statements in studies describe how researcher will meet human subjects' committee/IRB guidelines:
      a. Protection of subjects from harm
      b. Maintaining confidentiality of subject information
      c. Guaranteeing subject anonymity

K. Instrument(s)
   1. Operationally define or measure concepts of interest in study, thereby transforming them into variables
      a. For example, body temperature is a concept and can be operationally defined with a thermometer, thereby transforming it into a variable
   2. Can be equipment (e.g., thermometer, weight scale) or pencil and paper tests, questionnaires, and interview forms

L. Reliability of instruments
   1. Defined as dependability of instrument in measuring variables
   2. If equipment is used to operationalize variables, must discuss how equipment was calibrated before study
   3. If instrument is paper and pencil, four types of reliability can verify its dependability:
      a. Internal consistency reliability: determines how all items in pencil and paper test consistently measure concept
         (1) For example, instrument to measure anxiety must contain items that exclusively reflect the concept of anxiety
         (2) Can be calculated with Cronbach's coefficient alpha (normal range, 0.0 to 1.0, where >0.70 is desired) for data derived from rating scales (1–5)
         (3) Kuder-Richardson 20 (KR-20) can be used to calculate internal consistency of dichotomous data (yes/no)
         (4) For instruments with few questions, split-half reliability can be calculated in which items are selected (odd/even) and compared
         (5) Must be calculated each time instrument is used with subjects
      b. Equivalence reliability determines whether two or more tests that measure same concept are equal
         (1) For example, two tests that measure nurse competence could be compared
         (2) Frequently used when developing a new instrument and comparing it with an existing instrument that is reliable
         (3) Calculated with Pearson's *r* or Spearman's rho correlations (range of −1.0 to +1.0; >0.70 desired)
      c. Interrater reliability: form of equivalence where more than one researcher is interviewing subjects
         (1) Calculated as percent agreement; >80% is desired
      d. Intrarater reliability: also calculated to determine whether one researcher is consistent in rating subjects on some variables; 95% to 100% agreement is desired
      e. Stability reliability: commonly known as test-retest or "is the instrument stable over time?"
         (1) Conducted when at least 2 weeks must elapse between first and second testing
         (2) Tested using Pearson's *r* correlation (range of −1.0 to +1.0; >0.80 is desired)

M. Validity: extent that an instrument measures what it intends to measure; four types:
   1. Content validity: adequacy that items in an instrument measure a concept
      a. Established during instrument development by five content experts on the basis of percent agreement among experts on each test item; percent agreement should be >80%
   2. Construct validity: extent that items in an instrument measure construct of interest
      a. Established through correlation matrix in which test items are expected to correlate (>0.50) or by factor analysis to determine which test items measure which construct (factor loadings >0.40)
   3. Criterion validity: relationship between instrument and some other criterion; consists of:
      a. Predictive validity to determine adequacy that data from an instrument predict performance on some future criterion
         (1) For example, NCLEX scores to predict how well PACU nurses will perform on certification examination

b. Concurrent validity: refers to how well data from an instrument measure some present criterion
(1) For example, preadmission surgical patient albumin values as predictor of risk for surgery

N. Data analysis methods: should reflect how hypotheses or research questions will be answered within a specific design
1. In a descriptive study, data will be analyzed using means, median, mode, percentage, frequency, etc.
a. Descriptive statistics: may also be used to profile data from other types of designs
2. In correlational study, data analyzed using Pearson's *r* or Spearman's rho correlations
3. In quasi-experimental and experimental studies, data analyzed in several ways:
a. Analysis of variance (ANOVA): used to test effect of treatment on two or more groups by comparing variability between and within the groups
b. Multiple analysis of variance (MANOVA): used to test effect of treatment on two or more groups or two or more dependent variables
c. ANOVA with repeated measures: used to test effect of two or more groups on repeated measures of same variables
d. Factorial analysis: used to test main effects of several variables and interactions of one variable on another
e. Discriminant function analysis: used to classify and analyze data and to predict group membership
f. Canonical correlation: used to test relationships between two or more independent variables and two or more dependent variables
g. Multiple regression analysis: used to test effects of two or more independent variables on a dependent variable

O. Results of statistical analysis of data begin with a description of subjects in study
1. Demographic data about subjects: may be narrative or in tables, figures, or graphs; usually derived from descriptive statistics
a. For example, "subjects in the study had a mean age of 56 years (standard deviation ±7.1)"
2. Data collected by using instruments; either equipment, laboratory data, or pencil and paper tests are then presented
a. For example, "the mean hemoglobin was 12.3 (SD ±2.8)"
b. "Subject's anxiety scores indicated significantly higher levels for same-day admit subjects without preoperative teaching (mean score 88, SD ±15, $P<0.05$) than for subjects who were same-day admit with preoperative teaching (mean score 55, SD ±11, $P<0.05$)"

P. Discussion, conclusions, implications for nursing, and recommendations for future research
1. Discussion of data then linked back to literature, theory/conceptual framework, or model
2. Conclusions can be derived from the study and how results confirm or refute results and conclusions from other studies and theories
a. For example, using anxiety data above, it could be concluded that "same-day admit patients experienced a decrease in anxiety as a result of preoperative teaching"
3. Implications for nursing then derived from results and conclusions
a. For example, using example above, it can be concluded that same-day admit nurses need to incorporate patient teaching into their plan of care to decrease patient anxiety
4. Future studies: recommendations identified from analysis of the meaning of the data; derived from discussion and conclusions; should reflect what was learned from conducting the study
a. For example, future studies are needed to determine which teaching method is most effective in decreasing same-day admit patient's anxiety

## BIBLIOGRAPHY


Burns N, Grove SK: *The Practice of Nursing Research: Conduct, Critique and Utilization.* Philadelphia, Saunders, 1993.

Goode CJ, Titler M, Rakel B, et al: A meta-analysis of effects of heparin flush and saline flush: Quality and cost implications. *Nurs Res* 40:324–330, 1991.

Nieswiadomy RM: *Foundations of Nursing Research.* Los Altos, Calif, Appleton & Lange, 1998.

Polit DF, Hungler BP: *Nursing Research Principles and Methods.* Philadelphia, JB Lippincott, 1995.

Streubert HJ, Carpenter DR: *Qualitative Research in Nursing.* Philadelphia, JB Lippincott, 1995.

Summers S: Reviewing the research process for post anesthesia care unit studies. *J Post Anesth Nurs* 5:421–424, 1990.

Summers S: Defining components of the research process needed to conduct and critique studies. *J Post Anesth Nurs* 6:50–55, 1991.

Summers S: Level of measurement: Key to appropriate data analysis. *J Post Anesth Nurs* 6:143–147, 1991.

Summers S: Selecting the sample for a research study. *J Post Anesth Nurs* 6:355–358, 1991.


## REVIEW QUESTIONS

**1. The purpose of PACU nursing research is to:**

A. Validate cost-effectiveness of nursing care
B. Validate PACU nursing practice
C. Apply the steps of the scientific method to answer questions relevant to nurses and nursing practice
D. Determine patient satisfaction with nursing care

**2. PACU nursing studies are important to:**

A. Document nursing's role in society
B. Add to the scientific basis for nursing practice
C. Validate students' attitudes toward nursing education
D. Substantiate medical practice

**3. Institutional approval of research proposals assures:**

A. The study will be important for nursing
B. The study will advance knowledge
C. Subjects will be fully informed before participation
D. The researcher is free to change the study protocol

**4. Research questions are usually used for:**

A. Experimental studies
B. Quasi-experimental studies
C. Correlational studies
D. Descriptive studies

**5. Hypotheses are usually used for:**

A. Experimental studies
B. Qualitative studies
C. Historical studies
D. Descriptive studies

**6. Independent variables are described as the:**

A. Intervention
B. Outcome
C. Concept
D. Construct

**7. Dependent variables are described as the:**
A. Intervention
B. Outcome
C. Concept
D. Construct

**8. Studies should be guided by a theory, conceptual framework, or model:**
A. To help in seeking funding for the study
B. To help in describing, explaining, predicting, and controlling phenomena
C. To help in publishing the study
D. To explain the findings to medical staff

**9. Research designs serve to:**
A. Establish a blueprint for the study
B. Allow the researcher to select the sample
C. Describe the risks and benefits of the study
D. Select the variables

**10. Samples that are less likely to be biased are:**
A. Convenience
B. Randomized
C. Cluster
D. Purposive

**11. Instruments are used to operationally define:**
A. Propositions
B. Concepts
C. Theories
D. Conceptual frameworks

**12. Reliability is defined as:**
A. Construct validity
B. Content validity
C. Internal consistency
D. Predictive validity

**13. Validity is defined as:**
A. Construct validity
B. Dependability
C. Internal consistency
D. Interrater reliability

**14. The purpose of descriptive statistics is to:**
A. Summarize data
B. Determine relationship
C. Measure differences in variables
D. Calculate correlations

**15. Implications for nurses should describe:**
A. The meaning of the study for medicine
B. How nurses can apply the findings
C. Future studies
D. The meaning of the study for patients

**ANSWERS:** 1. B, 2. B, 3. C, 4. D, 5. A, 6. A, 7. B, 8. B, 9. A, 10. B, 11. B, 12. C, 13. A, 14. A, 15. B

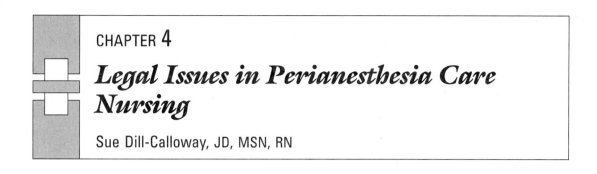

CHAPTER 4

# Legal Issues in Perianesthesia Care Nursing

Sue Dill-Calloway, JD, MSN, RN

## OBJECTIVES

**Study of the information represented by this outline will enable the learner to:**

1. List the four elements of negligence that must be proven by the plaintiff.
2. Identify aspects of documentation to minimize liability risks.
3. Explain the difference between case law and statutory law.
4. Describe the doctrine respondeat superior.
5. Explain the elements of informed consent.
6. Identify common areas of nursing negligence.
7. List practices to aid in the prevention of liability in the perianesthesia care unit (PACU).

## LEGAL TERMINOLOGY

**Plaintiff** Person who brings a claim or lawsuit

**Defendant** Person against whom the lawsuit is brought (e.g., nurse, physician or hospital, or facility)

**Standard of care** A measure against which the nurse's conduct is compared to determine whether there is negligence; acts performed that an ordinary, reasonable, and prudent nurse would have performed under the same or similar circumstances; standards come from many sources, including national specialty nursing standards (e.g., American Society of PeriAnesthesia Nurses [ASPAN], American Nurses' Association [ANA], hospital policies and procedures, state and federal laws, Joint Commission on Accreditation of Healthcare Organizations [JCAHO] standards, expert witnesses, and nursing articles and texts)

**Burden of proof** It is generally the plaintiff's job to prove that the nurse or defendant was negligent

**Complaint** Paper the plaintiff files to initiate a lawsuit

**Answer** Response the nurse files when a complaint is received

**Negligence** Failure to act as a reasonably prudent nurse that results in injury to the patient (e.g., there must be duty, breach of duty, direct or proximate cause, and damages)

**Respondeat superior** Latin term for "let the master answer"; holds the hospital liable for the negligent acts of its nurses while they act within the scope of employment

**Statute of limitation** Time period by which you can sue the nurse or defendant

**Res ipsa loquitur** A Latin term for "the thing speaks for itself"; invoked when a patient is injured and when the nurse or defendant has exclusive control of the thing that caused the harm; burden shifts to the nurse to prove there was no negligence (e.g., the patient had a laparoscopic cholecystectomy and awakens in PACU with a fractured femur)

**Negligence per se** Finding of negligence that is made by showing that a statute (law) was violated

**Practice parameter or clinical practice guideline (CPG)** A systematically developed statement to help practitioners decide about appropriate health care for specific conditions

## INTRODUCTION

1. The patient is called the plaintiff in a lawsuit.
2. The nurse, hospital, or employer is called the defendant.
3. The plaintiff can sue the nurse, hospital, or both.
4. The doctrine of respondeat superior means that the hospital is legally responsible for the nurse's negligent act that is performed while the nurse is acting within the scope of employment. Therefore the hospital must defend and pay a judgment if the PACU nurse is negligent.
5. The burden of proof requires the plaintiff to prove that the nurse was negligent.
6. The United States uses a tripartite governmental system with separate legislative, judicial, and executive branches, and uses both common or judge-made law, and statutory or legislative-made law.
7. Two important sources of laws are the statutory or legislature-made laws and *case* or judge-made laws.
8. Types of law include
   a. Contract law: a private law involving an agreement between two or more parties
   b. Constitutional law: a type of public law based on an individual's rights and responsibilities under the federal or state constitution
   c. Administrative law: a type of public law concerning administrative agencies and boards

**I. Negligence and Intentional Acts**
   A. Negligence: conduct that falls below the standard established by law for the protection of others against an unreasonable risk of harm
   B. Plaintiff must prove each of the four elements of *negligence*
      1. Duty: PACU nurse has a legal duty to provide good nursing care to all the patients in the postanesthesia care unit
      2. Breach of duty or breach of the standard of care: failure to conform to the acceptable standard of care
         a. Nursing standard of care: what an ordinary, prudent nurse would have performed in the same or similar manner (There are many standards on a national, state, or local level as discussed below.)
         b. The standard of care owed to a patient is the same whether the PACU nurse is certified in postanesthesia nursing or not, and regardless of the nurse's basic educational preparation such as associate's degree (AD), bachelor of science in nursing (BSN), or diploma (However, the fact that the nurse was a CPAN can be brought to the jury's attention and goes to improve the nurse's credibility.)
      3. Direct or proximate cause: the nurse's negligent action must have caused the problem; there must be a reasonably close connection between the nurse's conduct and the patient's resultant injury. For example, the PACU nurse hangs a 500 ml bag of $D_5W$ with 20,000 units of heparin by mistake; the patient does not have any bleeding problems, but postoperatively a wound infection develops; the nurse is not liable because the mistake that was made did not cause the patient's problem
      4. Damages: must be present for the patient-plaintiff to prevail in a malpractice suit; the plaintiff must prove actual damage or that the act or omission damaged the plaintiff in some way (e.g., a PACU nurse fails to timely notify the physician that a postoperative patient who had an abdominal hysterectomy had been hemorrhaging; as a result of the nurse's negligence, the patient got one unit of packed cells and acquired hepatitis from the transfusion; typical damages include compensation for the additional medical bills, time lost from work, pain and suffering, and money spent to pay a babysitter during prolonged hospitalization; spouse may also have a claim for loss of consortium, an action filed for loss of conjugal relations because of the spouse's injury)
   C. Standard of care
      1. Standards of care for the PACU nurse may be established by the following
         a. State law, including the nurse practice act

b. Federal laws, including the U. S. Occupational Safety and Health Administration (OSHA) bloodborne pathogen law
c. JCAHO or other applicable accrediting agency
d. ANA
e. Internal hospital policies and procedures
f. Expert witnesses (most common and required in most cases)
g. Specific state, case law
h. Board of nursing and specialty organization standards and position statements (e.g., the perianesthesia care standards of practice)
i. Custom (usual nursing practice)

D. Intentional acts

Negligence refers to conduct as opposed to state of mind; intentional act requires a specific state of mind, usually an intention to do the wrongful act; many insurance companies will not cover damages from intentional acts; assault and battery, slander, false imprisonment, defamation, and invasion of privacy are examples of intentional acts

1. Assault: an act that puts another in apprehension of being touched in a manner that is offensive or provoking; battery: the unlawful touch of another without consent
2. False imprisonment: the intentional and unjustifiable detention of patients against their will
3. Defamation: injury to a person's reputation or character through oral or written communication to a third person; oral defamation is called slander, and written defamation is called libel
4. Invasion of privacy: an unwarranted exploitation of one's personality or private affairs (e.g., publishing pictures of patients in a journal without their permission); disclosure of any confidential patient information to an unauthorized source can result in a claim of invasion of privacy

E. Types of liability

1. Respondeat superior: employer is liable for the employee's negligence done within the scope of their responsibility; if the PACU nurse makes a mistake, the hospital is responsible for the nurse's action; generally, the hospital must defend the nurse and pay any judgment
2. Independent contractor exception: many states recognize an exception to respondeat superior for independent contractors; if an agency nurse makes a mistake, the hospital may not be liable
3. Apparent authority or ostensible agency theory: several states hold hospital or employer liable for the negligent actions of anesthesiologists, even if they are independent contractors
4. Corporate liability: some states recognize the corporate liability doctrine, which imposes liability on the hospital because it has failed to meet some duty recognized by law (e.g., duty to maintain proper medical equipment and supplies); may also include a duty to exercise reasonable care to provide safe premises; hospitals should adopt internal, reasonably calculated policies and procedures to protect the safety and interest of patients; there is a duty to exercise reasonable care in the selection and retention of hospital employees and in the granting of staff privileges
5. Servant doctrine and captain-of-the-ship doctrine: captain-of-the-ship doctrine mostly used in the operating room and held the surgeon liable for the acts of the nurses; abandoned by most states

F. Defenses

1. Certain defenses (based on state law and case law, so there are variations from state to state) will negate liability even if the plaintiff has proven each of the four elements of negligence
2. Statute of limitation: time period in which a patient has the right to bring an action; recent trend has been to use the discovery rule: statute or law starts to run when the patient discovers or, in the exercise of reasonable care, should have discovered the alleged negligence

3. Comparative negligence: allows negligence of plaintiff to be weighed with that of the defendant; allows the comparison of fault; this is why it is especially important to document patient education, discharge instructions, and incidences where patients fail to follow instructions
4. Assumption of risk: still recognized by some states; does not allow a plaintiff to win when a known or understood risk was ignored

## CONSENT LAW

**I. General Provision**

A. Law of informed consent differs from state to state, generally derived from two sources, statutory law and case law; most states now have a written law (called a statute) that guides nurses as to what is required; also cases, or judge-made laws, that discuss informed consent; note that consent is a *process* and not just the handing of a form to a patient; patient must be provided sufficient information, understand the information, and voluntarily give consent before consent is informed and valid

**II. Typical Elements**

A. Nature and purpose of proposed procedure set out
B. Expected outcome and the likelihood of success
C. Material risks
D. Alternatives

**III. Typical Exceptions May Include**

A. Emergency doctrine
B. Medical contraindications
C. Therapeutic privilege (very restricted; in certain circumstances some states allow a physician to withhold information for which more harm would result by disclosing that information)
D. Prior patient knowledge
E. Waiver of right to consent (most states allow a patient to specifically request not to be informed)
F. Duty of third-party disclosure (most states recognize a duty to warn others of potential harm in certain circumstances; may arise if a patient has communicated an immediate threat of physical violence; must be coupled with the apparent intent and ability to carry out the threat against a clearly identified victim)

**IV. Types**

A. Expressed consent (e.g., patient states he or she wants the surgery)
B. Implied consent (e.g., patient holds his or her arm out for a tetanus injection)
C. Written consent (e.g., patient signs a consent form; should disclose all the elements required by law)

## COMMON AREAS OF NEGLIGENCE

**I. Common Areas of Negligence for PACU**

A. Errors in the administration of medications
B. Patient falls
C. Failure to monitor and observe patient's condition
D. Failure to notify physician timely of a change in patient's condition
E. Failure to monitor use of restraints
F. Administering medication when the patient is allergic
G. Failure to defer improper orders

H. Failure to keep abreast of nursing knowledge
I. Mistaken identity of patient
J. Failure to remove foreign bodies from patients
K. Burns to patients (from K-Pads, electric warming blankets, or other warming device)
L. Misplaced endotracheal tubes
M. Use of defective equipment
N. Abandonment
O. Loss or damage to patient's property
P. Failure to perform cardiopulmonary resuscitation (CPR) timely
Q. Failure to follow policies and procedures
R. Failure to document adequately and promptly
S. Failure to communicate concerns to anesthesiologists, surgeons or other physicians, nursing supervisors, and other health care practitioners
T. Failure to adhere to aseptic technique and universal precautions
U. Improper delegation or floating
V. Practicing outside scope of nurse practice act

## DOCUMENT CONSIDERATIONS IN THE PACU

Generally, the decision to sue the PACU nurse is based on the plaintiff's expert's review of the charting done during the postanesthesia care period. Therefore optimal documentation is one of the best ways to stay out of the courtroom. Optimal documentation increases the likelihood that the case, if filed at all, will be dismissed or otherwise favorably disposed of without going to trial. If the case is not dismissed, the nurse may use the documentation at trial.

**I. Documentation Requirements (Examples)**
A. JCAHO
B. ASPAN *Standards of Perianesthesia Nursing Practice*
C. American Hospital Association
D. State nurse practice act
E. State specific regulations
F. AAAHC for ambulatory care

**II. Purpose of Documentation**
A. To serve as a basis for planning patient's care and for continuity in evaluating patient's condition and treatment
B. To furnish documentary evidence of course of the patient's medical evaluation, treatment, and change in condition
C. To document communication between the practitioners responsible for the patient's care and any other health care professional who contributes to patient's care
D. To provide data for use in continuity, education, and research
E. To provide data for use in quality improvement and peer review studies
F. To provide documentation to obtain reimbursement
G. To create a legal record for the patient, institution, and health care practitioner

**III. Recommendations for Improving Documentation**
A. Ambulatory nurses who call patients back for follow-up information should be sure all information is documented
B. Charting errors corrected appropriately (no erasures, no White-out, no obliterations): single line can be drawn through entry and "delete" marked above; correct documentation can then be recorded followed by nurse's initials
C. Legible PACU notes
D. Date and time

E. Correct spelling
F. Omitted entries: if an entry is inadvertently omitted, omitted entry should be clearly marked as a late entry
G. Proper abbreviations used
H. Properly signed chart
I. Inclusion of recommendations made in ASPAN *Standards for Perianesthesia Nursing Practice*
J. Incident reports completed according to hospital policy
K. PACU nurse's notes should never mention that an incident report has been completed
L. Transfer of any patient directly from PACU to another facility should comply with COBRA laws
M. All pertinent patient and family communication documented
N. When restraints are used, types of restraint and time of the circulation checks should be clearly documented
O. If patient has cardiac or respiratory arrest, chart should clearly reflect that CPR was started promptly
P. If a patient is intubated in PACU, nurse's notes should reflect that breath sounds were present bilaterally
Q. Any telephone call to a physician should reflect what information was relayed to physician
R. Nurse's notes should reflect any time chain of command is used
S. Optimal documentation during codes; should include name and dose of every drug given and response; should record everything that transpired during code (e.g., CPR, pulse oximetry, monitor on, defibrillation, external pacemaker); code sheet should include names of all team members who responded to code
T. Patient noncompliance with any procedure or treatment documented
U. Initial PACU nursing assessment documented
V. Prompt recording and notification of physician whenever patient's condition changes
W. Any time a question about an order is discussed with the physician, it should be documented
X. Any abnormal test result and physician notification recorded in the PACU nurse's notes
Y. Aldrete scale, if used, should be documented

## PREVENTION OF LIABILITY IN THE PACU

**I. Recommendations**

A. Ensure all appropriate internal policies and procedures are followed
B. Inappropriate policies and procedures corrected
C. New nurses should have orientation that includes information on policies and procedures
D. Use of restraints according to hospital protocol and their use documented
E. Appropriate staffing according to JCAHO, acuity scale adopted, and ASPAN standards
F. Nurses familiar with the common causes of nursing liability
G. Optimal documentation: relevant, timely, specific, objective, and accurate
H. PACU nurse familiar with and complies with the state's living will and durable power of attorney law
I. PACU nurses familiar with state's specific laws (e.g., nurse practice act, acquired immune deficiency syndrome [AIDS] law)
J. Incident reports filled out appropriately
K. Nurses must protect the patient's right to confidentiality
L. Appropriate informed consent obtained before surgical procedures
M. Minimize use of verbal orders; physicians who are present in PACU should be encouraged to write their own orders

N. PACU nurses familiar with and comply with federal laws such as the OSHA bloodborne pathogen law, Americans with Disabilities Act, Patient Right to Self-Determination Act, COBRA, OBRA, and Safe Medical Devices Act
O. PACU nurses familiar with patient's bill of rights under JCAHO, American Hospital Association's 1992 Patient Bill of Rights, and any internal policy and procedure on patient rights
P. PACU nurse courteous to patients and families; good public relations (PR) is one of the best mechanisms for preventing litigation
Q. Appropriate, written discharge instructions

## LEGAL ISSUES IN PRACTICE GUIDELINES

**I. Tips to Minimize Liability in Drafting CPGs**

A. Use a disclaimer: a statement to convey that the CPG does not reflect all medical consideration
B. Know specific state's law, if applicable
C. Be familiar with AHCPR's document on Using CPGs to Evaluate Quality of Care (*http://www.ahcpr.gov* or call 800.358.9205—publication Nos. 95-0045 and 95-0046)
D. Know the eight attributes of good CPGs; validity, reliable/reproducible, clinically applicable, flexible, clear, multidisciplinary, periodically reviewed, and documented
E. Maintain an archive
F. Know its intended purpose; generally to improve care
G. Be aware of customary practice in adopting common CPGs
H. Use to improve communication and public relations
I. Avoid negligence per se liability by following state specific law, if applicable
J. Regularly review and update
K. Avoid antitrust claims; CPGs may violate antitrust law if they selectively favor one profession over another (e.g., both general surgeons and obstetricians can perform hysterectomy)
L. Follow institution's own policies and procedures
M. Educate defense attorney on the issue of CPGs if a lawsuit is ever filed (to date, no lawsuits have been filed regarding the use of CPGs)
N. Be aware of the accepted minority defense issue where medical literature recognizes that there is more than one acceptable method or care
O. Be realistic in claims about CPGs (e.g., success or cost-savings)
P. CPGs can decrease unacceptable variations in practice and prevent lawsuits
Q. Make sure CPG is consistent with the acceptable standard of care
R. Do not try to cover every situation
S. Avoid inconsistent guidelines as topics for CPGs (e.g., treatment for breast cancer)
T. Good documentation of both the CPG in the medical record and in drafting CPG
U. Always do a literature search
V. Train and educate staff in developing and applying CPGs
W. Avoid defensive medicine

## PROFESSIONAL LIABILITY INSURANCE

**I. Types of Policies**

A. Occurrence: covers alleged incident that occurred within policy period, regardless of when the event was reported; preferred type, and most nursing policies are occurrence coverage
B. Claims made: only covers claims reported during the policy period; if the policy is canceled, future claims, even if they occurred during the time the insurance was in effect, are not covered unless a "tail" policy is purchased

**II. Issues to Consider in Deciding Whether to Purchase a Policy**

A. Increasing number of lawsuits are filed against nurses
B. Nurses are responsible for their own acts of negligence
C. Protection of nurse's best interest
D. Nurses exposed to greater risks because more sophisticated procedures (arterial lines, pulse oximetry, balloon pumps, pacers)
E. Affordable rates
F. Tax deductible
G. Peace of mind if employer's liability company goes bankrupt
H. Liability exposure outside health care facility
I. An act outside nurse's job description

**III. Policy Limits**

A. Each policy specifies maximum amount of money the company will pay

## NURSES IN LEGAL ACTIONS

**I. Initial Steps**

A. Patient-plaintiff usually initiates a lawsuit by filing complaint
B. Nurse-defendant must file an answer (or something called a preanswer motion); answer will list any defenses

**II. Discovery**

A. This time period is when information is obtained surrounding circumstances of lawsuit; discovery tools include
   1. Interrogatories: written questions
   2. Request for production of documents: written request for materials, medical records, or documents
   3. Admissions of facts: written statements asking party to affirm or deny statements
   4. Deposition: question-and-answer session where the witness or party is under oath; either videotaped or recorded word by word by court reporter

**III. Some States Have Prelitigation Panels or Medical Review Panels (Patient Compensation Funds)**

**IV. Trial**

A. Jury selection
B. Opening statement
C. Plaintiff's presentation of case
D. Defendant's presentation of case
E. Closing argument
F. Jury instructions
G. Jury deliberations and verdict
H. Appeals process

## BIBLIOGRAPHY

Calfee B: *Staying Out of Court: A Self-Assessment Guide for Nurses.* Beachwood, Calfee and Associates, 1990.

Creighton H: Recovery room nurses: Legal implications. *Nurse Management* 18:1, 22–23, 1986.

Dill-Calloway S: *Legal Issues in Supervising Nurses.* Eau Claire, Wis, Professional Education Systems, 1993.

Dill-Calloway S: *Ohio Nursing Law.* Cleveland, Banks-Baldwin, 1990.

Dill-Calloway S: *Nursing and the Law.* Eau Claire, Wis, Professional Education Systems, 1986.

Douglas S, Larson E: There's more to informed consent than information. *Focus Crit Care* 13:2, 43–48, 1991.

*Hospital Risk Control ERCI.* Pennsylvania, 1990.

Orlikoff J: *Malpractice Prevention and Liability Control for Hospitals,* 2 d Ed. Chicago, American Hospital Association, 1988.

Schouten R: Informed consent: Resistance and reappraisal. *Crit Care Med* Dec 1989.

Strodel R: *Securing and Using Medical Evidence.* Englewood Cliffs, NJ, Prentice Hall, 1988.

Veach M: *Risk Management Handbook for Healthcare Facilities.* Chicago, American Hospital Association, 1990.

## REVIEW QUESTIONS

1. **The four elements of negligence are:**
   A. Tort, statutes, case law and expert testimony
   B. Duty, breach of standard of care, direct cause, and damage
   C. Standard of care, deviation from standard, tort liability, and respondeat superior
   D. Negligence, standard of care, damages, and deviation from acceptable practices

2. **Respondeat superior means:**
   A. Hospital is liable for the negligent acts of PACU nurses created within scope of their employment
   B. If a foreign object is retained, burden shifts to hospital
   C. If nurse falls below standard of care there must be damages
   D. Expert testimony is required

3. **What is the most common source for determining whether the nurse has met the acceptable standard of care?**
   A. Respondeat superior
   B. Res ipsa loquitur
   C. Hospital policies and procedures
   D. Expert testimony

4. **A lawsuit is generally initiated by the filing of a (an):**
   A. Deposition
   B. Answer
   C. Complaint
   D. Interrogatory

5. **The patient in a lawsuit is called the:**
   A. Plaintiff
   B. Defendant
   C. Presiding party
   D. Tort feasor

6. **A type of law based on an individual's rights and responsibilities under federal or state constitution is:**
   A. Contract law
   B. Constitutional law
   C. Administrative law
   D. Malpractice law

7. **The following are examples of standards of care that may have an impact on the PACU nurse:**
   A. State nurse practice act
   B. ASPAN *Perianesthesia Standards of Practice*
   C. Hospital policies and procedures
   D. All of the above

8. **Which of the following is not a potential defense to a malpractice action?**
   A. Comparative negligence
   B. Statute of limitation
   C. Assumption of risk
   D. Respondent superior

9. **Informed consent requires:**
   A. Patient comprehension
   B. Voluntary participation
   C. Disclosure of information
   D. All of the above

10. **The preferred type of nursing insurance is:**
    A. Claims made
    B. Occurrence
    C. Specified policy limit
    D. Aggregate coverage

**ANSWERS:** 1. B, 2. A, 3. D, 4. C, 5. A, 6. B, 7. D, 8. D, 9. D, 10. B

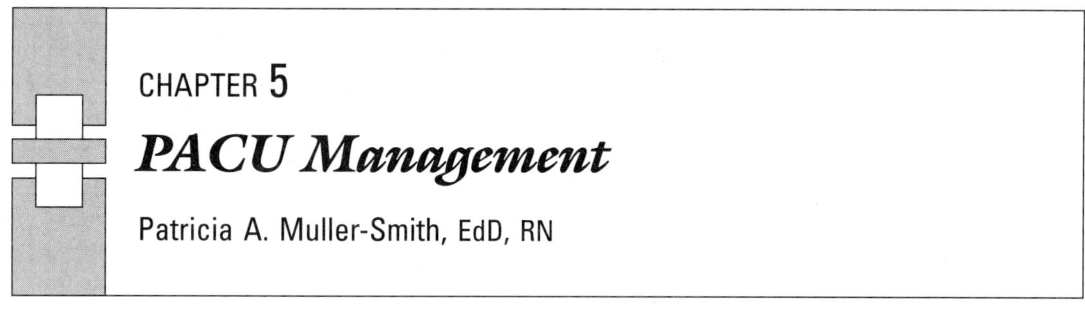

CHAPTER 5

# PACU Management

Patricia A. Muller-Smith, EdD, RN

## OBJECTIVES

**Study of the information represented by this outline will enable the learner to:**

1. Identify the components of the management process.
2. List the minimum requirements for selection as a manager in a postanesthesia care unit (PACU).
3. Identify the major responsibilities of the head nurse in PACU.
4. List some skills necessary to carry out the head nurse's role in each component of the management process.
5. Differentiate between management and leadership.

Management is planning, organizing, directing, and evaluating the use of resources to achieve goals through other people.

## NURSE MANAGER IN PACU

**I. Minimum Requirements**
   A. Registered nurse (RN) with appropriate education
   B. Proficient in nursing practice and management
   C. Demonstrated interpersonal skills

**II. Role Responsibility**
   A. 24-hour accountability for those management activities necessary to ensure patients receive optimal care in PACU
   B. Administratively responsible to a designee of the department of nursing
   C. Medically responsible to chairperson of department of anesthesia or medical director

**III. Planning**
   A. Purpose: clarifies purpose of organization or unit and identifies values, beliefs, strengths, weaknesses, and resources needed to achieve goals
   B. Types
      1. Strategic: long range; less specific
      2. Operational: short range; specific to unit maintenance and improvement goals for coming year; developed in conjunction with budget
   C. Decision making: selection from alternatives
      1. Steps in decision making
         a. Define problem
         b. Identify possible alternatives
         c. Choose best or most desirable alternative
         d. Implement decision
         e. Evaluate results

2. Critical skills
   a. Creativity
   b. Critical thinking
   c. Use of consultation process
3. Ethics
   a. Judging relationship of means to ends
   b. Influenced by values
   c. Focus on intent
4. Tools
   a. Probability theory: assumes factors occur in accordance with predictable patterns
   b. Gantt chart: highly developed schedule that defines tasks to be done, who is responsible for task, and time frames involved in completing task
   c. Decision trees: graphic method to visualize alternatives available, outcomes, risks, and information needs for a specific problem over a particular period
   d. PERT (program evaluation and review technique): identifies key activities in a project, shows sequence of activities, and assigns a duration for each phase of project
   e. Critical path method: calculates a single time estimate for each activity, the longest possible time

D. Budget: plan for allocation of resources
1. Types
   a. Operational: revenue and expense
   b. Capital: equipment, physical changes
   c. Labor: cost of labor needed to meet objectives

E. Marketing: plan for voluntary exchange of resources considered valuable by parties involved

**IV. Organizing**

A. Purpose
1. Establish formal structure to provide coordination of resources needed to accomplish objectives

B. Types
1. Formal
   a. Defined by executive decision
   b. Can be diagramed to show relationships among people and positions
   c. Describes positions, task responsibilities, and relationships
   d. Can be bureaucratic or adaptive
2. Informal
   a. Comprises personal and social relationships
   b. Provides social control of behavior
   c. Has its own channel of communication (grapevine)
   d. Helps members meet personal objectives

C. Organizational chart
1. Defines formal relationships, areas of responsibility, person to whom one is accountable, and channels of communication
2. Types
   a. Flat vs. tall: number of management levels in organization
   b. Decentralized vs. centralized: degree to which decision making is diffused throughout organization
3. Authority
   a. Line: direct command relationship between manager and employee
   b. Staff: supports line manager and is advisory

D. Organization culture: customary ways of thinking and behaving that express values that demonstrate basic organizational beliefs

E. Policies
    1. Explain how goals will be achieved
    2. Define general course of action
    3. Establish scope of activities permissible to achieve goals
    4. Affect whole organization
F. Procedures
    1. Specific guides to action
    2. Enumerate chronologic sequence of steps
    3. Unit or department specific

**V. Staffing**

A. Purpose: to ensure that necessary human resources are available to provide optimal patient care
B. Types (assignment systems)
    1. Case method: RN assigned total care
    2. Functional: RN directs care using personnel available
    3. Team: RN plans, supervises, and evaluates nursing care and assigns team members to carry out tasks, matching skill levels with patient needs
    4. Primary nursing: puts patient needs as focus of nursing activities; RN works with other providers to achieve patient outcomes
    5. Case management: plan for entire episode of illness; defines patient needs in various settings where patient will receive nursing care
C. Selection based on:
    1. Educational preparation
    2. Experience and skill level
    3. Interpersonal skills
    4. Compatibility of values, professional goals, and current personal situation
    5. Availability
D. Orientation
    1. Job description, roles, and responsibilities
    2. Skill competency: general, unit-specific, and ASPAN standards
        a. Airway management to include insertion of pediatric and adult airways
        b. Management of patient during altered states of consciousness
        c. Management of monitoring and respiratory equipment
        d. Management of fluid lines
        e. Management of tubes, drains, and catheters
        f. Basic life support review annually with biannual certification through American Heart Association or American Red Cross; ACLS desirable
        g. Administration of drugs and drug-related problems
        h. Knowledge of anesthetic agents, reversal agents, techniques, actions, and interactions to include patients of all ages
        i. Subsequent epidural analgesia dosing of patient by PACU nurse when this is an accepted practice by individual state board of nursing; will include:
            (1) Acquiring and maintaining level of knowledge and skill needed to carry out role safely
            (2) Written protocol that complies with state board of nursing requirements, maintained by each employer, that includes procedure guidelines, use of monitoring equipment, use of infusion pumps, availability of naloxone and resuscitation equipment, and course of instructions
        j. Arrhythmia recognition and treatment
        k. Assessing learning needs and patient education as appropriate per unit policy
        l. Knowledge of normal growth and developmental stages
        m. Fire safety, patient and staff safety, infection control: ASPAN standards

3. Occupational Safety and Health Administration (OSHA) requirements
   a. Infection control
      (1) Body substance isolation
      (2) Universal precautions
      (3) Exposure policy
   b. Hazardous communication (Haz Com)
      (1) Chemical groupings
      (2) Material safety data sheets (MSDSs)
      (3) Right to know
   c. Other safety issues for training of personnel
      (1) Fire and disaster
      (2) Body mechanics
      (3) Electrical
      (4) Mechanical
      (5) Modes of transportation
      (6) Ambient gas monitoring
      (7) Latex sensitivity

E. Staff development
   1. Goes beyond orientation
   2. Continuing education
   3. Encourages development of latent potential

F. Scheduling (Table 5–1)
   1. Patient volume
   2. Acuity: patient classification
      a. Phase I
         (1) Class 1:3—one nurse to three patients who are awake, stable, and have no complications
         (2) Class 1:2—one nurse to two patients who are (a) unconscious, stable, without artificial airway, and older than 9 years of age or (b) awake, stable, 11 years of age or younger, and with family or support staff present
         (3) Class 1:1—one nurse to one patient who is (a) at the time of admission, (b) requiring mechanical life support or artificial airway, or (c) any unconscious patient 9 years of age or less; a second nurse must be available to assist as necessary
      b. Phase II
         (1) Class 1:5—one nurse to five patients who are (a) more than 5 years of age and ready for discharge or (b) 5 years of age or less and ready for discharge, and with family present
         (2) Class 1:4—one nurse to four patients who are (a) more than 5 years of age, awake, and stable or (b) 5 years of age or less, awake, and stable with family present
         (3) Class 1:3—one nurse to three patients who are (a) more than 5 years of age and within ½ hour of procedure/discharge from phase I or (b) 5 years of age or less and within ½ hour of procedure/discharge from phase I with family present
         (4) Class 1:2—one nurse to two patients who are (a) 5 years of age or less without family or support staff present or (b) at initial admission of patient after procedure
         (5) One nurse to one patient who is an unstable patient of any age requiring transfer
      c. Phase III
         (1) Class will vary depending on scope of care provided—intent of the phase is to provide ongoing care for patients requiring extended observation or intervention after transfer or discharge from phase I or phase II with the intention of preparing patient for self-care or family care
   3. Staff mix

**TABLE 5–1 Formula for Determining Daily Staffing Needs**

Number of patients scheduled in each class × Hours of care required for each class (average time in PACU for each class) × Nurse/patient ratio required for each class, with minimum of 2 nurses present for each classification

EXAMPLE: Class III patients schedules = 4 × 2 (nurse/patient ratio of 1 : 1, minimum 2 nurses)
Average PACU stay for class III = 2 hr
4 × 2 = 8
8 × 2 = 16 hr, or 2 full-time equivalents (FTEs)

To schedule staff according to patient acuity use the average hours of PACU care patients in each classification required.

For example, class I patients require an average of 1 hr in PACU, and class II patients stay in PACU an average of 1½ hr. Class III patients may average 2 or more hr in PACU, depending on the types of procedures (cardiovascular, organ transplant, etc.) most often performed that require transfer to the intensive care unit (ICU) after stabilization in PACU.

Use the number of patients in each class times the hours of care required to obtain the nursing care hours required. Divide the nursing hours required by 6.5 to obtain the number of full-time equivalents (FTEs) needed. FTEs calculated at 6.5 hr represent 100% productivity based on an 8-hr shift, allocated as follows:

| | |
|---|---|
| Breaks | 2 @ 15 min = 30 min |
| Meal | 1 @ 30 min = 30 min |
| Clothing changes | 2 @ 5 min = 10 min |
| Discharge, transport, or report | 10 min |
| Maintenance of supplies/equipment | 10 min |

TOTAL . . . . . . . . . . 1.5 hr per 8-hr shift per nurse

4. Environmental factors
   a. PACUs, phases I and II, will be in close proximity to area in which anesthesia is to be administered
   b. Recommended that phase-I PACU and phase-II PACU be two separate rooms or areas; also recommended that preoperative patients not be present when patients are recovering from anesthesia; if possible, it is advantageous that pediatric patients recover in a separate area from adult postanesthesia patients
   c. One and one-half beds will be available in PACU for every one operating room; two beds will be available in PACU for every one operating room when dealing with short, simple procedures on relatively healthy patients
   d. Each patient care unit will be equipped to provide:
      (1) Various means of oxygen delivery
      (2) Constant and intermittent suction
      (3) Means to monitor blood pressure
      (4) Adjustable lighting
      (5) Capacity to ensure patient privacy
   e. Phase I PACU will have:
      (1) One electrocardiogram (ECG) monitor and one pulse oximeter for every patient care unit
      (2) Monitors for arterial, central venous, and pulmonary artery pressure for those patients requiring these measures
      (3) Means to monitor temperature
   f. Phase II PACU will have:
      (1) One ECG monitor
      (2) One pulse oximeter
      (3) One emergency cart with defibrillator
   g. Patients requiring strict isolation or respiratory precautions must be housed in a private room as required by the infection control department; if a private room with

needed ventilation requirements is not available in PACU, continuous postanesthesia care will be provided elsewhere in the facility; quality of care in this situation will be equal to that available in PACU

h. Method of calling for assistance in emergency situations shall be provided in all areas

i. Plan for transport of patients from a freestanding facility to a full-service hospital must be in place for emergency situations

**VI. Directing**

A. Purpose: to achieve organizational goals and objectives through other people

B. Critical skills

1. Leadership style
   a. Great person theory: leaders are well rounded and simultaneously display instrumental (planning, organizing, and controlling) and supportive (participation and consultation from staff) leadership behaviors
   b. Charismatic theory: inspires others through emotional commitment; arouses strong feelings of loyalty and enthusiasm in staff
   c. Trait theory: suggests leadership traits are inherited
   d. Situational theory: style of leadership would vary according to situation; would depend on performance requirements, time pressures, physical environment, needs of leader and followers, culture of organization, and outside pressure
   e. Contingency theory: style is effective or ineffective on the basis of the situation; must always look at (1) leader-member relations, (2) task structure, and (3) position power
   f. Transformational leadership: motivates through values, vision, and empowerment; looks for what is effective, not just efficient; builds trust
2. Management
   a. Negotiation: decides issues on merits, looks for mutual gains, and insists on fair standards
      (1) Separate people from problem
      (2) Focus on interests instead of positions
      (3) Generate variety of options
      (4) Select option made on basis of objective criteria
   b. Motivation: internal needs that cause employee to behave in certain ways to achieve goals
      (1) Maslow's hierarchy of needs theory: people have five basic needs: physiologic, safety, love, esteem, and self-actualization
      (2) Alderfer's modified need hierarchy: ERG theory: existence, relatedness, and growth needs
      (3) Herzberg's motivation hygiene theory: motivators include achievement growth, responsibility, advancement, and recognition; lack of expected hygiene factors distracts from motivation; lack of fair pay, benefits, and good interpersonal relationships will create dissatisfaction
      (4) McGregor's theory X and theory Y
         (a) Theory X: assumes people will avoid work if possible and therefore need to be managed; uses fear and threats to motivate
         (b) Theory Y: assumes people like and enjoy work, are self-directed, and seek responsibility; uses praise and recognition to reward
      (5) Theory Z: Japanese form of participative management; cooperation and collective decision making stressed

C. Communication: all management functions involve communication

1. Steps in communication
   a. Ideation

b. Encoding
c. Transmission
d. Receiving
e. Decoding
f. Response
2. Types
a. Downward: traditional from manager down
b. Upward: from staff up
c. Lateral: between peers
d. Diagonal: between different levels in different departments
e. Grapevine: informal, rapid, and usually distorted
3. Barriers
a. Faulty reasoning and poorly expressed messages
b. Lack of clarity: use of jargon
c. Lack of appropriate feedback mechanisms
d. Physical and environmental restraints
e. Preconceptions of receiver and sender

D. Assertiveness: ability to communicate expectations clearly from an adult ego state; components:
1. Use of direct statements with clear meaning
2. Use of "I" messages
3. Eye contact and spontaneous verbal expression of caring
4. Honest description of feelings
5. Focus on issues not people

E. Conflict resolution: ability to negotiate win-win outcomes when differences occur
1. Sources of conflict
a. Differences in facts
b. Differences in goals
c. Competition for scarce resources
2. Types
a. Interdepartment: between departments
b. Interpersonal: between personnel
c. Intradepartmental: within department
d. Intrapersonal: within person
3. Stages of conflict
a. Anticipation: expected because conditions exist for it to occur
b. Perceived: known but unexpressed differences
c. Discussion: differences expressed openly
d. Open dispute: conflict acknowledged
e. Open conflict: rigid positions are assumed
4. Approaches to conflict resolution
a. Avoiding: seen as uncooperative and unassertive; no outcome but may be useful when issue is trivial or other party is more powerful; cost of resolution is too high
b. Accommodating: seen as cooperative but unassertive; neglect of personal needs; useful when you are wrong or issue is more important to other party; does not resolve issue
c. Compromising: seen as assertive and cooperative; all concerned get some needs met; useful when issue is moderately important and power is equal
d. Collaborating: seen as assertive and cooperative; really leads to win-win outcome; search for mutually satisfactory outcome; seen as most effective strategy
e. Competing: seen as assertive but uncooperative; power oriented; create win/loss situation; may be necessary to implement unpopular decision; creates hostility in loser

## VII. Control

A. Purpose: to set standards to measure performance against and provide methods for reporting results and taking corrective action
B. Types
  1. Performance appraisal
    a. To determine job competence
    b. To enhance staff development and motivate staff toward higher achievement
    c. To recognize employee accomplishment
    d. To improve communication
    e. To determine professional development needs of individual staff
    f. To identify unsatisfactory employee performance
  2. Disciplinary action
    a. Investigate carefully
    b. Be prompt and judicious
    c. Protocol for employees' privacy
    d. Focus on act
    e. Be consistent in enforcement of policies
    f. Take corrective, constructive action
    g. Check that employee understands what change is expected
    h. Follow-up to determine that behavior change took place
  3. Quality improvement: hospital (health care facility)-wide interdisciplinary program that evaluates patient care, makes recommendations, and does follow-up to ensure corrective action has been taken on the basis of professional standards for structure, process, and outcome; uses specifically identified aspects of care
  4. Quality management: natural evolution of quality assurance process with specific interest to:
    a. Improve quality
    b. Decrease cost
    c. Improve productivity
    d. Capture market share
    e. Stay in business
    f. Provide jobs

## BIBLIOGRAPHY

American Society of PeriAnesthesia Nurses: *Standards of Perianesthesia Nursing Practice*. Richmond, Va, The Society, 1998.

Binkerton SE, Schroeder P: *Commitment to Excellence*. Rockville, Md, Aspen Publications, 1988.

Garner JF, Smith HL, Piland NE: *Strategic Nursing Management*. Rockville, Md, Aspen Publications, 1990.

Marriner-Tomey A: *Guide to Nursing Management*. St Louis, Mosby, 1992.

Pugh JB, Woodward-Smith MA: *Nurse Manager*. Philadelphia, WB Saunders, 1989.

Simendinger CA et al (eds): *The Successful Nurse Executive*. Management Series, American College of Healthcare Executives, Ann Arbor, Mich, Health Administration Press, 1990.

## REVIEW QUESTIONS

**1. Operational planning activities:**
A. Are long range and general
B. Focus on physical changes and equipment
C. Cover 5- to 10-year spans
D. Are specific goals for the coming year developed in conjunction with budget

**2. An organizational chart defines all but:**
A. Customary ways of thinking and behaving
B. Formal relationships
C. Areas of responsibility
D. Channels of communication

**3. Policies are used in the organizational component of management to:**
   A. Promote unit-specific direction
   B. Determine the chronologic sequence of steps
   C. Explain how goals will be achieved
   D. Control behavior

**4. In phase I of the PACU, the recommended nurse/patient ratio when patients are admitted requiring mechanical life support or artificial airway is:**
   A. 1:4
   B. 1:2
   C. 1:1
   D. 1:3

**5. In phase II of the PACU, it is within the American Society of Perianesthesia Nurses (ASPAN) standards to have a staffing ratio of 1:5 in all situations except:**
   A. Patients more than 5 years of age and ready for discharge
   B. Patients less than 5 years of age and ready for discharge with a family member present
   C. Patients less than 5 years of age but awake and stable with family present
   D. There are no acceptable conditions for a 1:5 staffing ratio

**6. Negotiation that decides issues on merits and looks for mutual gain requires that the manager does all but:**
   A. Separate people from problem
   B. Focus on interests instead of position
   C. Have a solution in mind
   D. Select option based on objective criteria

**7. The Japanese form of participative management that stresses cooperation and collective decision making is called:**
   A. Theory X
   B. Theory A
   C. Theory Y
   D. Theory Z

**8. The ability to communicate expectations clearly from an adult ego state is called:**
   A. Avoiding
   B. Assertiveness
   C. Accommodation
   D. Aggressiveness

**9. The hospital or health care facility interdisciplinary program that evaluates patient care, makes recommendations, and does follow-up to ensure that corrective action has been taken is referred to as:**
   A. Auditing
   B. Management by objective
   C. Strategic planning
   D. Quality improvement

**10. The conflict resolution strategy that is seen as assertive and cooperative because all concerned get some needs met is called:**
   A. Compromising
   B. Collaborating
   C. Competing
   D. Avoiding

**ANSWERS:** 1. D, 2. A, 3. C, 4. C, 5. C, 6. C, 7. D, 8. B, 9. D, 10. A

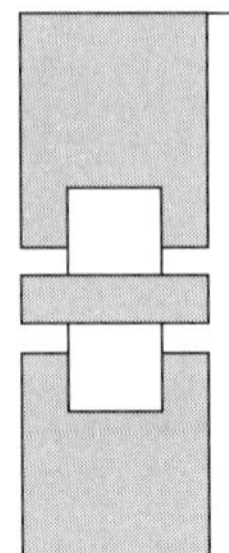

CHAPTER 6

# A Systems Approach to Education of the Surgical Patient

Mary E. Watson, MSCP, EdD, RRT

## OBJECTIVES

**Study of the information represented by this outline will enable the learner to:**

1. Describe the systems approach to patient teaching.
2. Identify elements of a needs assessment.
3. Develop goals for patient education.
4. Write objectives for instruction in three domains of learning.
5. Develop teaching strategies that meet the needs of patients with different learning styles.
6. Identify barriers to learning.
7. Identify methods to provide psychologic comfort to patients and families.
8. Develop methods for evaluation of patient education.
9. Use evaluation outcomes to make changes in the educational process.

**I. Using a Systems Approach to Patient Education** (Fig. 6–1)
- A. Provides a logical approach to designing instruction for patient interventions
- B. Provides a process for making changes in the intervention when learning outcomes are not met
- C. Can also be used for other training/education needs, such as designing staff education or for clinical instruction

**II. Instructional Design Begins With the Learner (Patient)**
- A. The needs of the patient are assessed first
- B. Consider the patient as an individual with specific needs, abilities, values, knowledge, and skills
  1. Start with what the learner knows
  2. Determine learning style
- C. As soon as possible:
  1. Use a collaborative approach with the patient
  2. Empower the patient, even if in small ways, e.g., encourage patient to set up a schedule for deep-breathing exercises
  3. Give patient choices whenever possible, e.g., making decisions about when teaching might take place

**III. Perform a Needs Assessment** (see Fig. 6–1): sources of information are:
- A. Statistics from the literature or experience, such as who is most likely to develop specific complications
- B. Patient history
- C. Consider the age of the patient
- D. Educational background and primary language
- E. Cultural background
- F. What knowledge, skills, values, and attitudes does the patient have?

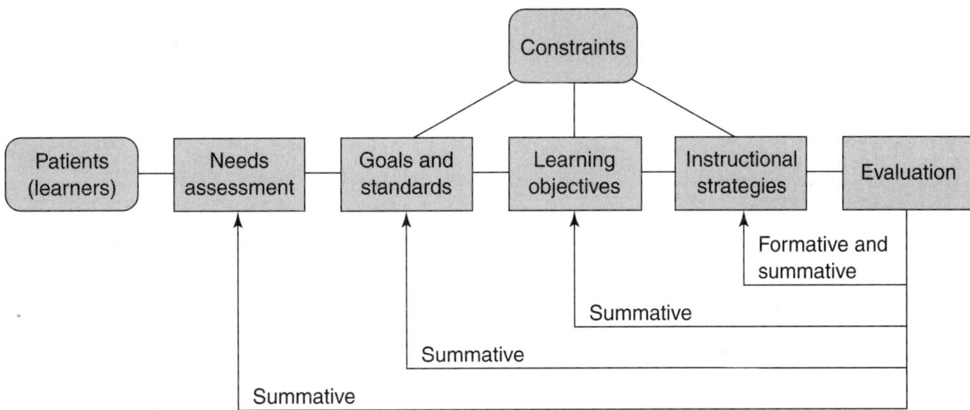


**FIGURE 6–1** Systems approach to patient education. (© ME Watson, 1998.)

1. Assess what patient already knows and needs to know
2. Gather data, using patient, family, other health professionals, chart, discharge instructions

G. Any faulty learning that needs to be corrected?

H. What knowledge, skills, and attitudes will need to be reinforced?

I. What are previous health practices?

J. Physical assessment data to include the stress response that may impose barriers to learning or interfere with learning readiness (see Chapter 27)

**IV. Develop Goals for Patient Learning** (see Fig. 6–1)

A. Definition of goals
1. Broad statements of direction
2. General statements of learning outcomes
3. General knowledge, skills, or attitudes that the learner will have after instruction takes place
4. They provide direction for writing objectives that further define the goals in specific terms

B. Examples of goals in patient teaching:
1. The patient will understand the importance of deep breathing to prevent atelectasis during postoperative care
2. The patient will function independently

C. Consider the purposes of patient teaching when setting goals
1. Forewarn: provide information e.g., what happens after PACU
2. Teach skills: e.g., how to do a dressing change
3. Assist in decision making
4. Reinforce what may already be known
5. Explain procedures, follow-up, medications
6. Instruct about home health follow-up, ways to manage at home
7. Change: provide alternative behaviors or thoughts
8. Maximize current level of functioning

D. From where are goals derived?
1. Results of needs assessments
2. From the health care team
    a. Nurses, physicians and other health professionals involved with patient care
    b. Patient and his or her family as appropriate
3. Philosophy of the unit and health care facility
4. Professional guidelines for standards of care
5. Health care facility or unit procedures for care

6. In some situations goals are developed first and then a needs assessment follows, e.g.:
   a. To decrease the incidence of postoperative atelectasis in cardiac surgical patients
   b. To increase patient compliance with prescribed medications

**V. Design Standards Related to the Goals** (see Fig. 6–1)
- A. Criteria for acceptable individual patient performance
- B. Criteria for determining whether overall program was successful
- C. Examples of standards related to the previously stated goals:
  1. On a follow-up survey, it will be reported (by nurses, therapists, patients, etc.) that 100% of the patients performed deep-breathing exercises after being instructed on the new protocol (refer to goal in IVB1)
  2. On a follow-up survey (to patient by visiting nurse etc.), 95% of the patients were able to function independently 4 weeks after discharge (refer to goal in IVB2)

**VI. Objectives for Instruction Are Developed from Goals** (see Fig. 6–1)
- A. Definition of objectives:
  1. Statements of *specific* learning outcomes, e.g.:
     a. The patient will be able to state signs and symptoms of wound infection
     b. The patient will be able to demonstrate management of an indwelling urinary catheter
  2. Objectives are written with more detail than goals
  3. They specify the *observable* knowledge, skills, or attitudes that the learner will exhibit
  4. They communicate the instructor's intent for the outcome of learning
- B. Objectives are written in *three domains* of learning as appropriate for the patient situation
  1. *Cognitive:* intellectual skills, learner's knowledge and understanding
  2. *Affective:* learner's values, attitudes, emotions, and ways of adjusting to illness
  3. *Psychomotor:* skills requiring neuromuscular coordination
- C. Steps in writing objectives
  1. State the *terminal* behavior: what the learner will be able to do after the instruction; e.g., the patient will *perform an inspiratory capacity* with the incentive spirometer
  2. State the *conditions* placed on the learner; e.g., add to the above objective—*without assistance*
  3. State the *standards* of performance
     a. How well the learner must perform
     b. Requirements such as how often, how many times, how accurate
     c. Example: add to the above objective—*10 times per hour at 80%* of preoperative inspiratory capacity
  4. Complete objective: the patient will perform an inspiratory capacity at 80% of preoperative inspiratory capacity with the incentive spirometer without assistance 10 times per hour
- D. Common *errors* in writing or using objectives
  1. Ignoring an essential domain, e.g.,
     a. Writing the objective in the cognitive domain when the important part is for the learner to *perform (psychomotor domain)*
     b. Underestimating the need to challenge the values and belief systems of the learner *(affective domain)* to accomplish a goal
  2. Emphasizing what will be taught instead of what the learner is expected to be able to do

**VII. Develop Learning Strategies for Instruction** (see Fig. 6–1)
- A. Consider that individuals have different learning styles (see Sonbuchner, 1991)
  1. *Visual learners:* learn if they can see it, picture something in mind
     a. Videotapes, charts, diagrams, tours of unit or environment where care will take place

2. *Auditory learners:* learn easily by listening
   a. Give explanations of information, audiotapes
3. *Readers:* cognitive learners who take in information when they can read it
   a. Have available written information
4. *Verbal learners:* learn when they can talk about information
   a. Give time for questions/discussions
5. *Writers:* learn through writing things down
   a. Give opportunity to take notes on information
6. *Manipulation:* learn through touching, handling
   a. Use models, games, let them handle equipment/supplies etc.
   b. Will benefit from psychomotor teaching strategies

B. Types of learning appropriate for patients
   1. Individual instruction
   2. Self-directed strategies
   3. Lecture
   4. Discussion (individual and small group)
   5. Audiovisual aids and models
   6. Written materials
   7. Group teaching
   8. Demonstration/repeat demonstration
   9. Role-playing
   10. Tours/visits
   11. Games

## VIII. Eliminate or Decrease Barriers That Interfere With Effective Teaching and Communication

A. Consider barriers and make adjustments whenever possible, e.g.,
   1. Patient may have cognitive or psychomotor limitations
   2. Stress may cause difficulties in processing information
   3. Patient may have difficulty transfering learning from the health care facility to the home environment

B. Choose appropriate time: do not compete with other things

C. Use appropriate environment: consider privacy, room temperature, noise distractions

D. Decrease physiologic distraction: pain, nausea, vomiting, cold

E. Consider patient readiness to process information
   - Assess cognitive, psychomotor, and affective ability before instruction (learning requires perception, i.e., the ability to hear and understand)
   - Senses may be impaired from anesthesia, postoperative drugs
   - Fear of outcome of surgery, fear of unfamiliar surroundings, etc. will impact ability to take in information
   - Learning will be more effective if the patient sees a need for it

F. Provide different strategies for delivering information for initial teaching and for reinforcement
   1. Allow sufficient time: do not rush
   2. Consider age and developmentally appropriate learning strategies, e.g., games for children
   3. Feedback must be given during the learning process
   4. Learning must be reinforced
   5. For learning to be retained, information must be put to immediate use
   6. Base learning on real life experiences
   7. Make instruction application oriented: use what is to be learned
   8. Eliminate the use of technical language that patient does not understand

## IX. Providing Psychologic Comfort

A. Acknowledge feelings and behavior of individual

1. Verbalizations and behaviors may be uncomfortable for patient, family, and staff
2. Do not minimize or ignore feelings
3. Really listen to the patient

B. Develop trusting relationship
   1. Foundations
      a. Consistency
      b. Nonjudgmental approach
      c. Honesty: give accurate information and don't provide false reassurance
      d. Confidentiality: do not violate the patient's trust

C. Involve family and significant others
   1. Build on support system
   2. Will be important for outpatients

## X. Develop and Implement Methods of Evaluation

A. *Formative evaluation:* assessment of learning throughout the process
   1. Ask questions to determine understanding
   2. Give self-assessment materials to patient
   3. Observe and document patient behaviors
   4. Ask patient to document behaviors
      a. How new knowledge or skills have been used
      b. Attitudes about behaviors or situations encountered
      c. Problem areas that need attention
      d. Self-perceived abilities, skills, and attitudes

B. Types of evaluation methods
   1. Objective written assessments
   2. Oral questioning
   3. Direct observation: rating scales, anecdotal records, checklists
   4. Self-evaluation
   5. Physical assessment data
   6. Laboratory data

C. Analyze and use information from formative evaluation
   1. What has been learned?
   2. What skills need to be reinforced?
   3. Plan and implement alternative teaching strategies where needed

D. *Summative evaluation:* evaluation at the end of instruction to assess long-term results
   1. Is more comprehensive than formative
   2. Evaluation to assess mastery of learning and to determine readiness to progress, e.g.,
      a. To leave the unit
      b. To go home
      c. To live independently
   3. Were goals achieved?
   4. Assess long-term success where appropriate
   5. May use some methods as in formative evaluations
   6. Includes evaluation information about the patient related to success of instruction, e.g.,
      a. Follow-up surveys to patients, families, caregivers
      b. Follow-up surveys to units where patients are discharged
      c. Determine long-term success of teaching where appropriate
      d. Assess patient satisfaction
      e. Ask for suggestions
   7. Gather information in aggregate about success of patient instruction over a period of time, e.g.,
      a. Statistics on specific postoperative complications

b. Morbidity and mortality rates
c. Emergency room visits
8. Use this information to adjust parts of the process where needed, e.g.,
a. Make changes in goals
b. New considerations in performing needs assessment
c. Modify or add to objectives
d. Develop more effective strategies for teaching and reinforcement
e. Evaluate and assess outcomes
f. Again, make adjustments in the patient teaching system on the basis of analysis of results

E. General considerations for evaluation
1. Assure content validity: the extent to which an evaluation measures the intended content
a. Occurs during the evaluation construction
b. Match the objectives to the questions
2. Assure criterion validity: the extent that an evaluation predicts a specific outcome, e.g.,
a. Does the evaluation predict long-term success of patient?
b. Does successful performance of a skill in the hospital result in the ability to do the same at home?
3. Assure the best possible reliability: consistency of evaluation results
a. Reliability is effected by, for example,
(1) Quality of evaluation or survey items
(2) Number of items
(3) Physical and emotional state of patient
(4) What directions are given to patient
(5) Environmental factors
(6) Experience or knowledge of the evaluator or practitioner
(7) Rapport between the patient and practitioner
b. Develop assessment instruments and surveys that go through a critiquing process by expert professionals
c. Train the practitioners to use the evaluation instruments
d. Review evaluation instruments periodically

## BIBLIOGRAPHY


Bordens KS, Abbott BB: *Research Design and Methods: A Process Approach.* Mountain View, Calif, Mayfield, 1988.

Gronlund NE: *How to Write and Use Instructional Objectives,* 5th Ed. Upper Saddle River, NJ, Prentice-Hall, 1995.

Harrison L: A health promotion model for wellness education. *MCN* 15:191, 1990.

Kruger S: A review of patient education in nursing. *J Nurs Staff Dev* 6:71, 1990.

Sonbuchner GM: *Finding Your Best Learning Style and Study Environment.* Rochelle Park, NJ, The Peoples Publishing Group, 1991.

Timmreck TC: *Planning, Program Development, and Evaluation. A Handbook for Health Promotion, Aging, and Health Services.* Boston, Jones and Bartlett, 1995.

Watson ME: *A Systems Approach to Education and Program Planning for Health Professionals.* Boston, Northeastern University, 1998.


## REVIEW QUESTIONS

**1. The systems approach to patient teaching:**

A. Assures that goals will be met if enough strategies are used
B. Provides a process for changes if outcomes are not successful
C. Can only successfully be used for patient education
D. Does not require evaluation until the patient is discharged

**2. Sources of information for a needs assessment could include:**

A. Statistics from the literature
B. Patient history
C. Knowledge, skills, and values of the patient
D. All of the above

**3. Goals for patient teaching are:**

A. Broad statements of direction
B. General statements of learning outcomes
C. Provide direction for writing specific objectives
D. All of the above

**4. Which of the following is an example of a patient goal? The patient will:**

A. State three symptoms of infection
B. Function independently
C. Demonstrate the ability to use crutches
D. All of the above

**5. The aspect of learning most influenced by a learner's attitudes and emotions is:**

A. Affective
B. Cognitive
C. Psychomotor
D. Experiential

**6. Which of the following is an example of a psychomotor objective? The patient will:**

A. Understand the need to cough post-operatively
B. Describe the appropriate process of coughing
C. Demonstrate effective coughing techniques
D. Develop a good attitude about coughing

**7. Which of the following is an example of a cognitive objective? The patient will:**

A. State the signs and symptoms of infection
B. Demonstrate the ability to walk with crutches
C. Develop a good attitude about the result of surgery
D. All of the above

**8. Which of the following is an example of an affective objective? The patient will:**

A. Develop a good attitude about learning
B. Respond to teaching by attending to the protocol
C. Define atelectasis
D. Describe the reasons for deep breathing and coughing

**9. Videotapes, charts, and diagrams are effective strategies for:**

A. Auditory learners
B. Verbal learners
C. Visual learners
D. Readers

**10. Barriers to effective communication and teaching include:**

A. Invading and lack of privacy
B. Noisy and cold environment
C. Not listening and minimizing feelings
D. All of the above

**11. Auditory learners will benefit from:**

A. Careful explanations of the information
B. Reinforcement of the learning with audiotapes
C. Both A and B
D. None of the above

**12. Physiologic distractions that interfere with learning are:**
A. Pain
B. Nausea
C. Cold
D. All of the above

**13. Formative evaluation methods during the process of patient teaching include:**
A. Oral questions
B. Direct observation
C. Physical assessment data
D. All of the above

**ANSWERS:** 1. B, 2. D, 3. D, 4. B, 5. A, 6. C, 7. A, 8. B, 9. C, 10. D, 11. C, 12. D, 13. D

PART TWO

# Life Span Considerations in PACU Practice

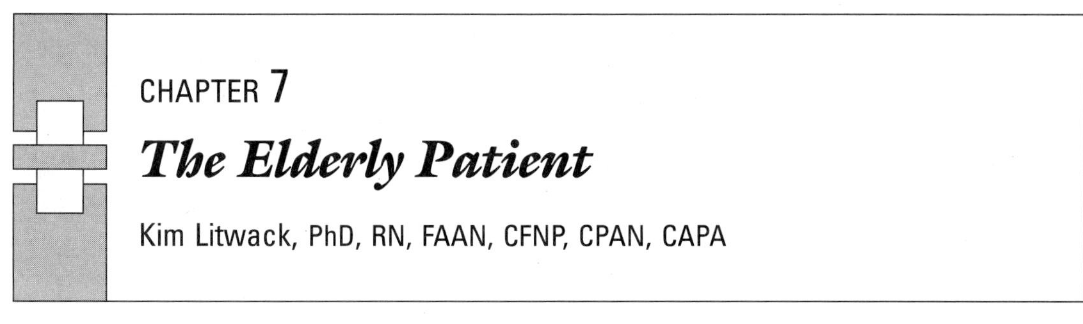

# CHAPTER 7
# *The Elderly Patient*

Kim Litwack, PhD, RN, FAAN, CFNP, CPAN, CAPA

## OBJECTIVES

**Study of the information represented by this outline will enable the learner to:**

1. Use a systems approach to identify changes that occur with aging.
2. Identify potential problems that may occur after a surgical procedure.
3. Discuss the purpose of a preoperative assessment.
4. Identify postoperative priorities in consideration of the physiologic changes that occur with aging.

Elderly patients present a unique challenge for the perianesthesia care unit (PACU) nurse. Physiologic changes of aging combined with pathologic conditions necessitating surgical intervention mandate careful assessment, planning, and implementation of the nursing process and PACU care plan.

**I. Definition of Elderly**
- A. Greater than 65 years old
  - 1. 65 to 75 years: "young-old"
  - 2. 75 to 85 years: "old"
  - 3. 85+ years: "old-old"
- B. Life expectancy
  - 1. Men: 74 years
  - 2. Women: 78 years
- C. Number of elderly in United States is increasing
  - 1. By 2030, 22% of population >age 65
  - 2. 5000 Americans celebrate 65th birthday each day
  - 3. Elderly account for one third of all health care costs

**II. Theories of Aging (Proposed)**
- A. Random mutation of DNA
- B. Cumulative abnormalities of DNA
- C. Damage to tissues by free radicals
- D. Biologic clock
- E. Genetic program of life expectancy
- F. Failure of growth substance
- G. Production of an "aging factor"

**III. Physiologic Changes of Aging: Changes in Both Structure and Function**
- A. Cardiovascular changes
  - 1. Arteriosclerotic changes: calcification
    - a. Loss of large artery elasticity
      - (1) Coronary
      - (2) Aorta
      - (3) Carotid

                (4) Iliac
                (5) Femoral
                (6) Popliteal
                (7) Renal
            b. Decreased organ perfusion and decreased compensatory regulation from loss of elasticity
            c. Vessel fragility
        2. Myocardial changes
            a. Left ventricular hypertrophy
            b. Increased myocardial irritability, leading to dysrhythmias
            c. Fibrosis of endocardial lining, leading to endocardial thickening and rigidity, decreased contractility
            d. Calcification of valves, leading to valve incompetence
        3. Altered hemodynamics
            a. Decreased cardiac output (1% per year after 30 years of age)
            b. Decreased stroke volume
            c. Increased blood pressure
            d. Slowed circulation time, leading to slower onset of drug effects
            e. Decreased cardiac reserve; stressors:
                (1) Fever
                (2) Tachycardia
                (3) Exertion
                (4) Anxiety
                (5) Hypoxemia
                (6) Pain
        4. Orthostatic hypotension
            a. Decreased blood vessel tone, leading to peripheral pooling of blood, increased risk for DVT
            b. Baroreceptor failure
            c. Medications (most common cause)
                (1) Antihypertensives
                (2) Diuretics
                (3) Tricyclic antidepressants
                (4) Phenothiazines
                (5) Alcohol
            d. Decreased tolerance to volume changes
        5. Slowed conduction
            a. Decreased heart rate
                (1) Resulting from increased parasympathetic activity
                (2) Resulting from degenerative changes in conduction system
            b. Can lead to central nervous system (CNS) changes
    B. Respiratory changes
        1. Anatomic changes
            a. Increased anteroposterior (AP) diameter
            b. Progressive flattening and decreased muscle strength of diaphragm
            c. Increased chest wall rigidity
                (1) Arthritic changes in rib cage
            d. Reduction in alveolar surface
            e. Narrowing of intervertebral disks
                (1) Reduces total lung capacity by 10%
            f. Loss of skeletal muscle mass, leading to wasting of diaphragm and skeletal muscles
            g. Loss of teeth changes jaw structure, leading to difficult airway maintenance

2. Physiologic changes
   a. Reduction in pulmonary elasticity
   b. Decreased chest wall mobility
   c. Loss of alveolar septa, leading to air trapping
   d. Decreased pulmonary compliance
   e. Increased airway resistance
   f. Decreased cough and gag reflex, leading to risk of aspiration
   g. Ventilation/perfusion ($\dot{V}/\dot{Q}$) alterations develop
      (1) Decreased tidal volume
      (2) Decreased vital capacity
      (3) Decreased inspiratory reserve
      (4) Decreased cardiac output
      (5) Decreased aerobic capacity
      (6) Increased dead space
      (7) Decreased $O_2/CO_2$ exchange
      (8) Decreased oxygen content of blood
         (a) $Pao_2 = 100 - (0.4 \times \text{Age in years}) = \text{mm Hg}$
         (b) For example, in an 80-year-old: $Pao_2 = 100 - (0.4 \times 80) = 68$ mm Hg (vs. normal $Pao_2$ of 100 mm Hg)

C. CNS changes
   1. Decrease in neuronal density and nerve conduction
      a. Resulting from neurogenic atrophy/loss of peripheral nerve fibers
      b. Results in slowed reflexes
      c. Increased CNS side effects of drugs
   2. Decline in sympathetic response
      a. Resulting from decreased synthesis of neurotransmitters
      b. Decreases ability of body to face stressors
         (1) Decreased cardiac reserve and responsiveness
   3. Compromised thermoregulation secondary to decreased hypothalamic perfusion
   4. Compromised perfusion due to arteriosclerotic changes
      a. Increased incidence of organic brain syndrome
      b. Increased incidence of cerebrovascular accidents (strokes)
      c. Increased incidence of microemboli
      d. Decreased cerebral blood flow
      e. Decreased cerebral metabolic oxygen consumption
      f. Decreased CNS activity

D. Gastrointestinal changes
   1. Decreased salivation
   2. Decreased peristalsis
      a. Gastric emptying delayed
      b. Increased risk of aspiration
      c. Increased problem of constipation
   3. Decreased hepatic blood flow resulting from arteriosclerotic changes
   4. Decreased microsomal enzyme activity
      a. Delayed drug metabolism, e.g., fentanyl, vecuronium
   5. Decreased absorption of orally administered drugs/nutrients, e.g., ferrous sulfate (iron) and calcium
   6. Malnutrition possible
      a. Can increase perioperative morbidity
      b. Can compromise postoperative recovery and wound healing
      c. Most reliable indicator of malnutrition is hypoalbuminemia

E. Genitourinary changes
   1. Decreased bladder capacity (200 ml)

2. Decreased muscle tone and weakened sphincters
   a. Especially in women after multiple obstetric deliveries
   b. May result in incontinence
   c. Increased residual urine
3. Enlarged prostate (men)—may result in urinary incontinence and retention
4. Decreased glomerular filtration rate
   a. Resulting from decreased blood flow
   b. Decreases 1% to 1.5% per year after 30 years of age
   c. Results in decreased renal metabolism
      (1) Decreased clearance of medications/metabolites
      (2) Examples: fentanyl, vecuronium, midazolam
5. Response time to correct fluid/electrolyte balance increased
   a. May increase risk of fluid overload
   b. Decreased ability to concentrate urine
   c. Inability to conserve sodium, leading to hyponatremia
   d. Decreased activity of renin or aldosterone, leading to hyperkalemia

F. Musculoskeletal changes
1. Osteoporosis
   a. Leads to decline in bone matrix
   b. Skeletal support compromised
   c. Bone resorption exceeds bone formation
   d. Increased risk of fractures, pain, skeletal deformities
      (1) Repair of hip fractures is one of top five surgeries done in elderly patients
   e. Decrease in flexibility
2. Degenerative changes in vertebrae increase difficulty of spinal anesthesia and intubation
3. Atrophy of muscles
4. May compromise intraoperative positioning

G. Endocrine changes
1. Decreased ability to metabolize glucose
   a. Results in glucose intolerance
   b. Pancreatic function declines
      (1) Increased incidence of adult-onset diabetes mellitus
      (2) Greatest between 60 and 70 years of age
   c. Plasma renin concentrating ability decreases 30% to 50%

H. Dermatologic changes
1. Loss of subcutaneous fat
   a. Compromises thermoregulation
   b. Increased risk of hypothermia
   c. Loss of padding for bony prominences
2. Increase in overall body fat (especially women)
   a. Increased availability of lipid-storage sites
      (1) Reservoir for lipid (fat)-soluble drugs: diazepam, midazolam, enflurane
      (2) Prolongs drug action
3. Loss of sweat glands
4. Decreased skin pigmentation caused by decreased production of melanocytes; pallor does not equal anemia
5. Epidural atrophy and loss of collagen
   a. Increases risk of skin breakdown and injury
   b. Decreases skin elasticity and turgor

I. Sensory changes
1. Visual changes
   a. Decreased visual acuity
   b. Decreased peripheral vision

c. Decreased accommodation (presbyopia)
d. Retinal vascular changes
e. Cataract formation
f. Increased incidence of glaucoma
2. Auditory changes
a. Decreased sensitivity to sound (presbycusis)
b. Loss of high-pitched sound perception
c. Impairment of sound localization
3. Tactile changes
a. Decreased sensation
b. Decreased response to pain
4. Taste and smell acuity decreases

J. Laboratory changes
1. Decreased potassium
a. Medications—diuretics
b. Diet deficient in potassium
2. Decreased sodium
a. Dilutional
b. True decrease
c. Renal failure
3. Decreased hemoglobin
a. Blood loss (GI and postmenstrual uterine bleeding)
b. Malabsorption of iron
c. Malnutrition

K. Neuropsychiatric changes
1. Acute brain syndrome
a. Physiologic
b. Rapid-onset
c. Reversible
d. Possible causes—always rule out hypoxemia first!
(1) Medication intolerance
(2) Metabolic disturbance
(3) Electrolyte imbalance
(a) Hypernatremia/hyponatremia
(4) Nutritional deficit
(5) Depression
(6) Stress, fear, anxiety
2. Chronic brain syndrome
a. Associated with arteriosclerosis
b. Degenerative changes
(1) Alzheimer's disease
(2) Cerebrovascular accident (CVA; stroke)
(3) Dementia
3. Depression
a. Causes: isolation, illness, loss, biochemical changes
b. Symptoms: fatigue, insomnia, anorexia, somatic changes

**IV. Pharmacologic Alterations in Aging**

A. Alterations in organs responsible for drug metabolism and clearance
1. Lungs
2. Kidneys
3. Liver

B. Protein binding of medications impaired
1. Increases amount of available (free/unbound) drug
a. Free drug is active drug, increasing drug effects

- C. Storage of lipid-soluble medications increased
  - 1. Unpredictable clearance and elimination
- D. Prolonged action and elimination of medications
  - 1. Require decreased doses of medications
  - 2. Increase risk of cumulative drug effects
  - 3. Increase risk of adverse drug reactions

**V. Pathophysiologic Conditions in Elderly:** 86% of people >75 years old have one or more chronic conditions

- A. Organ system changes—organ system dysfunction
  - 1. Cardiovascular: hypertension, atherosclerosis, dysrhythmias, valve disease
  - 2. Cerebral: cerebrovascular accident, cognitive degeneration
  - 3. Pulmonary: chronic obstructive pulmonary disease (COPD), asthma
  - 4. Endocrine: diabetes mellitus, hypothyroidism
  - 5. Neurologic: Parkinson's disease
  - 6. Musculoskeletal: arthritis
  - 7. Sensory: visual and hearing loss
  - 8. Hepatic: cirrhosis
- B. Physical status changes increase anesthetic and surgical risk
  - 1. Medications for treatment may increase risk

**VI. Common Surgical Procedures**

- A. Ophthalmic: cataract, vitrectomy
- B. Genitourinary: cystoscopy, TURP
- C. Orthopedic: ORIF—hip, joint replacement
- D. Cardiovascular: pacemaker, carotid endarterectomy
- E. General: herniorrhaphy, cholecystectomy

**VII. Considerations Before Surgery**

- A. Preoperative assessment (purposes)
  - 1. To obtain precise baseline
    - a. Consider physiologic not chronologic age
    - b. Age alone does not determine risk
  - 2. To obtain information about preexisting disease
    - a. Especially with ambulatory patients
    - b. Includes medications used and appropriateness of use
    - c. Acute vs. chronic conditions
    - d. Evaluation of risk
  - 3. To review or obtain laboratory information
    - a. Anemia common
    - b. Electrolyte imbalance
      - (1) Hypokalemia resulting from diuretics
      - (2) Hyponatremia resulting from inability to conserve sodium
      - (3) Glucose levels in diabetic patients
  - 4. To identify special needs
    - a. Prostheses
    - b. Language and communication barriers
    - c. Mobility aids
    - d. Barriers to ambulatory patient returning home
      - (1) Transportation
      - (2) Caregiver availability—ability to care for self
      - (3) Access to follow-up care
  - 5. To anticipate postoperative sequelae and to reduce risk factors
  - 6. To begin patient teaching

7. To maximize preoperative physical status
   a. Pulmonary function
   b. Nutritional status, including hydration
   c. Medication protocol

B. Multidisciplinary assessment
   1. PACU nurse
   2. Anesthesiologist
   3. Surgeon
   4. Medical consultation as needed

## VIII. Anesthetic Options for Elderly Patient

A. General anesthesia
   1. Smooth induction/rapid recovery
   2. Inhalation requirements less
      a. Minimum alveolar concentration (MAC) decreases by 4%/yr after 40 years of age
   3. Delayed clearance/metabolism of intravenous anesthetic agents
      a. Decrease dose of barbiturates, benzodiazepines, opioids
   4. Increased risk of hypothermia
   5. If edentulous, may be difficult to ventilate by mask
   6. Arthritis may limit cervicospinal mobility for intubation

B. Regional anesthesia
   1. Minimal physiologic alterations
   2. Decreased cardiopulmonary complications
   3. Less postoperative confusion
   4. Provides postoperative analgesia
   5. Spinal anesthesia
      a. Lower abdomen and lower extremity surgery
      b. Duration prolonged in elderly
      c. Hypotension may be pronounced
      d. May be complicated by musculoskeletal changes
      e. Low incidence of spinal headaches
   6. Epidural anesthesia
      a. Less hypotension
      b. Greater cardiovascular stability
      c. Reduced anesthetic dose requirements

C. Intravenous conscious sedation (IVCS)
   1. Increased sedating effects of benzodiazepines
   2. Increased respiratory depressant effects of narcotics
   3. Because of coexisting diseases, may not be appropriate for RN to administer IVCS

D. Ambulatory surgery
   1. Minimizes separation from family/environment
   2. May be appropriate depending on type of surgery
      a. Must consider risks of anesthetic, surgery, home care

## IX. Postoperative Priorities for Elderly Patient

A. Reduction of morbidity and mortality

B. Ventilation
   1. Promote optimal gas exchange
      a. Provide high-humidity oxygen
      b. Promote deep breathing
      c. Prevent atelectasis
      d. Elevate head of bed to facilitate lung expansion

2. Prevent respiratory infections
   a. Sterile suctioning of endotracheal tube
   b. Protect patient from aspiration
   c. Promote deep breathing (prevent pneumonia)
3. Monitor for compromised function
   a. Observe for residual drug effects
   b. Maintain artificial airways
   c. Use pulse oximetry monitoring
   d. Consider preexisting disease

C. Fluid balance
1. Correct preoperative dehydration
   a. NPO status
   b. Diuretic therapy
   c. Poor nutritional status
   d. Presence of nausea and vomiting
2. Prevent fluid overload
   a. Assess preexisting cardiopulmonary disease
   b. Monitor intake and output
   c. Assess breath sounds
3. Monitor urine output
   a. Decreased bladder capacity
   b. Urinary retention (men); incontinence (women)
   c. Perioperative diuretics
   d. Perioperative fluid intake
   e. Decreased awareness of distension

D. Activity—"stir-up" routine
1. Promotes circulation and ventilation
2. Permits assessment of neurologic status
   a. Deviations from preoperative status
3. Monitor for orthostatic hypotension when mobilizing outpatients
   a. Mobilize more slowly than younger adults

E. Thermoregulation
1. Rewarm patient
2. Document temperature
3. Normothermia promotes cardiovascular stability

F. Comfort
1. Positioning
   a. Care in turning; turn frequently
   b. Anatomic and surgical alignment
   c. Pad bony prominences
2. Skin care
   a. Avoid excessive tape application
   b. Remove tape and electrocardiogram (ECG) leads carefully
   c. Dry wet skin promptly
   d. Hold venipuncture sites after removal of needle
   e. Remove skin prep solutions to decrease irritation
3. Pain management
   a. Titrate narcotics
   b. Pain increases myocardial oxygen demand
   c. Consider decreased sensory response to pain
   d. Evaluate presence of residual preoperative/anesthetic drugs
4. Psychologic support
   a. Reorientation
   b. Avoid sensory deprivation and overload

c. Avoid use of restraints
d. Continue verbal and tactile communication
e. Provide hearing aids, glasses, and dentures
f. Provide simple, clear instructions—ascertain patient's level of understanding
g. Rule out hypoxemia as cause of postoperative agitation
h. Maintain dignity and respect

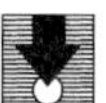

**NURSING DIAGNOSIS**

Examples of related nursing diagnostic categories include:

- Impaired gas exchange
- Potential for infection
- Ineffective breathing pattern
- Alteration in fluid volume (excess or deficiency)
- Ineffective thermoregulation: hypothermia
- Knowledge deficit: preoperative/postoperative information
- Alteration in comfort: pain
- Sensory-perceptual alteration
- Ineffective airway clearance
- Impaired physical mobility
- Self-care deficit

## BIBLIOGRAPHY

Callahan L: General considerations in planning anesthetic care for the geriatric patient. *Anesth Today* 3(1):10–14, 1991.

Litwack K: The elderly patient in the post anesthesia care unit. *Nurs Clin North Am* 28(3):507–518, 1993.

Litwack K: *The Elderly Surgical Patient.* Sacramento, Calif. CME Resource, 1995.

Martin-Sheridan D: Geriatrics and anesthesia practice. In Nagelhout J, Zaglaniczny K (eds): *Nurse Anesthesia* (pp 981–987). Philadelphia, Saunders, 1997.

McLeskey C: Pharmacokinetic and pharmacodynamic differences in the elderly patient undergoing anesthesia. *Anesth Today* 3(1):1–9, 1991.

McLeskey C, Nibel D: Anesthesia for the geriatric outpatient. In White P (ed): *Outpatient Anesthesia.* New York, Churchill-Livingstone, 1990.

Norman J: *Gerontological Nursing.* Sacramento, Calif, CME Resource, 1994.

Roy R, Price A: Geriatric patients. In McGoldrick K (ed): *Ambulatory Anesthesiology: A Problem-Oriented Approach* (pp 111–126). Baltimore, Williams & Wilkins, 1995.

Stiff J: Evaluation of geriatric patient. In Rogers M, Tinker J, Covino B, et al (eds): *Principles and Practice of Anesthesia* (pp 480–492). St Louis, Mosby, 1993.

## REVIEW QUESTIONS

**1. Which of the following cardiovascular changes occur with aging?**

A. Large artery elasticity, decreased myocardial irritability, increased cardiac reserve
B. Left ventricular hypertrophy, slowed circulation time, decreased blood vessel tone
C. Increased organ perfusion, right ventricular hypertrophy, decreased blood pressure
D. Increased compensatory regulation, increased stroke volume, increased cardiac output

**2. Which of the following is not a respiratory change seen in the elderly?**

A. Increased airway resistance
B. Reduction in pulmonary elasticity
C. Loss of alveolar septa
D. Increased pulmonary compliance

**3. There is an increased incidence of adult-onset diabetes mellitus in the elderly because of:**
A. Enhanced pancreatic function
B. Increased tolerance to elevated glucose levels
C. Decreased ability to metabolize glucose
D. Increased plasma renin concentrations

**4. All of the following organs are responsible for drug metabolism, clearance, or both except the:**
A. Lungs
B. Kidney
C. Spleen
D. Liver

**5. A preoperative assessment is important in:**
A. Establishing a baseline
B. Obtaining information about preexisting disease
C. Identifying special needs
D. All of the above

**6. Which of the following statements about the use of general anesthesia in the elderly is true?**
A. Smooth induction, rapid recovery
B. Increased inhalation requirements
C. Lower risk of hypothermia
D. Increased intravenous drug requirements

**7. Postoperative agitation in the elderly patient is most likely due to:**
A. Medication intolerance
B. Hypoxemia
C. Alzheimer's disease
D. Organic brain syndrome

**8. Laboratory changes that might be seen in the elderly patient include:**
A. Hyperkalemia resulting from diuretics used to treat hypertension
B. Increased hemoglobin and hematocrit
C. Hypoglycemia resulting from chronic respiratory alkalosis
D. Hyponatremia resulting from the inability to conserve sodium

**9. Barriers to the elderly patient being a candidate for ambulatory surgery include:**
A. Lack of access to transportation
B. Lack of access to follow-up care
C. Lack of a companion
D. All of the above

**10. The most common cause of orthostatic hypotension in the elderly patient is:**
A. Sensitivity to medications
B. Decreased blood vessel tone
C. Baroreceptor failure
D. Peripheral pooling of blood

**ANSWERS:** 1. B, 2. D, 3. C, 4. C, 5. D, 6. A, 7. B, 8. D, 9. D, 10. A

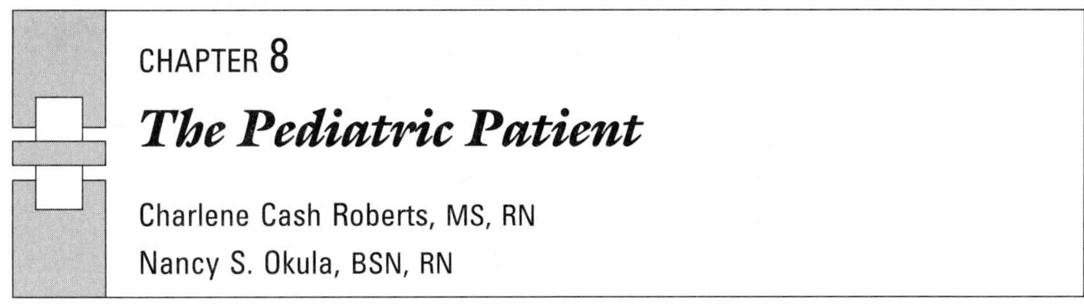

# CHAPTER 8
# *The Pediatric Patient*

Charlene Cash Roberts, MS, RN
Nancy S. Okula, BSN, RN

## OBJECTIVES

**Study of the information represented by this outline will enable the learner to:**

1. Identify the anatomic differences between the pediatric patient and the adult patient with emphasis on the airway.
2. Identify common pediatric airway problems and appropriate nursing management modalities.
3. Discuss extubation of the pediatric patient.
4. Assess and evaluate pain and its management for the pediatric patient.
5. Discuss pediatric medications.
6. Discuss the importance of monitoring vital signs in the pediatric patient with particular attention to the blood pressure.
7. Engage in crisis intervention and manage postanesthesia complications for the pediatric patient in the perianesthesia care unit (PACU).
8. List various items needed for a pediatric crash cart and their importance.
9. Manage fluid and electrolyte balance in the pediatric patient.
10. Understand postanesthesia nursing implications in caring for the premature infant.
11. Identify important aspects of specific surgical procedures for the pediatric patient and particular nursing interventions.
12. Discuss the impact of surgery and postanesthesia care on the growth and development of the pediatric patient.
13. Incorporate family dynamics in the care of the pediatric postanesthesia patient.
14. Discuss the significance of postoperative or postanesthetic home care instructions and their relevance to the pediatric population.

Providing safe, effective, and appropriate postanesthesia nursing care to the pediatric patient is a unique challenge. Pediatric patients are not miniature adults, although the goal of nursing care for these postanesthesia patients is the same as that for their adult counterparts—a safe return to their preanesthesia state. Obviously, parental anxiety is high during the pediatric patient's surgery. The PACU nurse deals not only with the child as patient but also with the integrity of the family unit during the child's care.

Infants and children can tolerate a much greater alteration of homeostatic state than adults. Drastic fluctuation is a hallmark of pediatric illness. This section provides a review for PACU nurses who do not care exclusively for pediatric patients.

## GROWTH AND DEVELOPMENT

**NURSING DIAGNOSIS**

Examples of related nursing diagnostic categories include:
- Anxiety
- Altered family processes
- Hypothermia
- Ineffective thermoregulation
- Ineffective breathing pattern

**I. Physiologic**
- A. Important contrasts between child and adult
  1. Normal 7-pound newborn is:
     - a. 1/3 the size of adult in length
     - b. 1/9 the size of adult in body surface area
     - c. 1/21 the size of adult in weight
  2. Differences in proportion and relative body size sometimes less obvious
     - a. Child's head is large at birth
     - b. Child's head outgrows all other areas throughout early infancy
  3. Infants are obligatory nose breathers first several months of life
  4. Larynx location
     - a. At C3 to C4 in infant
     - b. At C4 to C5 in adult
     - c. Cross-sectional diameter of adult larynx is 8 mm
     - d. Cross-sectional diameter of infant larynx is 4 mm
  5. Epiglottis
     - a. Short, narrow, stiff, U shaped in infant
     - b. Flexible, flat in adult
  6. Trachea
     - a. 22 to 29 cm long in child
     - b. 74 to 76 cm long in adult
  7. Tongue
     - a. Proportionately larger for mouth in child and lacking in muscle tone
     - b. Adult tongue considered to be proportionately smaller than child's
  8. Neck
     - a. Infant's neck is very short, almost nonexistent
  9. Chest
     - a. Relatively small in infant
     - b. Thorax and sternum small
     - c. Intercostal muscles of normal respiration poorly developed
  10. Abdomen
     - a. Protuberant in infant
     - b. Muscles poorly developed
- B. Anatomic differences and the implications of these differences in the postanesthesia period for child and adult
  1. Differences must be considered when evaluating child vs. adult
     - a. Respiratory effort or functional reserve
     - b. Appropriately sized mask
     - c. Metabolism ability

## II. Psychosocial or Emotional

A. PACU nurse must be prepared to allay fears of child and parents
   1. Separation anxiety
   2. Fear of unknown
   3. "Oddly" dressed people with masks covering faces
   4. Fear of pain, disfigurement

B. Infants frequently cry postoperatively for various reasons
   1. Pain
   2. Hunger
   3. Lack of security

C. Calm, caring voice, touch, and smile helpful in relieving anxiety

D. Talking on child's level is important

E. Children 12 months to 3 years who are separated from parents feel deserted and may be frightened

F. Children 3 to 7 years often act out their fears through anxiety, hostility, or aggression

G. Children 7 to 11 years are in their "quiet years"
   1. Usually able to respond to questions about fears
   2. May also be "good" child and not complain
   3. May think "good" behavior will get them back to parents sooner (i.e., do not cry, even when in pain)

H. After 13 years, children understand separation is temporary

I. Be alert to evidence of pain
   1. Preteens and teenagers may exaggerate pain
      a. Pain sometimes not the problem
      b. Fear and not being in control of the situation are usually root of problem
   2. Pain scales appropriate to age of child helpful in determining degree of pain

J. Determine preoperatively whether "traditional" family is intact
   1. Children who have lost one or both parents may not have accepted the fact
   2. Could cause problems on emergence from anesthesia for child who is greeted with, for example, "Do you want to see your mom now?"

K. Keep explanations simple and to the point

L. Children who ask questions usually need simple, honest, direct answers

## III. Special Concerns of Premature Infant

A. Generally much more unstable than other infants

B. Temperature regulation possibly most critical problem
   1. Keeping these patients warm cannot be stressed too strongly
      a. Keep head covered
   2. Status can change from second to second

C. Respiratory pattern is a critical monitoring measurement
   1. Premature infants generally breathe rapidly for a few seconds, and pause, appearing apneic
   2. PACU nurses must be alert for changes in breathing patterns, such as "periodic" (altered pattern) breathing without evidence of bradycardia

D. In institutions not exclusively pediatric, consultation with neonatal nursing unit (if available) is prudent

## IV. Time and Timing Important When Dealing with Children

A. Children change rapidly
   1. PACU nurse must act quickly, anticipate possible problems
   2. Rapid intervention and preparation for unexpected are two essential tasks

B. Pediatric PACU is multifaceted; multiskilled nurses required

C. Family dynamics play a crucial part in pediatric care

**V. Anesthetic Implications**
  A. Halothane commonly used for mask induction
    1. Well tolerated, less pungent
    2. Less airway irritation or laryngospasm
  B. Regional anesthesia (spinal, caudal, or epidural block) may be used as adjunct to general anesthesia to provide for postoperative pain control
  C. Intraoperative narcotics or other analgesics may not be part of anesthetic administered but are important considerations when assessing pain postoperatively
  D. Ketamine may be used, particularly in developmentally handicapped children, during surgical and diagnostic procedures (magnetic resonance imaging; computed tomography)
  E. If intravenous (IV) line is placed, important to maintain postoperatively until oral fluid intake is assured
  F. Preoperative medications may decrease anesthetic requirements
  G. Infants respond to intubation with bradycardia because of immature sympathetic innervation (adults—tachycardia because of mature parasympathetic innervation)
    1. Atropine may be used preoperatively before intubation
    2. Short procedures may be done with mask or laryngeal mask airway (LMA) without intubation

## PREOPERATIVE SEDATION

**I. Considerations**
  A. Calm, quiet child entering surgical suite is generally better equipped for surgery
  B. "All or nothing" response to anxiety and fear is tendency in children
  C. Wide range of thought regarding preoperative medication (generally is a regional or institutional bias)

**II. Atropine Sulfate Used to Inhibit Production of Secretions in Infants**

**III. Midazolam (Versed) Used Successfully in Some Areas**
  A. Given intramuscularly (IM) or IV
  B. May be given orally (PO) in small amount of flavored syrup or juice

**IV. Use or Avoidance of Preoperative Medication Highly Individualized in Pediatrics**

**V. Preoperative Teaching and Play Therapy**
  A. Used to calm child before surgery
    1. Generally includes a visit to hospital and a tour of area
    2. Opportunity given to children to play with stethoscopes and masks to decrease mystery and fear of hospital equipment
  B. Does not always work
    1. Some children are fearful and cannot be calmed, need active parental participation

## AIRWAY MANAGEMENT

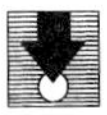

**NURSING DIAGNOSIS**

Examples of related nursing diagnostic categories include:
- Ineffective airway clearance

**I. Extubation of Pediatric Patient**
  A. Complications
    1. Airway obstruction most common after extubation
    2. Dangerous in any postanesthesia patient

B. Extubation "readiness"
   1. Controversial in medical and nursing communities
   2. Varies according to institution, anesthesiologist
      a. Child sits up, tries to pull tube out
      b. Child coughs on tube
   3. No set rule when dealing with children
   4. General considerations regarding extubation
      a. Child is awake
      b. Can lift head off bed
      c. Swallowing reflex present
      d. Coughing on endotracheal tube
         (1) Excessive coughing may cause postextubation stridor, croup
         (2) Can disrupt delicate surgery (some plastic surgery procedures, ear grafts, and some ophthalmologic procedures)

## II. Common Respiratory Problems

A. Tongue obstruction
   1. Most common problem
   2. Tongue may adhere to roof of infant's mouth
      a. Pinching cheeks may alleviate
      b. Holding child in sitting position may solve problem
      c. Turn child's head to side or place child in lateral position
   3. Tongue obstruction in infants treated differently than in older child
      a. Infant has shorter tongue base
      b. Obstruction can be relieved by pulling chin forward
      c. Hyperextension of jaws of infant generally results in obstruction of airway rather than opening airway as with adults
      d. Pacifier can help maintain patent oral airway in infant
         (1) Particularly if infant wakes long enough to clear airway, goes back to sleep, and obstructs again
         (2) Pacifier keeps tongue from roof of mouth; also provides for child's sucking need
      e. Placement of neck or shoulder roll
   4. Oral airways
      a. Frequently used in children
      b. Child will usually tolerate oral airway longer than adult will at similar levels of anesthesia
      c. Tongue obstruction often relieved by verifying position of oral airway, manipulating jaw
   5. Nasal airways
      a. Alternative if other manipulations ineffective
      b. Range in size from No. 16F to No. 38F
      c. Are soft and pliable
      d. Will not harm delicate mucosa when lubricated properly
      e. Contraindicated with tonsillectomy, adenoidectomy, or cleft palate repair

B. Secretions
   1. Excessive secretions cause respiratory problems
      a. Can rapidly obstruct airway
      b. Atropine sulfate or glycopyrrolate helpful if given preoperatively or intraoperatively
   2. Suctioning
      a. Variety of sizes of suction catheters should be available
      b. Catheters range in size from No. 5F to No. 16F
      c. Correct size should be used for suctioning endotracheal tubes (Table 8–1)
      d. Nonintubated child with excessive secretions must be carefully suctioned
         (1) Suctioning too deeply may trigger laryngospasm

**TABLE 8–1 Endotracheal Tube/Catheter Size for Suctioning**

| TUBE SIZE (mm) | CATHETER SIZE (Fr) |
|---|---|
| 2.0–2.5 | No. 5 |
| 3.0–3.5 | No. 6.5 |
| 4.0–4.5 | No. 8 |
| 5.0–6.5 | No. 10 |
| 7.0 and up | No. 14 |

C. Stridor
 1. Stridor (or crowing) most often seen postoperatively in children who have been intubated
  a. Crowing respirations sometimes begin with emergence from anesthesia
  b. Usually caused by irritation, edema from intubation
  c. Oral airway; LMA can cause stridor
  d. Excessive amount of loose auricular tissue around glottis area is susceptible to edema
 2. Treatment
  a. Moisturized oxygen
  b. Administration of racemic epinephrine through nebulizer with oxygen
   (1) Use is physician practice or regional bias
   (2) Most frequent concentration is 0.5 ml racemic epinephrine and 3 ml normal saline given by nebulizer
 3. Assess child's voice by asking his or her age or name
  a. Confirm hoarseness
  b. Ascertain orientation

D. Croup
 1. Postintubation croup
  a. Frequent complication
  b. Increasing tendency in 1- to 4-year-old age group
  c. Usually accompanies stridor
 2. Factors causing croup
  a. Traumatic intubation
  b. Long duration of intubation
  c. Too large an endotracheal tube causing edema of vocal cords
  d. Prolonged, excessive coughing on endotracheal tube
  e. Surgical trauma
 3. Treatment
  a. Same as for stridor
  b. Mist generally recommended overnight
  c. Observation for signs of increased respiratory difficulty of paramount importance

E. Laryngospasm
 1. Treated essentially same in child as in adult
  a. Positive pressure with oxygen
  b. Immediately call for help from anesthesiologist
  c. Administration of muscle relaxant and reintubation if spasm unrelieved by positive pressure
 2. Warm blankets often prevent, sometimes stop, impending laryngospasm
  a. Children respond rapidly to temperature changes
  b. Warming lights and other rewarming devices may be used to facilitate rewarming effort

F. Other source of respiratory difficulty—teeth
 1. Loose teeth often overlooked as important aspect of airway obstruction

2. PACU nurse has responsibility to ensure loose teeth are still intact on arrival in PACU
3. Notify anesthesiologist of teeth likely to fall out
   a. Removed tooth must be given to child's parent
   b. Document in PACU nursing notes

G. Partial or complete respiratory paralysis
1. Seen when effects of muscle relaxant have not worn off or when they are inadequately reversed
2. Edrophonium (Tensilon) or neostigmine (Prostigmin) usually used to reverse effects of nondepolarizing relaxants
   a. Both drugs are short acting
   b. Respiratory depression can recur when these agents have been metabolized
3. Notation of time that reversal agent was given is important
   a. Reparalyzation usually takes place 15 to 20 minutes after administration of reversal agent
4. Close observation of color, oxygen saturation, and respiratory effort is critical

H. Hypoventilation
1. Narcotics
   a. Drug overdose is common source of respiratory depression
      (1) Titration of narcotics of utmost importance when medicating children

I. Aspiration
1. Aspiration and its complications much the same in child as in adult
2. Aspiration of acidic gastric secretions may cause irritation of trachea and bronchi

J. Atelectasis
1. Can be reduced by aggressive PACU nursing interventions
2. Chest physiotherapy and postural drainage aid lung expansion
3. Meticulous pulmonary toilet very important for intubated patient
4. Assure that each patient is ventilating and is free from airway obstruction
5. Suctioning
   a. Instill 0.5 to 1 ml normal saline solution into endotracheal tube
   b. Ventilate with 100% oxygen
   c. Sterile suctioning will help loosen thick secretions
      (1) Suctioning decreases oxygen concentration
      (2) Child needs rest between suctioning to return $Sao_2$ to normal

## PAIN ASSESSMENT AND MANAGEMENT

**I. Many Studies Done Regarding Pain and Children**

A. Infants and children do experience pain, extent unknown

B. Indications that pain relief is needed
1. Crying that is not alleviated by comfort measures (i.e., cuddling, rocking, feeding if appropriate)
2. Increases in heart rate, respiratory rate, and blood pressure, particularly at rest
3. "Guarding" site of injury
4. Verbal complaints
5. Behavioral indicators most reliable in preverbal child

C. Children 4 to 10 years old may be stoic
1. Too frightened to admit experiencing pain
2. Fear and anxiety contribute greatly to pain
3. Experience of pain often difficult to express
   a. Pain scale can be helpful
   b. Patient-controlled analgesia (PCA) pump may be useful for older children
   c. Input from parents helpful for older children

4. IV administration of pain medication preferable to IM injection (Table 8–2)
   a. Easily tolerated
   b. Effectiveness can be readily evaluated
   c. Monitor respiratory effort, adequacy of ventilation, and oxygen saturation when titrating pain medication
5. Suppositories
   a. Appropriate for small children and infants
   b. Effective mode for patient with nausea or vomiting
      (1) Acetaminophen (Tylenol)
         (a) Most effective when given intraoperatively
         (b) Onset of action 30 to 60 minutes
      (2) Promethazine (Phenergan)

**II. Nonpharmacologic Interventions**

A. Child not responding to pain control interventions may respond to:
   1. Pacifier
   2. Bottle of clear liquid; if using juice, dilute to one-half strength if allowed or tolerated
   3. Rocking
   4. Warmth from blankets
   5. Being held
      a. Instill feeling of security in frightened infant or young child
      b. Child will rest more comfortably with pain and anxiety alleviated

B. Abdominal distension can be source of pain in infant
   1. Burping will often relieve distension
   2. Medication may no longer be necessary

C. Efforts may not be successful
   1. Some children are inconsolable
   2. Some will not respond to any measure other than return to parents

D. Report to nurses on receiving unit:
   1. Whether child has been medicated
   2. Response to pain medication
   3. Need for reassessment

## VITAL SIGNS

**I. Importance of Monitoring All Vital Signs in Pediatric Patient Cannot Be Stressed Strongly Enough**

A. Respiratory parameters (Table 8–3)
   1. Use stethoscope to count respiratory and apical pulse rates

**TABLE 8–2 Examples of Pain Medications and Recommended Dosages**

| PAIN MEDICATION | ROUTE | DOSAGE |
|---|---|---|
| Acetaminophen (Tylenol) | PO or PR every 4 hr | 10–15 mg/kg |
| Morphine sulfate | IM or IV | 0.05–0.1 mg/kg every 2–4 hr; or 1–2 hr if IV needed; usually titrated to effect in PACU |
| Fentanyl | IV | 1–2 μg/kg every 1–2 hr; usually titrated to effect in PACU |
| Ketorolac (Toradol) | IV, IM | 0.5 mg/kg |
| Meperidine (Demerol) | IV, IM, PO | 1–1.5 mg/kg every 3–4 hr; more frequently if IV; usually titrated to effect in PACU |
| Promethazine (Phenergan) | IV, IM, PR | 0.25–0.5 mg/kg every 4–6 hr |

**TABLE 8–3 Age-Specific Respiratory Rates**

| AGE | RATE/min |
|---|---|
| Premature infant | 50–65 |
| Newborn infant | 30–50 |
| 2 yr | 24–32 |
| 6 yr | 22–28 |
| 10 yr | 20–26 |
| 12 yr | 18–24 |
| Adult | 16–22 |

2. Other problems regarding pulmonary and cardiac function can be determined by auscultation
   a. Depth, character, and respiratory patterns can be assessed
   b. Particularly important in patient with compromised pulmonary function

B. Heart rate
   1. Varies greatly in pediatric patients (Table 8–4)
   2. Can be difficult for inexperienced professional to count rapid heart rate in infant
      a. Particularly one who is crying
      b. To aid in counting child's heart rate:
         (1) Listen and count while keeping two fingers on a strong pulse
         (2) Match heart rate and pulse

C. Temperature
   1. Important, often overlooked parameter in pediatric patients
   2. Infants can become quite cool if temperatures are not monitored closely
      a. Bradycardia in children commonly caused by hypothermia
      b. Hypothermia may interfere with reversal of muscle relaxants
   3. Children respond very quickly to rewarming
      a. Total body surface is smaller than that of adult
      b. Infant's (premature and term) temperature-regulating mechanism is immature
   4. Drastic change in temperature can affect oxygen consumption and cardiac output
      a. Removal of blankets for short periods results in heat loss
      b. Further warming will be required
      c. Recovery time will be delayed
      d. Causes discomfort for patient

**TABLE 8–4 Age-Specific Heart Rates**

| AGE | RATE (Mean/min) | RATE (Range/min) |
|---|---|---|
| 0–24 hr | 119 | 100–150 |
| 1–7 days | 133 | 100–175 |
| 7–30 days | 163 | 115–190 |
| 1–3 mo | 154 | 124–190 |
| 3–6 mo | 140 | 111–179 |
| 6–12 mo | 140 | 112–177 |
| 1–3 yr | 126 | 98–163 |
| 3–5 yr | 98 | 65–132 |
| 5–8 yr | 96 | 70–115 |
| 8–12 yr | 79 | 55–107 |
| 12–16 yr | 75 | 55–102 |

**TABLE 8–5 Age-Specific Blood Pressure Readings**

| AGE | READING* |
|---|---|
| Newborn to 4 yr | 85/60 |
| 5 yr | 87/60 |
| 6 yr | 90/60 |
| 7 yr | 92/62 |
| 8 yr | 95/62 |
| 9 yr | 98/64 |
| 10 yr | 100/65 |
| 11 yr | 110/60 |
| 12 yr | 114/60 |
| 13 yr | 116/60 |
| 14 yr | 118/64 |

*May be plus or minus 10 to 15 points.

5. Heat loss in premature or small infant can be minimal if warming caps and booties are used
    a. Infant's head is largest surface compared with rest of body
    b. Usually warms more quickly if head is covered
    c. Keep infant in preheated Isolette or use temperature-regulated radiant warmers

D. Blood pressure (Table 8–5)
1. Blood pressure (BP) monitoring crucial during immediate postoperative phase
2. BP very important parameter in assessing status of children
    a. Choose correct cuff size
    b. Cuff should be two-thirds size of upper arm
3. If infant's BP difficult to obtain and other means are unavailable, obtain by palpation

E. Monitoring
1. Best practice is to monitor temperature, heart rate, respiratory rate, blood pressure, and oxygen saturation on all pediatric patients in PACU
2. Constant monitoring especially needed for:
    a. Newborn and premature infants
    b. Infants with history of prematurity
    c. Pediatric patients who have had long periods of anesthesia
3. Pulse oximetry should be used on all pediatric patients
4. Nursing personnel must be alert: pediatric patient condition undergoes rapid changes

## PEDIATRIC CRISIS INTERVENTION

### NURSING DIAGNOSIS

Examples of related nursing diagnostic categories include:
- Decreased cardiac output
- Impaired gas exchange
- Fluid volume excess or deficit

**I. Equipment and Supplies**

A. Infants' and children's conditions are labile

B. Anticipatory plans should be standard

1. Crash cart should be equipped with appropriate size equipment
   a. Small cardiac board
   b. Small-size IV access needles
   c. Appropriate size endotracheal tube (Table 8–6)
   d. Small laryngoscope blades and handles
2. Flip chart
   a. Listing of code drugs, dosages, calculations
   b. Extremely valuable in PACU with limited pediatric population
   c. Standard procedure appropriate with right size equipment

**II. Considerations for Oxygen Delivery**

A. Maintaining calmness important during pediatric emergency
B. Child usually becomes apneic and cyanotic before heart rate decrease and cardiac arrest
C. Children generally respond to IV atropine and ventilation with 100% oxygen
   1. Unlike adults, healthy children have not developed coronary artery disease and other physiologic problems
   2. Neonates receiving high oxygen concentrations are at risk for retinopathy of prematurity developing
      a. Current literature states lower oxygen concentration, with concomitant risk of hypoxia and brain sequelae, is more detrimental
      b. During resuscitation, after neonate's saturation has returned to optimal $Sa_{O_2}$ of 96% to 98%, prudence dictates lowering oxygen concentration
         (1) On basis of arterial blood gas sampling, $O_2$ saturations
         (2) Pulse oximetry
         (3) To limit possible retinopathy

**III. Vascular Access**

A. Emergency drugs may be given by endotracheal tube to patients with no vascular access
   1. Absorbed through mucosa
   2. Include atropine, epinephrine, lidocaine, naloxone (Narcan)
B. Intraosseous access highly favored:
   1. Physician may place 13- or 15-gauge needle directly into tibia or femur to give life-sustaining fluids until other means are established
   2. If venous access is not established in 3 to 4 minutes
   3. If patient has gone into cardiac arrest

**IV. Fluid Therapy**

A. Pediatric parameters
   1. Metabolic rate in infants and children two to three times higher than in adults
   2. Fluid and electrolyte balance must be observed
      a. Infants and children cannot tolerate heavy sodium load
      b. Increased susceptibility to fluid overload
      c. Use mini- or microinfusion sets and/or infusion pumps to regulate IV fluid intake

**TABLE 8–6** Appropriate Size of Endotracheal Tubes

| AGE | SIZE (mm) |
|---|---|
| Premature | 2.5–3.0 |
| 0–6 mo | 3.0–3.5 |
| 6–12 mo | 3.5–4.0 |
| 12–18 mo | 4.0–4.5 |
| 2–4 yr | 4.5–5.5 |
| 4–6 yr | 5.5–6.5 |
| 6 yr | 6.5–7.5 |

3. Congestive heart failure and pulmonary edema can develop rapidly from fluid overload
4. Children can also become dehydrated easily

B. Cardiac and pulmonary status assessment
1. Skills in identification of "wet" breath and heart sounds
2. Recognition of clinical signs that signal possibility of fluid-related problems
   a. Change in skin color
   b. Labored breathing
   c. Flaring nostrils
   d. Excessive crying or weak and labored crying
   e. Chest retractions
   f. Significant decrease or absence of urine
   g. Tachycardia
   h. Tachypenia

C. Guidelines for fluid administration (Table 8–7)
1. Many theories and recommendations regarding appropriate IV solution, rate, and quantity of fluid for children
2. Follow regimen of institution
3. Maintain catheter patency and security

D. Urine output
1. Should be at least 0.5 ml/kg/hr
2. Notify anesthesiologist if less
3. Initiate proper treatment

E. Blood loss
1. Monitoring blood loss extremely important in child
   a. Blood volume approximately 10% of total body fluid
   b. Remaining 90% consists of intracellular and extracellular fluid
2. Evaluate blood loss in milliliters and as percentage of total blood volume to determine replacement therapy
3. Wide difference between loss of one third of blood volume in adult compared with infant
   a. Insignificant percentage of blood loss in adult
   b. Same percentage loss to infant is critical, requiring replacement
4. Electrolyte monitoring will help determine proper fluid intervention therapy

## OTHER COMPLICATIONS

### NURSING DIAGNOSIS

Examples of related nursing diagnostic categories include:
- Potential for suffocation
- Altered thought processes

**TABLE 8–7 General Guidelines for Fluid Calculation**

| WEIGHT (kg) | AMOUNT |
|---|---|
| 0–10 | 4 ml/kg/hr |
| 10–20 | 40 ml + 2 ml/kg/hr for each kg over 10 |
| >20 | 60 ml + 1 ml/kg/hr for each kg over 20 |

**I. Emesis**
- A. Nausea and vomiting
  1. Frequent in children; intolerable to some
  2. Particularly with ophthalmologic, otologic, and abdominal procedures
- B. Medicate with antiemetic for comfort and rest
  1. Slowly advance ice chips or Popsicles, to clear liquids

**II. Aspiration**
- A. Threat that always accompanies vomiting
  1. May occur with endotracheal tube in place
  2. Turn child onto one side, if possible
- B. Auscultate lungs for any damage immediately
- C. Obtain chest film if indicated

**III. Delirium**
- A. Emergence delirium
  1. Excitement phase after anesthesia
  2. Usually manifests itself with incoherent moaning, crying, kicking, or thrashing
  3. Common in children 1 to 4 years of age
- B. Protecting child from injury is most important
  1. Side rails padded with foam or blankets are helpful
  2. Flumazenil useful in managing sedation or delirium induced by midazolam
- C. Patients are often unaware of their actions during these transitional phases
  1. Generally, patients who try to bite or have very purposeful movement are likely to be more "awake"
     - a. To err on the doubtful side and protect the patient is better
     - b. These children require psychologic support and extra "TLC"
  2. Operative pain
     - a. Can be incorporated with excitement phase
     - b. Should be treated

**IV. Abdominal Distension**
- A. Very common
  1. Infants and young children cry or swallow air
  2. Burping required to relieve this discomfort
  3. Parents are often fearful of holding their infant or young child after surgery
     - a. PACU nurse can teach parents how to hold and burp child after surgery
     - b. Sometimes a simple task of burping infant can help allay parent's feelings

## PACU CONSIDERATIONS FOR SPECIFIC SURGICAL PROCEDURES

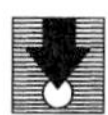

### NURSING DIAGNOSIS

Examples of related nursing diagnostic categories include:
- Potential for injury
- Altered cerebral tissue perfusion (increased intracranial pressure)
- Pain

**I. Urologic Procedures**
- A. Can include ureteral reimplantation, hypospadias repair, orchiopexy, repair of torsion of the testicle
- B. Provide privacy
  1. Restraining may be necessary to prevent injury

2. Observe and record urine output
3. Check for patency of drainage tubes
4. Children will feel urge to void
    a. Need to be reminded that it is acceptable to void "in the tube"
    b. Some children will have problems with this explanation
        (1) Especially those who have recently undergone toilet training
        (2) Those who have problems with nocturnal enuresis may try to hold back flow of urine
    c. Painful bladder spasms
        (1) B & O (belladona and opium) suppositories may be used to relieve spasms
5. Patience, understanding, and reassurance will help alleviate this problem

C. Increased use of regional adjuncts to general anesthesia, i.e., continuous epidural or caudal, narcotic caudal

## II. Neurosurgical Procedures

A. Can include myelomeningocele repair, craniotomy, craniectomy, placement of ventricular peritoneal shunts

B. Close observation essential
1. Generally not allowed to lie on operative site
2. Document pupillary response, size, and equality on all neurosurgical patients
3. Continually monitor intracranial pressure (ICP) if monitoring device is in place
4. Watch for signs of increasing ICP
    a. Decreased level of consciousness, lethargy
    b. Pupillary changes
        (1) Size
        (2) Reflexes
    c. Nausea
    d. Abnormal posturing or motor activity
        (1) Restlessness
        (2) Seizures
5. Check extremities for strength and purposeful movement
6. Elevate head of bed 10 to 30 degrees if not contraindicated, to facilitate venous return
7. Avoid hyperventilation and hyperemia
    a. Cause cerebral edema
    b. Increase ICP
    c. Impair autoregulation
8. Hyperoxygenate with 100% oxygen before and after suctioning
    a. Limit each suctioning time to no more than 10 to 15 seconds
    b. Avoid child's coughing and bucking on endotracheal tube
9. Administer glucocorticoids as ordered
10. Monitor and control temperature

## III. Ophthalmologic Procedures

A. Corneal transplants, scleral buckle, strabismus repair
1. Nausea and vomiting common with these procedures
    a. Elevation of head may decrease some nausea
    b. Encourage older children to deep breathe through mouth (helps eliminate feeling of nausea)
2. Medical immobilization devices placed on upper extremities in PACU to prevent injury

B. Preoperative teaching and postoperative emotional and psychologic support
1. Essential components of care for child having any surgical procedure
2. Especially when eye patch is necessary

## IV. Head and Neck Procedures

A. Include thyroglossal duct cyst, parathyroidectomy, cervical node biopsy

B. Concerns include integrity of airway and facial nerve
   1. Observe for facial inequality, facial nerve paralysis
      a. Ask child to smile widely, showing all teeth
      b. Note whether smile is symmetric
   2. Observe for swelling; edema or hematoma can quickly close pediatric airway
   3. Listen for stridor, hoarseness

**V. Herniorrhaphy**

A. Hernias in childhood are congenital
   1. Not the result of strain or pull, as in adult
   2. Result from weakness in muscular wall
B. Umbilical hernias more frequent in children
C. Indirect inguinal hernias among the more common
   1. Section of intestine or ovary can pass through inguinal ring into canal
   2. Can descend into scrotum
D. Hernias may not show up until child begins new exercise, such as gymnastics
E. In infants, hernias generally protrude and thus alarm parents
   1. Are usually reducible
   2. Generally can be electively scheduled procedures
F. Allow child to lie in position of comfort, generally more comfortable in semi-Fowler's position
G. When lifting a child after a herniorrhaphy, support lower extremities with hand under buttocks
   1. Allowing legs to dangle places stress and pressure on operative site causing pain
   2. Infants naturally raise their legs to relieve this distress
H. Regional anesthesia or ileoinguinal/ileohypogastric nerve block, local anesthetic injected into wound site may be adjunct to general anesthesia

**VI. Tonsillectomy/Adenoidectomy**

A. Common outpatient procedure
B. Frequent swallowing may indicate bleeding
   1. Check oropharynx (look for red bubbles at base of tongue)
C. Swallowed blood may cause nausea and vomiting
D. Crying increases bleeding
   1. Assess pain status
   2. Medicate prn
E. Steroids or ice collars may be used to decrease swelling
F. Maintain patent IV until tolerating PO fluids well

## POSTOPERATIVE HOME CARE INSTRUCTIONS

**I. Pediatric Patients and Particularly Their Parents Need Much Reassurance Regarding Home Care**

A. Clear and concise instructions, written at an appropriate level of general adult understanding
B. Be age-specific regarding patient
C. Give specific information regarding expected outcomes of procedure performed
   1. Expected drainage, if any, and how to deal with it
   2. Importance of monitoring intake and output
   3. Medication information
   4. Activity level and when to expect return to normal state
D. Give specific information (or parameters) regarding physician notification
   1. Temperature greater than 101° F
   2. Uncontrolled, frequent emesis
   3. Increased drainage or bleeding

4. Breathing problems
5. Insufficient or lack of pain medication response

**II. Telephone Follow-Up and Documentation of Patient Record Important**

A. Present opportunity for feedback and assessment
B. Proactive approach to problem solving

## ACKNOWLEDGMENT

PACU Nursing Staff, Egleston Children's Hospital at Emory University, Atlanta.

## BIBLIOGRAPHY

Addleman CD: What do you look for in the pediatric postanesthesia patient? *J Post Anesth Nurs* 3(1): 3–10, 1988.

Badgwell JM: *Clinical Pediatric Anesthesia.* Philadelphia, Lippincott-Raven, 1997.

Bell C, Kain Z: *The Pediatric Anesthesia Handbook,* 2nd Ed. Philadelphia, Harcourt Brace, 1997.

Broadman LM: Regional anesthesia for the pediatric outpatient. *Anesthesiol Clin North Am* 5(1):53–72, 1987.

Cote CJ et al: *A Practice of Anesthesia for Infants and Children,* 2nd Ed. Philadelphia, WB Saunders, 1993.

Drain CB: *The Post Anesthesia Care Unit,* 3rd Ed. Philadelphia, Saunders, 1994.

Finucane B, Santora A: *Principles of Airway Management.* Philadelphia, FA Davis, 1989.

Hollinger IB: Management of postanesthetic pediatric problems. *Anesthesiol Clin North Am* 8(2):323–353, 1990.

Junge C: Development and evaluation of parental visitation in the PACU. *J Post Anesth Nurs* 2(3):166–170, 1987.

Litwack K: *Post Anesthesia Care Nursing,* 2nd Ed. St Louis, Mosby, 1995.

Motoyama EK, Davis P, Smith RM: *Smith's Anesthesia for Infants and Children,* 6th Ed. St Louis, Mosby, 1996.

Oldham K, Colombani P, Foglia R: *Surgery of Infants and Children: Scientific Principles and Practice.* Philadelphia, Lippincott-Raven, 1997.

Patel RI: Discharge criteria and postanesthetic complications following pediatric ambulatory surgery. *J Post Anesth Nurs* 3(2):114–117, 1988.

Wilson TA, Graves SA: Pediatric considerations in a general postanesthesia care unit. *J Post Anesth Nurs* 5(1):16–24, 1990.

## REVIEW QUESTIONS

**1. What is the difference between the adult and pediatric epiglottis?**

A. Adult: round, L shaped; pediatric: flexible, flat
B. Adult: short, round; pediatric: long, stiff
C. Adult: stiff, flat; pediatric: long, flexible
D. Adult: flexible, flat; pediatric: short, stiff, U shaped

**2. What is the most common pediatric respiratory problem observed in the PACU?**

A. Croup
B. Tongue obstruction
C. Pacifier; pull chin forward
D. Pinching nose, pulling chin down

**3. What method(s) can help maintain a patent airway in the infant?**

A. Lay child flat, face up
B. Hyperextension of jaw
C. Pacifier; pull chin forward
D. Pinching nose, pulling chin down

**4. What is the usual cause of stridor?**
A. Irritation, edema from intubation
B. Excessive secretions
C. Intraoral suctioning
D. Premature extubation

**5. Which one is not the appropriate treatment of stridor?**
A. Racemic epinephrine
B. Dexamethasone
C. Atropine
D. Warmed oxygen mist

**6. The postanesthetic complication of croup is frequently seen in which age group?**
A. 3 to 10 months of age
B. 1 to 4 years
C. 6 to 8 years
D. 10 to 12 years

**7. Which respiratory rate would be abnormal for a 2-year-old?**
A. 24
B. 18
C. 32
D. 28

**8. What is the appropriate urine output in the pediatric patient?**
A. 0.5 ml/kg/hr
B. 3 ml/kg/hr
C. 0.1 ml/kg/hr
D. 2 ml/kg/hr

**9. In what age child is separation anxiety a problem?**
A. 6 to 24 months
B. 3 to 6 years
C. 7 to 9 years
D. 12 months to 3 years

**10. What is the appropriate size for a pediatric blood pressure cuff?**
A. ½ the size of the upper arm
B. ¼ the size of the upper arm
C. ⅓ the size of the upper arm
D. ⅔ the size of the upper arm

**ANSWERS:** 1. D, 2. B, 3. C, 4. A, 5. C, 6. B, 7. B, 8. A, 9. D, 10. D

PART THREE

# The Conceptual Basis for PACU Practice

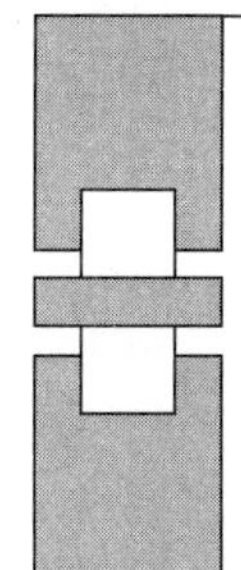

CHAPTER 9

# *Anesthetic Agents and Adjuncts*

Ronald E. Harbut, PhD, MD

## OBJECTIVES

**Study of the information in this chapter will enable the learner to:**

1. Understand the mechanism of action of inhalation anesthetics.
2. Identify properties specific to each inhalation anesthetic.
3. Discuss implications for the postanesthesia care unit (PACU) nurse in caring for patients who have received an inhalation agent.
4. Describe the physiologic and pharmacologic differences between depolarizing and nondepolarizing muscle relaxants.
5. Understand the mechanism of action of anticholinesterase reversal agents.
6. Discuss the differences between thiopental, methohexital, etomidate, ketamine, and propofol as intravenous (IV) anesthetics.
7. Identify common pharmacologic properties of opioids.
8. Discuss the use of local anesthetics for regional anesthesia.
9. Discuss the PACU nursing care implications for patients who have received epidural and spinal anesthetics.
10. Discuss the use of anticholinergic agents in anesthesia.
11. Identify the PACU nursing care implications for patients who have received benzodiazepines.
12. Describe the differences between common antiemetics.

NOTE: Dosage guidelines presented in this chapter are for healthy adults unless otherwise stated.

## I. Volatile Inhalational Anesthetics

A. Common properties

1. General facts
    a. Exist as liquids that evaporate at room temperature
    b. Amount of liquid evaporated is controlled by a device called a vaporizer
    c. Concentration of vapor administered determines the patient's depth of anesthesia
    d. The term *minimum alveolar concentration (MAC)* defines the concentration (vol%) of anesthetic vapor (at 1 atmosphere of pressure) that prevents skeletal muscle movement in 50% of the patients given a painful stimulus (surgical skin incision). The MAC is determined only after the anesthetic has had time to equilibrate throughout the body
2. Administration route and dosage
    a. "Simple" inhalational anesthesia
        (1) Volatile agent is used by itself with no adjuncts
        (2) Either halothane or sevoflurane are used because they are pleasant smelling; these two agents are recommended for mask inductions and maintenance anesthesia

(3) Enflurane, isoflurane, and desflurane are used only for maintenance anesthesia because they are too irritating to inhale for mask inductions; with these agents general anesthesia is commenced with a short-acting IV induction agent (see below, Intravenous Anesthetic Induction Agents)

b. "Balanced" inhalational anesthesia

(1) Intravenous adjuncts (narcotics, $N_2O$, muscle relaxants) are added to enhance the effects of the volatile agents, thus reducing the doses of the inhalational agents required

3. Pharmacokinetics

a. Uptake into the capillary blood (from alveoli) is directly proportional to the lipid-solubility of the anesthetic vapor

b. The amount of anesthetic agent distributed to each region of the body is directly proportional to the amount of blood each region receives; those regions receiving the greatest amounts of blood will be anesthetized first

(1) Highly perfused regions
(a) Brain
(b) Heart
(c) Kidney
(d) Liver

(2) Moderately perfused regions
(a) Muscle
(b) Skin

(3) Mildly perfused regions
(a) Fat
(b) Bone marrow

(4) Poorly perfused regions
(a) Tendons
(b) Ligaments
(c) Bone

c. Vapor elimination from various regions of the body (back to the lungs) is also determined by the regional rates of blood flow; elimination is slowest from the regions with the poorest blood supply

(1) Poorly perfused regions serve as storage sites for volatile anesthetics—the extent of this "storage" being a function of the time allowed these regions to absorb anesthetic agent and their size (i.e., obese patients have a larger capacity to store volatile anesthetics than slender patients)

4. Pharmacodynamics

a. Dose-dependent central nervous system (CNS) depression

(1) Several sites and mechanisms of action are under consideration; all of these are not completely understood

(2) Overall, it can be stated simply that general anesthetics "anesthetize" by impairing CNS synaptic transmission

5. CNS effects

a. Impairs CNS synaptic transmission

b. Decreases cerebral metabolism

c. Increases cerebral blood flow

(1) Effect occurs within minutes

(2) Cerebral blood flow (CBF) is variably increased by each agent

(3) Intracranial pressure (ICP) is also variably increased

(4) Increases in intracranial swelling and ICP are serious concerns in cases involving head trauma; note that the above deleterious effects of volatile agents can be attenuated by intentionally hyperventilating the patient to achieve hypocarbia

6. Cardiovascular effects
   a. Sensitization of the myocardium to dysrhythmogenic actions of catecholamines:
      (1) Halothane > isoflurane ≥ enflurane
      (2) Ventricular ectopy, tachycardia, or fibrillation are all possible
7. Respiratory (ventilatory) system
   a. Dose-dependent depression of spontaneous ventilation
   b. Dulls ventilatory responsiveness to hypoxemia and hypercarbia
   c. Obtunds laryngeal and pharyngeal reflexes
      (1) Some of the agents can be used to facilitate intubation (i.e., halothane and sevoflurane)
      (2) Depressed laryngeal reflexes increase the risk for aspiration (if gastric contents are present)
   d. Bronchodilation
      (1) There is a direct relaxing effect on bronchial smooth muscles
      (2) All the volatile agents can be useful in unconscious patients, but only halothane and sevoflurane are useful in initiating anesthesia by mask (the others are too irritating to inhale by awake patients)
8. Renal effects
   a. Dose-dependent decreases in renal blood flow, glomerular filtration, and urine output can be offset by adequate prehydration
9. Hepatic effects
   a. Dose-dependent reductions in total hepatic blood flow can lead to impaired hepatocyte oxygenation and a self-limiting form of hepatic dysfunction (can be more significant with halothane)
   b. Although all volatile anesthetics can cause a rare form of severe hepatitis, certain adults exposed to halothane appear to be at greater risk (see below, Halothane)
10. Gastrointestinal effects
    a. Relaxes smooth muscle and motility
11. Uterine effects
    a. Dose-dependent relaxation of uterine smooth muscle
       (1) Greater degrees of relaxation may cause greater amounts of uterine bleeding during cesarean sections
       (2) A safe rule of thumb is to administer volatile anesthetics at a dose equal to 0.5 MAC (a dose that should only inhibit uterine contractility by about 80%); supplemental analgesia can be provided by the coadministration of nitrous oxide with oxygen in a 50 : 50 mixture (see below, Nitrous oxide)
12. Drug interactions that *potentiate* the effects of volatile anesthetics (some of these drugs can also introduce some of their own unique problems)
    a. Acute ethanol intoxication
    b. Ketamine
       (1) May enhance the occurrence of dreams and hallucinations
       (2) When used in patients with asthma receiving aminophylline, it may induce seizures (i.e., combinations of ketamine and aminophylline can lower the seizure threshold)
    c. Nitrous oxide (see below, Gaseous Inhalational Anesthetics)
    d. Narcotics (morphine, fentanyl, sufentanil)
       (1) Cause a dose-dependent desensitization in the normal ventilatory response to increases in plasma $CO_2$; narcotics upwardly reset the concentration of plasma $CO_2$ that is considered to be "normal" by the medullary chemoreceptors
       (2) Higher than normal concentrations of plasma $CO_2$ eventually will restore "normal" spontaneous tidal volumes, but this assumes that ventilation is sufficient in the meantime to maintain an adequate supply of oxygen

(3) As a consequence of this dose-dependent narcotic-induced hypercapnia, carbon dioxide levels will continue to rise until the catecholamines released trigger cardiac dysrhythmias or until the hypercapnia becomes so severe that the CNS becomes progressively depressed

(4) Patients who have received narcotics must be monitored closely to ensure that their ventilatory patterns are sufficient to maintain adequate oxygenation and exhalation of carbon dioxide; supplemental oxygen and ventilatory equipment must be available.

e. Sedatives (benzodiazepines and barbiturates)

(1) As with narcotics, sedatives decrease chemoreceptor sensitivities to plasma $CO_2$, but unlike narcotics, sedatives also depress the maximal response that can be achieved to increase ventilation; i.e., no increase in plasma $CO_2$ will ever be sufficient to stimulate the chemoreceptors enough to restore normal tidal volumes; thus the excessive use of sedatives (more so than narcotics) threatens a patient with irreconcilable hypercapnia

(2) Patients must also be monitored closely to ensure adequate oxygenation and exhalation of carbon dioxide; supplemental oxygen and ventilatory equipment must be supplied as needed

f. Acute tetrahydrocannabinol (marijuana) intoxication

13. Drug interactions that ***antagonize*** the effects of volatile anesthetics (increase the amount of volatile anesthetics required)
    a. Amphetamines
    b. Cocaine
    c. Chronic ethanol intoxication
    d. Naloxone
    e. Chronic tetrahydrocannabinol (marijuana) intoxication
14. Toxicities
    a. Respiratory depression
    b. Respiratory arrest (apnea)
    c. Cardiovascular depression
    d. Malignant hyperthermia: see Nursing considerations below
15. Nursing considerations
    a. Impairment of spontaneous ventilation
        (1) CNS response to hypercapnia may be depressed
        (2) CNS response to hypoxemia may be depressed
    b. Depression of laryngeal and pharyngeal reflexes
        (1) Aspiration risks are increased
        (2) WARNING: be vigilant!
    c. Volatile anesthetics have dysrhythmogenic effects (to varying degrees); these effects are worsened by the concomitant use of epinephrine (in mixture with local anesthetics)
    d. Volatile anesthetics offer no residual analgesic effect
        (1) When general anesthesia is discontinued, a patient will awaken into an awareness of the pain of his surgery (unless IV analgesics, regional anesthetics, or local anesthetics are used before his emergence from general anesthesia)
        (2) The rapidity with which a patient awakens into pain is determined in part by how fast his anesthetic wears off (see Nursing Concerns for each specific volatile anesthetic)
    e. Be vigilant for malignant hyperthermia (see Chapter 17); its onset is sometimes delayed and may first be recognized in the PACU
    f. Monitoring vital signs will trace the waning residual effects of anesthesia
    g. Monitoring urine output will assess the patient's volume status, renal blood flow, glomerular filtration rate, and the overall health of the kidney

h. Hypothermia
   (1) Results from marked intraoperative heat loss
   (2) May lead to marked peripheral vasoconstriction
      (a) If the skin appears blanched, suspect vasoconstriction
      (b) If skin appears hyperemic, vasoconstriction is less likely
   (3) Temperature of patient must be normalized
      (a) Administer warmed IV fluids
      (b) Use active rewarming methods (warmed blankets or air)
   (4) May lead to profound shivering
i. Shivering
   (1) Increases oxygen consumption (important in anemic patients or in patient with poor pulmonary or cardiac reserve)

B. Halothane
1. General facts
   a. Brand name: various manufacturers
      (1) Oldest agent currently in use; commonly used in pediatric anesthesia
   b. Its vapor is pleasant smelling and nonirritating
      (1) Commonly used for mask inductions
      (2) Not likely to cause coughing and laryngospasm
      (3) Can be used for maintenance anesthesia
2. Administration route
   a. Inhalation only
3. Pharmacokinetics
   a. Metabolism: by hepatic microsomal enzymes
   b. Elimination
      (1) Unmetabolized drug: lungs (80%)
      (2) Metabolized drug: kidneys (20%)
4. CNS effects
   a. Cerebral vasodilation
      (1) Greatest with halothane
      (2) Can induce an increase in ICP
      (3) Hypocapnia, if induced before exposure, will blunt the increase in ICP
5. Cardiovascular effects
   a. Myocardial depression: decreased heart rate, contractility, stroke volume, and cardiac output
   b. Systemic vasodilation: decreased systemic vascular resistance (SVR) by direct relaxant effect on vascular tone
   c. Impairs normal function of AV node
      (1) Bradycardia
      (2) Nodal rhythms
      (3) Wandering pacemaker
   d. Dysrhythmias
      (1) Sensitization of the myocardium (by volatile anesthetics) to exogenously administered epinephrine is the highest seen (i.e., halothane > isoflurane = desflurane > enflurane)
         (a) Dose of exogenously administered epinephrine (e.g., found in some local anesthetics) should be kept to less than 2 μg/kg body weight
         (b) The above sensitization to epinephrine can be lessened by the coadministration of lidocaine
6. Renal effects
   a. Decreased renal blood flow and glomerular filtration may be offset by adequate prehydration

7. Hepatic effects
   a. Reversible reduction in hepatic blood flow is possible
   b. Reversible decrease in hepatic function and self-limited hepatotoxicity is possible
   c. Halothane hepatitis
      (1) Rare (1:20,000 to 200,000); less likely in children
      (2) Can lead to massive hepatic necrosis and death
      (3) Occurs 5 to 6 days after exposure
      (4) Risk factors may include enzyme induction, female gender, genetic predisposition, hypoxemia, hypermetabolic states, multiple exposures, middle age, and obesity
      (5) Appears to be caused by the covalent binding of oxidative metabolites to liver parenchyma:
         (a) The binding of these metabolites to the liver deranges its molecular architecture in such a way that the body does not recognize the liver as "self" anymore (thus, neoantigens are formed) and the immune system begins to attack the "nonself" liver with antibodies
      (6) The disease presents with marked increases in serum ALT, AST, and bilirubin; other findings include hepatomegaly, hepatic encephalopathy, fever, jaundice, malaise, and nonspecific gastrointestinal symptoms
8. Sympathetic nervous system effects
   a. Sensitizes heart to dysrhythmogenic action of catecholamines
9. Skeletal muscle effects
   a. Causes mild relaxation
   b. Can augment overall effect of muscle relaxants
10. Toxicities (by two different mechanisms)
   a. Self-limited mild hepatotoxicity (related to decreased blood flow) that presents with low-grade fever, nausea, lethargy, and mild transient elevations of liver aminotransferase enzymes (ALT, AST)
   b. "Halothane hepatitis" is a much rarer but more severe toxicity (see above, Hepatic effects)
11. Drug interactions
   a. Adrenergic blockers
      (1) Hypotension as a result of decrease in heart rate and contractility

C. Enflurane
1. General facts
   a. Brand name: Ethrane
      (1) Older agent used with decreasing popularity, in part because of its slow onset and offset of anesthetic action
   b. Volatile liquid with pungent and irritating odor
      (1) Not useful for mask inductions; may cause breathholding, coughing, and laryngospasm
      (2) Used only for maintenance anesthesia after general anesthesia has been initiated with intravenous induction agents
   c. In an unwanted reaction, enflurane can be degraded into carbon monoxide as it passes through the $CO_2$ absorbent of the anesthesia machine. Normally, enflurane passes through the anesthesia machine unchanged and does not interact with the soda lime or Baralyme of the $CO_2$-absorbing canisters. However, if enflurane is exposed to excessively dry soda lime or Baralyme, it can be chemically degraded and released as carbon monoxide gas
2. Administration route
   a. Inhalation only
3. Pharmacokinetics
   a. More resistant to metabolism than halothane
   b. Some liver metabolism (2%)

c. Metabolites excreted by kidneys
d. Primarily eliminated as unchanged exhaled vapor (80% to 95%)

4. CNS effects
   a. Motor hyperactivity in 2% of patients
      (1) May see electroencephalographic (EEG) seizure patterns
      (2) May progress to tonic-clonic seizures
5. Cardiovascular effects
   a. Hypotension possible
      (1) Mild depression of cardiac output
      (2) Mild relaxation of vascular resistance
   b. Dysrhythmias
      (1) Stable heart rate
      (2) Sensitization of the myocardium (by volatile anesthetics) to exogenously administered epinephrine is minimal (i.e., halothane > isoflurane = desflurane > enflurane)
      (3) Dose of exogenously administered epinephrine (e.g., found in some local anesthetics) should be kept to less than 11 μg/kg body weight
6. Respiratory effects
   a. See above, Common Properties
7. Hepatic effects
   a. Less likely when compared with halothane but still may cause syndrome like "halothane hepatitis" (see above, Halothane)
8. Skeletal muscle effects
   a. Promotes and potentiates neuromuscular blockade, although it is not a true nondepolarizing or depolarizing muscle relaxant (see below, Nondepolarizing Muscle Relaxants)
9. Drug interactions
   a. See above, Common properties
10. Nursing considerations
    a. May enhance seizure activity
    b. Patients are more hemodynamically stable than with halothane
    c. Enflurane, which is slowly eliminated, is the most likely of all volatile anesthetics to produce a lingering CNS depressant effect in PACU

D. Isoflurane
   1. General facts
      a. Brand name: Forane
         (1) Clinically useful anesthetic for maintenance of general anesthesia
      b. Volatile liquid with a strongly pungent and irritating odor
         (1) Not useful for mask inductions; may cause breathholding, coughing and laryngospasm
         (2) Used only for maintenance anesthesia after general anesthesia has been initiated with intravenous induction agents
      c. In an unwanted reaction, isoflurane can be degraded into carbon monoxide as it passes through the $CO_2$ absorbent of the anesthesia machine (see carbon monoxide discussion, Enflurane: General facts)
   2. Administration route and dosage
      a. Inhalation only
   3. Pharmacokinetics
      a. More resistant to metabolism than enflurane and halothane
      b. Eliminated primarily by exhalation as an intact molecule
      c. Some metabolism (0.2%) by liver
      d. Metabolites excreted by kidneys
   4. CNS effects
      a. See above, Common properties

5. Cardiovascular effects
   a. Myocardial function only slightly affected
      (1) Weak negative inotrope
   b. Peripheral vasodilation
   c. Dysrhythmias
      (1) No bradycardia
      (2) Possible tachycardia
      (3) Sensitization of the myocardium (by volatile anesthetics) to exogenously administered epinephrine is less than that seen with halothane (i.e., halothane > isoflurane = desflurane > enflurane)
         (a) Dose of exogenously administered epinephrine should be kept to less than 7 μg/kg body weight
6. Respiratory effects
   a. See above, Common properties
7. Hepatic effects
   a. Historically, a possible carcinogenic effect was reported
      (1) Original study and results not reproducible
      (2) Clinical use now widely accepted
8. Skeletal muscle effects
   a. Promotes and potentiates neuromuscular blockade
9. Toxicity: rare
10. Drug interactions
    a. See above, Common Properties
11. Nursing considerations
    a. Commonly used inhalational agent
    b. Postoperative shivering may be caused by increased heat loss from intraoperative vasodilation

E. Desflurane
1. General facts
   a. Brand name: Suprane
      (1) Newer clinically useful anesthetic for maintenance of general anesthesia
   b. Volatile liquid with pungent and irritating odor
      (1) Not useful for mask inductions; may cause breathholding, coughing and laryngospasm
      (2) Used only for maintenance anesthesia after general anesthesia has been initiated with intravenous induction agents
   c. In an unwanted reaction, desflurane can be degraded into carbon monoxide as it passes through the $CO_2$ absorbent of the anesthesia machine (see carbon monoxide discussion, Enflurane: General facts).
   d. Solubility in blood extremely low and similar to nitrous oxide
      (1) Allows for very fast onset and offset of CNS effects
2. Administration route and dosage
   a. Inhalation only
3. Pharmacokinetics
   a. Extremely resistant to metabolism
   b. Most chemically inert of all volatile anesthetic agents
   c. Eliminated primarily by exhalation as an intact molecule
4. Cardiovascular effects
   a. May have coronary arteriolar vasodilator effects that promote "coronary steal" and myocardial ischemia; this concern is controversial clinically but should not be a problem perioperatively as long as the oxygen supply to the myocardium is maintained and its oxygen demand is minimized
   b. During sudden increases in inspired gas concentrations, desflurane stimulates a transient sympathetically mediated increase in heart rate and blood pressure (to a

lesser extent this is also observed with isoflurane); this response can be blunted by the preadministration of narcotics like fentanyl

c. Dysrhythmias
   (1) Sensitization of the myocardium (by volatile anesthetics) to exogenously administered epinephrine is comparable to that seen with isoflurane (i.e., halothane > isoflurane = desflurane > enflurane)
      (a) Dose of exogenously administered epinephrine should be kept to less than 7 μg/kg body weight

5. Respiratory effects
   a. See above, Common properties
6. Hepatic and renal systems
   a. Hepatic and renal blood flow appear to be well preserved
7. Skeletal muscle effects
   a. Promotes and potentiates neuromuscular blockade
8. CNS effects
   a. Remarkably fast onset/offset of anesthesia
      (1) Solubility in blood is very low (like nitrous oxide)
   b. Preliminary evidence suggests that desflurane at 1 MAC significantly increases cerebrospinal fluid (CSF) pressure more so than 1 MAC isoflurane
9. Nursing considerations
   a. Commonly used for maintenance anesthesia in adults and in ambulatory surgery settings
   b. Extremely rapid onset and offset of CNS effects; rapid offset leaves no lingering analgesia; the requirement for supplemental analgesia must be anticipated

F. Sevoflurane
   1. General facts
      a. Brand name: Ultane
         (1) Newest inhalational anesthetic
      b. Because of chemical configuration it *cannot* be broken down into carbon monoxide even if it does pass through dry carbon dioxide absorbents (see above, Enflurane: General Facts)
         (1) Sevoflurane *can,* however, be converted into other toxic products, including Compounds A and B (see below, Breakdown Products)
      c. Its vapor is pleasant smelling and nonirritating
         (1) Very useful for mask inductions
         (2) Also useful for maintenance anesthesia as long as certain criteria are followed (see below, Breakdown Products)
   2. Administration route
      a. Inhalation only
   3. Pharmacokinetics
      a. Up to 5% of administered dose is metabolized by liver
   4. Cardiovascular effects
      a. Has less potent coronary arteriolar vasodilator effects and does not appear to cause "coronary steal"
      b. During sudden increases in inspired gas concentrations, it does not result in transient sympathetically mediated increases in heart rate and blood pressure (i.e., like desflurane and to a lessor extent isoflurane)
      c. Dysrhythmias
         (1) Unlike the other volatile agents, sevoflurane does not appear to sensitize the myocardium to the dysrhythmogenic effects of exogenously administered catecholamines
   5. Respiratory effects
      a. Dose-dependent depression of ventilation

b. Pleasant smelling and nonirritating; of all the volatile agents, it is least likely to cause coughing, breathholding, excessive salivation, or laryngospasm

6. Hepatic and renal systems
   a. Hepatic and renal blood flow appear to be well preserved
   b. Hexafluoroisopropanol, one of the metabolites, is conjugated in the liver with glucuronic acid and excreted by the kidney into the urine
   c. Fluoride ion, the other metabolite, may be associated with renal impairment if allowed to accumulate (see below, Toxicity of metabolites)
7. Skeletal muscle effects
   a. Promotes and potentiates neuromuscular blockade
8. CNS effects
   a. Solubility in blood is very low (like desflurane and nitrous oxide)
      (1) Allows for fast onset/offset of CNS effects
      (2) Speed of onset/offset slightly slower than desflurane and nitrous oxide
   b. Is not associated with convulsive or epileptic activity (like enflurane)
   c. Causes minimal increases in intracranial pressure over the 0.5 to 1 MAC range
9. Toxicity of metabolites
   a. Fluoride ion can be nephrotoxic if levels are allowed to rise high enough
      (1) The peak concentration of fluoride ion appears to be similar to that after enflurane use
      (2) No clinical demonstration of nephrotoxicity has yet been described, even though moderately elevated plasma levels of fluoride ion have been seen
      (3) Caution is advised in using sevoflurane in patients with known renal impairment
   b. Hexafluorisopropanol: is potentially hepatotoxic if not eliminated rapidly by glucuronidation (beware in patients with hepatic disease); glucuronide metabolite is excreted by the kidneys (be wary in patients with renal impairment)
10. Breakdown product
   a. Sevoflurane can be broken down by exposure to Baralyme or soda lime; the rate of this breakdown is increased by certain conditions
   b. Several breakdown products can be formed
      (1) Compounds A, B, C, D, and E
      (2) Note, only compound A (and to a lessor extent compound B) is likely to be clinically relevant
      (3) Compound A causes renal, hepatic, and cerebral damage in animal studies
11. Nursing considerations
   a. Pediatric use is becoming more common and is competing with halothane usage
   b. Adult use in ambulatory surgery settings is becoming more common
   c. Least irritating of all the volatile agents used
   d. Extremely rapid onset and offset of CNS effects; rapid offset leaves no lingering analgesia; the requirement for supplemental analgesia must be anticipated
   e. May not be useful in patients with hepatic or renal insufficiency

## II. Gaseous Inhalational Anesthetic

A. Nitrous oxide ($N_2O$)

1. General facts
   a. Exists as a gas at atmospheric pressure
   b. Brand name: various manufacturers
      (1) Odorless to sweet-smelling inorganic gas
   c. Nonflammable but will support combustion
   d. Prominent analgesic effects
      (1) Reduces amount of volatile agents required
      (2) Analgesic effect is further enhanced by narcotics

   e. Weak anesthetic effects
      (1) Is not potent enough to provide anesthesia
   f. Minimal muscle relaxant properties
2. Administration route
   a. Administered by inhalation
   b. Clinically useful doses range between 50% and 70%
      (1) Use of greater concentrations may cause hypoxia
      (2) Clinical doses at 50% to 70% provide limited analgesic effects
      (3) The limited analgesia provided may be enhanced by the coadministration of opioids
3. Pharmacokinetics
   a. Quick onset of effects occurs over minutes
      (1) Quick onset is related to its very low solubility in blood
      (2) Quick onset is also related to high concentrations used
   b. Metabolism is negligible
   c. Offset of effects
      (1) 5 to 10 minutes (assuming adequate ventilations)
      (2) Related to its very low solubility in blood
      (3) Assumes adequate ventilation of fresh oxygen into lungs
   d. Diffusion hypoxia/anoxia
      (1) When a $N_2O$-$O_2$ blend is being delivered into patients' lungs, the $N_2O$ cannot accumulate in the alveoli more than the 50% to 70% being given; however, when the external delivery of $N_2O$ is stopped, the entire amount of $N_2O$ that accumulated within the patient can diffuse back into the alveoli at a concentration approaching 100% if the patient is poorly ventilated
      (2) The back diffusion of $N_2O$ dilutes alveolar $O_2$ and ultimately causes hypoxemia
      (3) Accumulating alveolar $N_2O$ must be ventilated out of lungs and replaced with a fresh supply of 100% oxygen
4. CNS effects
   a. Mild amnesia (incomplete CNS depression)
   b. Very good analgesic effects
   c. May increase cerebral blood flow (CBF) and intracranial pressure (ICP)
5. Cardiovascular system
   a. May initially increase heart rate, systemic vascular resistance (SVR), and cardiac contractility indirectly by evoking release of catecholamines
   b. However, it ultimately decreases heart rate, SVR, and cardiac contractility by a direct depressant effect
      (1) Depressant effect is seen when catecholamine stores in sympathetic nerve endings are depleted because of prolonged hypovolemia, cardiac failure, shock, or trauma
6. Pulmonary/ventilatory system
   a. Chemoreceptor response to hypercapnia decreased
   b. High inhaled concentrations (50% to 70% ) are required for analgesia
      (1) Must mix this agent with 100% oxygen, not air (21% oxygen)
      (2) Must be vigilant for possible development of hypoxemia
7. Uterine effects
   a. Does not alter contractility in doses used for analgesia
8. Untoward effects
   a. Diffusion hypoxia (see above)
   b. Nausea may be related to diffusion of nitrous oxide into middle ear
   c. Undesirable expansion by $N_2O$ of closed gaseous spaces (within the body) filled with nitrogen

(1) Room air is approximately 80% nitrogen
(2) When nitrous oxide is introduced into the lungs, it (like all gases) will begin to evenly distribute itself (through the bloodstream) throughout the body's fluid space, and also, into any collections of air or nitrogen
(3) As it moves down its concentration gradient into the blood and any collections of air, it will be met by the opposite movement of nitrogen down its concentration gradient (from the collections of air) toward the lungs full of nitrous oxide (and oxygen) but very little nitrogen
(4) Given enough time, these two gases will equilibrate down their gradients
(5) Because nitrous oxide is 34 times more soluble in blood than nitrogen, nitrous oxide equilibrates first and thus tends to expand any pockets of air trapped within the body until the nitrogen eventually equilibrates "out"
(6) In the interim (while nitrogen is trying to leave), there can be a tremendous increase in the volume and pressure of these pockets of gases, which leads to the undesirable gaseous expansions
(7) Examples of trapped air that can expand (with consequent dilemmas) include middle ear (nausea; a ruptured tympanic membrane), small air pneumothoraces (tension pneumothorax), air emboli in blood (myocardial infarction; stroke), and air emboli in CSF (tension pneumoencephaly)

d. Undesirable collapse of closed gaseous spaces (within the body) filled with nitrous oxide
(1) The exact opposite of the above can occur after a patient has been under general anesthesia with nitrous oxide for a long period; in this case, an eardrum can be severely retracted until room air nitrogen equilibrates back into the gaseous vacuum left behind in the middle ear space after the nitrous oxide equilibrated "out"

9. Drug interactions
   a. Narcotics enhance analgesia and may enhance circulatory depression (see above)
10. Nursing considerations
   a. Be wary of diffusion hypoxemia in patients who have received intraoperative nitrous oxide; on their initial arrival in the PACU patients may have some degree of diffusion hypoxia if $N_2O$ was not adequately eliminated from their bodies before their departure from the operating room
   b. Be wary of the potential for increased nausea
   c. Be wary of the potential for expanded or retracted pockets of air

## III. Nondepolarizing Muscle Relaxants (NDMRs)

A. Common properties
1. Physiology of the neuromuscular junction (NMJ) (Fig. 9–1)
   a. Anatomy and physiology
      (1) Presynaptic nerve terminal
         (a) Releases "packets" of neurotransmitter
      (2) Neurotransmitter
         (a) Acetylcholine (ACh)
         (b) Transmits a chemical signal across the synaptic cleft
      (3) Synapse (synaptic cleft)
         (a) Extremely narrow, extracellular interconnection point between a nerve ending and a muscle cell
      (4) Postsynaptic ACh receptors (on muscle cells)
   b. Presynaptic activity
      (1) Impulse is conducted down the presynaptic neuron
      (2) Presynaptic nerve ending is depolarized
      (3) Nerve ending releases ACh into synapse

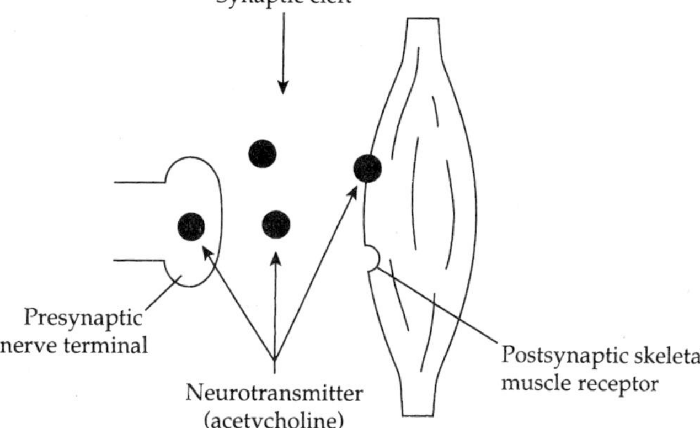


**FIGURE 9–1** Neuromuscular junction.

c. Synaptic activity
   (1) Released ACh diffuses across the synapse to postsynaptic receptors on muscle cell
d. Postsynaptic activity
   (1) ACh binds to receptors on muscle cell
   (2) Postsynaptic membrane of muscle cell is depolarized
   (3) Membrane depolarization triggers a mechanism within muscle cell that leads to contraction
e. Termination of skeletal muscle contraction
   (1) Impulses are no longer conducted down presynaptic neuron
   (2) Presynaptic nerve ending repolarizes
   (3) ACh release into synapse is reduced
   (4) Cholinesterase in synapse hydrolyzes previously released ACh
   (5) Insufficient ACh remains in synapse to continue depolarization of the postsynaptic side of the neuromuscular junction
   (6) Muscle cells return to noncontracted state

2. Pharmacokinetics
   a. Absorption
      (1) Poorly absorbed from gastrointestinal tract
      (2) Typically given by IV injection
      (3) Onset of paralysis by IV injection is 1 to 2 minutes
   b. Elimination
      (1) First, redistribution occurs
      (2) Next, hepatic or renal excretion or both
3. Pharmacodynamics
   a. NDMRs block the binding of ACh to postsynaptic receptors of skeletal muscle, impairing skeletal muscle contraction (Fig. 9–2)
      (1) NDMRs bind to postsynaptic receptors
      (2) ACh is still released from presynaptic terminals
      (3) However, NDMRs compete with ACh for postsynaptic receptor sites
      (4) Degree of competition (i.e., the extent of muscle paralysis) depends on dose of NDMR given
   b. Sequence of paralysis
      (1) Advances from fine to gross motor impairment (eyes → jaw → hands → limbs and neck → intercostal muscles → diaphragm)
   c. Sequence of recovery is in the *reverse* order of the sequence of paralysis
   d. Reversal of NDMR effects

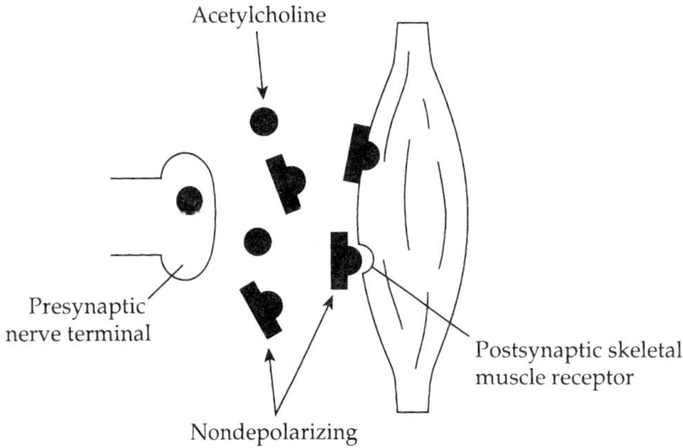


**FIGURE 9–2** Nondepolarizing muscle relaxants compete with acetylcholine for skeletal muscle receptor site.

(1) Various mechanisms lead to a "natural decay" in the concentration of NDMR within the synapse (thus restoring the ability of "naturally" released ACh to reach postsynaptic muscle receptors)
   (a) Redistribution
   (b) Metabolism
   (c) Renal excretion
   (d) Biliary excretion

(2) Reversal can be enhanced or expedited by "pharmacologic intervention" to exaggerate amount of ACh "naturally" found within synapse during blocked neuromuscular transmission; increased amounts of ACh can compete more easily with NDMRs for postsynaptic muscle receptors (see information on NDMR reversal agents)

4. CNS effects
   a. NDMRs do not cross blood-brain barrier
      (1) No CNS effects
      (2) Patient can be paralyzed and not speaking but be fully awake and alert!
5. Toxicity
   a. Ventilatory paralysis requires ventilatory support
   b. *Recurarization* (i.e., reblockade) occurs when some condition or factor invigorates a previously attenuated neuromuscular blockade (this effect requires the presence of "subtherapeutic" amounts of NDMR that would not normally cause skeletal muscle paralysis)
      (1) Can be induced when respiratory acidosis occurs because of the injudicious use of narcotic analgesics
      (2) Can occur when long-acting NDMRs are "reversed" with short-acting NDMR reversal agents (see Reversal agents)
6. Interactions
   a. NDMR paralysis can be enhanced by drugs
      (1) Aminoglycosides
      (2) Calcium channel blockers
      (3) Clindamycin
      (4) Lithium
      (5) Magnesium
      (6) Tetracyclines
      (7) Volatile anesthetics
   b. NDMR paralysis can be enhanced by physiologic imbalances
      (1) Respiratory acidosis
      (2) Dehydration

(3) Hypercapnia
(4) Hypokalemia
(5) Hyponatremia
(6) Hypermagnesemia
(7) Hypothermia

c. NDMR paralysis can be antagonized by drugs
(1) NDMR reversal agents (increase synaptic ACh)
(2) Caffeine
(3) Epinephrine
(4) Norepinephrine
(5) Theophylline

d. NDMR paralysis can be antagonized by physiologic imbalances
(1) Hypocapnia
(2) Hyperkalemia
(3) Hypernatremia
(4) Respiratory alkalosis

7. Nursing considerations
a. CNS
(1) Never assume a paralyzed patient is asleep
(2) A paralyzed patient may be fully awake and feeling pain
b. Paralysis may be potentiated by many drugs or conditions (see above)
c. Hypothermia
(1) Can prolong recovery from a neuromuscular block
d. WARNING: watch for "reparalysis" in patients that may be inadequately reversed or may still have unacceptably high residual amounts of long-acting NDMRs
(1) Need to clinically assess each patient's muscle strength
(2) Inquire as to *if, how much,* and *when* a long-acting NDMR was given
(3) NOTE: Be familiar with the long-acting NDMRs by name: doxacurium, pancuronium, pipecuronium, and tubocurarine

B. Atracurium
1. General facts
a. Brand name: Tracrium
(1) Classified as an intermediate-acting NDMR
b. Commonly used
c. Drug spontaneously "self-destructs" systemically by a process known as Hoffman elimination
(1) No enzyme systems required
(2) Occurs only in mildly alkaline solutions or blood at its normal pH of 7.4
(3) Process can still occur when hepatorenal systems are impaired
(4) Hoffman elimination is slower and paralysis lasts longer if blood is acidotic
d. Drug can also be degraded by ester hydrolysis in an otherwise healthy patient
2. Administration route and dosage
a. IV doses: 0.4 to 0.5 mg/kg for intubation
3. Pharmacokinetics
a. Onset: 3 to 5 minutes
b. Duration: 20 to 35 minutes
c. Elimination
(1) Hoffman elimination normally eliminates 33% of a given dose with the production of two metabolites: laudanosine and a monoacrylate compound
(a) Laudanosine does not have NDMR properties, but in high concentrations has been shown to cause vasodilation, cerebral excitation and seizure activity in animals
(b) Laudanosine is principally eliminated by the kidneys; theoretically it may accumulate in patients with renal failure

(2) Under normal conditions spontaneous recovery from paralysis can occur in 40 to 60 minutes
(3) Even with hepatic or renal system failure, complete recovery can still occur (albeit slower) by way of Hoffman elimination

4. Cardiovascular effects
   a. Histamine release: may cause hypotension and tachycardia
      (1) Depends on dose and rate of IV injection
      (2) More likely to occur if dose is injected rapidly
      (3) More likely to occur if dosage exceeds 0.4 to 0.5 mg/kg
5. Effect of physiochemical extremes on elimination
   a. Hypothermia and acidemia: may lengthen the time of paralysis by slowing Hoffman degradation
   b. Hyperthermia and alkalemia: may shorten the time of paralysis by hastening Hoffman degradation
6. Nursing considerations
   a. Eliminated by nonrenal and nonhepatic pathways
   b. Hypothermia and acidemia prolong paralysis/weakness
   c. Residual paralysis or weakness is easily reversed with NDMR reversal agents

C. Cisatracurium
1. General facts
   a. Brand name: Nimbex
      (1) Classified as an intermediate-acting NDMR
   b. Is one of 10 stereoisomers of atracurium
   c. It is three times more potent than atracurium
   d. In contrast to atracurium it is primarily eliminated (80%) by the process known as Hoffman elimination
   e. In sharp contrast to atracurium it is not significantly degraded by nonspecific plasma esterases
   f. Clinically, less laudanosine is generated
   g. Overall it may offer advantages over atracurium when used during very long operations or in the ICU for patients being chronically ventilated (especially those with renal failure)
2. Administration route and dosage
   a. IV doses: 0.15 to 0.2 mg/kg for intubation
3. Pharmacokinetics
   a. Onset: 1.5 to 2 minutes
   b. Duration: 50 to 60 minutes
   c. Elimination
      (1) Hoffman elimination: 80% of a given dose
      (2) Plasma esterase hydrolysis: not significant
      (3) Renal and hepatic excretion: 20% of a given dose
      (4) Even with hepatic or renal system failure complete recovery can still occur by way of Hoffman elimination
4. Cardiovascular effects
   a. Histamine release is less of a concern than with atracurium
5. Effect of physicochemical extremes on elimination
   a. Hypothermia and acidemia: may lengthen the time of paralysis by slowing Hoffman degradation
   b. Hyperthermia and alkalemia: may shorten the time of paralysis by hastening Hoffman degradation
6. Nursing considerations
   a. May be considered an improved form of atracurium
   b. Greater use for long OR cases or mechanically ventilated ICU patients

D. Curare (*d*-tubocurarine, DTC)
   1. General facts
      a. Brand name: various manufacturers
         (1) Classified as a long-acting NDMR
         (2) It is the oldest NDMR in clinical use
         (3) Not commonly used clinically anymore as a primary NDMR
      b. Has the greatest potential of all NDMRs to release histamine
      c. Some preparations contain sulfite preservatives
         (1) Ascertain sulfite presence in brand to be used
         (2) Allergic reactions may occur in susceptible patients
      d. Reversal of blockade should not be attempted unless some spontaneous recovery has begun (this point applies to all NDMRs, especially the long-acting NDMRs)
   2. Administration route and dosage
      a. IV dose: 0.6 mg/kg for intubation
   3. Pharmacokinetics
      a. Onset: 3 to 5 minutes
      b. Duration: 60 to 90 minutes
      c. Hepatic metabolism: not significant
      d. Biliary excretion (unchanged drug): 10% to 40%
      e. Renal excretion (unchanged drug): 45%
      f. Uptake: Some drug may be taken up into inactive tissue sites for a prolonged period (longer than 24 hours)
   4. Cardiovascular effects
      a. Hypotension
         (1) Caused by release of histamine from mast cells
         (2) Amount of histamine released depends on the curare dose and its rate of injection
         (3) Can be caused by the blockade of autonomic ganglia if the predominant autonomic tone is sympathetic
         (4) More pronounced in presence of hypovolemia
      b. Bradycardia/decreased contractility
         (1) Can be caused by the blockade of autonomic ganglia if the predominant autonomic tone is sympathetic
      c. Tachycardia
         (1) Can be caused by the blockade of autonomic ganglia if the predominant autonomic tone is parasympathetic
         (2) May be potentiated by a reflex response secondary to above mentioned hypotension
   5. Gastrointestinal effects
      a. Impaired peristaltic activity
         (1) Can be caused by the blockade of autonomic ganglia if the predominant tone is parasympathetic (peristaltic)
   6. Side effects
      a. Secondary to histamine release
         (1) Wheals
         (2) Pruritus
         (3) Erythema
         (4) Hypotension
         (5) Bronchospasm
         (6) Bronchial and salivary secretions
         (7) Decreased coagulability: caused by concomitant release of heparin from mast cells

- b. Secondary to ganglionic blockade
  - (1) Affects many systems but is usually incomplete (see above)

7. Toxic effects
   - a. Cardiovascular collapse
     - (1) Excessive histamine release
     - (2) Ganglionic blockade of a dominant sympathetic tone
   - b. Some preparations contain benzyl alcohol preservatives
     - (1) Toxicity may occur in neonates
8. Nursing considerations
   - a. Hypotension
     - (1) More profound in presence of hypovolemia
     - (2) Rehydrate and support blood pressure as needed
   - b. History of allergies, asthma, and/or anaphylactic reactions
     - (1) Avoid curare
   - c. Use not recommended in patients with renal disease
     - (1) Decreased renal elimination causes slower recovery from paralysis

E. Doxacurium

1. General facts
   - a. Brand name: Nuromax
     - (1) Classified as a long-acting NDMR
   - b. Most potent NDMR currently available: 2.5 to 3 times more potent than pancuronium
   - c. Recommended for use during long surgical cases
   - d. Useful in cases requiring cardiovascular stability (minimal drug-related changes in blood pressure and heart rate)
   - e. Reversal of blockade should not be attempted unless some spontaneous recovery has begun (this point applies to all NDMRs, especially the long-acting NDMRs)
2. Administration route and dosage
   - a. IV dose: 0.04 to 0.08 mg/kg for intubation
3. Pharmacokinetics
   - a. Onset: 4 to 6 minutes
   - b. Duration: 60 to 90 minutes
   - c. Hepatic metabolism: unknown
   - d. Biliary excretion (unchanged drug): unknown
   - e. Renal excretion (unchanged drug): 70%
4. Cardiovascular effects
   - a. Does not cause clinically significant hemodynamic effects; slight decrease in heart rate, central venous pressure, or pulmonary artery pressure is possible
5. Side effects uncommon but can include
   - a. Flushing
   - b. Urticaria
   - c. Hypotension
   - d. Bronchospasm
6. Nursing considerations
   - a. Very long-acting NDMR
   - b. Elimination depends on renal and biliary excretion
   - c. Renal and hepatic disease: slows recovery from paralysis
   - d. Requires adequate reversal or long spontaneous recovery period
     - (1) WARNING: be watchful for a downward trend in minute ventilation in the PACU
     - (2) A return of paralysis can be due to the administration of inadequate amounts or inappropriate selections of NDMR reversal agents
     - (3) A return of paralysis can also be due to the administration of excessive amounts of this long-acting NDMR given too close toward the end of surgery
     - (4) NOTE: Additional reversal agent may be required in PACU

F. Gallamine
  1. General facts
    a. Brand name: various manufacturers
      (1) Classified as a long-acting NDMR
    b. Not commonly used clinically
    c. Substantial "vagolytic" (antimuscarinic) effect
      (1) May cause tachycardia
    d. Histamine release occurs only with excessive doses
  2. Administration route and dosage
    a. IV dose: 3 to 4 mg/kg for intubation
    b. Not suitable for prolonged surgery because of its solubility in fat
      (1) Repetitive dosing may lead to accumulation of drug in fat tissue
      (2) Weakness or paralysis may be prolonged in obese patients
  3. Pharmacokinetics
    a. Onset: 3 to 5 minutes
    b. Duration: 60 to 90 minutes
    c. Hepatic metabolism: not significant
    d. Biliary excretion (unchanged drug): ~0%
    e. Renal excretion (unchanged drug): ~100%
  4. Drug interactions: same as with curare
  5. Nursing considerations
    a. Excreted entirely by kidneys
    b. Useful in patients with hepatic impairment
    c. Not useful in patients with renal impairment
    d. Moderate solubility in fat
      (1) WARNING: reparalysis or prolonged weakness may occur in obese patients

G. Metocurine
  1. General facts
    a. Brand name: various manufacturers
      (1) Classified as a long-acting NDMR
    b. Not commonly used anymore
    c. Small amount of histamine release (dose dependent)
  2. Administration route and dosage
    a. IV dose: 0.3 to 0.4 mg/kg for intubation
  3. Pharmacokinetics
    a. Onset: 3 to 5 minutes
    b. Duration: 60 to 90 minutes
    c. Hepatic metabolism: not significant
    d. Biliary excretion (unchanged drug): 1% to 2%
    e. Renal excretion (unchanged drug): ~43%
    f. Uptake: Some drug may be taken up into inactive tissue sites for a prolonged period
  4. Cardiovascular effects: negligible
  5. Drug interactions: same as with curare
  6. Nursing considerations: same as with curare

H. Mivacurium
  1. General facts
    a. Brand name: Mivacron
      (1) Classified as a short-acting NDMR
    b. Administered as a continuous infusion or with frequent boluses
    c. Drug does not usually accumulate
    d. Reversal of neuromuscular blockade is frequently not necessary
    e. Succinylcholine (SCh) is still the best choice for emergency intubations
  2. Administration route and dosage
    a. IV dose: 0.25 mg/kg for intubation (in two divided doses)

3. Pharmacokinetics
   a. Onset: 2 to 3 minutes
   b. Duration: 12 to 20 minutes
   c. Metabolism: by plasma cholinesterase (PChE)
      (1) Typical homozygous PChE (most common variant)
         (a) "Normal" condition
         (b) No "abnormal" reduction in rate of PChE metabolism
      (2) Atypical heterozygous PChE
         (a) Not usually clinically significant
         (b) Mild reduction in rate of PChE metabolism
         (c) Small reduction in dosage may be required
      (3) Atypical homozygous PChE
         (a) Clinically significant
         (b) Dosage reduction required
         (c) Occurs infrequently: 1:2500 patients
         (d) Seriously impairs metabolism and prolongs paralysis/weakness
         (e) "Abnormality" seriously impairs role of PChE metabolism
      (4) Burn patients require reduction in dosage because of reduced levels of typical homozygous PChE
      (5) Hepatic disease requires dosage adjustment because of decreased synthesis of typical homozygous PChE
      (6) Full-term and postpartum women
         (a) Mild prolongation of paralysis/weakness may occur
         (b) Patients have reduced levels of typical homozygous PChE
         (c) Dosage adjustment not typically required
   d. Biliary excretion (unchanged drug): not significant
   e. Renal excretion (unchanged drug): not significant
4. Cardiovascular effects
   a. Some histamine-related effects possible
      (1) Hypotension and tachycardia: determined by dose and rate of IV injection
5. Side effects
   a. Apnea or hypoventilation
   b. Some related to histamine release
6. Nursing considerations
   a. Short-acting NDMR
   b. Residual paralysis or weakness is not likely to be seen but is easily reversed with a little time or NDMR reversal agents
   c. With prudent dosing, use of NDMR reversal agents is rarely needed in patients with typical homozygous PChE

I. Pancuronium
1. General facts
   a. Brand name: Pavulon and others
      (1) Classified as a long-acting NDMR
   b. Commonly used
   c. Potential histamine release with excessive doses
   d. Reversal of blockade should not be attempted unless some spontaneous recovery has begun (this point applies to all NDMRs, especially the long-acting NDMRs)
2. Administration route and dosage
   a. Dose: 0.08 to 0.10 mg/kg for intubation
3. Pharmacokinetics
   a. Onset: 3 to 5 minutes
   b. Duration: 60 to 90 minutes
   c. Hepatic metabolism: 10% to 40%

d. Biliary excretion (unchanged drug): 5% to 10%
e. Renal excretion (unchanged drug): 80%
4. Cardiovascular effects
a. Anticholinergic/vagolytic action: may cause tachycardia
b. Sympathomimetic actions
(1) Enhances release of norepinephrine from adrenergic nerve endings
(2) Inhibits reuptake of norepinephrine from adrenergic nerve endings
(3) Overall sympathetic effect may increase heart rate and blood pressure
5. Nursing considerations
a. Requires adequate reversal or a long spontaneous recovery period
(1) WARNING: Be watchful for a downward trend in minute ventilation in the PACU
(2) A return of paralysis can be due to the administration of inadequate amounts or inappropriate selections of NDMR reversal agents
(3) A return of paralysis can also be due to the administration of excessive amounts of this long-acting NDMR given too close toward the end of surgery
(4) NOTE: Additional NDMR reversal agent may be required in PACU

J. Pipecuronium
1. General facts
a. Brand name: Arduan
(1) Classified as a long-acting NDMR
b. Recommended for use during prolonged surgery
c. Recommended for cases requiring cardiovascular stability
d. Reversal of blockade should not be attempted unless some spontaneous recovery has begun (this point applies to all NDMRs, especially the long-acting NDMRs)
2. Administration route and dosage
a. IV dose: 0.07 to 0.085 mg/kg for intubation
(1) Onset within 5 minutes
(2) Recovery usually begins in 45 to 120 minutes
3. Pharmacokinetics
a. Onset: 3 to 5 minutes
b. Duration: 60 to 90 minutes
c. Hepatic metabolism: 10%
d. Biliary excretion (unchanged drug): 20%
e. Renal excretion (unchanged drug): 70%
4. Cardiovascular effects
a. Does not cause clinically significant hemodynamic effects
5. Side effects
a. Rash and urticaria: possibly related to histamine release
b. Hypoventilation and apnea: caused by effects of residual NDMR
6. Nursing considerations
a. Long-acting NDMR
b. Elimination depends on renal excretion; dose should be reduced in patients with renal impairment
c. Requires adequate reversal or a long spontaneous recovery period:
(1) WARNING: inadequate reversal may have been given in OR
(2) WARNING: watch for downward trend in minute ventilation
(3) Paralysis may recur once effect of reversal agent has worn off; additional reversal may be required in PACU

K. Rocuronium
1. General facts
a. Brand name: Zemuron
(1) Classified as a short-acting NDMR
b. No histamine release
c. Appears devoid of cardiovascular effects

d. Very fast onset of muscle relaxation
e. However, in certain situations SCh may still be the best choice for emergency intubations
2. Administration route and dosage
a. IV dose: 0.5 mg/kg for intubation
3. Pharmacokinetics
a. Onset: 1 minute
b. Duration: 15 to 20 minutes
c. Metabolism: does not appear to be significant
d. Elimination: unchanged by liver and kidney
4. Nursing considerations
a. Similar to vecuronium: see below
L. Vecuronium
1. General facts
a. Brand name: Norcuron
(1) Classified as an intermediate-acting NDMR
b. No histamine release (even at high doses)
c. Generally speaking, no cardiovascular effects
(1) Minimal, if any, effects on blood pressure and heart rate
(2) Occasional reports of histamine-like reactions
2. Administration route and dosage
a. IV dose: 0.08 to 0.1 mg/kg for intubation
3. Pharmacokinetics
a. Onset: 3 to 5 minutes
b. Duration: 20 to 35 minutes
c. Hepatic deacetylation: 20% to 30%
d. Biliary excretion (unchanged drug): 40% to 75%
(1) Elimination can be prolonged with severe liver disease
e. Renal excretion (unchanged drug): 15% to 25%
4. Nursing considerations
a. Lack of cardiovascular effects; useful in cardiac surgery
b. Hepatobiliary excretion: prolonged effect with severe liver disease

## IV. Depolarizing Muscle Relaxant (DMR)

A. Succinylcholine (SCh) (only drug of this class in the U.S.A.)
1. General facts
a. Brand names: Anectine, Quelicin, and others
(1) Classified as ultrashort-acting DMR
(2) Very rapid onset and offset
(3) Frequently used when intubating conditions are needed rapidly
b. WARNING: Its use in children is controversial and potentially dangerous; its use may be appropriate if the benefits of promptly intubating the trachea are greater than the risks of using SCh:
(1) NOTE: If used in children, be wary of sudden cardiac standstill caused by a SCh-induced sudden release of intracellular skeletal muscle potassium (which abruptly establishes a hyperkalemic crises and depolarizes all the contractile tissue of the heart); should this occur (in addition to providing any requisite basic life support) the hyperkalemic crisis is treated initially with titrated doses of calcium chloride (which helps to stabilize and repolarize the resting membrane potential of the cardiac cells) and subsequently with the administration of insulin, glucose, and bicarbonate (which helps pump extracellular potassium back into skeletal muscle cells)
c. WARNING: Contraindicated in patients after the acute phase (after 2 to 4 days) of certain types of neuromuscular injury (because of the potential for the release of

life-threatening amounts of intracellular potassium from denervated skeletal muscle subsequently exposed to SCh):
(1) Major burns
(2) Multiple trauma
(3) Upper motor neuron injury
(4) Lower motor neuron injury
(5) Cerebral vascular accidents
(6) Extensive denervation of skeletal muscle

d. WARNING: May also be contraindicated in patients with chronic illnesses (after several days) because of an excessive release of intracellular potassium from skeletal muscle that has been in a state of chronic disuse:
(1) Disuse atrophy
(2) Critical illness
(3) Severe infection
(4) Prolonged immobilization
(5) Recent discontinuation of prolonged NDMR use in a critical care setting

e. WARNING: Use in children with muscular dystrophies or myotonias is particularly ill-advised; these children may be more likely to develop a life-threatening type of prolonged skeletal muscle spasm, or malignant hyperthermia (see Chapter 17)

2. Administration route and dosage
a. Usually as single IV bolus
(1) About 1.6 mg/kg for intubation
(2) Infusion "titrated to effect" may be used to prolong relaxation
b. Phase I block (occurs after a brief single-dose exposure to SCh)
(1) This is the type of neuromuscular paralysis typically associated with DMRs
(a) Caused by single doses of SCh not exceeding 3 mg/kg
(b) Relaxant effect wears off quickly (usually within minutes) after SCh is rapidly metabolized and the neuromuscular junction completely repolarizes (see exceptions below, Atypical PChE)
(c) If a nerve stimulator is used minutes after administering SCh, a brief sustained (tetanic) stimulation to the nerve of a muscle (being tested for recovery) will produce a contraction of *low* but *sustained* amplitude. Over time, as the effects of the DMR block continues to wear off, each subsequent tetanic stimulation (allowing for rest periods in between) will continue to produce *sustained* amplitudes of contraction (within each test) but with *increasing* amplitudes overall
(d) If an anticholinesterase drug is given during the drug recovery period (a practice not recommended), there will be an augmentation of the DMR block (now due to an increase in synaptic ACh rather than SCh concentrations) and a return of neuromuscular paralysis; a brief tetanic stimulation will produce a sustained contraction of decreased (or no) amplitude
c. Phase II block (acts more like a NDMR block)
(1) This is a type of neuromuscular paralysis similar to that caused by NDMRs
(a) Occurs after a single bolus dose of >3 mg/kg or after a continuous infusion (total dose) of >7 mg/kg
(b) The postsynaptic ACh-receptor appears to change the way it interacts with SCh. SCh still binds to the ACh receptor, but depolarization no longer occurs. Thus under the conditions of chronic exposure to SCh, the ACh-receptor appears to protect itself (from continuing depolarization) by responding to SCh as if it was an NDMR. General anesthetics may facilitate this phenomenon
(c) Note that the phase-II relaxant effect of SCh does *not* wear off quickly and completely; thus prolonged apnea, slow recovery from paralysis, and prolonged intubation and mechanical ventilation may be observed

(d) A brief tetanic stimulation to the nerve of a muscle recovering from a phase-II block will produce contractions of *low* and *unsustained* amplitude. As the effects of the NDMR block wear off, each subsequent tetanic stimulation (allowing for rest periods in between) continues to produce *unsustained* amplitudes of contraction (within each tetanic period) but with ever-increasing amplitudes overall. As the effects of phase-II block completely resolve, the *unsustained* amplitudes (seen during a tetanic stimulation) ultimately become *sustainable*

(e) If an anticholinesterase drug is given during the drug recovery period, there will be a beneficial antagonism of the phase-II block and a return of neuromuscular function; edrophonium, 0.1 mg/kg IV, may be used to briefly test if a phase-II type block exists (the effects of this small dose are short-lived if a phase-I type block is actually present)

3. Pharmacokinetics
   a. Absorption
      (1) Must be given by IV or IM injection
      (2) Onset of paralysis after IV injection occurs in about 1 minute
   b. Duration
      (1) Generally short (about 5 minutes), after a single intubating dose
      (2) Complete recovery normally occurs in about 15 minutes
   c. Metabolism
      (1) Normally hydrolyzed by plasma cholinesterase (PChE)
      (2) Not hydrolyzed by acetylcholinesterase (AChE)
      (3) Decreases in the quantity (concentration) or quality (i.e., molecular defects) of PChE will prolong the effects of an administered dose of SCh
      (4) See information on plasma cholinesterase below
   d. Renal excretion (unchanged drug): 10%
4. Plasma cholinesterase (PChE)
   a. Also called pseudocholinesterase
   b. Produced by liver
   c. Serum albumin and PChE levels
      (1) Tend to be directly related
      (2) Hypoalbuminemic patients tend to have PChE deficiency
   d. Role of PChE
      (1) No clearly understood physiologic role
      (2) Responsible for metabolism of SCh, local anesthetics (esters), and trimethaphan (an antihypertensive medication)
   e. Typical homozygous PChE
      (1) Majority of population has this genetic variant
      (2) SCh metabolized with rapid rate of ester hydrolysis
   f. Atypical heterozygous PChE
      (1) 4% of population
      (2) SCh metabolized with mildly reduced rate of hydrolysis
      (3) Mild prolongation of intraoperative apnea possible if SCh given
   g. Atypical homozygous PChE
      (1) 0.03% of population
      (2) SCh metabolized with severely reduced rate of hydrolysis
      (3) Severe prolongation of postoperative apnea possible if SCh given
5. Acquired changes in plasma cholinesterase activity
   a. Decreased activity (decreased quantity of active enzyme molecules)
      (1) Advanced age
      (2) Renal failure
      (3) Malnutrition
      (4) Severe anemia

(5) Severe hepatic disease
(6) Bronchogenic carcinoma
(7) Prolonged cardiopulmonary bypass
(8) Postpartum period (levels lowest on third postpartum day)
(9) Inquire as to the recent administration of NDMR reversal agents (i.e., neostigmine/pyridostigmine)

b. Increased activity (increased quantity)
(1) Obese have more activity than nonobese patients
(2) Whole blood, packed red blood cells (RBCs), and fresh frozen plasma (FFP) are an exogenous source of PChE

6. Pharmacodynamics
a. SCh depolarizes the NMJ of skeletal muscle as endogenous ACh does (Fig. 9–3)
(1) Normally, ACh binds to the nicotinic receptors of the NMJ, but this binding is short-lived because ACh is rapidly hydrolyzed by the presence of acetylcholinesterase (AChE)
(2) SCh also binds to the nicotinic receptors of neuromuscular junction and, notably, does so more effectively; SCh's binding and depolarization of the NMJ lasts longer than that caused by ACh

b. Sequence of SCh-induced paralysis
(1) Advances from fine to gross motor impairment
(2) Eyes, jaw, and hands → limbs and neck → intercostal muscles → diaphragm

c. Initial depolarization causes transient fasciculations
(1) May or may not cause postoperative myalgia
(2) Myalgia can be reduced by pretreatment with small dose of NDMR
(3) May transiently increase intraocular pressure (possibly involves transient contraction or fasciculation of extraocular muscles)
(4) Use of SCh may cause extrusion of eye contents in "open globe" cases

7. CNS effects
a. Does not cross blood-brain barrier
(1) No CNS effects
(2) Patient can be paralyzed (and not speaking) but be fully awake and alert!

8. Cardiovascular effects
a. Stimulation of vagal nuclei and nerve (the vagus nerve innervates the atria and the SA/AV nodes) leads to
(1) Bradycardia/supraventricular dysrhythmias
(2) "Digitalized patients" may manifest exaggerated bradycardia

b. Stimulation of sympathetic ganglia
(1) Hypertension/tachycardia may follow usual doses because of the initial (phase I) effects of SCh on ganglionic nicotinic receptors

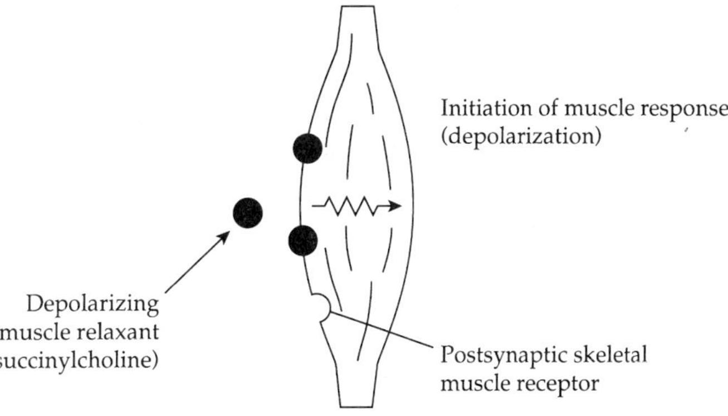


**FIGURE 9–3** Paralysis with succinylcholine: Initiation of skeletal muscle response. First, depolarization initiates uncontrolled random contractions (fasciculations); then during the next several minutes, persisting receptor depolarization leads to muscle paralysis/relaxation.

c. Inhibition of sympathetic ganglia
   (1) Hypotension/bradycardia may subsequently follow extremely high doses of SCh because of its phase II blockade of ganglionic nicotinic receptors
9. Respiratory effect
   a. Ventilation must be artificially supported during muscle paralysis
10. Gastrointestinal effects
   a. Increases intragastric and intraabdominal pressure
   b. But also increases lower esophageal sphincter pressure
      (1) Therefore risk of regurgitation is lower than expected
      (2) "Aspiration precautions" should still be maintained
11. Hepatic effects (none)
12. Renal effects
   a. Direct: not likely
   b. Indirect: excessive fasciculations may cause myoglobinuria, however, myoglobinuria is most likely seen in children or adults in whom malignant hyperthermia develops (see Chapter 17)
13. Histamine release
   a. Occasionally causes mild reaction: rash on arms and upper chest
14. Eye effect (transiently raises IOP)
   a. Contracts extraocular muscles
   b. Contraindicated in patients with eye injuries (i.e., "open globe") because the eye contents may be extruded during the initial SCh-induced fasciculations of the extraocular muscles
15. Induced hyperkalemia
   a. Depolarization of skeletal muscle causes release of intracellular potassium into the extracellular fluid (ECF):
      (1) Normally amounts to about 0.5 mEq/L
      (2) Effect peaks in 5 minutes; normalizes in 10 to 15 minutes
      (3) Excessive increases in serum potassium can cause cardiac arrest
   b. As mentioned above, SCh-induced depolarization of denervated skeletal muscle causes an copious release of potassium into the ECF (effect is observed initially 2 to 4 days after denervation and is maximal after 14 days); this unusual release of potassium occurs because denervated skeletal muscle increases (i.e., "up regulates") its population of nicotinic receptors in the hope of "reestablishing contact" with its formerly attached and functioning nerve endings
   c. Conditions that can lead to some form of skeletal muscle denervation:
      (1) Severe burns
      (2) Denervation injuries
      (3) Massive muscle or soft tissue trauma
      (4) Spinal cord injury (up to 6 months after initial insult)
      (5) Upper motor neuron lesions: stroke, encephalitis
   d. Muscle fasciculations
      (1) Related to the wholesale depolarization of skeletal muscles throughout the human body
      (2) Very small and judicious doses of NDMRs (administered before the use of SCh) are used by some clinicians to reduce these fasciculations
16. Concurrent hyperkalemia
   a. As stated above, SCh releases potassium into the ECF
   b. The use of SCh may be inadvisable with some conditions
      (1) Renal disease
      (2) Severe intraabdominal infections
      (3) Patients experiencing congestive heart failure (CHF) or receiving digoxin
17. Toxic effects
   a. Prolonged apnea

b. Cardiac arrest
c. Malignant hyperthermia (see Chapter 17)

18. Interactions
    a. Enhancement of DMR effects by drugs:
        (1) Calcium channel blockers
        (2) NDMR reversal agents inhibit PChE
            (a) NOTE: If SCh is administered in the PACU, a patient who has been given the NDMR reversal agent neostigmine or pyridostigmine (not edrophonium) can have an unanticipated period of prolonged muscle paralysis (see below, NDMR Reversal Agents)
    b. Drugs that inhibit PChE can prolong the effects of SCh
        (1) Trimethaphan
        (2) Local anesthetic esters (procaine, chloroprocaine, and tetracaine)
    c. DMR paralysis can be enhanced by physiologic imbalances:
        (1) Respiratory alkalosis
        (2) Hyperkalemia
        (3) Hypermagnesemia
        (4) Hypothermia
        (5) Decreased renal function
        (6) Dehydration
        (7) Lithium pharmacotherapy
        (8) Low quantity or abnormal quality of PChE
    d. DMR paralysis can be antagonized by physiologic imbalances
        (1) Respiratory acidosis
        (2) Hypokalemia
        (3) Decreased peripheral perfusion
19. Nursing considerations
    a. SCh has no effect on mentation; thus never assume that a paralyzed patient is asleep or pain free
    b. Malignant hyperthermia
        (1) May or may not occur during anesthesia
        (2) It may first manifest itself in the PACU
    c. Postoperative myalgia
        (1) Caused by SCh-induced fasciculations
        (2) Can be lessened by a very small dose of NDMR before SCh
    d. If a slow recovery occurs from SCh-induced paralysis
        (1) Check serum albumin level; if albumin low, PChE level may also be low
    e. Treatment of phase-II block
        (1) Careful clinical correlation required
        (2) Reversal of paralysis is attempted with an anticholinesterase drug
    f. SCh use after patient has received an anticholinesterase drug
        (1) Acceptable if SCh is used to treat postoperative laryngospasm
        (2) Acceptable if SCh is used to reintubate patient in PACU
        (3) Remember that relaxation of skeletal muscle will be prolonged if PChE is inhibited
        (4) NOTE: Neostigmine and pyridostigmine will inhibit PChE as well as AChE (see below, NDMR Reversal Agents)
        (5) NOTE: Edrophonium inhibits AChE but *not* PChE

## V. NDMR Reversal Agents (Anticholinesterases)

A. Common properties
1. Physiology
    a. Physiology of neuromuscular junction (NMJ) (see p. 100)

b. Released ACh depolarizes skeletal muscle by binding to postsynaptic nicotinic receptors at the NMJ
   (1) Contraction of skeletal muscle is initiated in this manner
   (2) Contraction ceases when neural release of ACh ends and when residual ACh in synapse is destroyed: such destruction of ACh is performed rapidly by a synaptic enzyme called acetylcholinesterase (AChE)
c. NDMRs prevent released ACh from reaching the nicotinic receptors of skeletal muscle
   (1) Molecules of NDMRs bind to and block these receptors
   (2) Voluntary control of skeletal muscle contraction is thereby weakened or lost

2. Pharmacodynamics
   a. NDMR reversal agents provide a means of overpowering the effects of NDMRs
      (1) This is done by inhibiting synaptic AChE and thus increasing the synaptic levels of ACh
      (2) Greater amounts of NDMR are displaced from nicotinic receptors as the synaptic concentration of ACh exceeds that of NDMR
      (3) The return of neuromuscular control can thusly be hastened as the synaptic concentration of ACh is artificially increased concurrent with the progressive reduction in the concentration of NDMR (by breakdown, metabolism, excretion, and discontinuing its administration)
   b. NDMR reversal agents exert a *desired* effect by increasing the synaptic levels of ACh at the nicotinic receptors of skeletal muscle
   c. However, NDMR reversal agents exert an *undesired* effect by increasing the synaptic levels of ACh at muscarinic receptors in the following organs
      (1) Eyes: miosis
      (2) Heart: bradycardia
      (3) Lungs: bronchospasm
      (4) Gastrointestinal tract: enhanced peristalsis
      (5) Secretory glands: enhanced secretions
   d. The undesired effects of NDMR reversal agents can be minimized by the coadministration of antimuscarinic agents (atropine or glycopyrrolate)
   e. If excessive doses of NDMR reversal agents are administered, an excessive increase in synaptic ACh will occur; this will result in synaptic depolarization (by ACh) and resulting skeletal muscle weakness

3. CNS effects
   a. NDMR reversal agents have no direct effects (they do not cross blood-brain barrier)

4. Toxicities
   a. Minimal if dosed properly and combined with the appropriate antimuscarinic drug (see below)

B. Neostigmine
   1. General facts
      a. Brand name: various manufacturers
         (1) Commonly used reversal agent for NDMRs
      b. Binds to synaptic AChE
         (1) Prevents AChE from breaking down ACh
            (a) Half-life of neostigmine-AChE binding: 30 minutes
            (b) Half-life of ACh-AChE binding: 42 microseconds
         (2) Synaptic levels of ACh accumulate
            (a) Competitive antagonism between ACh and NDMR occurs
         (3) Bound neostigmine eventually hydrolyzes spontaneously
            (a) Thereafter AChE is available to bind more ACh

c. Inhibits PChE and will prolong the effects of other drugs metabolized by PChE
   (1) SCh
   (2) Mivacurium
   (3) Trimethaphan
   (4) Local anesthetic esters (i.e., procaine, chloroprocaine and tetracaine)

2. Administration route and dosage
   a. IV dose: 0.05 mg/kg
      (1) Must be given concurrently with IV glycopyrrolate (0.01 mg/kg)
      (2) Should not be given unless some spontaneous recovery of the NMJ is evident (assess motor strength before dosing)
3. Pharmacokinetics
   a. Onset (IV injection)
      (1) 50% of peak activity within 3.5 minutes
      (2) 100% of peak activity within 7 minutes
   b. Duration: 60 minutes
   c. Metabolism: ester hydrolysis by AChE and PChE
   d. Excretion: renal (50%)
   e. Elimination: primarily renal (75%)
      (1) Metabolites from hydrolysis
      (2) Unchanged drug, small amount
4. Pharmacodynamics
   a. Reversibly inhibits synaptic AChE
      (1) Dose-dependent increase in synaptic ACh
      (2) ACh competitively antagonizes presence of NDMRs
   b. ALERT: Neostigmine also reversibly inhibits PChE
      (1) Effect may last up to 4 hours
      (2) This will prolong the effects of drugs metabolized by PChE
         (a) SCh
         (b) Mivacurium
         (c) Trimethaphan
         (d) Local anesthetics, esters
   c. NOTE: Excessive neostigmine can actually cause neuromuscular paralysis
      (1) A "depolarization block" can occur (as with SCh)
      (2) Caused by the effects of excessive doses (>0.075 mg/kg)
         (a) Direct effects: in excessive doses neostigmine can directly depolarize nicotinic receptors
         (b) Indirect effects: maximally increased levels of ACh in synapse may also cause a depolarization block of the NMJ
5. Cardiovascular effects
   a. Bradycardia
      (1) Caused by increased ACh at sites of vagal innervation: SA and AV nodes
      (2) Can profoundly lower heart rate and cardiac output
   b. Peripheral vasodilation: may cause hypotension
      (1) Caused by activation of vascular muscarinic receptors
6. Drug combinations
   a. Neostigmine with atropine
      (1) Not a preferred combination
      (2) The onset and effect of atropine precedes that of neostigmine
         (a) More tachycardia
         (b) More dysrhythmias
   b. Neostigmine with glycopyrrolate
      (1) Preferred combination for neostigmine

(2) Onset time of glycopyrrolate better matches that of neostigmine
(a) Less tachycardia
(b) Fewer dysrhythmias
(3) In addition, neither drug crosses blood-brain barrier; therefore CNS effects are minimal
7. Nursing considerations
a. Commonly used reversal agent for NDMRs
b. Monitor vital signs and $Spo_2$ when reversal agents are given
C. Edrophonium
1. General facts
a. Brand name: Enlon
(1) Frequently used anticholinesterase for NDMRs
b. ALERT: Onset of effects is rapid; a profound increase in vagal tone (muscarinic tone) on the heart will occur if atropine is not coadministered; severe bradycardia, or even asystole, may result
c. It is good reversal agent if used correctly (atropine *must* be coadministered with edrophonium)
d. Does not inhibit PChE (neostigmine and pyridostigmine will)
2. Administration route and dosage
a. Intravenously: 0.5 to 1 mg/kg:
(1) Not given unless some spontaneous recovery is evident
(2) Given in combination with IV atropine (7 to 14 μg/kg)
3. Pharmacokinetics
a. Onset (IV injection)
(1) 50% of peak activity within 0.5 minutes
(2) 100% of peak activity within 1 minute
b. Duration: 60 minutes
c. Metabolism: conjugation to glucuronide
d. Elimination: primarily renal (75%)
(1) Tubular secretion
(2) Metabolites from hydrolysis
(3) Small amount of unchanged drug
4. Drug combinations
a. Edrophonium with atropine
(1) Preferred combination for edrophonium
(2) Onset time of atropine matches that of edrophonium
(a) Less bradycardia
(b) Fewer dysrhythmias
(c) Much less likely to see asystole
(3) Atropine does cross blood-brain barrier
b. Edrophonium with glycopyrrolate
(1) Potentially dangerous combination
(2) Onset time of glycopyrrolate lags behind that of edrophonium: severe bradycardia, asystole, and cardiovascular collapse can occur
5. Nursing considerations
a. Formerly was not a popular reversal agent because it was not regarded as being very potent
(1) This was true historically; however, inadequate doses were given
(2) Dosage should be 0.5 to 1 mg/kg (in combination with atropine)
b. Currently is used more
(1) Edrophonium is available in solution by itself (Enlon); use atropine concurrently
(2) Edrophonium also comes premixed with atropine (Enlon Plus)

c. ALERT: Edrophonium still not recommended for reversing a dense block; neostigmine (in combination with glycopyrrolate) will be more effective

D. Pyridostigmine
1. General facts
a. Brand name: various manufacturers
(1) Less commonly used reversal agent for NDMRs
b. Less potent reversal agent than neostigmine; only 20% of the reversal activity of neostigmine
c. Duration of action (4 to 5 hours) 40% longer than that of neostigmine
d. Fewer muscarinic effects
e. Profound depression of PChE
(1) Longer lasting than neostigmine
(2) Will prolong effects of drugs metabolized by PChE
(a) SCh
(b) Mivacurium
(c) Trimethaphan
(d) Local anesthetics, esters
2. Administration route and dosage
a. IV dose: 0.25 mg/kg
(1) Not given unless some spontaneous recovery is evident
(2) Given in combination with IV glycopyrrolate (0.01 mg/kg); administer slowly to diminish side effects
3. Pharmacokinetics
a. Onset (IV injection)
(1) 50% of peak activity in 4 minutes
(2) 100% of peak activity in 12 minutes
b. Duration: about 90 minutes
c. Metabolism: hydrolysis by AChE and PChE
d. Elimination: primarily renal (75%)
4. Drug combinations
a. Pyridostigmine with atropine
(1) Not a preferred combination
(2) Onset time of atropine precedes that of pyridostigmine
(a) More tachycardia
(b) More dysrhythmias
b. Pyridostigmine with glycopyrrolate
(1) Preferred combination for pyridostigmine
(2) Onset time of glycopyrrolate better matches that of pyridostigmine
(a) Less tachycardia
(b) Fewer dysrhythmias
(c) Neither crosses blood-brain barrier
5. Cardiovascular effects
a. Fewer autonomic side effects
b. Fewer dysrhythmias in elderly
6. Nursing considerations
a. Less commonly used NDMR reversal agent
b. Longer onset time than edrophonium or neostigmine

## VI. Intravenous Anesthetic Induction Agents

A. Common properties
1. General facts
a. IV administration
b. Good patient acceptance

c. Quick onset
d. Very brief duration
e. Quick offset because of redistribution
f. IV administration quickly and reversibly induces anesthesia
   (1) CNS depression occurs
   (2) Spontaneous ventilation is arrested
   (3) Laryngeal reflexes are lost
   (4) Increased risk for aspiration can occur
g. Patients generally recover within 5 to 10 minutes after a single dose
h. Specific agents have variable side effects depending on circumstances

2. Elimination
   a. See information on pharmacokinetics of liquid inhalational anesthetics
   b. Although metabolism does occur for most of these drugs, plasma levels are initially reduced, primarily by redistribution (below)
   c. Redistribution occurs very quickly with IV induction agents
      (1) On IV injection (single dose) the injected drug is diluted into the primary vascular space, i.e., central compartment (the concentration of drug in blood is now at its maximum)
      (2) Next (and very quickly) the central compartment distributes the drug first to those organs richly supplied by the vasculature
         (a) Because the brain and heart are small, only minor amounts of drug are distributed here
         (b) At this time the concentration of drug in the central compartment is still near its peak level
         (c) Note that drug's effects on the CNS and cardiovascular system are now maximal
      (3) As time proceeds, drug in the central compartment is redistributed into larger organs and tissue less richly supplied by the vasculature, i.e., muscle, skin, fat, and bone marrow
         (a) If monitored, the concentration of drug in the vascular space would now appear to decline
         (b) Clinically, the effects of the drug on the CNS and cardiovascular system begin to wane
3. Respiratory effects
   a. Respiratory, laryngeal, and pharyngeal reflexes are blunted
   b. Upper airway obstruction can be caused by relaxation of surrounding soft tissue muscle tone
   c. Ventilatory depression is usually guaranteed
4. Immune response effect
   a. Initial studies suggest that T-lymphocyte proliferations are inhibited by most of the induction agents (thiopental > methohexital = etomidate) except propofol
   b. Propofol may be one of the least T-lymphocyte-inhibiting drugs to use for patients who are immunocompromised
5. Nursing considerations
   a. Ventilation will need to be supported until the effects of these agents wear off
   b. If gastric contents are present, the airway and lungs will need to be protected until the protective airway reflexes return
      (1) Be vigilant
      (2) Maintain proper positioning of airway
      (3) Be prepared for immediate suctioning of the airway if vomiting occurs

B. Thiopental
   1. General facts
      a. Brand name: Pentothal and others
         (1) Used as anesthetic IV induction agent: generally rapid and pleasant

- b. Dose-dependent depression of CNS function: effects range from sedation through coma

2. Administration route and dosage
   - a. Individuals with adequate cardiovascular stability
     - (1) 2.5 to 5 mg/kg, titrated to effect
   - b. Individuals without adequate cardiovascular stability
     - (1) Induction dosage of thiopental must be reduced
     - (2) Consider alternate IV agents: etomidate or ketamine
3. Pharmacokinetics
   - a. Onset <30 seconds
   - b. Duration 5 to 10 minutes
   - c. Metabolism
     - (1) Hepatic microsomal enzymes
     - (2) Chronic use causes predictable enzyme induction
   - d. Elimination
     - (1) Termination of action is primarily by redistribution
     - (2) Multiple dosing saturates this process and will delay clinical recovery
     - (3) Thiopental is largely eliminated in urine as water-soluble metabolites
4. Pharmacodynamics
   - a. Dose-dependent depression of CNS function
     - (1) Depresses polysynaptic responses
     - (2) Thought to potentiate effect of inhibitory neurotransmitter (GABA)
     - (3) Important locus of depression is reticular activating system (required for wakefulness)
   - b. Hyperalgesic effect at low blood levels; patient may perceive more pain
5. Hepatic effects
   - a. With liver disease metabolism is impaired, drowsiness is prolonged, and ventilation is depressed
6. Nursing considerations
   - a. Reconstituted solution is very alkaline (pH >10) and incompatible with acidic solutions
     - (1) Infiltrated injections may need special attention: apply warm compresses

C. Methohexital

1. General facts
   - a. Brand name: Brevital and others
     - (1) Used as anesthetic induction agent
   - b. Dose-dependent depression of CNS function: effects range from sedation through coma
   - c. Potency: twice that of thiopental
   - d. Action: similar to thiopental at equianesthetic doses but has less effect on respiratory depression
2. Administration route and dosage
   - a. IV induction: 1 to 2 mg/kg
   - b. Rectal doses
     - (1) 20 to 30 mg/kg
     - (2) Used in pediatric patients
     - (3) Onset in about 7 minutes
     - (4) Recovery usually begins in about 45 minutes
3. Pharmacokinetics: see information on thiopental
4. Pharmacodynamics: see information on thiopental
5. Nursing considerations
   - a. Several side effects on injection: pain, myoclonus, hiccoughs

D. Etomidate

1. General facts

a. Brand name: Amidate
   (1) Used as anesthetic induction agent
b. Agent of choice in patients with cardiovascular disease
c. Excellent cardiovascular stability
   (1) Less likely to cause hypotension than thiopental
   (2) Heart rate and cardiac output tend to remain constant; negative inotropic effects are minimal
   (3) Slight decrease in blood pressure possible because of slight peripheral vascular relaxation
d. Dose-dependent suppression of adrenal steroidogenesis
   (1) Up to 24 hours after one induction dose
   (2) Also occurs after prolonged infusions
      (a) Use contraindicated in critically ill patients
      (b) May cause reversible adrenal insufficiency
e. Dissolved in propylene glycol: pain and venoirritation may occur on injection

2. Administration route and dosage
   a. IV induction: 0.2 to 0.4 mg/kg
3. Pharmacokinetics
   a. Onset: 15 to 45 seconds
   b. Duration: 3 to 12 minutes
   c. Metabolism: hepatic microsomal enzymes and plasma esterases; hydrolysis of this drug is nearly complete
   d. Elimination
      (1) Action is terminated primarily by redistribution
      (2) Rapid metabolism also contributes to prompt awakening
      (3) Overall, clearance is five times faster than with thiopental
4. Pharmacodynamics
   a. Hypnotic without analgesic effect
   b. Unconsciousness occurs in 1 minute or less
5. Cardiovascular effects: see general facts (above)
6. Respiratory effects
   a. Dose-dependent hypoventilation and apnea
   b. Rapid return of spontaneous ventilation
7. Skeletal muscle effects
   a. Myoclonus is occasionally seen on induction
   b. Premedication with narcotic or benzodiazepine diminishes myoclonus
8. Nursing considerations
   a. Several side effects on injection
      (1) Dose-dependent suppression of adrenal function
         (a) Etomidate inhibits cortisol synthesis
         (b) Circulating levels of cortisol are depressed
         (c) Circulating levels of ACTH are increased
         (d) Effects may last up to 24 hours after a single dose
      (2) Myoclonus
      (3) Pain when rapidly injected into small vein
      (4) Nausea or vomiting is common
   b. Use of etomidate infusions in ICUs leads to adrenocortical suppression with increased morbidity and mortality
      (1) Adrenal insufficiency possible
      (2) Use contraindicated in critically ill patients

E. Ketamine
   1. General facts
      a. Brand name: Ketalar
         (1) Used as anesthetic induction agent

b. Intense analgesic properties
c. Useful in minor surgical procedures
   (1) Burn debridement
   (2) Oral surgery where intense analgesia is necessary
d. Related to phencyclidine, PCP, and LSD; vivid hallucinations are possible during and after surgery

2. Administration route and dosage
   a. IV doses
      (1) Induction: 1 to 2 mg/kg
         (a) Rapid onset
         (b) Recovery usually begins in about 5 to 10 minutes
      (2) Maintenance: 0.5 to 1 mg/kg every 5 to 30 minutes
      (3) Infusion: 1 mg/kg/hr (may have fewer after effects)
   b. IM dose: 5 to 10 mg/kg
      (1) Onset within 3 to 5 minutes
      (2) Recovery usually begins in about 10 to 20 minutes
3. Pharmacokinetics
   a. Onset: 15 to 45 seconds
   b. Duration: 3 to 12 minutes
   c. Metabolism: occurs extensively by hepatic microsomal enzymes
   d. Elimination
      (1) Action is terminated primarily by redistribution
      (2) Largely eliminated in urine
4. Pharmacodynamics
   a. Depresses neocortex
   b. Produces excellent analgesia
   c. Stimulates limbic system
   d. Does not depress reticular activating system
   e. Produces dissociation of thalamoneocortical and limbic systems
   f. Produces dissociative anesthesia
      (1) No recollection of surgery
      (2) Patient appears to be awake
      (3) Minimal respiratory depression
5. CNS effects
   a. Increases cerebral blood flow; has been reported to increase intracranial pressure
   b. Emergence from anesthesia can be associated with delirium
      (1) Alterations in mood and body image
      (2) Vivid dreams, sometimes progressing to hallucinations
      (3) Out-of-body experiences or psychomotor activity
   c. Recurrent illusions or flashbacks (may occur up to several weeks after anesthesia)
   d. Strategies to reduce or eliminate "emergence" phenomena
      (1) Use diazepam as premedicant
      (2) Preoperatively mention possibility of dreams
      (3) Recovery in dark, quiet environment has no beneficial effect
6. Cardiovascular effects
   a. Increases heart rate, blood pressure, and cardiac output (probably mediated by CNS effects)
7. Respiratory effects
   a. Respiratory, laryngeal, and pharyngeal reflexes remain nearly normal
   b. Spontaneous ventilation tends to be maintained
   c. Ventilatory depression and obstruction indicate overdosage
   d. Potential for *increased salivary gland secretion* may require patient premedication with a antisialogogue like glycopyrrolate

8. Skeletal muscle effects
   a. Usually causes increase in muscle tone
9. Contraindications
   a. Hypertension
   b. Previous stroke
   c. Psychiatric disorders
   d. Elevated intracranial pressure
10. Nursing considerations
   a. Can produce vivid hallucinations in PACU; patient may need to be restrained or require benzodiazepine sedation
   b. Incidence of delirium
      (1) Greater in adults than in children
      (2) 50% of adults older than 30 years experience excitement and delirium
   c. Preanesthetic visit should mention potential for dreamlike effects that may be experienced on emergence and during first day after ketamine exposure
   d. Can produce irritability and compromise suck in infants

F. Propofol
1. General facts
   a. Brand name: Diprivan
      (1) Used as anesthetic induction agent
   b. Formulated in a milky white emulsion of glycerin, lecithin (from egg yolks), and soybean oil
   c. May cause hypotension if injected too rapidly; more pronounced in hypovolemic patients
   d. No analgesic effects
   e. Rapid and alert emergence
   f. High incidence of pain on IV injection
      (1) Distal veins: 40%
      (2) Larger veins: 10%
      (3) IV lidocaine used to decrease this pain
   g. No preservatives: cannot be stored after opening ampules (opened ampules can support vigorous growth of microorganisms)
2. Administration route and dosage
   a. IV doses
      (1) Reduce dosage in elderly, premedicated, and hypovolemic patients
      (2) Induction: 1.5 to 2.5 mg/kg
      (3) Maintenance: vary infusion from 50 to 150 μg/kg/min
         (a) Propofol can be used as primary anesthetic
         (b) Narcotics and nitrous oxide may be added as adjuncts
         (c) Infusion discontinued 10 to 15 minutes before case ends
3. Pharmacokinetics
   a. Onset: 15 to 45 seconds
   b. Duration: 5 to 10 minutes
   c. Metabolism: extremely rapid
   d. Elimination
      (1) Action is terminated primarily by redistribution; prolonged administration, however, can saturate this process
      (2) Largely eliminated in urine
      (3) Clearance 5 to 10 times faster than with thiopental
      (4) Clearance significantly greater than liver blood flow
4. Nursing considerations
   a. Lower incidence of postoperative side effects
      (1) Less hangover

(2) Less nausea and vomiting
(3) Less psychomotor impairment
b. Earlier ambulation and discharge after outpatient surgery
(1) Time in PACU decreased
(2) Outpatients ready to go home earlier
(3) Patients resume day-to-day activities earlier
(4) Patients are more alert and drink fluids and eat earlier
(5) Patients often more responsive and in elevated mood
c. Rapid emergence from anesthesia may hasten pain awareness
(1) Propofol does not provide any residual postanesthetic analgesic effect
(2) Intraoperative or postoperative analgesics may need to be administered

**VII. Intravenous Opioid Anesthetics**

A. Common properties
1. General facts
a. Synthetic opioids:
(1) Used as analgesic or anesthetic induction agents
(2) Also used as premedicant: sedative, analgesic, or anesthetic adjunct
(3) Intraoperative use will decrease requirement for general anesthesia
2. Pharmacokinetics
a. Onset: rapid
b. Duration of analgesia: 30 minutes
c. Redistribution half-life: 15 minutes
d. Metabolized by liver
e. Elimination
(1) Lower doses: termination of action primarily by redistribution; multiple doses or large doses will saturate this process; see information on intravenous anesthetic induction agents for more information on "redistribution" phenomena
(2) Higher doses: primarily by metabolism; various half-lives
(a) Alfentanil: 1.5 hours
(b) Sufentanil: 2.5 hours
(c) Fentanyl: 3.5 to 4 hours
3. Pharmacodynamics
a. Appears to modulate intracellular production of cyclic AMP
b. May inhibit transmembrane calcium currents
(1) Effect appears to be potentiated by calcium channel blockers
(2) Effect at presynaptic neurons may decrease release of neurotransmitters
c. Overall, opioids inhibit pain by modulating synaptic impulse transmission
d. Opioids decrease perception of and response to pain by
(1) Effects at level of dorsal horn cells of spine
(2) Activation of descending inhibitory pathways from brain stem
(3) Altering emotional response to pain in limbic cortex
(4) Opioids relieve continuous "dull" pain better than intermittent sharp pain
4. Side effects
a. Miosis: stimulation of oculomotor nerve; reversed by naloxone, atropine, or glycopyrrolate
b. Bradycardia: stimulation of vagus nerve is treatable with atropine or glycopyrrolate
c. Muscle rigidity: alfentanil is worst offender; more pronounced when injected rapidly
d. Nausea and vomiting: use antiemetics
e. Hypotension
(1) May be caused by bradycardia and/or a decrease in sympathetic tone
(2) Exaggerated in patients who are anxious, hypovolemic, or in pain

f. Delayed awakening
g. Respiratory depression: background $Pa_{CO_2}$ required to stimulate normal ventilation is increased
5. Nursing considerations
a. Observe for respiratory depression in PACU
(1) Assess need for ventilatory support
(2) Naloxone should be readily available

B. Alfentanil
1. General facts
a. Brand name: Alfenta
(1) Used as analgesic and anesthetic adjuvant
b. Synthetic narcotic analgesic
(1) 1/10 as potent as fentanyl
(2) 10 times more potent than morphine
2. Administration route and dosage
a. Guidelines for IV loading dose (titrated to effect)
(1) Perioperative analgesia: 10 to 25 μg/kg
(2) Balanced anesthesia: 50 to 150 μg/kg
b. Guidelines for continuous IV infusion (titrated to effect)
(1) Perioperative analgesia: 0.25 to 1 μg/kg/min
(2) Balanced anesthesia: 0.5 to 3 μg/kg/min

C. Fentanyl
1. General facts
a. Brand name: Sublimaze
(1) Used as analgesic and anesthetic adjuvant
b. Synthetic narcotic analgesic: 100 times more potent than morphine
c. Duration of analgesia: 30 to 60 minutes
2. Administration route and dosage
a. Guidelines for IV loading dose (titrated to effect)
(1) Perioperative analgesia: 1 to 3 μg/kg
(2) Balanced anesthesia: 5 to 15 μg/kg
b. Guidelines for continuous IV infusion (titrated to effect)
(1) Perioperative analgesia: 0.01 to 0.03 μg/kg/min
(2) Balanced anesthesia: 0.03 to 0.1 μg/kg/min

D. Remifentanil
1. General facts
a. Brand name: Ultiva
(1) Used as analgesic and anesthetic adjuvant
b. Newer synthetic narcotic with an extremely short half-life
c. After an initial loading dose, the effects of this drug must be continued by continuous infusion
d. The abrupt discontinuation of infusions of this drug can cause the sudden onset of extreme pain and related adverse effects
e. Because remifentanil by itself cannot assure unconsciousness, its exclusive use in general anesthesia is not recommended
f. Spinal or epidural use is not recommended because of the motor dysfunctions that might occur from its glycine vehicle (glycine is a spinal cord neurotransmitter)
2. Administration route and dosage
a. Guidelines for IV loading dose (titrated to effect)
(1) Balanced anesthesia: 0.5 to 2 μg/kg
b. Guidelines for continuous IV infusion (titrated to effect)
(1) Balanced anesthesia: 0.25 to 0.5 μg/kg/min

3. Nursing considerations
   a. The sudden discontinuation of infusions of this drug after surgery may bring on the sudden onset of intense pain; the supplemental use of longer lasting analgesics must be anticipated and administered without delay
   b. Because of its high potency, remifentanil not administered by nursing personnel

E. Sufentanil
1. General facts
   a. Brand name: Sufenta
      (1) Used as analgesic and anesthetic adjuvant
   b. Synthetic narcotic analgesic
      (1) 500 to 1000 times more potent than morphine
      (2) 5 to 10 times more potent than fentanyl
   c. Used in balanced general anesthesia
      (1) For induction and maintenance
      (2) In major surgical procedures
2. Administration route and dosage
   a. Guidelines for IV loading dose (titrated to effect)
      (1) Balanced anesthesia: 1 to 3 μg/kg
   b. Guideline for continuous IV infusion (titrated to effect)
      (1) Balanced anesthesia: 0.01 to 0.05 μg/kg/min

## VIII. Local and Regional Anesthetic Agents

A. Common properties
1. General facts
   a. Agents that impair conduction of neurally mediated impulses
   b. Two chemical groups
      (1) Amides: prilocaine, lidocaine, mepivacaine, bupivacaine, etidocaine
      (2) Esters: procaine, chloroprocaine, tetracaine
2. Administration route
   a. Brachial plexus agents
      (1) Lidocaine
      (2) Mepivacaine
      (3) Bupivacaine
   b. Epidural anesthetic agents
      (1) Lidocaine
      (2) Bupivacaine
      (3) Mepivacaine
      (4) Chloroprocaine
   c. Intravenous agents: Bier block
      (1) Lidocaine
      (2) Mepivacaine
   d. Nerve block: all agents
   e. Spinal anesthetic agents
      (1) Lidocaine
      (2) Bupivacaine
      (3) Procaine
      (4) Tetracaine
   f. Subcutaneous infiltration: all agents
3. Physiology: three major classes of nerves (Table 9–1)
   a. A fibers: myelinated somatic nerves
   b. B fibers: myelinated preganglionic autonomic nerves
   c. C fibers: lightly myelinated postganglionic autonomic nerves

**TABLE 9–1 Classification of Nerve Fibers**

| FIBER TYPE | MYELIN | DIAMETER (μm) | FUNCTION |
|---|---|---|---|
| Aα | +++ | 10–20 | Motor neurons (efferent: to skeletal muscle) |
| Aβ | ++ | 5–10 | Touch, pressure, and proprioception neurons (afferent: from skin) |
| Aγ | ++ | 5–10 | Motor neurons (efferent: to muscle spindles) |
| Aδ | ++ | 1–5 | Pain (sharp/fast) and temperature neurons (afferent: from skin) |
| B | + | 1–2.5 | Preganglionic sympathetic neurons (efferent: to vascular smooth muscle) |
| C | ± | 0.5–1 | Pain (dull/slow) and temperature neurons (afferent: from skin)<br>Postganglionic sympathetic neurons (efferent: to vascular smooth muscle) |

4. Pharmacodynamics
   a. Impair conduction of impulses along axons
      (1) Effect mediated by blocking sodium channels
      (2) Communication between CNS and peripheral nervous system is impaired
      (3) Block is reversible and dose dependent
   b. Rank order of nerve fiber sensitivity to local anesthetic blockade:
      (1) B > C and Aδ > Aγ > Aβ > Aα
   c. Rank order of nerve fiber diameters:
      (1) C < B < Aδ < Aβ and Aγ < Aα (thinnest/least myelinated nerves blocked first)
   d. Two separate pain-conducting pathways (both blocked by same tissue concentration of agent)
      (1) C fibers (slow pain)
      (2) Aδ fibers (fast pain)
5. Pharmacokinetics
   a. Amides: metabolized in liver
   b. Esters: hydrolyzed by plasma cholinesterase
6. Side effects
   a. Determined by rate of systemic absorption, which is related to vascularity of site of injection; most to least vascularity: intercostal < caudal < lumbar epidural < brachial plexus < spinal
   b. Cardiovascular system
      (1) Arterial vasodilation
      (2) Negative inotropic and dromotropic (impulse conduction) effects
      (3) Cardiovascular collapse occurs with severe toxicity
   c. Respiratory system
      (1) Ventilatory depression caused by CNS depression
      (2) Progresses from hypopnea to apnea to death
   d. CNS
      (1) Initial stimulation results in restlessness and tremors
      (2) Increasing absorption leads to drowsiness and CNS depression
      (3) May progress to convulsions
   e. Muscle
      (1) Paralysis of skeletal muscle by effect on neuromuscular junction
      (2) Directly depresses contraction of smooth muscle
   f. Plasma cholinesterase: esters inhibit this enzyme, prolonging effects of SCh and mivacurium

g. Hypersensitivity reaction: dermatitis, asthma, anaphylactic shock:
   (1) More common with esters because of their metabolite—PABA
   (2) If allergic to esters, amides may be used
   (3) Preservatives in some multiuse vials may be allergenic

7. Nursing considerations
   a. Hypotension frequently results from epidural or spinal use
      (1) Adult patients usually given 1000 to 2000 ml of crystalloid intravenously before dosing
      (2) Consider additional IV fluid challenges as needed
      (3) Consider IV ephedrine (5 mg) or phenylephrine (50 to 100 μg) doses as needed.
   b. Potential for systemic toxicity influenced by vascularity of area where agent is injected
   c. Persons with liver disease metabolize amide local anesthetics more slowly
   d. Atypical or inhibited PChE may prolong effects of ester local anesthetics

B. Procaine
   1. General facts
      a. Brand name: Novocaine and others
         (1) Short-acting local anesthetic of ester class
   2. Administration route
      a. Local infiltration
      b. Peripheral nerve block
      c. Spinal anesthesia
   3. Pharmacokinetics
      a. Absorption
         (1) Vasoconstrictors prolong local anesthetic action: slower absorption diminishes chance for systemic toxicity
      b. Metabolized by plasma cholinesterases, which include PChE

C. Chloroprocaine
   1. General facts
      a. Brand name: Nesacaine
         (1) Short-acting local anesthetic of ester class
      b. Two times more potent than procaine but shorter acting
      c. Low toxicity
      d. Thrombophlebitis is frequent side effect
      e. Notoriety of causing spinal neuropathy has limited its use
         (1) Toxicity traced to bisulfite preservative and acidic pH of its solution
         (2) Toxic combination of preservative and acidic solution is now removed
   2. Administration route
      a. Local infiltration
      b. Peripheral nerve block
      c. Epidural anesthesia (lumbar and caudal routes)
   3. Pharmacokinetics: metabolized by plasma cholinesterases (including PChE)
   4. Pharmacodynamics: blocks sensory more than motor nerves

D. Tetracaine
   1. General facts
      a. Brand name: Pontocaine
         (1) Long-acting local anesthetic of ester class
      b. 10 times more potent and toxic than procaine
      c. Longer acting
      d. Causes extensive motor and sympathetic blockade
   2. Administration route
      a. Topical anesthesia
      b. Spinal anesthesia

3. Pharmacokinetics
   a. Readily absorbed from all routes
   b. Metabolized by plasma cholinesterases (including PChE)
4. Pharmacodynamics
   a. Blocks sensory and motor nerves equally well

E. Cocaine
1. General facts
   a. Brand name: various manufacturers
      (1) Long-acting local anesthetic of ester class
   b. Sympathomimetic properties
      (1) Causes accumulation of synaptic norepinephrine
      (2) Inhibits reuptake of norepinephrine released from adrenergic nerve endings
      (3) Increased synaptic norepinephrine thus facilitates sympathomimetic responses
      (4) WARNING: cocaine can cause severe increases in heart rate and blood pressure
   c. CNS stimulant, especially cerebral cortex, because of accumulating synaptic norepinephrine
   d. Pyrogenic activity: potential side effect
2. Cardiovascular effects
   a. Tachycardia/hypertension
   b. Vasoconstriction
      (1) Decreases its own absorption: prolongs its local anesthetic effect
3. Administration route and dosage
   a. Topical use as 4% to 10% solution for mucous membrane anesthesia, especially nasopharynx
   b. No other uses because of side effects and toxicities
4. Pharmacokinetics
   a. Well absorbed from all routes
   b. Hydrolyzed by plasma cholinesterases
5. Drug interaction: causes myocardium to be more responsive/sensitive to catecholamines
6. Nursing considerations
   a. Potential for toxicity
   b. High potential for abuse: powerful cortical stimulant

F. Lidocaine
1. General facts
   a. Brand name: Xylocaine
      (1) Medium-acting local anesthetic of amide class
   b. Quick, potent and longer lasting than procaine
   c. High incidence of sleepiness and dizziness
   d. IV lidocaine depresses laryngeal and tracheal reflexes
   e. Notable antidysrhythmic properties on the myocardium
   f. When infiltrated as a local anesthetic, its vasodilator activity facilitates its rate of absorption
      (1) Epinephrine (coadministered with lidocaine) decreases this vasodilation and absorption
      (2) Mepivacaine (another local anesthetic, see below) does not have this vasodilator effect and thus can be a substitute for lidocaine with epinephrine when epinephrine's use is not desirable
2. Administration route and dosage
   a. Local infiltration, 0.5% to 2% (with or without epinephrine)
   b. Peripheral nerve block, 1% to 2% solutions (with or without epinephrine)
   c. Epidural anesthesia, 1.5% to 2% solutions
      (1) Average dose: 15 to 20 ml of 1.5% to 2% solution
      (2) Duration: 0.75 to 1.5 hours

d. Spinal anesthesia, hyperbaric, 1.5% or 5% solutions (with or without dextrose)
   (1) Average dose: 50 to 80 mg (1 to 1.6 ml)
   (2) Duration: 0.75 to 1.5 hours
   (3) NOTE: Because of a possible association with transient radicular irritation (TRI), it is now recommended that the 5% lidocaine solution be diluted with CSF to a final concentration of 2% before injection
e. Topical anesthesia, 2% jelly or 4% solution
f. Intravenous (Bier) block, 40 to 50 ml of 0.5% solution

3. Pharmacokinetics: metabolized by hepatic microsomal enzymes
4. Pharmacodynamics: blocks sensory and motor nerves equally well
5. Nursing considerations
   a. Lidocaine (topical or IV) is useful in anesthetizing the trachea prior to intubation
   b. Topical or IV lidocaine will depress laryngeal and tracheal reflexes

G. Mepivacaine
1. General facts
   a. Brand name: Carbocaine
      (1) Medium-acting local anesthetic of amide class
      (2) Longer duration of action than lidocaine
      (3) Does not cause vasodilation like lidocaine
   b. Moderate potency and toxicity
2. Administration route and dosage
   a. Local infiltration, 1% to 2% solutions
   b. Peripheral nerve block, 1% to 2% solution
   c. Epidural anesthesia (lumbar and caudal routes), 1% to 2% solutions
      (1) Average dose: up to 25 ml of 2% solution
      (2) Duration: 1 to 2 hours
   d. Not for use in spinal anesthesia
3. Pharmacokinetics: longer acting than lidocaine
4. Pharmacodynamics: similar to lidocaine (and other amide local anesthetics) except it does not cause vasodilation (alternative to lidocaine with epinephrine)

H. Bupivacaine
1. General facts
   a. Brand names: Marcaine, Sensorcaine
      (1) Long-acting local anesthetic of amide class
   b. Slow onset and prolonged duration
   c. Residual analgesia outlasts anesthetic effects
   d. Cardiac toxicity
      (1) WARNING: Excessive dosing or accidental IV injection can cause ventricular dysrhythmias that are difficult to correct; do not exceed the maximally allowed dose (see below, Nursing Considerations)
2. Administration route and dosage
   a. Epidural or caudal anesthesia, 0.25% to 0.5% solutions
      (1) Average dose: 15 to 20 ml of 0.5% solution
      (2) Duration: 2 to 4 hours
   b. Spinal anesthesia, 0.75% solution (with or without dextrose)
      (1) Average dose: 7.5 to 12 mg (1 to 1.6 ml)
      (2) Duration: 2 to 4 hours
3. Pharmacokinetics: metabolized by hepatic microsomal enzymes
4. Pharmacodynamics: blocks sensory more than motor nerves
5. Nursing considerations
   a. Has a prolonged anesthetic and analgesic action
   b. Frequently infiltrated during surgery as a postoperative analgesic for incision pain (analgesia lasts about 4 to 8 hours)
   c. May cause ventricular dysrhythmias when local anesthetic doses become excessive

or are injected intravenously by accident. Treatment must be with bretylium or amiodarone. Lidocaine will be ineffective or may worsen condition

I. Ropivacaine
   1. General facts
      a. Brand name: Naropin
         (1) New, longer acting local anesthetic of the amide class
      b. Chemically very similar to bupivacaine
      c. Similar onset and duration of action to bupivacaine
      d. Similar anesthetic properties to bupivacaine, i.e., both have more of an effect on sensory nerves than on motor nerves (although ropivacaine may have slightly less effect on motor nerves)
      e. Appears to be somewhat less cardiotoxic than bupivacaine, however, cardiotoxicity may still be of concern with slightly larger doses
      f. Preliminary clinical experience suggests a dosing schedule similar to that of bupivacaine's
      g. Ropivacaine's practical clinical utility over bupivacaine will have to be determined

**IX. Neuroaxial (NA) Anesthesia**

A. Common properties for spinal and epidural blocks (i.e., anesthetics)
   1. Typically used for surgical cases involving the abdomen, perineum, and the lower extremities
   2. Dermatomes
      a. Used in the assessment of the evolution and extent of a NA anesthetic
      b. Nerve roots exiting the spinal cord innervate the skin in contiguous sensory bands or stripes (1 to 2 inches wide); these bands arise posteriorly (from the spinal column) and typically radiate away laterally, anteriorly, or caudally (looking like zebra stripes, if they could actually be seen)
      c. Each sensory stripe (dermatome) corresponds to a specific nerve root
      d. Each sensory stripe (dermatome) has been investigated, mapped, and standardized in such a manner as to portray the idealized person
      e. The anatomic relationships of representative dermatomes (Fig. 9–4) are listed below
         (1) Neck → C3
         (2) Clavicles → C5
         (3) Nipples → T4
         (4) Xiphoid → T6
         (5) Navel → T10
         (6) Groin → L1
         (7) Knees → L4
         (8) Dorsum of foot → L5
         (9) Lateral ankles → S1
      f. Evolution of a NA anesthetic
         (1) The evolution of a NA anesthetic is influenced by a number of factors: amount of agent given (dose), the volume of the solution, the position of the patient after injection (i.e., sitting, supine, Trendelenburg, reverse Trendelenburg), the baricity of the solution (spinal blocks), and anatomic and physiologic considerations (height, hormonal influences, obesity, and the coincident pregnancy)
         (2) After NA injection, the evolution of the anesthetic block is monitored closely (as it moves cephalad) by assessing the loss of sensation along the above-mentioned dermatomal levels
         (3) The patient's loss of sensation to "sharp" (point of a sterile needle) or "dull" (blunt hub of a sterile needle) is commonly used in the assessment process

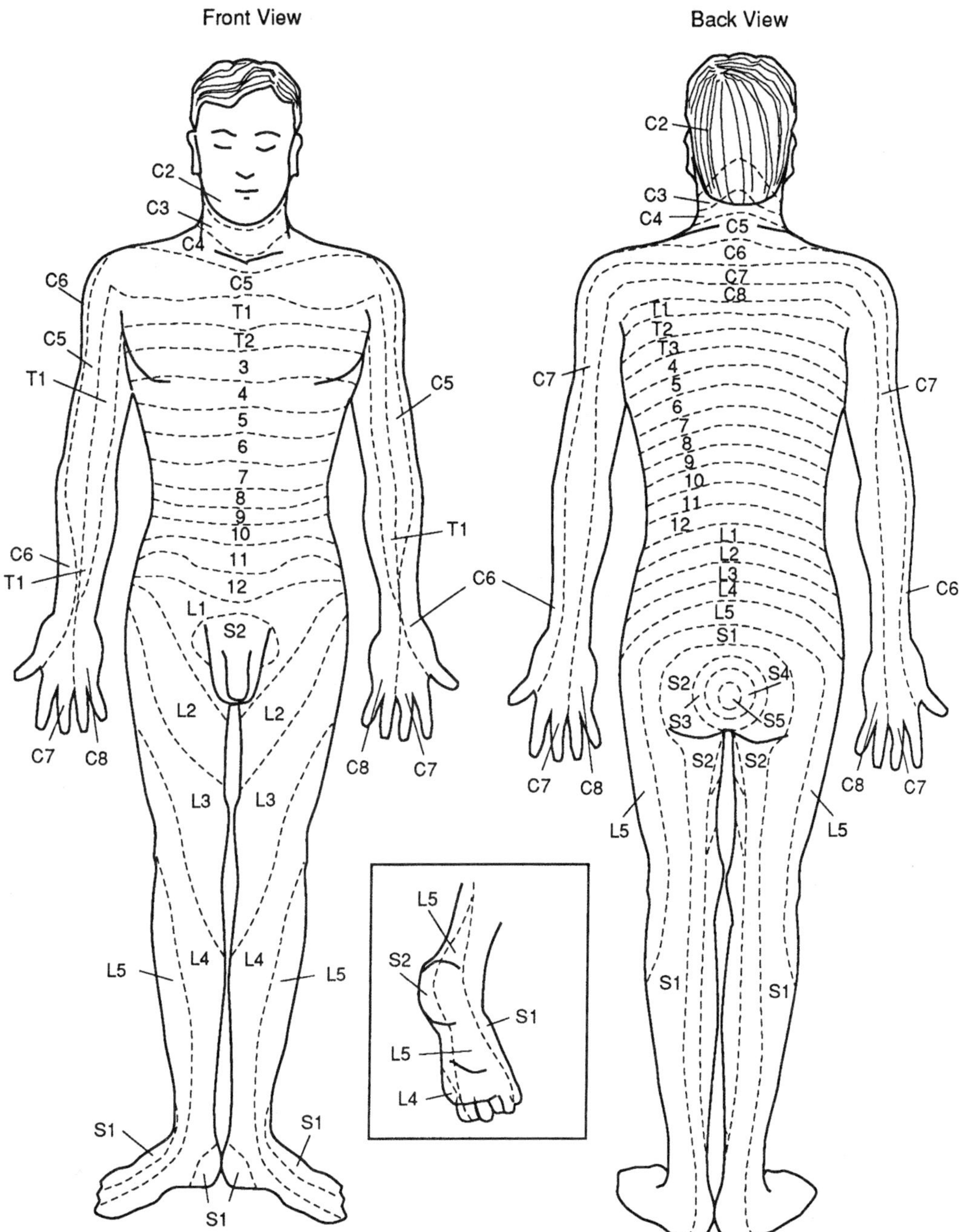


**FIGURE 9–4** Dermatomes. (From Cardona VD, Hurn PD, Mason PJB, Scanlon AM, Veise-Berry SW: Trauma Nursing from Resuscitation through Rehabilitation, 2nd ed. Philadelphia, WB Saunders, 1994, p. 444.)

(4) Typically, a NA anesthetic is noted to first take effect in the feet and then move cephalad (the degree of cephalad movement being influenced by the factors mentioned above)

3. Side effects
   a. Sympathetic blockade is more likely to be caused by a spinal rather than an epidural block (i.e., anesthetic)
      (1) Hypotension is more likely with a NA block higher than T6 (but less than T3) because such blocks tend to impair the sympathetic vasoconstrictor outflow

from the spinal cord (T6 to L2) to the blood vessels of the mesentery and lower extremities; this effect can lead to
   (a) Reduction in venous tone
   (b) Reduction in venous return to heart
   (c) Decrease in cardiac filling and cardiac output
   (d) Decrease in arterial blood pressure
   (e) Reflex increase in heart rate
   (f) Potential for a decrease in coronary blood flow
   (g) Probable increase in myocardial oxygen consumption
 (2) Bradycardia is more likely with a block higher than T3 because such blocks tend to impair the sympathetic cardioaccelerator outflow (T1 to T4) to the SA and AV nodes of the myocardium; this effect leaves the cardiodecelerator effects of the vagus nerve (cranial nerve X) unrestrained
   (a) Treat with atropine as needed
b. Precautionary treatments that may be considered before the potential development of hypotension due to sympathetic blockade include
 (1) Preblock fluid loading: use 20 to 25 ml/kg of normal saline or Lactated Ringers
 (2) Prophylactic administration of IM ephedrine, 25 to 50 mg
 (3) Not using excessive amounts of NA anesthetics
c. Treatment options for hypotension after there has been an excessive NA sympathetic block
 (1) Simple elevation of the patient's legs (this does not necessarily mean placing the patient in Trendelenburg's position; under some circumstances, Trendelenburg's position if initiated too early can worsen a high NA block)
 (2) IV fluid boluses as needed to fill dilated venous capacitance vessels
 (3) Vasopressors to support poor vascular tone (i.e., hypotension) until block resolves
   (a) Consider IV phenylephrine if heart is tachycardic (incremental IV doses of 100 μg). CAUTION: phenylephrine may cause reflex bradycardia
   (b) Consider IV atropine if heart is bradycardic; incremental IV doses of 0.5 to 1 mg per ACLS protocol
   (c) Do not hesitate to use incremental doses of IV epinephrine if cardiovascular collapse appears imminent
   (d) Consider infusion of dopamine if severe cardiovascular depression has occurred
   (e) Consider the placement of an arterial line for blood pressure monitoring if it is needed
d. "High" sensory block
 (1) Block higher than T1 may cause severe cardiopulmonary collapse
 (2) Hydration, vasopressors/vagolytics, intubation, and CPR may be needed as the NA blockade moves closer toward the brainstem
 (3) See information on respiratory effects below

4. Neurologic complications
 a. Postdural puncture headache (PDPH)
  (1) Incidence
   (a) Directly related to size of hole made in dura by the spinal or epidural needle used: larger needles make larger holes
   (b) Inversely related to age of patient: older patients are less likely to experience postdural puncture headaches
   (c) With regard to spinal anesthesia, blunt (spreading-tip) needles are less likely than sharp (cutting-tip) needles, to produce headaches; Whitacre, Sprotte, and Gertie-Marx needles are examples of the "blunt tip" category; Quincke needles are an example of the "cutting-tip" type

(2) Symptoms of a PDPH
(a) The headache typically is felt in a frontal or occipital location or both (worsened by sitting or standing up); if it is to occur, it usually does so after 24 to 72 hours
(b) Associated symptoms include neck ache or stiffness (57% ), backache (35%), and nausea (22%)
(c) Less commonly associated symptoms include shoulder pain, blurred vision, vomiting, tinnitus, or auditory difficulties, and diplopia (i.e., cross-eyed, from a bilateral abducens nerve palsy)
(d) The severity of the PDPH may be relieved by pressure on jugular veins or worsened by pressure on carotid arteries
(3) Symptomatic treatment includes hydration, analgesics, and caffeinated beverages
(4) Definitive treatment, if symptoms persist, includes an epidural blood patch that may be given 24 hours after a PDPH develops

b. Adhesive arachnoiditis
(1) Caused by introduction of foreign materials into intrathecal space
(2) Results in chronic inflammation of the arachnoid
(3) Progressive weakness and sensory loss of perineum or lower limbs
(4) May advance to paraplegia

c. Cauda equina syndrome
(1) May be due to adhesive arachnoiditis
(2) Persistent paresis of legs
(3) Sensory loss in perineum
(4) Bowel and bladder dysfunction
(5) Effects usually permanent and may slowly deteriorate
(6) In some cases, slow regression of symptoms occurs over months

d. Peripheral nerve palsy is usually temporary but can be permanent from nerve root damage

e. Septic meningitis
(1) Symptoms appear within 24 hours of intrathecal contamination
(a) Fever
(b) Headache
(c) Neck rigidity
(d) Kernig's sign: with the patient in the supine position, the thigh is flexed to a right angle with the trunk; Kernig's sign is present if the same-sided leg cannot be extended completely because of severe neck pain
(2) Good outcome if diagnosed early; must be treated immediately with antibiotics

5. Respiratory effects
a. Effects on the ventilatory system increase as the NA block moves in the cephalad direction
b. First, the ability to cough is weakened from paralysis of the abdominal muscles; the inability to cough can impair the patient's capacity to clear airway secretions
c. Next, the progressive cephalad anesthesia of the intercostal nerves increasingly impairs
(1) The intercostal *sensory* nerves and the patient's ability to perceive that he or she is breathing by the usual sensory cues from the skin (i.e., that the chest wall is moving normally with each breath)
(2) The intercostal *motor* nerves and the patient's ability to take deep breaths (the patient's inspiratory capacity is also progressively lost)
(3) NOTE: Some deprivation of chest wall sensation can be unavoidable under ordinary circumstances; reassurance is helpful in allaying patient anxiety
(4) WARNING: With a complete loss of chest wall sensation and patient complaints of increasing difficulty breathing, the possibility of a NA block progressing

toward complete phrenic nerve paralysis (C3 to C5) should be suspected: emergent intubation of trachea may be immediately necessary!

d. Finally, a high enough NA block to cause paralysis of the phrenic nerve (C3 to C5) is rarely seen if reasonable attention to technique is provided; however, if apnea does occur, patient will require assisted ventilation and possibly intubation to protect the airway from secretions or the aspiration of possible gastric contents

B. Spinal anesthesia
   1. Specific facts
      a. Anesthetic solution is injected into the intrathecal space
         (1) Nerve roots and part of spinal cord anesthetized
         (2) WARNING: Spinal cord usually ends at L1-2 interspace; agent should be injected below this level to avoid possible cord trauma
   2. Systemic toxicity: rare because of small doses given
   3. Baricity
      a. Addition of 5% to 10% glucose makes solution heavier than CSF
         (1) Solution tends to "sink" within CSF according to pull of gravity
         (2) Level of anesthesia influenced by body's position
         (3) Trendelenburg's position will hasten cephalad spread of local anesthetic

C. Epidural anesthesia
   1. Specific facts
      a. Anesthetic solutions can be administered into the epidural space by
         (1) Single injection
         (2) Repetitive bolus injections (by catheter)
         (3) Continuous infusion (by catheter)
      b. Produces nerve root, spinal cord, and paravertebral nerve anesthesia
      c. Produces less sympathetic blockade than intrathecal (spinal) block
      d. Higher chance for systemic toxicity than spinal block
         (1) Greater amount of drug needs to be administered for epidural anesthesia (in contrast to spinal anesthesia)
         (2) Greater amount of drug administered is systemically absorbed
      e. Because of the procedural use of a larger needle, an increased risk for a more pronounced headache is present if an inadvertent dural puncture occurs

D. Nerve block
   1. General facts
      a. Anesthetic is injected into or around a nerve or nerve plexus
         (1) Requires a knowledge of anatomy
         (2) Absorption of excessive doses can lead to systemic toxicity
         (3) Epinephrine-containing solutions will delay systemic absorption and thus decrease systemic toxicity

E. Local infiltration and field blocks
   1. General facts
      a. Anesthetic is injected directly into tissue
      b. Field block: anesthetic injected into surrounding tissue
         (1) Blocks transmission of sensory impulses
      c. WARNING: epinephrine-containing solutions should not be infiltrated into confined areas (fingers, toes, ears, nose, penis); gangrene may develop

F. Topical or surface anesthesia
   1. General facts
      a. Anesthetic is applied directly to skin or mucous membrane
      b. Systemic absorption occurs after application to mucous membranes
         (1) Increases the risk of toxicity if excessive doses are applied
         (2) Especially true of the vascular tracheobronchial tree

G. Preservative-free morphine
  1. General facts
    a. Brand names: Duramorph, Astramorph, and others
    b. Used as an adjunct for NA anesthesia
    c. Epidural administration provides pain relief for extended periods
      (1) No loss of motor or sensory functions
      (2) Some dose-dependent decreases in sympathetic function may occur
      (3) Respiratory depression is always possible but not likely if conservative doses are given
    d. Onset occurs 15 to 60 minutes after NA administration; analgesia may last 12 to 36 hours
    e. Initial adult dose is 2 to 5 mg
    f. Delayed respiratory depression is possible
      (1) Patient should be monitored for 18 to 24 hours after administration, depending on dose given
    g. Resuscitation equipment and naloxone should be available to counteract any potential respiratory depressant effects
    h. Nausea and vomiting possible; need for antiemetics should be anticipated
    i. Prophylactic antiemetics may be best defense against nausea and vomiting induced by NA administered morphine

## X. Intravenous Anesthetic Adjuncts

A. Droperidol
  1. General facts
    a. Brand name: Inapsine and others
      (1) In small doses this antipsychotic agent is widely used in anesthesia for its antiemetic properties
    b. Moderate antiemetic effects; dose: 0.0625 to 0.125 mg IV
    c. Neuroleptic anesthesia (Innovar)
      (1) Combines properties of droperidol with those of fentanyl in a 50:1 mixture
      (2) Primary effects
        (a) Ataraxia
        (b) Some amnesia
        (c) Reduced motor movement
        (d) Patient arousable and responsive but indifferent
    d. Additional effects
      (1) Alpha-adrenergic blocking activity produces vasodilation and mild to moderate hypotension
      (2) Elevates threshold for myocardial dysrhythmias but may also prolong the QT interval
      (3) Anticonvulsant action
      (4) Slight respiratory depression
  2. Pharmacokinetics: Metabolized by the liver
  3. Pharmacodynamics: Works within the CNS as dopamine antagonist
  4. Side effects
    a. Dystonic reaction: Muscle spasm of face, neck, tongue, or upper back
      (1) Occurs in about 1% of patient population
      (2) May also be caused by metoclopramide
      (3) Treatment: diphenhydramine (Benadryl), 25 to 50 mg by slow IV
      (4) Alternate treatment: benztropine (Cogentin), 1 to 2 mg IV
    b. Postanesthetic dysphoria (internalized overwhelming fear)
      (1) May occur when droperidol (a psychotropic drug) is given alone without the beneficial effect of narcotics like fentanyl

(2) May occur if the beneficial effect of a coadministered narcotic wanes
(3) Effect of droperidol usually persists longer than that of narcotics
(4) Patients and their families may require some reassurance if the dysphoric effect occurs

B. Anticholinergics
1. Atropine
a. 0.5 to 1 mg IM or IV
b. Inhibits salivary and respiratory tract secretions
c. Causes bronchodilation
d. Counteracts bradycardia and related dysrhythmias
e. Given with anti-AChE agents at end of general anesthesia
f. Crosses blood-brain barrier, causes CNS stimulation
g. Can produce central anticholinergic syndrome
(1) Restlessness, irritability, disorientation, delirium
(2) Can be major cause of postoperative dysphoria
(3) Central effects can be reversed by physostigmine
2. Scopolamine
a. Same preoperative use as atropine
b. Dose is 0.3 to 0.6 mg IM or IV
c. Causes CNS depression, drowsiness, amnesia, euphoria, fatigue
d. May cause paradoxical excitation
e. Less effective at preventing bradycardia
f. Higher incidence of postoperative dysphoria and delirium
g. May cause short-term amnesia when given with morphine
3. Glycopyrrolate (Robinul)
a. Longer acting than atropine
b. More potent antisialagogue than atropine
c. Dose: 0.1 to 0.2 mg IM or IV
d. More potent inhibitor of gastric acid secretion than atropine
e. Does not cross blood-brain barrier
f. Does not produce sedation
g. Does not produce central anticholinergic syndrome
h. More rapid postoperative awakening than with atropine
i. Prevents bradycardia and less likely to cause tachycardia than atropine

C. Benzodiazepines
1. General facts
a. Administered by oral, IM, or IV routes
(1) Absorbed from gastrointestinal tract
b. Metabolized by hepatic oxidative microsomal enzymes; inactive metabolites excreted in urine
c. Lack of analgesic properties
d. Dose-related depression of ventilation
e. WARNING: ventilatory rate must be monitored closely after IV sedation; use pulse oximetry to confirm patient's return to normalcy
f. Exhibits amnestic, anxiolytic, hypnotic, and sedative properties
g. Also exhibits anticonvulsant and muscle relaxant properties
h. Bind to modulating sites on GABA receptors in CNS
(1) Leads to hyperpolarization of postsynaptic membranes; highest density of benzodiazepine receptors is in cerebral cortex, where there is an inhibitory effect on excitation of neurons
i. Mild cardiovascular depressant effects: mild vasodilation
(1) Minor direct myocardial depression
(2) Midazolam < diazepam and lorazepam

j. Skeletal muscle relaxation reflects action on spinal internuncial neurons
    (1) Skeletal muscle tone reduced
    (2) Benzodiazepines do not reduce surgical requirements for muscle relaxants
k. Recovery of fine motor skills
    (1) More rapid with midazolam than with diazepam or lorazepam
l. Can markedly attenuate cardiostimulatory effects of ketamine; also minimizes emergence sequelae of ketamine

2. Diazepam
    a. Brand name: Valium and others
        (1) Used as a sedative and anesthetic adjunct
    b. Insoluble in water
        (1) Parenteral formulation contains propylene glycol; injection may be associated with venous irritation and pain
    c. Dosing schedule
        (1) Sedation
            (a) IV: 2.5 to 5 mg
            (b) PO: 5 to 10 mg
        (2) Induction of general anesthesia: 0.25 to 0.5 mg/kg IV
        (3) Treatment of seizures: 0.10 mg/kg IV and titrate to effect
    d. Onset
        (1) IV: rapid
        (2) PO: 30 to 60 minutes
    e. Duration: IV, 15 minutes to 3 hours
    f. Low hepatic clearance rates: elimination half-life is 20 to 40 hours
3. Lorazepam
    a. Brand name: Ativan
        (1) Used as sedative and anesthetic adjunct
    b. Insoluble in water
        (1) Parenteral formulation contains propylene glycol; injection may be associated with pain and venous irritation
    c. Dosing schedule for sedation
        (1) IV: 1 to 2 mg
        (2) PO: premedicant, 0.05 mg/kg (not to exceed 4 mg)
    d. Onset
        (1) May be slow and somewhat unpredictable
            (a) May be marked lag between peak blood concentration and clinical effect
            (b) Clinical effect may be difficult to titrate
        (2) IV: 5 to 20 minutes
        (3) IM: 0.5 to 2 hours
        (4) PO: 1 to 2 hours
    e. Duration
        (1) IV: 4 to 6 hours
        (2) IM: 8 hours
        (3) PO: 8 hours
    f. Elimination half-life is 10 to 20 hours
4. Midazolam
    a. Brand name: Versed
        (1) Used as sedative and anesthetic adjunct
    b. Water-soluble formulation
        (1) Minimal local irritation on injection
    c. Midazolam has a steep dose-response curve; careful titration very important
    d. Dosing schedule
        (1) Sedation

(a) IV: 1 to 4 mg
(b) IM: 0.05 to 0.1 mg/kg
(2) Induction of general anesthesia: 0.1 to 0.2 mg/kg IV

e. Onset
(1) IV: 15 minutes
(2) IM: 10 to 30 minutes

f. Duration
(1) IV: 2 to 6 hours (induction dose)
(2) IM: 1 to 2 hours

g. Rapid and extensive hepatic metabolism and renal excretion; elimination half-life is 2 to 4 hours

D. Benzodiazepine antagonist
1. Flumazenil
a. Brand name: Romazicon
(1) Only drug available in this class
(2) Specific benzodiazepine receptor antagonist
(3) Blocks CNS effects of benzodiazepines
b. Dosing schedule: IV doses of 0.1 mg increments to maximum of 1 mg
c. Onset (IV): within 1 minute
d. Duration: 1 to 2 hours
e. Hepatic metabolism and renal excretion
(1) Redistribution half-life: about 5 minutes
(2) Elimination half-life: about 60 minutes

E. Antiemetics (most commonly used agents presented)
1. Droperidol (Inapsine)
a. Antagonizes emetic effects of narcotic analgesics
b. Alpha-adrenergic blocking effects (mild to moderate) may cause some vasodilation; vasodilation may lead to hypotension and tachycardia in hypovolemic patients
c. May cause drowsiness and delay discharge of outpatients
d. IV dose is 0.625 to 1.25 mg; onset, 3 to 10 minutes; duration, 3 to 6 hours
e. Infrequently, it may cause an acute spasm (dystonic reaction) of one of the muscles innervated by the cranial nerves (i.e., muscles in the face or neck); this dystonic reaction is typically treated with diphenhydramine, 25 to 50 mg by slow IV push ("slow IV push" because diphenhydramine [i.e., Benadryl] is perceived by many patients to burn intensely on injection)

2. Metoclopramide (Reglan)
a. Dopamine antagonist; gastrointestinal stimulant enhances the tone on the lower esophageal sphincter and facilitates gastric emptying
b. Commonly used with outpatients because drug has few side effects in therapeutic doses
c. Large ratio between therapeutic and toxic effects
d. IV dose, 10 to 20 mg; IV onset, 1 to 3 minutes; duration, 1 to 2 hours
e. IM dose, 5 to 20 mg; IM onset, 10 to 15 minutes; duration, 1 to 2 hours
f. Metabolized by liver
g. Infrequently, like droperidol, it may cause an acute spasm (dystonic reaction) of one of the muscles innervated by the cranial nerves (see droperidol)

3. Ondansetron (Zofran)
a. Works on chemoreceptor trigger zone (central) and vagus nerve terminals (peripheral)
b. Serotonin (5-hydroxytryptamine$_3$, 5-HT$_3$) blocker
c. IV dose: 4 mg by slow IV injection over 30 to 90 seconds
d. Given prophylactically (before anesthesia) or in PACU to treat nausea and vomiting
e. Half-life is 4 hours (metabolized in liver)
f. Side effects include headache

4. Prochlorperazine (Compazine)
   a. Antiemetic; antipsychotic; neuroleptic
   b. Used to control severe nausea and vomiting
   c. Depresses cough reflex: watch for and prevent aspiration
   d. IM route preferred; IV route may cause hypotension
   e. IM dose, 12.5 to 25 mg, 3 to 4 times daily as needed; do not repeat within 4 hours
   f. PO dose, 25 mg, every 10 to 12 hours
   g. Drug effects may last 12 hours
   h. May cause sedation and may potentiate sedation from other drugs
   i. Infrequently, like droperidol, it may cause an acute spasm (dystonic reaction) of one of the muscles innervated by the cranial nerves (see Droperidol)
5. Scopolamine (Transderm-Scop)
   a. Useful as an antiemetic and antinauseant
   b. Is an anticholinergic drug that inhibits neural input from the vestibular apparatus to the CNS
   c. Results in inhibition of the vomiting reflex
   d. Also useful in the prophylaxis of motion sickness
   e. Should not be used with children
   f. Side effects include dry mouth, drowsiness, disorientation, and confusion
   g. Wash hands after applying and avoid hand-to-eye contact (may result in mydriasis and blurred vision)
   h. The transdermal patch contains 1.5 mg of scopolamine and is applied behind the ear; the patch delivers 0.5 mg of scopolamine over 3 days
   i. NOTE: Use in patients with glaucoma is contraindicated
   j. NOTE: Use during pregnancy is not recommended (category C)
   k. NOTE: Should be applied 4 hours before anesthetic exposure for maximum effectiveness. Not practical in many circumstances
6. Trimethobenzamide (Tigan)
   a. Depresses chemoreceptor trigger zone
   b. Sedative; weak antihistamine effects
   c. IM route: onset within 15 minutes; duration, 2 to 3 hours
   d. Important to restore hydration and electrolytes as adjunct to therapy
   e. Monitor for hypotension
   f. IM and rectal dose, 200 mg 3 to 4 times daily
   g. PO dose, 250 mg 3 to 4 times daily

## ACKNOWLEDGMENT

Recognition is given to Karen Ginther Harbut, RPh, for her most appreciated suggestions and review of this manuscript.

## BIBLIOGRAPHY

Barash PG, Cullen BF, Stoelting RK: *Handbook of Clinical Anesthesia*. Philadelphia, JB Lippincott, 1991.

Bevan DR, Bevan JC, Donati F: *Muscle Relaxants in Clinical Anesthesia*. Chicago, Year Book, 1988.

Butterworth JF, Brownlow RC, Leith JP, et al: Bupivacaine inhibits cyclic-3′,5′-adenosine monophosphate production: A possible contributing factor to cardiovascular toxicity. *Anesthesiology* 79(1):88, 1993.

Collins VJ: *Principles of Anesthesiology/General and Regional Anesthesia*, 3rd Ed. Philadelphia, Lea & Febiger, 1993.

Cousins MJ, Bridenbaugh PO (eds): *Neural Blockade in Clinical Anesthesia and Management of Pain*, 2nd Ed. Philadelphia, JB Lippincott, 1992.

Datta S, Camann W, Bader A, VanderBurgh L: Clinical effects and maternal and fetal plasma concentrations of epidural ropivacaine versus bupivacaine for cesarean section. *Anesthesiology* 82(6):1346, 1995.

Devlin EG, Clarke RSJ, Mirakhur RK, McNeil TA: Effect of four i.v. induction agents on T-lymphocyte proliferations to PHA in vitro. *Br J Anaesth* 73(3): 315, 1994.

Drug Facts and Comparisons: Monthly Update. *Muscle Relaxants: Adjuncts to Anesthesia.* St. Louis, Wolters Kluwer, 1996.

Drug Facts and Comparisons: *Antiemetic/Antivertigo Agents.* St. Louis, Wolters Kluwer, 1998.

Donnelly AJ: *A Review of Neuromuscular Blockers.* Research Triangle, NC, Burroughs Wellcome, 1992.

Fragen RJ (ed): *Drug Infusions in Anesthesiology* (p. 270). Philadelphia, Lippincott-Raven, 1996.

Hardman JG, Limbird LE (eds): *Goodman and Gilman's The Pharmacological Basis of Therapeutics,* 9th Ed. New York, Macmillan, 1996.

Hasio J, Pitkaren MT, Kytta J, Rosenberg PH: Treatment of bupivacaine-induced cardiac arrhythmias in hypoxic and hypercarbic pigs with amiodarone or bretylium. *Reg Anesth* 15(4):174–179, 1990.

Katz AM: *Physiology of the Heart.* New York, Raven Press, 1977.

Kharasch ED, Armstrong AS, Gunn K, et al: Clinical sevoflurane metabolism and disposition: II. The role of cytochrome P450-2E1 in fluoride and hexafluoroisopropanol formation. *Anesthesiology* 82(6):1379, 1995.

Lebowitz PW, Cook CE: *Clinical Anesthesia Procedures of the Massachusetts General Hospital,* 3rd Ed. Boston, Little, Brown, 1988.

Martin JL, Plevak DJ, Flannery KD, et al: Hepatotoxicity after desflurane anesthesia. *Anesthesiology* 83(5):1125, 1995.

Martyn JJ: The acetylcholine receptor: How does it change response to relaxants? Lecture No. 206: Regional Refresher Course, American Society of Anesthesiology. Las Vegas, Nevada, February 7–8, 1998.

Miller RD, Cucchiara RF, Miller ED, et al: *Anesthesia,* 3rd Ed. New York, Churchill Livingstone, 1990.

Moore MA, Weiskopf RB, Eger EI, et al: Arrhythmogenic doses of epinephrine are similar during desflurane or isoflurane anesthesia in humans. *Anesthesiology* 79(5): 943, 1993.

Muzi M, Ebert TJ, Hope WG, Robinson BJ, Bell LB: Site(s) mediating sympathetic activation with desflurane. *Anesthesiology* 85(4):737, 1996.

Muzzi DA, Losasso TJ, Dietz NM, et al: The effect of desflurane and isoflurane on cerebrospinal fluid pressure in humans with supratentorial mass lesions. *Anesthesiology* 76(5):720, 1992.

Neil JM: *Clinical Dialogues on Regional Anesthesia: Management of Postdural Puncture Headache.* Larchmont, NY, Customized Medical Communications, Dec 1990.

Ray DC, Drummond GB: Halothane hepatitis. *Br J Anaesth* 67(1):84, 1991.

Rogers MC, Tinker JH, Covino BG, Longnecker DE: *Principles and Practice of Anesthesiology.* Chicago, Mosby–Year Book, 1993.

Rubin AP: Hazards of local and regional anesthesia. In Taylor TH, Major E (eds): *Hazards and Complications of Anaesthesia,* 2nd Ed. New York, Churchill Livingstone, 1993.

Santos AC, Arthur GR, Wlody D, et al: Comparative systemic toxicity of ropivacaine and bupivacaine in nonpregnant and pregnant ewes. *Anesthesiology* 82(3):734, 1995.

Smith I, Nathanson M, White PF: Sevoflurane: A long-awaited volatile anaesthetic. *Br J Anaesth* 76(3):435, 1996.

Stanec A: Three essential steps in the clinical use of relaxants. *Anesthesiol News* p 23, March 1993.

Stoelting RK: *Pharmacology and Physiology in Anesthetic Practice,* 2nd Ed. Philadelphia, JB Lippincott, 1991.

Tinker JH, Abram SA, Chestnut DH, et al: A two-center comparison of the cardiovascular effects of cisatracurium (Nimbex) and vecuronium in patients with coronary artery disease. *Yearbook of Anesthesiology and Pain Management,* 229:4–35, 1997.

Tinker JH, Abram SA, Chestnut DH, et al: Pharmacokinetics of cisatracurium in patients receiving nitrous oxide/opioid/barbiturate anesthesia. *Yearbook of Anesthesiology and Pain Management,* 230: 4–36, 1997.

Wark H, Elliot RH, Strunin L: Hepatotoxicity of volatile anesthetic agents. *Br J Anaesth* 71(4):610, 1993.


## REVIEW QUESTIONS

**1. Inhalation anesthetics will be best distributed into the:**

A. Tendons and ligaments
B. Muscle and skin
C. Fat and bone marrow
D. Liver, kidney, heart, and brain

**2. Agents that potentiate the effects of volatile anesthetics include:**

A. Ketamine and narcotics
B. Nitrous oxide and cocaine
C. Naloxone and verapamil
D. Amphetamines and chronic ethanol intoxication

**3. The inhalation agent associated with the least potential for laryngospasm on induction is:**

A. Halothane
B. Enflurane
C. Isoflurane
D. Desflurane

**4. Balanced anesthesia refers to:**

A. Use of 50% volatile anesthetic and 50% nitrous oxide
B. Combination of volatile anesthetic with narcotics, nitrous oxide, and muscle relaxants
C. Combining general anesthesia for intraoperative anesthesia with regional anesthesia for postoperative analgesia
D. Using an inhalation anesthetic by itself with only oxygen as an adjunct

**5. Which of the following statements is true of depolarizing muscle relaxants?**

A. They are pharmacologically reversible
B. They are extremely long acting and limited in their usefulness
C. They cause a transient surge in serum potassium
D. They are not potentiated by alkalosis

**6. The sequence of paralysis when using nondepolarizing muscle relaxants is:**

A. Eyes, jaw, hands, limbs, neck, intercostal muscles, diaphragm
B. Diaphragm, intercostal muscles, neck, limbs, hands, jaw, eyes
C. Peripheral muscles, respiratory muscles, cardiac muscle
D. Sympathetic tone, sensory tone, motor tone

**7. Which of the following statements is true?**

A. When paralyzed with a nondepolarizing muscle relaxant, patient requires no narcotics because they cannot feel pain
B. Because nondepolarizing muscle relaxants cross the blood-brain barrier, no sedative agents should be given to prevent clouding postoperative neurologic assessment
C. Nondepolarizing muscle relaxants may be potentiated by acidosis, hypokalemia, hypothermia, and hypermagnesemia
D. Patients who are paralyzed are always asleep and require no neurologic assessment

**8. Which of the following drugs will have a delayed elimination in the presence of a plasma cholinesterase deficiency?**

A. Pancuronium and atracurium
B. Mivacurium and succinylcholine
C. Vecuronium and gallamine
D. Curare and doxacurium

**9. Succinylcholine is contraindicated in all of the following cases except:**

A. Major burns
B. Upper motor neuron injury
C. Routine pediatric anesthetic procedures
D. Emergency intubations

**10. Reversal agents for neuromuscular blocking agents cause undesirable effects because of stimulation of:**

A. Nicotinic receptors
B. Muscarinic receptors
C. GABA receptors
D. Kappa receptors

**11. Reduction of serum levels of IV anesthetic induction agents occurs primarily via:**

A. Metabolism
B. Absorption
C. Redistribution
D. Hoffman degradation

**12. The anesthetic induction agent of choice for a patient with cardiovascular disease is:**

A. Methohexital
B. Thiopental
C. Midazolam
D. Etomidate

**13. Which of the following IV agents is most useful in ambulatory surgery?**

A. Ketamine
B. Propofol
C. Odansetron
D. Meperidine

**14. Fentanyl is ________ times more potent than morphine.**

A. 10
B. 100
C. 50
D. 1000

**15. Which of the following statements is true?**

A. Cocaine is a short-acting local anesthetic of the amide class
B. Cocaine inhibits the reuptake of norepinephrine
C. Cocaine is widely used for IV regional blocks
D. Cocaine causes profound vasodilation and hypotension

**16. The addition of a vasoconstrictor to a local anesthetic:**

A. Decreases the absorption of the local anesthetic, thereby prolonging the block
B. Promotes rapid absorption of the local anesthetic, thereby increasing the onset of the block
C. Decreases the potential of local anesthetic toxicity, thereby increasing the safety of the block
D. Increases the spread of the local anesthetic, thereby increasing the region of the block

**17. Which of the following statements is true?**

A. Postdural puncture headaches are more common in elderly patients
B. The use of an epidural technique eliminates the risk of spinal headache
C. Postdural puncture headaches are more common when large, sharp needles are used
D. The risk of spinal headache can be eliminated by keeping the patient flat in the PACU for 2 hours after injection

**18. When morphine is used for epidural anesthesia and analgesia, the PACU nurse should be aware of the potential for:**

A. Recurrence of pain because the drug is very short acting
B. Loss of motor, sensory, and sympathetic function
C. Vasodilation and hypotension on injection
D. Delayed respiratory depression

**19. Which of the following statements is true?**

A. Glycopyrrolate has the potential to cause central anticholinergic syndrome
B. Atropine causes bronchoconstriction
C. Scopolamine inhibits gastric acid secretion more effectively than atropine
D. Glycopyrrolate causes more rapid postoperative awakening than atropine

**20. Benzodiazepines:**

A. Are profound analgesics
B. May cause dose-related respiratory depression
C. Must be given in larger doses to the elderly patient
D. Are not pharmacologically reversible

**ANSWERS:** 1. D, 2. A, 3. A, 4. B, 5. C, 6. A, 7. C, 8. B, 9. D, 10. B, 11. C, 12. D, 13. B, 14. B, 15. B, 16. A, 17. C, 18. D, 19. D, 20. B

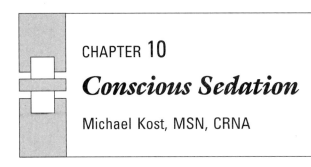

CHAPTER 10

# Conscious Sedation

Michael Kost, MSN, CRNA

## OBJECTIVES

**Study of the information represented by this outline will enable the learner to:**

1. Define conscious sedation, deep sedation, and light sedation.
2. Identify the statutory, regulatory, and promulgated professional standards of care for nurses administering conscious sedation.
3. State the components of preprocedural patient assessment.
4. List conscious sedation medications, dosing guidelines, and nursing considerations associated with their administration.
5. Identify required monitoring parameters for the patient receiving conscious sedation.
6. State postprocedural monitoring requirements for the patient receiving conscious sedation.
7. Identify risk management strategies used to reduce the incidence of complications associated with the delivery of conscious sedation.

## SEDATION

**I. Definitions**

A. Light sedation

1. The reduction of anxiety produced by the administration of oral medications. The following conditions should be present
   a. Normal respirations
   b. Normal eye movements
   c. Intact protective reflexes

B. Conscious sedation

1. Produced by the administration of amnestic, analgesic, and sedative pharmacologic agents. Patients receiving conscious sedation have a "depressed level of consciousness." They must, however, retain a patent airway and respond appropriately to physical and verbal stimuli. To satisfy the definition of conscious sedation, patients must
   a. Retain protective airway reflexes
   b. Independently and continuously maintain a patent airway
   c. Respond appropriately to physical and verbal stimuli

C. Deep sedation

1. A controlled state of depressed consciousness or unconsciousness accompanied by partial or complete loss of protective reflexes, such as the ability to respond purposefully to verbal or physical command. Characteristics of deep sedation include
   a. Unconsciousness
   b. Inability to cooperate
   c. Protective reflexes obtunded
   d. Amnesia always present
   e. Vital signs labile
   f. Perioperative complications in 25% to 75% of cases

2. Deep sedation predisposes the patient to respiratory depression, slowed response to the hypoxic drive, and cardiovascular depression

D. Goals and objectives of conscious sedation
   1. Maintain adequate sedation with minimal risk
   2. Relieve anxiety
   3. Produce amnesia
   4. Provide relief from pain and other noxious stimuli
   5. Overall goal: to allay patient fear and anxiety with a minimum of medication
   6. Mood alteration
   7. Enhanced patient cooperation
   8. Elevation of pain threshold
   9. Stable vital signs
   10. Rapid recovery
   11. Unconsciousness and unresponsiveness are not goals of conscious sedation

E. Indications for conscious sedation
   1. Diagnostic and therapeutic procedures not requiring general anesthesia, skeletal muscle relaxation, or major regional anesthesia
      a. Burn unit dressing changes
      b. Cardiology
      c. Cosmetic surgery
      d. Gastroenterology
      e. General surgery superficial procedures
      f. Gynecology
      g. Ophthalmology
      h. Oral surgery
      i. Orthopedic procedures
      j. Pulmonary biopsy and bronchoscopy
      k. Radiology
      l. Urology

## II. Legal Scope of Practice Issues

A. An understanding of the definition of conscious sedation and adherence to the criteria outlined are required for nurses to comply with the legal scope of practice issues in many jurisdictions
   1. Legal scope of practice issues related to nursing are delegated and administered through state boards of nursing
   2. It is imperative that nurses engaged in the administration of conscious sedation ascertain their state board of nursing's formal position or policy statement delineating the role and responsibility of the nurse engaged in the delivery of conscious sedation
   3. Most states have adopted guidelines. Some states, however, have not yet taken formal action on the issue or lack statutory authority to enact such legislation

## III. Joint Commission on Accreditation of Healthcare Organizations

A. JCAHO has taken an active role in the development of policies, standards, and intents related to the administration of conscious sedation

"1. Anesthesia care standards delineated under the 'Care of Patients' section are applied to patients receiving not only general, spinal, and other major regional anesthesia but also sedation (with or without analgesia), which in the manner used may be reasonably expected to result in the loss of protective reflexes

"2. It is the obligation of each institution to develop appropriate protocols for patients receiving conscious sedation

"3. The JCAHO further states that these protocols must be consistent with professional standards and address:

"a. Presence of sufficient qualified personnel

"b. Resuscitative equipment is present

"c. Appropriate monitoring of vital signs
"d. Care is properly documented" (JCAHO, 1998)

**IV. Professional Organizations**

A. In July 1991 the Nursing Organizations Liaison Forum in Washington, D.C., endorsed a position statement for the management of patients receiving intravenous conscious sedation for short-term therapeutic, diagnostic, or surgical procedures
   1. This position statement has been adopted by most professional nursing organizations

B. Professional organization guidelines, JCAHO recommendations, and statutory regulations require policy development that prepares the nurse participating in the delivery of conscious sedation to demonstrate
   1. Knowledge of anatomy, physiology, cardiac dysrhythmias, and complications related to the administration of sedative agents
   2. Knowledge of the pharmacokinetic and pharmacodynamic principles associated with conscious sedation medications
   3. Preprocedure assessment and monitoring of physiologic parameters, including
      a. Respiratory rate
      b. Oxygen saturation
      c. Blood pressure
      d. Cardiac rate and rhythm
      e. Level of consciousness
   4. An understanding of the principles of oxygen delivery and the ability to use oxygen delivery devices
   5. The ability to rapidly assess, diagnose, and intervene in the event of an untoward reaction associated with the administration of conscious sedation
   6. Proven skill in airway management
   7. Accurate documentation of the procedure and medications administered
   8. Competency validation for training and education conducted on a regular basis

## PREPROCEDURE ASSESSMENT AND PATIENT SELECTION

**I. Preprocedure Assessment Goals**

A. Identify preexisting pathophysiologic disease
B. Obtain baseline patient information
C. Take history and perform physical examination
D. Reduce patient anxiety through education and communication
E. Prepare a plan for the procedure
F. Obtain informed consent

**II. Components of Preprocedure Assessment**

A. Medical history
   1. Cardiac
      a. Angina
      b. Coronary artery disease
      c. Dysrhythmias
      d. Exercise tolerance
      e. Hypertension
      f. Myocardial infarction
   2. Pulmonary
      a. Asthma
      b. Bronchitis
      c. Dyspnea
      d. Exercise tolerance

    e. Cigarette smoking
    f. Recent cold or flu
  3. Hepatic
    a. Ascites
    b. Cirrhosis
    c. Hepatitis
  4. Renal
    a. Dialysis
    b. Renal failure
    c. Renal insufficiency
  5. Neurologic
    a. Convulsive disorders
    b. Headaches
    c. Level of consciousness
    d. Stroke
    e. Syncope
    f. Cerebrovascular insufficiency
  6. Endocrine
    a. Adrenal disease
    b. Diabetes
    c. Hyper/hypothyroidism
  7. Gastrointestinal
    a. Hiatal hernia
    b. Nausea
    c. Vomiting
  8. Hematology
    a. Anemia
    b. Aspirin, nonsteroidal anti-inflammatory drug (NSAID) use
    c. Excessive bleeding
  9. Musculoskeletal
    a. Arthritis
    b. Back pain
    c. Joint pain
B. NPO status
  1. Adult recommendations
    a. NPO after midnight for all solid food
    b. Clear liquids permitted up to 3 hours before the procedure
    c. Oral medications 1 to 2 hours before procedure with up to 150 ml of water
    d. Confirm institution policy
  2. Pediatrics
    a. No solid foods for 8 hours before scheduled procedure
    b. Clear fluids as wanted up to 3 hours before scheduled procedure
    c. Confirm institution policy

## PROCEDURAL CARE

**I. Monitoring**

A. The monitoring process during the procedure includes
  1. Observation and vigilance
  2. Interpretation of data
  3. Initiation of corrective action when required

B. Electrocardiogram (ECG)
   1. ECG monitoring during conscious sedation procedures is helpful in the detection of
      a. Dysrhythmias
      b. Myocardial ischemia
      c. Electrolyte disturbance
      d. Pacemaker function
   2. Cardiac rhythm and dysrhythmias that may be encountered during the administration of conscious sedation include
      a. Sinus tachycardia (ST)
      b. Sinus bradycardia (SB)
      c. Sinus arrhythmia (SA)
      d. Premature atrial contractions (PAC)
      e. Supraventricular tachycardia (SVT)
      f. Atrial flutter
      g. Atrial fibrillation
      h. Junctional rhythm
      i. Premature ventricular contractions (PVC)
      j. Ventricular tachycardia (VT)
      k. Ventricular fibrillation (V-Fib)
   3. See Chapter 16 for description, ECG criteria, and treatment protocol for specific dysrhythmias
C. Noninvasive blood pressure
   1. Hypotension
      a. A decrease in systolic arterial blood pressure of 20% to 30%. Hypotension may be caused by a variety of factors including
         (1) Hypovolemia
         (2) Myocardial ischemia
         (3) Pharmacologic agents
         (4) Acidosis
         (5) Parasympathetic stimulation (pain, vagal stimulation)
      b. Treatment
         (1) Administer oxygen
         (2) Administration of a fluid challenge (300 to 500 ml crystalloid)
         (3) Correction of acidosis or hypoxemia
         (4) Relief of myocardial ischemia
         (5) Titration of sympathomimetic medications
         (6) Titration of inotropic agents
   2. Hypertension
      a. Systolic blood pressure greater than 160 mm Hg or a diastolic blood pressure greater than 95 mm Hg. Hypertension
         (1) Increases bleeding
         (2) Predisposes the patient to hemorrhage
         (3) May lead to cardiac dysrhythmias
         (4) Increases systemic vascular resistance
         (5) Increases myocardial oxygen consumption
      b. Treatment
         (1) Diuresis for fluid overload
         (2) Noxious stimuli require analgesia or discontinuation of stimuli
         (3) Sympathetic nervous stimulation may require alpha and beta blockade
         (4) Myocardial ischemia requires nitrates and analgesia
D. Pulse oximetry
   1. Required for all conscious sedation procedures to monitor ventilatory status of the patient

2. Provides a noninvasive, continuous monitoring parameter to assess the percent of hemoglobin combined with oxygen
3. Pulse oximetry technology allows two light-emitting diodes (LEDs) to measure the intensity of transmitted light across the vascular bed

**II. Procedural Considerations**

A. All syringes labeled
B. Emergency medications and equipment immediately available
C. Adequate intravenous access established before the procedure

## AIRWAY MANAGEMENT AND MANAGEMENT OF RESPIRATORY COMPLICATIONS

**I. Evaluation of the Airway**

A. Oral cavity inspection
   1. Loose, chipped, capped teeth
   2. Dental anomalies
      a. Crowns
      b. Bridges
      c. Dentures
   3. Obstruction to airflow
      a. Tumors
      b. Edema
      c. Inflammatory processes
B. Temporomandibular joint examination
   1. Conducted with patient's mouth opened wide
      a. Normal distance between upper and lower central incisors is 4 to 6 cm
   2. Indications of reduced temporomandibular joint mobility
      a. A clicking sound when mouth is opened
      b. Pain associated with opening the mouth
      c. Reduced ability to open the mouth
C. Physical characteristics
   1. The following physical characteristics may indicate the potential for difficult airway management:
      a. Recessed jaw
      b. Protruding jaw (hypognathous)
      c. Deviated trachea
      d. Large tongue
      e. Short, thick neck
      f. Protruding teeth
      g. High, arched palate
D. Mallampati airway classification system
   1. Initially described in 1983, it offers the clinician a grading system for anticipation of difficult intubation
   2. Examination is conducted while the patient's head is maintained in a neutral position and the mouth is opened 50 to 60 mm. Classes I to IV are based on anatomical areas visualized
      a. Class I: uvula, tonsillar pillars, soft and hard palate visualized
      b. Class II: uvula, hard and soft palate visualized
      c. Class III: portion of uvula and hard palate visualized
      d. Class IV: portion of hard palate visualized

**II. Complications**

A. Sedative, hypnotic, and analgesic medications when used together have a potent synergistic effect

B. Decreased oropharyngeal muscle tone predisposes the patient to airway obstruction, leading to apnea and hypoxemia

C. Steps for restoration of airflow

1. Lateral head tilt
2. Chin lift
3. Jaw thrust
4. Nasal airway insertion
5. Oropharyngeal airway insertion
6. Endotracheal tube insertion

D. Oxygen delivery devices: because of the respiratory depressant effects associated with the administration of sedative, hypnotic, or opioid medications, it is strongly recommended that supplemental oxygen be administered to all patients receiving conscious sedation (see Chapter 11)

## PHARMACOLOGIC AGENTS

**I. Conscious Sedation Medications**

A. Benzodiazepines: see Chapter 9 for general facts, pharmacokinetics, and pharmacodynamics

B. Midazolam (Versed) conscious sedation dosing guidelines are individualized and titrated to effect. Do not administer by rapid injection. Titration to effect means administration of drug until somnolence, nystagmus, or slurred speech occurs

1. Healthy patients: before the procedure, small increments (0.5 mg) of midazolam are administered over 2 minutes. Initial intravenous dose should not exceed 2.5 mg. Some patients may respond to as little as 0.5–1 mg
2. Adults 60 years of age or older: elderly, debilitated, chronically ill patients or patients with reduced pulmonary reserve require small incremental (0.25 to 0.5 mg) doses administered over 2 minutes. Initial dose should not exceed 1.5 mg. If additional sedation is required, it is imperative to wait several minutes to evaluate the pharmacologic effect before administering additional sedation

C. Diazepam conscious sedation dosing guidelines: individualized and titrated to effect. Before the planned procedure, 1 to 2 mg of intravenous diazepam is titrated over 2 minutes. Additional 1 mg increments may be administered over several minutes during the procedure. Additional time must be allowed to evaluate pharmacologic effect in geriatric or debilitated patients or patients with decreased cardiac output. Do not administer by rapid or single bolus injection. Extreme care must be exercised when administering diazepam concurrently with opioids

D. Benzodiazepine antagonist: flumazenil (Romazicon)

1. Specific benzodiazepine antagonist. Reverses the central nervous system effects of benzodiazepines through competitive inhibition of the benzodiazepine receptor sites on the γ-aminobutyric acid (GABA) benzodiazepine receptor complex. The duration and degree of reversal is related to the total dose administered and plasma benzodiazepine concentration
   a. Dosage: 0.2 mg over 1 minute (4 to 20 μg/kg); may repeat at 20-minute intervals
   b. Onset: 1 to 2 minutes; an 80% response will be achieved within 3 minutes of administration
   c. Duration: 40 to 80 minutes
   d. Resedation: patients who have responded to flumazenil should be carefully monitored (up to 120 minutes) for resedation

E. Opioids
   1. Opioids bind to specific opiate receptors located within the central nervous system: the mu, kappa, delta, and sigma receptor subtypes
   2. See Chapter 9 for general facts, pharmacokinetics, and pharmacodynamics
   3. Dosing guidelines
      a. Fentanyl: 1 to 2 μg/kg titrated in 25 μg increments
      b. Meperidine: 0.5 to 1 mg/kg titrated in 25 mg increments
      c. Morphine: 0.05 to 0.2 mg/kg titrated in 1 to 2 mg increments

F. Sedatives, hypnotics, and dissociative anesthetic agents
   1. Sedative, hypnotic, and dissociative medications are added to deepen levels of sedation. The administration of these medications by registered nurses depends on statutory, regulatory, and recommended standards of care. Manufacturer recommendations generally advise that these agents be administered by anesthesia providers
   2. See Chapter 9 for general facts, pharmacokinetics, and pharmacodynamics

**II. Techniques of Administration**

A. The single-dose injection technique uses individual medications titrated slowly to effect. To establish an analgesic base, often opioids are administered before benzodiazepines. Two to three minutes before the procedure, intravenous opioids may be slowly administered to establish analgesia. Benzodiazepines are then added and titrated to patient effect
   1. Combining medications (narcotics, benzodiazepines, and hypnotics) reduces total dosage through synergistic action, assists the clinician in the maintenance of conscious sedation parameters, and provides rapid patient recovery

B. Bolus techniques have been popular in oral surgery and gastroenterology. Based on a predetermined dosage (mg/kg), the entire dose or a large percentage is administered in one single injection
   1. The technique is particularly popular for administration of benzodiazepines. One advantage of this technique is its ability to rapidly provide a therapeutic plasma level immediately before the procedure
   2. Disadvantages associated with the bolus technique include respiratory depression, unconsciousness, chest wall rigidity, and cardiovascular depression. The bolus technique eliminates the safety features of slow titration, which assesses for patient response and clinical sedation end points (nystagmus, slurred speech)
   3. Despite the speed with which a desired plasma concentration can be achieved, the risks associated with the bolus technique may outweigh the potential benefits. Small incremental doses allow therapeutic plasma levels to be reached slowly and produce the desired pharmacologic effect with a minimum of medication

C. Continuous infusion techniques produce a constant medication plasma level. The continuous infusion technique avoids the fluctuations in medication plasma levels associated with the bolus technique. Continuous infusion is a popular sedative technique in critical care units for mechanically ventilated or agitated patients
   1. Additional benefits include shorter recovery time, reduced medication requirement, and minimized side effects
   2. Careful titration based on predetermined clinical endpoints (nystagmus, slurred speech, sedation) allows a rapid return to an alert state after the infusion is discontinued at the conclusion of the procedure

## POSTPROCEDURE RECOVERY

**I. Monitoring**

A. Purpose
   1. Assure return of physiologic function
   2. Assess patient

3. Diagnose
4. Treat complications

B. Monitoring and discharge policies
1. Required by accrediting bodies
2. Recommended by professional organizations

C. Dependent on
1. Diagnostic or surgical procedure performed
2. Length of procedure
3. Preprocedure physiologic status
4. Intraprocedural complications
5. Medications administered
6. Quantities of medications administered

D. Documentation of recovery parameters
1. Use of a postprocedure objective scoring tool. Objective parameters must assess
   a. Activity
   b. Respiration
   c. Circulation
   d. Level of consciousness
   e. Oxygenation
2. Upon completion of the procedure, all patients must be monitored until all institution-approved discharge criteria are met. These discharge criteria must be developed in conjunction with statutory, regulatory, and professional organization standards

**II. Postprocedure Teaching**

A. Instruction
1. Must be conducted in the presence of a responsible adult assuming care of the patient on discharge
2. Written discharge instructions addressing medications, diet, and procedure-specific information must be reviewed with each patient
3. Conscious sedation medication discharge instructions identify medication used, side effects, and specific postprocedural guidelines to protect the patient

B. Conscious sedation postprocedure follow-up
1. A mechanism to ascertain postprocedure status is recommended for patients discharged on the day of the procedure. Inpatient information may be gathered by the conscious sedation practitioner following the procedure. Methods of gathering data include the following
   a. Patient questionnaire
   b. Telephone interview
   c. Satisfaction survey
2. The purpose of postprocedure assessment is to evaluate the following
   a. Incidence of complications related to the administration of conscious sedation
   b. Delayed recovery
   c. Procedural complication rate
   d. Return to function

## CONSCIOUS SEDATION RISK MANAGEMENT STRATEGIES

A. Quality is broadly defined as the comprehensive positive outcome of a product. Achievement of excellence in health care requires quality care and service evaluation

B. The quality of conscious sedation services is based on compliance with prescribed standards and recommended practice guidelines

C. Implementation of a successful conscious sedation program is based on the delivery of the highly technical aspects of care combined with positive outcomes

D. Unexpected events and complications may occur as a result of human error, periods of reduced observation, environmental factors, poor communication, haste, and lack of prepa-

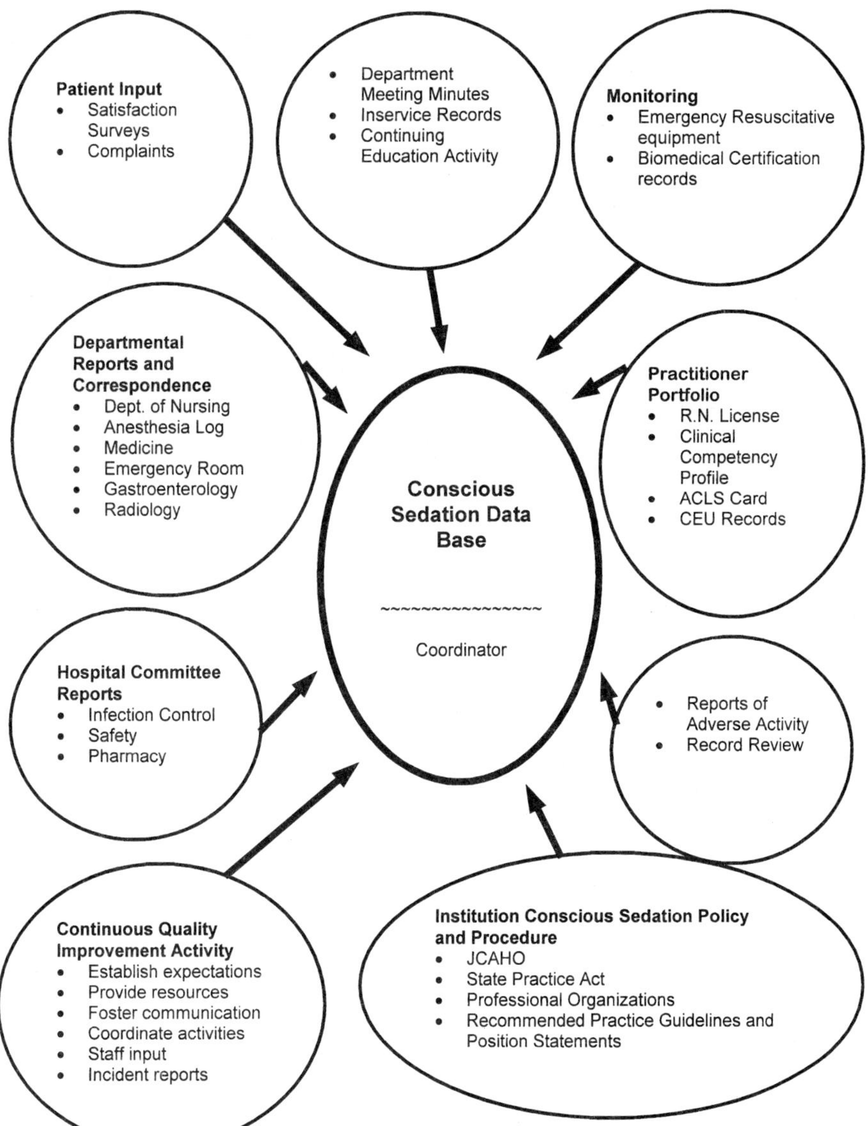


**FIGURE 10–1** Conscious sedation database program. (From Kost M: *Manual of Conscious Sedation.* Philadelphia, WB Saunders, 1998. © 1996, Specialty Health Consultants.)

ration. To prevent or reduce the number of adverse events, a risk reduction strategy should be implemented for all units and personnel engaged in the administration of conscious sedation. Individual injury prevention strategies include the following

1. Development of a complete conscious sedation plan
2. Preprocedure preparation and patient assessment
3. Application and use of required monitoring equipment
4. Selection of appropriate pharmacologic medications and techniques
5. Preparation and presence of emergency resuscitation equipment and personnel
6. Preparation for specific procedures and locations
7. Postprocedure monitoring and discharge planning

E. Ideally, individual risk reduction strategies prevent injury before an adverse incident or event takes place. Application of a risk management program on a department or institution basis requires development and implementation of mechanisms aimed at risk identification, analysis, and control. Creation of a conscious sedation database program as depicted in Figure 10–1 is essential. A coordinator guides input into the conscious sedation database. Once the database has been instituted, strategies to implement changes are used.

## BIBLIOGRAPHY


Aldrete J: Postanesthesia recovery score revisited. *J Clin Anesth* 7:84, 1995.

American Nurses Association: Nursing Liaison Forum: Policy Statement on Conscious Sedation. Washington, DC: The Association, 1991.

American Nurses Association: Policy Statement on Conscious Sedation. Washington, DC: The Association, 1991.

Association of Operating Room Nurses: Standards, recommended practices and guidelines. Denver, *AORN J* 65:149–154, 1997.

Clark B: A New Approach to Assessment and Documentation of Conscious Sedation During Endoscopic Examinations. Society of Gastroenterology Nurses and Associates, April, 1994.

Commonwealth of Pennsylvania: Pennsylvania Code Title 49. Professional and Vocational Standards. Department of State, Chapter 21.413. State Board of Nursing, 1997.

Cummins R: *Textbook of Advanced Cardiac Life Support*. Dallas: American Heart Association, 1994.

Gould K: Conscious sedation. *Crit Care Nurs Clin North Am* 9:3, 1997.

JCAHO: 1998 *Accreditation Manual for Hospitals,* vol 1: Standards. Oakbrook Terrace, Ill, JCAHO, 1998.

Kortbawi P: Developing a conscious sedation program: From policy development through quality improvement. *Gastroenterol Nurs* 20(2):34–41, 1997.

Kost M: *Manual of Conscious Sedation*. Philadelphia, WB Saunders, 1998.

Smith C: Preparing nurses to monitor patients receiving local anesthesia. *AORN J* 59:5, 1994.

White PF, Negua JB: Sedative infusions during local and regional anesthesia: A comparison of midazolam and propofol. *J Clin Anesth* 3:32, 1991.


## REVIEW QUESTIONS

**1. The primary goal of conscious sedation is to:**

A. Enhance patient cooperation
B. Amnesia
C. Rapid recovery
D. Allay fear and anxiety

**2. A state of depressed consciousness, accompanied by partial or complete loss of protective reflexes, including the inability to respond appropriately to verbal or physical command, is defined as:**

A. Anesthesia
B. Conscious sedation
C. Light sedation
D. Deep sedation

**3. The position statement on the Role of the Registered Nurse in the Management of Patients Receiving Intravenous Conscious Sedation, which is endorsed by most professional nursing organizations, was promulgated by:**

A. JCAHO sample policy
B. American Nurses Association
C. American Society of Anesthesiologists
D. Nursing Organizations Liaison Forum

**4. Current NPO recommendations for patients receiving conscious sedation include:**
A. NPO after midnight for all solids; clear liquids permitted up to 3 hours before the scheduled procedure
B. NPO for clear liquids after midnight with no solids after 6 AM on the morning of the planned procedure
C. No solid food on the day of surgery; however, clear liquids may be ingested up to 30 minutes before the procedure
D. No solid food for 2 hours before the procedure

**5. A mechanical maneuver used initially to restore airflow during respiratory obstruction is:**
A. Chin lift
B. Jaw thrust
C. Lateral head tilt
D. Finger sweep

**6. During the administration of conscious sedation a critical respiratory event requires the nurse to use a bag valve device. The oxygen flow required for the adult patient using a bag valve device is _______ liters per minute.**
A. 2–5
B. 6–9
C. 10–15
D. 16–20

**7. Use of individual medications titrated slowly to effect to achieve a state of conscious sedation is identified as which pharmacologic administration technique?**
A. Single-dose injection technique
B. Bolus technique
C. Continuous infusion technique
D. Multiple medication technique

**8. The primary purpose of postprocedure assessment following the administration of conscious sedation is to:**
A. Prevent malpractice claims
B. Evaluate the incidence of complications related to the administration of conscious sedation
C. Provide opportunity for provider-client social interaction
D. Satisfy JCAHO requirements

**9. The comprehensive positive outcome of a product has been broadly defined as:**
A. Excellence
B. Continuous quality improvement
C. Risk management
D. Quality

**10. Conscious sedation policies and procedures, mission statement, and clinical scope of services:**
A. Must be developed separately with no overlap
B. Are only to be developed by administrators
C. Require patient input
D. Must be readily available in all patient care areas where conscious sedation is administered

**ANSWERS:** 1. D, 2. D, 3. D, 4. A, 5. C, 6. C, 7. A, 8. B, 9. D, 10. D

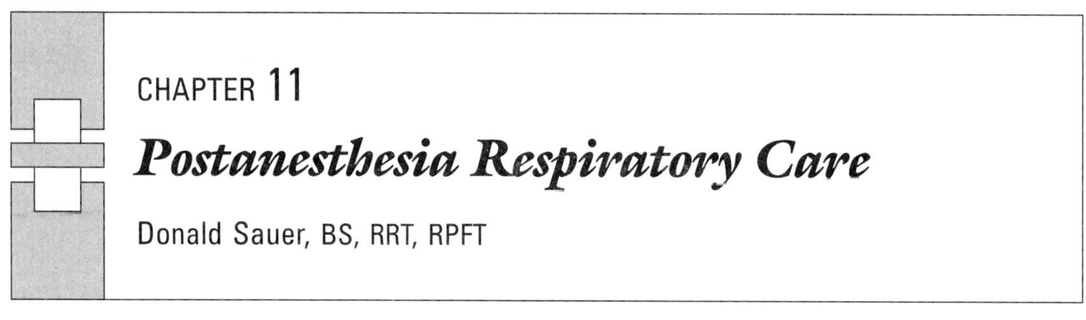


## OBJECTIVES

**Study of the information represented by this outline will enable the learner to:**

1. Describe the indications for $O_2$ therapy.
2. Describe the difference between and applications for low-flow and high-flow oxygen delivery systems.
3. Discuss the potential complications of inappropriate oxygen therapy.
4. Discuss the advantages and disadvantages of intermittent mandatory ventilation, assist/control, pressure assist, and pressure control ventilation.
5. Identify the extubation criteria for the postanesthesia care unit (PACU) patient.
6. Discuss the application of pulse oximetry and capnography.

## RESPIRATORY CARE TERMINOLOGY

**$\alpha$ effects** Sympathomimetic drug response: peripheral vasoconstriction

**$\beta_1$ effects** Sympathomimetic drug response: increase in heart rate, contractility, automaticity, and conduction velocity

**$\beta_2$ effects** Sympathomimetic drug response: relaxation of bronchial muscle (bronchodilation)

**Aerosol** Fine suspension of a substance in a carrier gas; an aerosol of $H_2O$ is not humidity, but it increases humidity of the inspired gas; for pulmonary application, aerosol size must be 1 to 5 μm

**Compliance** Measurement of the distensibility of the lung; the pressure required to maintain a given lung volume

**Dead space** Ventilation that does not participate in gas exchange; normally one third to one fourth of tidal volume

**Fractional concentration of inspired oxygen ($FIO_2$)** Amount of oxygen inspired by the patient expressed as a decimal; because room air is approximately 21% oxygen, the $FIO_2$ of room air is 0.21

**Humidity** Invisible moisture in the air expressed as a percentage

**Hypercapnia** Condition in which $PaCO_2$ is elevated; usually defined as >45 mm Hg (also known as hypercarbia)

**Hypoxemia** Condition in which $PaO_2$ is below normal; usually defined as <60 mm Hg

**Hypoxia** When cellular oxygen demand exceeds oxygen supply

**Negative inspiratory force (NIF)** Force exerted to achieve maximum inspiration; normal NIF is greater than −100 cm $H_2O$; an NIF of at least −20 cm $H_2O$ should be achieved before extubation

**Oxygen saturation** Oxygen content of hemoglobin divided by oxygen capacity and expressed as a percent; when measured by a cooximeter as part of arterial blood gases, it is abbreviated $SaO_2$; when measured by a pulse oximeter it is abbreviated $SpO_2$; normal (at sea level) is usually considered to be 96% to 100%

**Shunt** Portion of cardiac output that does not exchange with alveolar gas; normal shunt usually is defined as 4% or less

**Ventilation/Perfusion Ratio ($\dot{V}/\dot{Q}$)** Ratio at which pulmonary ventilation and cardiac perfusion are matched; alveoli may be adequately perfused but inadequately ventilated, or adequate alveolar ventilation may be present without appropriate pulmonary perfusion; normal $\dot{V}/\dot{Q}$ is usually defined as 0.8

## LUNG VOLUMES AND CAPACITIES

Lung volumes and capacities measure the divisions of ventilation as defined by the American Thoracic Society (Fig. 11–1). There are four *volumes,* which do not overlap, and four *capacities,* each of which contains two or more volumes.

**Expiratory reserve volume (ERV)** Maximal volume of gas that can be expired from the end expiratory level

**Functional residual capacity (FRC)** Volume of gas remaining in the lungs at the resting expiratory level

**Inspiratory capacity (IC)** Maximal volume of gas that can be inspired from the resting expiratory level

**Inspiratory reserve volume (IRV)** Maximal amount of gas that can be inspired from the end inspiratory position

**Residual volume (RV)** Volume of gas remaining in the lungs after maximum expiration

**Tidal volume (TV or $V_T$)** Amount of gas inspired or expired in a normal breath; normal is 10 to 15 ml/kg

**Total lung capacity (TLC)** Total amount of gas contained in the lungs at the end of a maximal inspiration

**Vital capacity (VC)** Maximal amount of gas that can be expelled from the lungs after a maximal inspiration

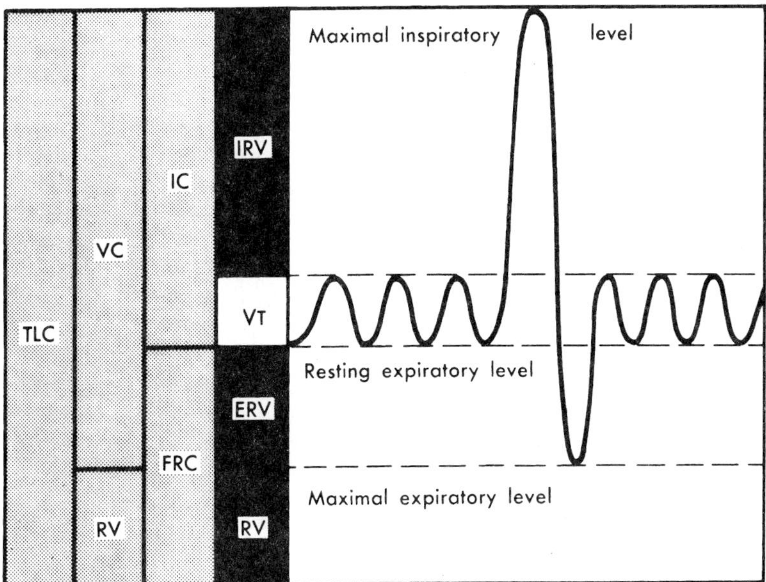


**FIGURE 11–1** Division of total lung capacity into lung volumes and lung capacities. (From Ruppel G: *Manual of Pulmonary Function Testing,* 4th Ed. St Louis, Mosby, 1986.)

## OXYGEN ADMINISTRATION

**I. Indications for Oxygen Therapy**

A. To prevent and treat hypoxemia
B. To decrease work of breathing
C. To decrease work of heart
D. To decrease pulmonary hypertension

**II. Oxygen Delivery Systems**

A. Low-flow systems: do not meet total patient demand because patient breathing patterns vary and more or less room air is inhaled, resulting in variable $FIO_2$
  1. Advantages
    a. Comfort (especially nasal cannula)
    b. Less expensive
    c. Convenient for patient transport
    d. Good for long-term stable patient or any short-term patient
  2. Disadvantages
    a. Humidity and temperature cannot be controlled
    b. $FIO_2$ varies with ventilatory pattern
  3. Types
    a. Nasal cannula: 1 to 8 L/min; $FIO_2$ 0.24 to 0.50; patient can eat and talk
    b. Simple mask: 5 to 10 L/min; $FIO_2$ 0.40 to 0.60; flow must be at least 5 L/min to flush out $CO_2$ from mask
    c. Partial nonrebreathing mask: $FIO_2$ 0.80 to 0.95; adjust flow so that reservoir bag does not deflate

B. High-flow systems: meet total breathing demands of the patient
  1. Advantages
    a. $FIO_2$ does not change with breathing patterns
    b. Humidity and temperature can be controlled (with aerosol devices)
  2. Disadvantages
    a. May be uncomfortable for some patients
    b. More expensive than low-flow devices
    c. Double oxygen setups (two $O_2$ flowmeters with a Y into one $O_2$ wall outlet) may be required for high $FIO_2$
    d. Difficult to use for patient transport
    e. High flow rates required will deplete oxygen "E" tanks quickly
  3. Types
    a. Air entrainment mask (often inaccurately called *Venturi* mask or *Venti-mask*)
      Flow rate of 4 L/min for $FIO_2$ of 0.24
      Flow rate of 6 L/min for $FIO_2$ of 0.28
      Flow rate of 6 L/min for $FIO_2$ of 0.30
      Flow rate of 8 L/min for $FIO_2$ of 0.35
      Flow rate of 12 L/min for $FIO_2$ of 0.40
    b. Aerosol devices: use flow rates of >8 L/min; $FIO_2$ from 0.30 to 1.00 (except face tent)
      (1) Aerosol mask
      (2) Tracheostomy mask (or collar)
      (3) T-piece (Briggs adapter)
      (4) Face tent: good for patients with facial deformities or burn victims

**III. Precautions**

A. Oxygen toxicity
  1. Can develop when high $FIO_2$ is maintained for several days; risk increases with
    a. Steroid use

b. Hyperthermia
c. Epinephrine use
2. Symptoms
a. Substernal pain
b. Alveolar edema or hemorrhage
c. Nausea or vomiting
d. Paresthesia
e. Decreased vital capacity, total lung capacity, and diffusing capacity
3. Prevention: keep $FIO_2$ as low as possible, preferably 0.40 or less; added positive end-expiratory pressure (PEEP) may allow reduction of $FIO_2$

B. Hypoventilation (patients on hypoxic drive)
1. Can occur in chronic $CO_2$ retainers
2. Prevention: try to maintain $PaO_2$ between 60 and 70 mm Hg

C. Absorption atelectasis (high $FIO_2$ can cause alveolar collapse)
1. Can result within minutes when patient is retaining mucus
2. Prevention: keep $FIO_2$ as low as possible while still maintaining adequate $SpO_2$

D. Retrolental fibroplasia (premature infants)
1. Can occur in neonates when $PaO_2$ >100 mm Hg is maintained
2. Prevention: maintain $PaO_2$ between 60 and 80 mm Hg

E. Dehydration
1. Oxygen as delivered from a tank or hospital system is 0% humidity
2. Prevention: do not rely on humidification or aerosol therapy; give the patient fluids orally (PO) or intravenously (IV)

F. Fire
1. Oxygen supports combustion; do not use near oil-based products such as petroleum jelly (Vaseline); do not use near electrical sparks such as an electric razor; do not use near a fire, such as from cigarettes

G. Infection
1. Less effective cillia
2. Drying of airways
3. Increased adherence of bacteria

**IV. Contraindications** (none)

**V. Nursing Considerations**

A. Never use petroleum-based lubricants on face (i.e., Vaseline)
B. Do not allow use of electric razor
C. Masks should fit securely for proper $FIO_2$
D. Check and recheck to be sure that prongs of nasal cannula stay in nares
E. Monitor patient's vital signs and pulse oximetry to evaluate adequacy of oxygen therapy/ delivery

## HUMIDIFICATION AND AEROSOL THERAPY

**I. Indications**

A. Bronchial hygiene
B. To humidify inspired gas for long-term oxygen therapy
C. After inhalation anesthesia or intubation to maintain mucous blanket and promote expectoration

**II. Physiologic Effects**

A. Hydrate inspissated secretions
B. Maintain mucous blanket
C. Improve cough stimulation

D. Decrease airway inflammation
E. Promote expectoration

**III. Types of Humidifiers**

A. Bubble diffuser (Bubbler): used with low-flow devices; provides approximately 20% humidity—relatively ineffective
B. Cascade humidifier: used with ventilators or continuous positive airway pressure (CPAP) masks; can provide up to 100% humidity
C. Room humidifier (cool mist): adds humidity to room air; can provide 100% humidity in a closed room

**IV. Types of Aerosol Generators**

A. Jet nebulizer: the "bottles" used with aerosol masks; can deliver $FIO_2$ of 0.21 if used with compressed air instead of oxygen
B. Ultrasonic nebulizer and Babington nebulizer: used to mobilize thick secretions in lower airways; provide 100% humidity

**V. Precautions**

A. Bronchospasm
B. Obstruction from swelling of dried secretions
C. Overmobilization of secretions
D. Fluid overload
E. Contamination

**VI. Contraindications**

A. Patient intolerance

**VII. Nursing Considerations**

A. Humidity, especially from ultrasonic nebulizer, can cause bronchospasm or overmobilization of secretions
B. Do not depend on humidifiers or aerosols to help a dehydrated patient; give fluids either PO or IV
C. Cool mist humidifiers are relatively ineffective in a big room (e.g., a PACU)

## RESPIRATORY PHARMACOLOGIC THERAPY

**I. Indications**

A. Bronchoconstriction occurs in response to:
   1. Asthma
   2. Emphysema
   3. Smoke or other airborne irritants
   4. Spasm
   5. Suctioning
   6. Aspiration

B. Upper airway obstruction (i.e., stridor, croup)
C. Thick secretions

**II. Aerosolized Bronchodilators** (see Table 11–1)

**III. Other Aerosolized Drugs**

A. Cromolyn sodium: asthma prophylactic; not to be used during an acute episode
B. Acetylcystine (Mucomyst): breaks mucous bonds, helps patient clear thick secretions; can cause bronchospasm, so *must* be used in conjunction with a bronchodilator; use 1 to 10 ml

**IV. Nonaerosolized Respiratory Drugs**

A. Theophylline or aminophylline: xanthine drug; causes bronchodilation and pulmo-

**TABLE 11–1 Aerosolized Bronchodilators**

| | VASOCONSTRICTION | CARDIAC STIMULATION | BRONCHODILATION | DOSAGE | LENGTH OF EFFECT (HOURS) |
|---|---|---|---|---|---|
| **Sympathomimetic Drugs** | | | | | |
| Albuterol (Ventolin, Proventil) | None | Very minor | Strong | 0.5 ml + 3 ml NS | 4–6 |
| Metaproterenol (Alupent) | None | Minor | Medium | 0.3 ml + 3 ml NS | 3–5 |
| Isoetharine (Bronkosol) | None | Minor | Medium | 0.5 ml + 3 ml NS | 2–4 |
| Salmeterol* (Serevent) | None | Minor | Medium | 2 puffs MDI only | 12 |
| Racemic epinephrine (used mainly for upper airway obstructions) | Mild | Medium | Medium | 0.2 to 0.5 ml + 3 ml NS | 1–2 |
| **Parasympatholytic Drugs** | | | | | |
| Ipratropium bromide (Atrovent) | None | Very minor | Medium to strong | 0.5 mg (premixed) | 4–6 |
| Glycopyrrolate (Robinul) | None | Very minor | Medium to strong | 0.5 ml + 3 ml NS | 3–4 |

*Note: *not* used to reverse acute bronchoconstriction.

nary vasodilation; a cardiac stimulant; given IV, loading dose 6 mg/kg and maintain at 0.5 mg/kg/hr with a maximum of 1.15 g in 24 hours

B. Terbutaline (Brethine): strong $\beta_2$ effect, but virtually no $\beta_1$ effect; give 0.25 of 0.1% solution subcutaneously

## V. Delivery Devices

A. Nebulizer (also called NEB, hand-held nebulizer, small volume nebulizer): easy to use; requires only that patient be breathing; can be used on intubated patients

B. Intermittent positive pressure breathing (IPPB): "helps" aerosolized medicine into lungs with positive pressure; requires patient cooperation except in intubated patients

C. Metered dose inhaler (MDI): Mostly for home use; requires patient coordination; sometimes used preoperatively, especially for patients with asthma

## VI. Precautions

A. Theophylline blood levels must be kept less than 20 mg/L

B. Bronchodilators can cause ventricular tachycardia or other tachydysrhythmias

C. Inhaled corticosteroids can cause candidiasis

## VII. Contraindications

A. Heart rate >120 beats per minute (bpm)

B. Patient unable to ventilate (use IV drugs)

## VIII. Nursing Considerations

A. Check pulse before and after administration of bronchodilators

B. Monitor respiratory rate

C. If breath sounds *decrease* after NEB treatment, it could be that dried secretions are now hydrated and have swollen, obstructing lungs; suctioning or intubation may be needed

D. Have patient rinse out mouth after inhaling corticosteroids to prevent candidiasis

E. If patient appears dyspneic, get arterial blood gases (ABGs) regardless of reading of pulse oximeter

## PULSE OXIMETRY

### I. General Principles of Operation

The sensor, usually placed on patient's finger, consists of light-emitting diodes (LEDs) and a photodetector; the LEDs emit two specific wavelengths of light, which are absorbed selectively by oxyhemoglobin and reduced hemoglobin (dyshemoglobins, e.g., carboxyhemoglobin and methemoglobin, are not measured); ratio of oxyhemoglobin to total hemoglobin is then expressed in a percent ($Spo_2$)

### II. Indications for Pulse Oximetry

A. Whenever patient's oxygen status needs to be monitored without repeated sticks for ABGs

### III. Precautions

A. Ambient light such as radiant warming units and phototherapy lights can interfere with pulse oximeters; shield sensor from light
B. Very dark (dark purple, black) or metallic nail polish can interfere with correct readings; remove the nail polish if there is any question
C. Patient motion such as shivering or agitation can interfere with readings; hold patient's hand still while reading, or try alternative monitoring sites such as ear, forehead, or toe if proper sensors are available

### IV. Contraindications (obtain ABGs instead of using oximetry)

A. Low perfusion status of patient renders pulse oximeter unable to read
   1. Low cardiac output
   2. Vasoconstrictor therapy
   3. Hypothermia
B. Dyshemoglobinemias make saturation readings inaccurate
   1. Carboxyhemoglobin (from carbon monoxide)
   2. Methemoglobin (from amphetamines, heroin, and many other substances)
C. Low oxygen saturations ($Spo_2$ <70%)
D. Exogenous dyes can cause spurious decreases in readings
   1. Methylene blue
   2. Indigo carmine
   3. Indocyanine green

### V. Interpretation of Pulse Oximeter Readings/Nursing Implications

A. Pulse oximeter needs to be turned on and connected to patient for at least 1 minute before readings are taken
B. $Spo_2$ reads only the percent of saturated hemoglobin; it does *not* indicate oxygen content; if hemoglobin is low, a patient could have 100% $Spo_2$ and still be short of breath
C. $Pao_2$ can be estimated from $Spo_2$, using Figure 11–2

## CAPNOGRAPHY

### I. General Principles of Operation

Monitors partial pressure of end-tidal $CO_2$ ($P_{ETCO_2}$) to help evaluate adequacy of patient ventilation; uses infrared light of a wavelength that is absorbed by $CO_2$ but not water vapor (infrared light is not absorbed by oxygen, nitrogen, or most of the other components of the atmosphere); a detector compares amount of infrared light that passes through patient's exhaled gas to that of a reference chamber; difference between the two relates to amount of $CO_2$ in the patient's sample

### II. Indications

A. Monitoring the adequacy of mechanical ventilation
B. Monitoring airflow for polysomnography/apnea detection

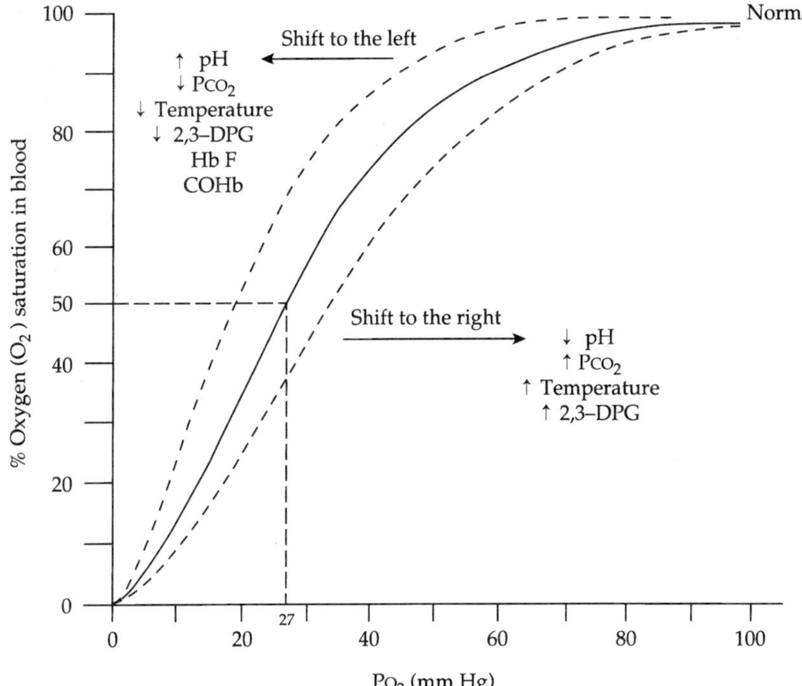


**FIGURE 11–2** Oxyhemoglobin dissociation curve, showing relationship between $Pao_2$ and $Sao_2$ and how that relationship can change (producing a curve shift) with factors such as patient arterial blood pH and patient temperature.

C. Regulating hyperventilation in craniocerebral trauma
D. Monitoring cardiopulmonary resuscitation
E. Monitoring anesthesia: disconnections, proper tube position, hypoventilation

**III. Types of Capnometers**

A. Direct sampling: monitor is in ventilator circuit as close to endotracheal tube as possible
  1. Advantage: very fast—gives breath-by-breath results
  2. Disadvantages
    a. Increased dead space in circuit
    b. Weight of monitor

B. Sidestream: siphons off a portion of expired gas
  1. Advantage: does not interfere with ventilator circuit
  2. Disadvantages
    a. Slow: gives results after they happened
    b. Water droplets in sampling port can interfere with readings

**IV. Precautions**

A. Correlation of $CO_2$ measured by capnography ($P_{ETCO_2}$) and arterial blood gases ($Paco_2$) is imprecise in patients with increased respiratory dead space (high $\dot{V}/\dot{Q}$) caused by
  1. Pulmonary embolism
  2. Hypotension
  3. Hemorrhage
  4. Pulmonary hypoperfusion
  5. Cardiac arrest

**V. Contraindications** (none)

**VI. Nursing Implications**

A. Capnometers must be recalibrated every 24 hours

## INTUBATION

I. **Indications**
   A. Ensure an unobstructed airway
   B. Protect patient's airway from aspiration
   C. Provide conduit for positive-pressure ventilation
   D. Provide conduit for suctioning
   E. Provide conduit for medication administration
   F. For general anesthesia

II. **Routes for Intubation**
   A. Oral/nasal
      1. Equipment needed
         a. Two laryngoscope handles with a variety of curved and straight blades
         b. Oral and nasal endotracheal tubes of various sizes
            (1) Cuffed: for adults
            (2) Uncuffed: for infants and small children
         c. 10 ml syringe: for inflating cuff
         d. Lubricant
         e. Suction devices
         f. McGill forceps
         g. Tape: for securing tube after placement
         h. Local anesthetic solution
         i. Oxygen source, flowmeter, and tubing
         j. Resuscitation bag
         k. Hypnotics and sedatives: if necessary
         l. Ventilator: if necessary
         m. Face mask with eye shields and rubber gloves
         n. Pulse oximeter
      2. Complications of tracheal intubation during tube placement
         a. Trauma
            (1) Facial (split lip, swelling)
            (2) Dental (tooth damage or dislodgement)
            (3) Nasal, oral, or pharyngeal soft-tissue injury
            (4) Laryngeal, including laryngospasm
            (5) Cervical spine and cord injuries
         b. Improper placement of tube: causing dyspnea or apnea
            (1) Esophageal intubation
            (2) Intubation of right main-stem bronchus
         c. Pulmonary aspiration
         d. Cardiac dysrhythmias (from vagal nerve stimulation)
         e. Hypertension
         f. Elevation of intracranial pressure
      3. Complications of intubation after tube placement
         a. Injury to larynx or subglottic airway
         b. Sinusitis
         c. Dislocation of tube
         d. Patient discomfort
         e. Nosocomial infection
   B. Tracheostomy: *not* an emergency procedure; done under sterile conditions, usually in an operating room
      1. Indications
         a. Provide patent airway

   b. Provide for prolonged mechanical ventilation
   c. Permit effective tracheal suctioning
2. Complications after placement of tracheostomy tube
   a. Infection
   b. Hemorrhage
   c. Air leak: pneumothorax or subcutaneous emphysema
   d. Tracheal injury, perforation, or tracheoesophageal fistula
   e. Pulmonary aspiration
   f. Displacement of tube
   g. Reduction in mucociliary transport
   h. Patient discomfort

C. Cricothyroidotomy: an emergency procedure; in the hospital setting, done only by a physician
   1. Indications
      a. Provide an open airway when upper airway is blocked
      b. Temporary airway only until intubation or tracheostomy is performed
   2. Precautions
      a. Does *not* allow mechanical or bag ventilation; use tracheostomy mask with as high an $FIO_2$ as possible; then intubate or perform a tracheostomy as soon as possible
   3. Complications
      a. Perforation of the esophagus
      b. Subcutaneous emphysema
      c. Pneumothorax
      d. Hemorrhage into the trachea
      e. Infection

## III. Precautions

A. Intubation must only be performed by trained and hospital-certified personnel

## IV. Contraindications

A. Ethical considerations (i.e., do not resuscitate [DNR])

## V. Nursing Implications

A. Suction as necessary to keep inner cannula free of blood and other secretions
B. Observe for hemorrhage
C. Auscultate breath sounds hourly (in the case of a cricothyroidotomy, auscultate continuously); listen for bilateral breath sounds present and equal
D. Obtain chest x-ray film for tube placement
   1. Tube too high will provide inadequate ventilation due to leakage
   2. Tube too low may intubate right main-stem bronchus
E. Observe chest frequently for bilateral synchronous and equal expansion
F. Check tube placement hourly to be sure that right main-stem bronchus is not intubated
G. Palpate for subcutaneous emphysema hourly
H. Be aware that metal tracheostomy tubes do not have cuffs or standard fittings: they cannot be used for mechanical ventilation or resuscitator bags
I. Keep dressing clean and dry; keep twill tape or foam strap snug
J. Check that balloon cuff on endotracheal tube is not overly inflated; inflate cuff until there is no leak on machine ventilation, then back off until a just barely audible leak is heard (minimal leak technique)
K. Establish and maintain communication with the patient to reduce anxiety level

## MECHANICAL VENTILATION

I. **Indications**
   A. Apnea
   B. Hypoventilation
   C. Disorders of pulmonary gas exchange
      1. Respiratory distress syndrome: mechanical ventilation with PEEP can greatly improve oxygenation
      2. Cardiac disease: mechanical ventilation can improve oxygenation and impede venous return to help reverse pulmonary edema
      3. Pulmonary embolism: mechanical ventilation with PEEP greatly improves oxygenation

II. **Criteria for Mechanical Ventilation** (see Table 11–2)

III. **Ventilation Modes in PACU**
   A. Assist/control (A/C): patient initiates ventilation and is also guaranteed a backup rate; each breath, whether initiated by machine or patient, will have a predetermined volume; patient's inspiratory flow triggers a breath
   B. Intermittent mandatory ventilation (IMV, synchronized IMV [SIMV]): ventilator delivers breaths at predetermined rate and volume, patient can breath between machine breaths at his or her own rate and volume
   C. Pressure support ventilation (PSV): patient initiates ventilation; each breath will have a predetermined amount of positive pressure added for support; can be used alone or with IMV; when used with IMV, machine breaths have a predetermined rate and *volume* and spontaneous breaths have a predetermined *pressure*
   D. Pressure-controlled ventilation (PCV): can be used either like A/C or IMV except breaths have a predetermined pressure (instead of a predetermined volume); used mainly for infants and adult respiratory distress syndrome (ARDS)

IV. **Expiratory Phase Options**
   A. Positive end-expiratory pressure (PEEP): a small amount of positive pressure (1 to 20 cm $H_2O$) is kept in the airways at all times
      1. Helps keep alveoli open (increases FRC) for better oxygenation
      2. When used with spontaneous breathing (no set rate, volume, or pressure) this is called continuous positive airway pressure (CPAP)
      3. Indication: use PEEP when patient's $Pa_{O_2}$ is less than 50 while the $F_{IO_2}$ is greater than 0.50 (50-50 rule)

**TABLE 11–2 Guidelines for Ventilatory Support in Adults with Acute Respiratory Failure**

| DATUM | NORMAL RANGE | TRACHEAL INTUBATION AND VENTILATION INDICATED |
|---|---|---|
| **Mechanics** | | |
| Respiratory rate (breaths per minute) | 12–20 | >35 |
| Vital capacity (ml/kg body weight) | 65–75 | <15 |
| $FEV_1$ (ml/kg body weight) | 50–60 | <10 |
| Inspiratory force (cm $H_2O$) | 75–100 | <25 |
| **Oxygenation** | | |
| $Pa_{O_2}$ (mm Hg) | 100–75 (air) | <70 (on mask) |
| $P(A - aD_{O_2})$ (mm Hg) | 25–65 | >450 |
| **Ventilation** | | |
| $Pa_{CO_2}$ (mm Hg) | 35–45 | >55 |
| VD/VT | 0.25–0.40 | >0.60 |

From Burton GG, Hodgkin JE, Ward JJ: *Respiratory Care,* 3rd Ed. Philadelphia, JB Lippincott, 1991.

4. Complications
   a. Decreased venous return and cardiac output
   b. Hypotension
   c. Increased work of breathing
   d. Pneumothorax
   e. Increased intercranial pressure
   f. Decreased urine output
   g. Barotrauma (in patients with ARDS)

**V. Initial Settings**

A. Tidal volume (TV): 10 to 15 ml/kg (ideal body weight)
B. Rate (f): 12 breaths per minute
C. $FIO_2$: 0.50 to 1.00 (titrate down with evaluation of arterial blood gases [ABGs])
D. Flow rate: 25 to 60 L/min; titrate to keep inspiratory time at one half to one third the expiratory time (inspiratory/expiratory [I/E] ratio ½ to ⅓)
E. Pressure alarms and limits
   1. High-pressure alarm: set 10 cm $H_2O$ higher than pressure caused by machine-initiated breath; alarm sounds when that pressure is reached and any additional volume is dumped; so, if alarm is constantly sounding, patient is not receiving set TV
   2. Low-pressure alarm: set 10 cm $H_2O$ lower than pressure caused by machine-initiated breath; alarm sounds when there is a circuit leak—most often from a disconnection

**VI. Nursing Implications**

A. Obtain ABGs 15 minutes after initial settings or change in settings and monitor with pulse oximeter
B. Monitor breath sounds and patterns; suction if rhonchi are heard
C. Monitor hemodynamics: cardiac rhythms, blood pressure, urine output
D. Keep stress off of ET tube by proper positioning
E. Low-pressure alarm on ventilator probably indicates a leak in the breathing circuit; check immediately for a disconnect or open port
F. High-pressure alarm on ventilator that just alarms on one breath and then quits probably indicates a patient cough; no action needed
G. High-pressure alarm that does not quit usually means the patient needs suctioning
H. Check sterile water level in humidifier for proper level. (There will be no water if using a *heat-moisture exchanger*—sometimes called an *artificial nose*)
I. Empty ventilator circuit and collection bottle of excess water; *never* let water run back into humidifier
J. Reposition patient every 2 hours
K. As patient wakes up, explain ventilator and offer reassurance
L. Restrain patient as needed to prevent accidental extubation
M. Offer pain medication, sedation, or paralysis if indicated

## WEANING FROM MECHANICAL VENTILATION

**I. Indications for Weaning**

A. Adequate reversal of anesthesia/muscle relaxants
   1. Return of protective laryngeal reflexes
   2. Head lift >5 seconds from horizontal
   3. Hand grip >5 seconds
B. Adequate ventilation
   1. Tidal volume ≥5 to 7 ml/kg
   2. Vital capacity ≥10 to 15 ml/kg
   3. Respiratory rate ≤25 breaths per minute (adult)
   4. Negative inspiratory force <–20 cm $H_2O$

C. Hemodynamically stable
D. Acceptable ABGs

**II. Post Weaning**

A. If patient is still intubated
1. Connect tube to aerosol T-piece with $F_{IO_2}$ of 0.05 to 0.1 more than the previous ventilator setting
2. Continue monitoring $Sp_{O_2}$, breath sounds, and hemodynamics

B. If patient has been extubated
1. Place patient on oxygen delivery system with $F_{IO_2}$ of 0.05 to 0.1 higher than previous ventilator setting. (Use nasal cannula, unless $F_{IO_2}$ needs cannot be met or humidification is needed)
2. Continue monitoring $Sp_{O_2}$, breath sounds, and hemodynamics

C. Extubation
1. Criteria for discontinuing ventilator/extubation: same as Indications for Weaning, above
2. Extubation technique
   a. Explain procedure to patient
   b. Suction trachea or nasopharynx or both
   c. Hyperoxygenate
   d. Deflate endotracheal tube cuff
   e. Have patient take a deep breath
   f. Tell patient to cough, and then remove tube
   g. Evaluate for shortness of breath, stridor, obstruction
3. Complications of extubation
   a. Laryngospasm
   b. Aspiration
   c. Sore throat
   d. Postintubation croup

**III. Nursing Implications**

A. Get baseline ABGs 15 minutes after extubation
B. Monitor $Sp_{O_2}$ continuously for at least 1 hour after extubation
C. Maintain general comfort measures
D. Auscultate and observe chest for bilateral, synchronous, and equal expansion
E. Encourage coughing and deep breathing to keep airway clear of mucus
F. Be aware of hospital or unit policy regarding who should extubate patient

## BIBLIOGRAPHY

Burton G, et al: *Respiratory Care,* 3rd Ed. Philadelphia, JB Lippincott, 1991.

Cummins R (ed): *Textbook of Advanced Cardiac Life Support.* Dallas, American Heart Association, 1994.

Dantzker D: *Cardiopulmonary Critical Care,* 2nd Ed. Philadelphia, WB Saunders, 1991.

DesJardins T: *Cardiopulmonary Anatomy and Physiology.* Albany, NY, Delmar, 1990.

Hess D: Capnometry and capnography: Technical aspects, physiologic aspects, and clinical applications. *Respir Care* 6:557–573, 1990.

Mitchell J: Lower respiratory problems. In Lewis S, Collier I (eds): *Medical-Surgical Nursing: Assessments and Management of Clinical Problems,* 3rd Ed. St Louis, Mosby, 1992.

Oakes D: *Clinical Practitioners Pocket Guide to Respiratory Care.* Old Town, Health Educator Publications, 1988.

Rau J: *Respiratory Care Pharmacology,* 3rd Ed. St Louis, Mosby, 1989.

Ruppel G: *Manual of Pulmonary Function Testing,* 6th Ed. St Louis, Mosby, 1991.

## REVIEW QUESTIONS

**1. Negative inspiratory force (NIF) should be at what level before attempting extubation?**
A. –20 cm $H_2O$
B. +10 cm $H_2O$
C. It is not important to measure NIF before extubation

**2. All the following are advantages to a high-flow oxygen delivery system except**
A. $FIO_2$ does not vary with breathing pattern
B. Humidity and temperature can be controlled
C. Can meet total breathing demands of patient
D. $FIO_2$ is variable, allowing for easier weaning of patients

**3. What do we wish to achieve with the drug albuterol, and what is its mechanism of action?**
A. Bronchoconstriction; $\beta_2$-antagonist
B. Bronchodilation; $\beta_2$-agonist
C. Cardiac stimulation; $\beta_1$-agonist
D. Control of inflammation; steroid

**4. After inhaling a corticosteroid, a patient should rinse out his/her mouth. Why?**
A. To minimize the bad taste
B. To decrease systemic absorption
C. To increase drug metabolism
D. To prevent candidiasis

**5. A patient has $SpO_2$ measured by a pulse oximeter of 90%, yet is visibly dyspneic. What should you do?**
A. Nothing, a 90% $SpO_2$ is normal
B. Administer an aerosol nebulizer treatment
C. Get ABGs and hemoglobin
D. Manually ventilate with 100% oxygen

**6. After intubating a patient, you auscultate the lungs and find breath sounds absent. What could be wrong?**
A. Cuff not inflated
B. Bilateral pneumothorax
C. Intubated the esophagus
D. Right mainstem intubation

**7. When pressure support ventilation (PSV) is used alone, is there a preset respiratory rate (f)?**
A. No
B. Yes

**8. Does assist control ventilation (A/C) deliver a preset volume of gas to the patient?**
A. Yes
B. No

**9. Can assist control (A/C) and pressure support ventilation (PSV) be used together?**
A. No (but PSV can be used with IMV)
B. Yes

**10. When is it advisable to add PEEP to a ventilator patient?**

A. When $PaO_2$ is less than 50 and $FIO_2$ is greater than 50
B. PEEP is never added to a ventilator
C. When $SpO_2$ is less than 90%
D. When the respiratory rate is <8 or >12 and the $SpO_2$ is <90%

**11. A low-pressure alarm on a ventilator most commonly indicates what?**

A. A leak in the breathing circuit
B. A disconnect of the circuit
C. The patient may be vomiting
D. The patient is assisting the ventilator

**ANSWERS:** 1. A, 2. D, 3. B, 4. D, 5. C, 6. C, 7. A, 8. A, 9. A, 10. A, 11. A

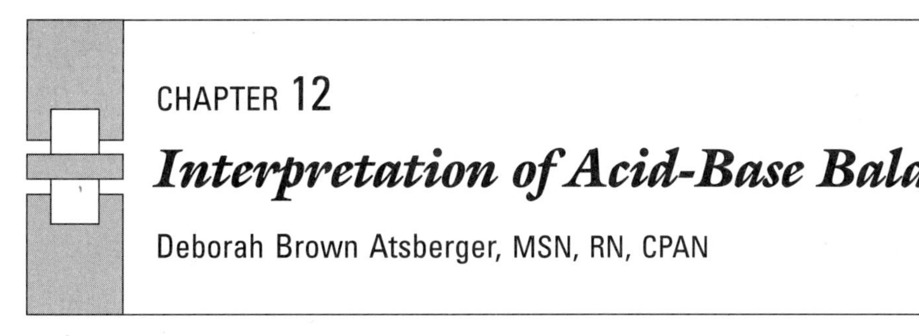

CHAPTER 12

# *Interpretation of Acid-Base Balance*

Deborah Brown Atsberger, MSN, RN, CPAN

**OBJECTIVES**

**Study of the information represented by this outline will enable the learner to:**

1. Determine from a set of arterial blood gas (ABG) results the direction of the pH, the primary cause of the disturbance, and whether compensation is occurring.
2. Distinguish between symptoms of acidosis and alkalosis.
3. Describe appropriate nursing interventions for each of the primary acid-base disturbances.

Abnormalities in ABG values are relatively common in the immediate postoperative period, and a normal recovery process can only occur if acid-base balance is maintained. Understanding ABG results in the postanesthesia patient is essential for the postanesthesia care unit (PACU) nurse. The PACU nurse is the front line of defense when it comes to recognizing symptoms of acid-base abnormalities, interpreting blood gas results, and applying appropriate nursing interventions.

## ELEMENTS OF ACID-BASE BALANCE

I. **pH Balance** (Fig. 12–1)
   A. Body cells are extremely sensitive to their environment
   B. Slight changes in acidity or alkalinity of body fluids can affect normal cellular function and may even lead to cellular death
   C. pH refers to measurement of relative balance between acids and bases in solution
   D. pH is defined as negative logarithm of hydrogen ion concentration; scale of 1 to 14, reflecting hydrogen ion ($H^+$) concentration of solution
      1. One acid to one base is neutral solution
         a. Example: $H^+ + OH^- = H_2O$
         b. pH = 7.00
      2. As acid is added to solution, pH will go down
         a. Acids donate $H^+$
         b. pH <7.00
         c. Solution acidotic
      3. As bases are added to solution, pH will go up
         a. Bases accept $H^+$, buffering acids
         b. pH >7.00
         c. Solution alkalotic
   E. Normal pH of arterial blood ranges from 7.35 to 7.45
      1. Considered to be slightly alkalotic (solution that contains more bases)
      2. Human arterial blood normally maintains ratio of 1 acid to 20 bases
         a. Primary acid is $CO_2$
         b. Primary base is $HCO^-_3$

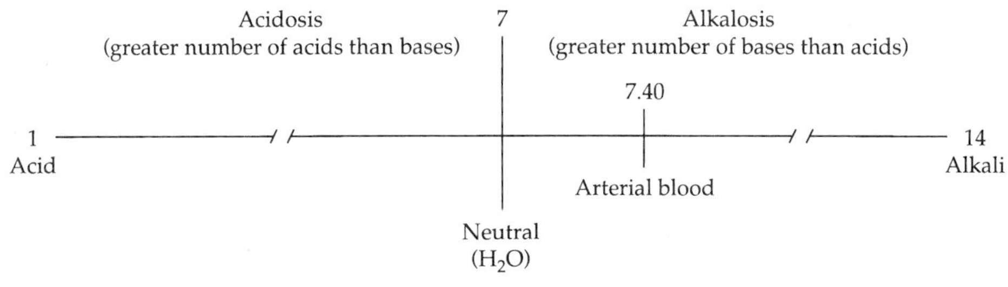


**FIGURE 12–1** pH scale.

3. Definitive therapy is indicated at a pH less than 7.15 or greater than 7.60
4. Death is imminent at pH below 6.90 or above 7.90

**II. Respiratory Component: $Paco_2$**
   A. Represents partial pressure of carbon dioxide in arterial blood
   B. Regulated by alveolar ventilation (lungs)
   C. Considered nonfixed (volatile) acid because it dissolves in plasma to create carbonic acid

**III. Metabolic Component: $HCO^-_3$**
   A. Represents amount of $HCO^-_3$ available to buffer acids
   B. Regulated by renal system (kidney)
   C. Influenced by amount of fixed (nonvolatile) acid in body

**IV. Reasons to Obtain ABGs**
   A. Determine status of alveolar ventilation and arterial oxygenation
   B. Determine acid-base status of patient
   C. Guide respiratory and metabolic treatment modalities

## ETIOLOGIES OF FOUR PRIMARY ACID-BASE DISTURBANCES

There are four primary acid-base disturbances: two respiratory and two metabolic.

**I. Respiratory Acidosis**
   A. Results from alveolar hypoventilation
   B. $Paco_2$ >45 and pH <7.35
   C. Clinical causes
      1. Depression of central respiratory centers
         a. Effects of residual anesthetic agents
         b. Oversedation from narcotics or sedatives
         c. Compression of medullary centers (increased intracranial pressure from edema or lesions)
         d. Hypothermia
      2. Interference with muscles of respiration
         a. Residual effects of neuromuscular blocking agents
         b. Neuromuscular diseases such as myasthenia gravis, poliomyelitis, and pickwickian syndrome
         c. Pain with splinting (especially common after thoracic and abdominal surgery)
         d. Physical limitation of chest expansion
            (1) Tight chest binders and dressings
            (2) Thick eschar from chest burns encasing chest wall

(3) Severe kyphoscoliosis
(4) Obesity (related to excess weight hampering lung expansion, especially accentuated in supine position)

3. Airway obstruction
   a. Excessive secretions in oropharynx
   b. Aspiration
   c. Relaxation of tongue
   d. Edema of pharyngeal soft tissues
   e. Subglottic or tracheal stenosis
   f. Laryngospasm or bronchospasm
   g. Endotracheal tube malpositioned in single bronchus with subsequent single lung ventilation
   h. Blockage of endotracheal tube by secretions or kinking of tube
4. Lung disease
   a. Chronic obstructive pulmonary disease (COPD)
   b. Pulmonary fibrosis
   c. Atelectasis and pneumonia
5. Inadequate mechanical ventilatory support (inadequate minute volumes or rates on mechanical ventilator)

**II. Respiratory Alkalosis**

A. Results from alveolar hyperventilation
B. $Paco_2$ <35 and pH >7.45
C. Clinical causes
   1. Tissue hypoxia
      a. Anemia
      b. Early pneumonia
      c. Pulmonary edema
      d. Pulmonary embolism
      e. Early stage of asthma attack
   2. Respiratory center stimulation
      a. Psychogenic causes: anxiety, pain
      b. Fever
      c. Thyrotoxicosis
      d. Hepatic failure
   3. Central nervous system (CNS) diseases
      a. Medullary or pons tumors
      b. Surgical manipulation of brainstem
   4. Excessive minute volumes from mechanical ventilation
   5. Pregnancy (normal finding)

**III. Metabolic Acidosis**

A. Results from accumulation of fixed acid or excessive depletion of base
B. $HCO^-_3$ <22 and pH <7.35
C. Clinical causes
   1. Overproduction of acids; high anion gap
      a. Diabetic ketoacidosis
      b. Starvation ketoacidosis
      c. Anaerobic metabolism (lactic acidosis)
      d. Overdoses of salicylic acid (aspirin poisoning)
      e. Overdoses of ferrous sulfate (iron poisoning)
      f. Renal failure, uremia
      g. Rhabdomyolysis

2. Severe body loss of bicarbonate; normal anion gap
   a. Diarrhea
   b. Small bowel fistulas
   c. Urinary diversion
   d. Pancreatic secretions lost through pancreatic fistulas
   e. Excessive acetazolamide (Diamox) or ammonium chloride
   f. Renal failure

## IV. Metabolic Alkalosis

A. Results from excessive depletion of fixed acid or accumulation of bases
B. $HCO^-_3$ >26 and pH >7.45
C. Clinical causes
   1. Loss of body acid
      a. Gastric suctioning
      b. Vomiting
      c. Gastric lavage
      d. Volume contraction due to dehydration
   2. Excessive circulating bicarbonate
      a. Excessive infusions of lactate solutions
      b. Excessive antacid ingestion
      c. Baking soda ingestion
   3. Overcorrection of acidosis with bicarbonate
   4. Excessive retention of base ions
      a. Diuretic therapy: furosemide (Lasix) and thiazides
      b. Excessive administration of corticosteroids
   5. Systemic diseases
      a. Cushing's disease
      b. Aldosteronism

## V. Mixed Acidosis or Alkalosis*

A. Results when two or more primary acid-base disorders are present simultaneously
B. pH may change more dramatically in direction of acidosis or alkalosis depending on specific disorders involved
C. Examples
   1. Renal failure + Narcotic-induced respiratory depression = Metabolic acidosis + Respiratory acidosis
   2. COPD + Diarrhea = Respiratory Acidosis + Metabolic acidosis
   3. Furosemide diuretic + Hypoxia = Metabolic alkalosis + Respiratory acidosis
   4. Nasogastric suction + Sedative-induced respiratory depression = Metabolic alkalosis + Respiratory acidosis
D. Salicylate poisoning
   1. Direct stimulation of respiratory chemoreceptors results in hyperventilation
   2. Salicylate metabolites result in increased fixed acids
   3. Results in respiratory alkalosis and metabolic acidosis
   4. Respiratory alkalosis predominates in adults
   5. Metabolic acidosis predominates in young children and infants

---

*Mixed acid-base alterations may be of the same or an opposing nature. The pH change will be dramatic with like disorders. However, pH change will be minor or less severe with opposing disorders because disorders balance each other.

## COMPENSATION

Compensation is the body's attempt to return the ratio of acid to base back toward 1:20 to maintain the pH at 7.40. The patient is not considered to be compensated unless pH is within normal range. If changes in that direction are noted either in $Paco_2$ or $HCO^-_3$ with minimal changes in pH, the patient is considered to be partially compensated.

**I. Respiratory Alteration Leads to Renal Compensation**

A. Slow but sustained response by kidneys (hours to weeks to years)

B. Compensation for respiratory acidosis

1. Reabsorption of bicarbonate ion
2. Excretion of hydrogen ion
3. Acidic urine

C. Compensation for respiratory alkalosis

1. Excretion of bicarbonate ion
2. Retention of hydrogen ion
3. Alkalotic urine

**II. Metabolic Alteration Leads to Respiratory Compensation**

A. Rapid response, but lungs may fatigue (minutes to days to weeks)

B. Compensation for metabolic acidosis

1. Hyperventilation
2. Eliminate carbon dioxide

C. Compensation for metabolic alkalosis

1. Hypoventilation
2. Accumulation of carbon dioxide

## ARTERIAL BLOOD GAS INTERPRETATION

Blood gas results must be interpreted in the context of the clinical picture. ABG results will substantiate initial clinical impression, direct initial treatment, and guide further intervention (Table 12–1).

**I. Normal Values**

| | |
|---|---|
| pH | 7.35–7.45 |
| $Paco_2$ | 35–45 mm Hg |
| $HCO^-_3$ | 22–26 mEq/L |
| $Pao_2$ | 80–100 mm Hg |
| $O_{2\ sat}$ | 95% or greater |
| Base excess | 0 ± 2 |

**II. Systematic Analysis of Arterial Blood Gas Components**

A. Step 1: assessment of pH

1. Normal: 7.35 to 7.45

**TABLE 12–1** Acid-Base Abnormalities

| | pH | $Paco_2$ | $HCO^-_3$ |
|---|---|---|---|
| Respiratory acidosis | ↓ (<7.35) | ↑ (>45) | Normal |
| Respiratory alkalosis | ↑ (>7.45) | ↓ (<35) | Normal |
| Metabolic acidosis | ↓ (<7.35) | Normal | ↓ (<22) |
| Metabolic alkalosis | ↑ (>7.45) | Normal | ↑ (>26) |
| Mixed acidosis | ↓ (<7.35) | ↑ (>45) | ↓ (<22) |
| Mixed alkalosis | ↑ (>7.45) | ↓ (<35) | ↑ (>26) |

2. Low: <7.35 = acidosis
3. High: >7.45 = alkalosis

B. Step 2: evaluation of components
1. Respiratory component: $Paco_2$
   a. Regulated by lungs
   b. Normal: 35 to 45 mm Hg
   c. Low: <35 mm Hg (respiratory alkalosis)
      (1) Hyperventilation
      (2) Decreased carbonic acid
      (3) Increase in pH
   d. High: >45 mm Hg (respiratory acidosis)
      (1) Hypoventilation
      (2) Increased carbonic acid
      (3) Decrease in pH
2. Metabolic component: $HCO^-_3$
   a. Regulated by kidneys
   b. Normal: 22 to 26 mEq/L
   c. Low: <22 mEq/L (metabolic acidosis)
      (1) Results from direct loss of base ions
      (2) Depleted when used to buffer excess fixed acids
   d. High: >26 mEq/L (metabolic alkalosis)
      (1) Results from retention of base ions
      (2) Excess when decline in fixed acids

C. Step 3: determine abnormality
1. Determine correlation of pH, $Paco_2$, and $HCO^-_3$
2. Acidosis/alkalosis determined by pH
3. Causes reflected by changes in $Paco_2$ and/or $HCO^-_3$
   a. $Paco_2$ reflects respiratory changes
   b. $HCO^-_3$ reflects metabolic processes
4. Acidosis
   a. Respiratory acidosis
      (1) pH <7.35
      (2) Increased $Paco_2$
   b. Metabolic acidosis
      (1) pH <7.35
      (2) Decreased $HCO^-_3$
   c. Mixed acidosis
      (1) pH <7.35
      (2) Increased $Paco_2$
      (3) Decreased $HCO^-_3$
5. Alkalosis
   a. Respiratory alkalosis
      (1) pH >7.45
      (2) Decreased $Paco_2$
   b. Metabolic alkalosis
      (1) pH >7.45
      (2) Increased $HCO^-_3$
   c. Mixed alkalosis
      (1) pH >7.45
      (2) Decreased $Paco_2$
      (3) Increased $HCO^-_3$

## III. Interpretation of Compensatory Mechanisms

A. Returns pH close to 7.40, rarely overcompensates

B. Differentiate between primary abnormality and compensatory process
   1. Step 1: assess pH
      a. "Leaning tendency": pH within normal range but not exactly 7.40
      b. Leans toward acidosis (7.35 to 7.39)
      c. Leans toward alkalosis (7.41 to 7.45)
   2. Step 2: determine processes of other components (refer to step 2 above)
      a. $Paco_2$
      b. $HCO^-_3$
   3. Step 3: assimilate and label
      a. Primary process: signified by component that supports leaning tendency of pH
      b. Compensation: signified by component that supports opposite tendency before treatment is initiated

C. Compensation vs. correction
   1. Compensation: natural attempts by body systems to return pH to within normal limits
   2. Correction: therapeutic attempts by health care team to correct imbalance, i.e., increasing rate on mechanical ventilator to correct hypoventilation as evidenced by respiratory acidosis (increased $Paco_2$)

## SIGNS AND SYMPTOMS

**I. Acidosis** (Table 12–2)

**II. Alkalosis** (Table 12–2)

**TABLE 12–2 Signs and Symptoms of Acidosis and Alkalosis**

| Acidosis | Alkalosis |
|---|---|
| **Respiratory Acidosis** | **Respiratory Alkalosis** |
| Decreased respiratory rate, depth | Increased respiratory rate, depth |
| Dyspnea | Light-headedness, syncope |
| Apnea | Irritability, belligerence |
| **Metabolic Acidosis** | **Metabolic Alkalosis** |
| Increased respiratory rate, depth (compensatory Kussmaul respirations) | Decreased respiratory rate, depth (as compensatory mechanism) |
| | Mental confusion, obtundation |
| **Respiratory or Metabolic Acidosis** | **Respiratory or Metabolic Alkalosis** |
| Early, transient signs | Paresthesias |
| Headache | Circumoral tingling |
| Tachycardia | Blurred vision |
| Hypertension | Chest tightness |
| Followed by: | Muscle twitching |
| Restlessness | Carpopedal spasm |
| Lethargy | Diaphoresis |
| Bradycardia | Decreased serum chloride |
| Hypotension | Decreased serum potassium |
| Nausea/vomiting | Dysrhythmias |
| Increased intracranial pressure | Increased urine pH |
| Twitching | Seizures |
| Asterixis (flapping tremors) | Tetany |
| Increased serum potassium | |
| Dysrhythmias | |
| Decreased urine pH | |

**NURSING DIAGNOSIS**

Examples of related nursing diagnostic categories include:

- Ineffective breathing pattern
- Ineffective airway clearance
- Impaired gas exchange
- Pain
- Anxiety

## NURSING INTERVENTIONS

**I. Interventions for Respiratory Acidosis**

A. Restore alveolar ventilation
   1. Increase ventilatory depth and/or rate
   2. Maintenance of patent airway
      a. Suctioning
      b. Oral-nasal airways
      c. Jaw thrust maneuvers
      d. Manual ventilation
      e. Intubation

B. Treat cause medically*

**II. Interventions for Respiratory Alkalosis**

A. Decrease ventilatory rate and/or depth
B. Provide emotional support
C. Treat cause medically

**III. Interventions for Metabolic Acidosis**

A. Support compensatory increase in ventilation
B. Administer sodium bicarbonate to replenish depleted $HCO^-_3$
C. Treat cause medically

**IV. Interventions for Metabolic Alkalosis**

A. Support compensatory decrease in ventilation
B. Administer chloride
C. Treat cause medically

*Not treated with sodium bicarbonate ($NaHCO^-_3$). $NaHCO^-_3$ increases osmolar concentration of blood, leading to fluid shifts into the vascular space. Increased vascular volume could further compromise respiratory function (Horn et al, 1991). $NaHCO^-_3$ contains and releases a large amount of $CO_2$ into the blood. The $CO_2$ released when sodium bicarbonate is given diffuses into the cells more quickly than does $HCO^-_3$, causing a paradoxical rise in intracellular $Paco_2$, a further fall in intracellular pH, and further impairment in cellular function (America Heart Association, 1987). Sodium bicarbonate therapy should be reserved for use when $HCO^-_3$ is depleted (identified by ABGs).

## BIBLIOGRAPHY


Alspach JG: *Core Curriculum for Critical Care Nursing.* Philadelphia, WB Saunders, 1991.

America Heart Association: *Textbook of Advanced Cardiac Life Support.* Dallas, The Association, 1994.

Anup AB: *Arterial Blood Gas Analysis made Easy.* USA, The Author, 1996.

Drain CB: *The Post Anesthesia Care Unit: A Critical Care Approach to Anesthesia Nursing,* 3rd Ed. Philadelphia, WB Saunders, 1994.

Horn MM, Heitz UE, Swearingen PL: *Fluid, Electrolyte and Acid-Base Balance: A Case Study Approach.* St Louis, Mosby–Year Book, 1991.

Litwack K: *Post Anesthesia Care Nursing,* 2nd Ed. St Louis, Mosby–Year Book, 1995.

Martin L: *All You Really Need to Know to Interpret Arterial Blood Gases.* Philadelphia, Lea & Febiger, 1992.

Rose BD: *Clinical Physiology of Acid-Base and Electrolyte Disorders,* 4th Ed. New York, McGraw-Hill, 1994.

Rothenberg D: Postoperative acid-base disorders: Recognition and management. In Vender J, Spiess B (eds): *Post Anesthesia Care.* Philadelphia, WB Saunders, 1992.

Shapiro B, Peruzzi W, Templin R: *Clinical Application of Blood Gases,* 5th Ed. St Louis, Mosby–Year Book, 1994

Taylor L, Stephens D: Arterial blood gases: Clinical application. *J Post Anesth Nurs* 5(4):264–272, 1990.


### Practice ABGs

| ABG RESULTS | | EVALUATION PROCESS | |
|---|---|---|---|
| 1. pH | 7.30 | Step 1 | pH signifies acidosis |
| $Paco_2$ | 50 | Step 2 | Respiratory component ($Paco_2$) increased; indicates increased acid production and acidosis |
| $HCO^-_3$ | 24 | | Metabolic component ($HCO^-_3$) within normal range |
| | | Step 3 | *Respiratory acidosis* with no compensation |
| 2. pH | 7.48 | Step 1 | pH signifies alkalosis |
| $Paco_2$ | 44 | Step 2 | Respiratory component ($Paco_2$) within normal range |
| $HCO^-_3$ | 32 | | Metabolic component ($HCO^-_3$) increased; indicates excess base and alkalosis |
| | | Step 3 | *Metabolic alkalosis* with partial compensation (pH not within normal range) from respiratory component |
| 3. pH | 7.26 | Step 1 | pH signifies acidosis |
| $Paco_2$ | 40 | Step 2 | Normal respiratory component |
| $HCO^-_3$ | 13 | | Decreased metabolic component, reduced base indicates acidosis |
| | | Step 3 | *Metabolic acidosis* with no compensation |
| 4. pH | 7.10 | Step 1 | pH signifies severe acidosis |
| $Paco_2$ | 50 | Step 2 | Increased respiratory component indicates increased acid production and acidosis |
| $HCO^-_3$ | 15 | | Decreased metabolic component, reduced base leads to acidosis |
| | | Step 3 | *Mixed acidosis* |
| 5. pH | 7.54 | Step 1 | pH signifies alkalosis |
| $Paco_2$ | 20 | Step 2 | Reduced respiratory component indicates reduced acids and alkalosis |
| $HCO^-_3$ | 26 | | Normal metabolic component |
| | | Step 3 | *Respiratory alkalosis* with partial compensation (pH not within normal range) from metabolic component |
| 6. pH | 7.33 | Step 1 | pH signifies mild acidosis |
| $Paco_2$ | 25 | Step 2 | Reduced respiratory component, reduced acid leads to alkalosis |
| $HCO^-_3$ | 20 | | Reduced metabolic component, reduced base leads to acidosis |
| | | Step 3 | *Metabolic acidosis* with partial compensation from respiratory component (pH not within normal range, $Paco_2$ reduced to level outside normal range) |

*Table continued on following page*

**Practice ABGs** *(Continued)*

| ABG RESULTS | | EVALUATION PROCESS | |
|---|---|---|---|
| 7. pH | 7.28 | Step 1 | pH signifies acidosis |
| $Paco_2$ | 54 | Step 2 | Increased respiratory component, increased acid leads to acidosis |
| $HCO^-_3$ | 20 | | Reduced metabolic component, reduced base leads to acidosis |
| | | Step 3 | *Mixed acidosis* |
| 8. pH | 7.52 | Step 1 | pH signifies alkalosis |
| $Paco_2$ | 48 | Step 2 | Increased respiratory component, increased acid leads to acidosis |
| $HCO^-_3$ | 36 | | Increased metabolic component, increased base leads to alkalosis |
| | | Step 3 | *Metabolic alkalosis* with partial compensation from respiratory component (pH outside normal range, $Paco_2$ increased from normal range) |
| 9. pH | 7.39 | Step 1 | Normal pH, leans toward acidosis |
| $Paco_2$ | 62 | Step 2 | Increased respiratory component, increased acid leads to acidosis |
| $HCO^-_3$ | 36 | | Increased metabolic component, increased base leads to alkalosis |
| | | Step 3 | Compensated respiratory acidosis (pH within normal range and both components outside normal range) |
| 10. pH | 7.37 | Step 1 | Normal pH, leans toward acidosis |
| $Paco_2$ | 29 | Step 2 | Decreased respiratory component, reduced acid leads to alkalosis |
| $HCO^-_3$ | 18 | | Decreased metabolic component, reduced base leads to acidosis |
| | | Step 3 | Compensated metabolic acidosis |

## REVIEW QUESTIONS

**1. Signs and symptoms of acidosis may include:**
A. Diaphoresis, tetany
B. Hypotension, lethargy
C. Muscle twitching, irritability
D. Belligerence, carpopedal spasm

**2. Which of the following indicates metabolic alkalosis?**
A. pH <7.35, $Paco_2$ normal, $HCO^-_3$ >24
B. pH >7.45, $Paco_2$ normal, $HCO^-_3$ <22
C. pH <7.35, $Paco_2$ normal, $HCO^-_3$ <22
D. pH >7.45, $Paco_2$ normal, $HCO^-_3$ >24

**3. Appropriate interventions for respiratory alkalosis include:**
A. Emotional support, analgesics
B. Discontinuing lactate infusions, electrolyte replacement
C. Administering sodium bicarbonate, continuing gastric suctioning
D. Encouraging deep breathing, placing patient in semi-Fowler's position

**4. Gastric suctioning and vomiting can result in:**
A. Metabolic acidosis
B. Respiratory acidosis
C. Metabolic alkalosis
D. Respiratory alkalosis

**5. Anaerobic metabolism from processes such as malignant hyperthermia will result in:**
A. Metabolic acidosis
B. Metabolic alkalosis
C. Respiratory alkalosis
D. Respiratory acidosis

**6. Respiratory acidosis may be caused by:**

A. Anxiety, pulmonary edema
B. Diuretic therapy, overdoses of salicylic acid
C. Diabetic ketoacidosis, renal failure
D. Residual anesthetic agents, hypothermia

**7. Which electrolyte imbalances will result in alkalosis?**

A. Hyponatremia, hypochloremia
B. Hyperkalemia, hypercalcemia
C. Hypochloremia, hypokalemia
D. Hypernatremia, hyperchloremia

**8. Arterial blood gases (ABGs) of pH 7.30, $Paco_2$ 50, $Pao_2$ 102, $HCO^-_3$ 24, base excess (BE) −1, and saturation (Sat) 97% reflect:**

A. Respiratory alkalosis
B. Respiratory acidosis
C. Metabolic alkalosis
D. Metabolic acidosis

**9. Values of pH 7.48, $Paco_2$ 44, $Pao_2$ 84, $HCO^-_3$ 32, BE +7, and Sat 96% are an example of:**

A. Respiratory alkalosis
B. Respiratory acidosis
C. Metabolic alkalosis
D. Metabolic acidosis

**10. Your analysis of ABG results of pH 7.26, $Paco_2$ 40, $Pao_2$ 98, $HCO^-_3$ 13, BE −12, and Sat 98% would be:**

A. Respiratory alkalosis
B. Respiratory acidosis
C. Metabolic alkalosis
D. Metabolic acidosis

**11. An example of respiratory alkalosis is:**

A. pH 7.49, $Paco_2$ 49, $Pao_2$ 94, $HCO^-_3$ 24, BE 0, Sat 96%
B. pH 7.54, $Paco_2$ 20, $Pao_2$ 98, $HCO^-_3$ 26, BE +1, Sat 99%
C. pH 7.33, $Paco_2$ 25, $Pao_2$ 74, $HCO^-_3$ 22, BE −3, Sat 94%
D. pH 7.28, $Paco_2$ 54, $Pao_2$ 104, $HCO^-_3$ 24, BE 0, Sat 98%

**12. Which compensatory mechanism will you see for ABG values of pH 7.54, $Paco_2$ 40, $Pao_2$ 98, $HCO^-_3$ 36, BE +11, and Sat 97%?**

A. Decreased $Paco_2$
B. Increased $HCO^-_3$
C. Decreased $Pao_2$
D. Increased $Paco_2$

**ANSWERS:** 1. B, 2. D, 3. A, 4. C, 5. A, 6. D, 7. C, 8. B, 9. C, 10. D, 11. D, 12. D

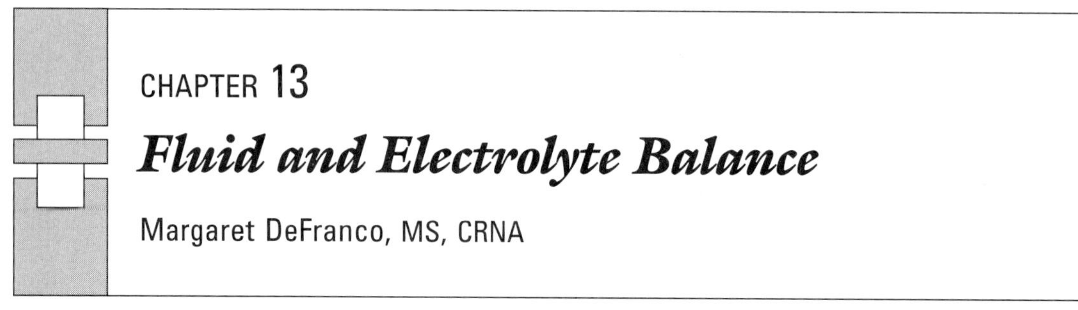

CHAPTER 13

# Fluid and Electrolyte Balance

Margaret DeFranco, MS, CRNA

## OBJECTIVES

**Study of the information represented by this outline will enable the learner to:**

1. Name and describe three fluid compartments.
2. Describe four factors that regulate water balance.
3. Name and describe the three primary control systems of acid-base balance.
4. Define the following: diffusion, osmosis, active transport, filtration.
5. State the causes, physiology, diagnosis, significance, treatment, and nursing actions involved with the following clinical problems: extracellular fluid volume deficit, extracellular fluid volume excess, third spacing.
6. List two general characteristics of each of the following electrolytes: sodium, potassium, chloride, calcium, phosphorus, magnesium.
7. State causes, symptoms, laboratory values, treatment, and nursing care involved in imbalances of each of the above electrolytes.

Under normal conditions the body maintains an exquisite fluid and electrolyte balance. Stressful events, the effects of food and fluid restriction, drug therapy, and fluid loss during surgery are only a few of the factors responsible for imbalances that may be evident in the postanesthesia patient. Understanding the causes, symptoms, laboratory values, treatment, and nursing care involved in states of fluid and electrolyte imbalance is an essential component of postanesthesia nursing practice.

## PHYSIOLOGY OF BODY FLUID

**I. Volume and Distribution**

- A. Intracellular fluid (ICF)
    1. Approximately 25 L
    2. 50% to 60% of adult body weight (75% of newborn and decreases rapidly in first year of life)
    3. Occupies space within cells
- B. Extracellular fluid (ECF)
    1. Intravascular: fluid within blood cells (plasma)
    2. Interstitial: fluid between cells
        - a. 12 L
        - b. 20% of adult body weight (45% of newborn)
    3. Transcellular: nonfunctioning fluid present in viscera
        - a. Gastric juices
        - b. Intraocular fluid
        - c. Cerebrospinal fluid (CSF)

## II. Composition of Fluid

A. Electrolytes: chemicals that have positive or negative charges when dissolved in solution
  1. Cations (positive ions)
    a. Potassium ($K^+$) and magnesium ($Mg^{++}$) more prevalent in intracellular fluid
    b. Sodium ($Na^+$) more prevalent in extracellular fluid
  2. Anions (negative ions)
    a. Phosphorus ($P^-$) and phosphate ($HPO^-_4$) more prevalent in ICF
    b. Chloride ($Cl^-$) and bicarbonate ($HCO^-_3$) more prevalent in ECF

B. Acids, bases, salts, buffers (see also Chapter 12)
  1. Acid: hydrogen ion donor
  2. Base: hydrogen ion acceptor
  3. pH: hydrogen ion concentration of ECF
  4. Buffer mechanism: regulates pH by maintaining bicarbonate/carbonic acid ratio of 20:1
  5. Respiratory mechanism: regulates pH by adjusting $CO_2$ through hypoventilation and hyperventilation
  6. Renal mechanism: regulates pH by secreting or reabsorbing bicarbonate or $H^+$ ions
    a. When acid-base disturbance is not compensated by buffer or respiratory mechanisms
    b. During alkalosis (excess base or decreased acid)
      (1) Kidneys retain $H^+$ (acid)
      (2) Kidneys excrete bicarbonate (base)
    c. During acidosis (excess acid or decreased base)
      (1) Kidneys excrete $H^+$
      (2) Kidneys retain bicarbonate
  7. Salts: electrolytes composed of a cation other than $H^+$ and an anion other than hydroxyl (such as NaCl)
  8. Nonelectrolytes: compounds (e.g., sugar) that do not dissociate in solution

## III. Dynamics of Water and Electrolytes

A. Diffusion: tendency of molecules of gaseous or liquid substance to move from a region of higher to a region of lower concentration until concentration is the same (Fig. 13–1, *A*)

B. Osmosis: movement of water through a semipermeable membrane from area of low to area of higher concentration of solute (a type of diffusion) (Fig. 13–1, *B*)

C. Osmotic pressure: pressure exerted during process of osmosis

D. Osmolality: total number of osmotically active particles that cause osmotic pressure per liter of solution; reflects status of body hydration; water diffuses from area of low to area of high osmolality; normal serum osmolality is 280 to 294 mOsm/kg
  1. Includes electrolytes and nonelectrolytes such as glucose, urea
  2. Isotonic: concentration of dissolved particles in ECF equals that of ICF
    a. Intravenous (IV) solutions with osmolality of 290 ± 50 (240 to 340) mOsm are isotonic
    b. Examples
      (1) 0.9 normal saline (NS) solution = 310 mOsm/L
      (2) 5% dextrose in water ($D_5W$) = 252 mOsm/L
      (3) 5% dextrose in 0.25 NS ($D_5$.25 NS) = 326 mOsm/L
      (4) Lactated Ringer's (LR) = 272 mOsm/L
  3. Hypertonic: extracellular concentration greater than intracellular
    a. Causes water to move out of cell
    b. Cell dehydrates, ECF volume expands
    c. Osmolality greater than 340
    d. Examples
      (1) 5% dextrose in lactated Ringer's ($D_5LR$) = 524 mOsm/L
      (2) 5% dextrose in 0.45 normal saline ($D_5$.45 NS) = 406 mOsm/L
      (3) 10% dextrose in water ($D_{10}W$) = 505 mOsm/L

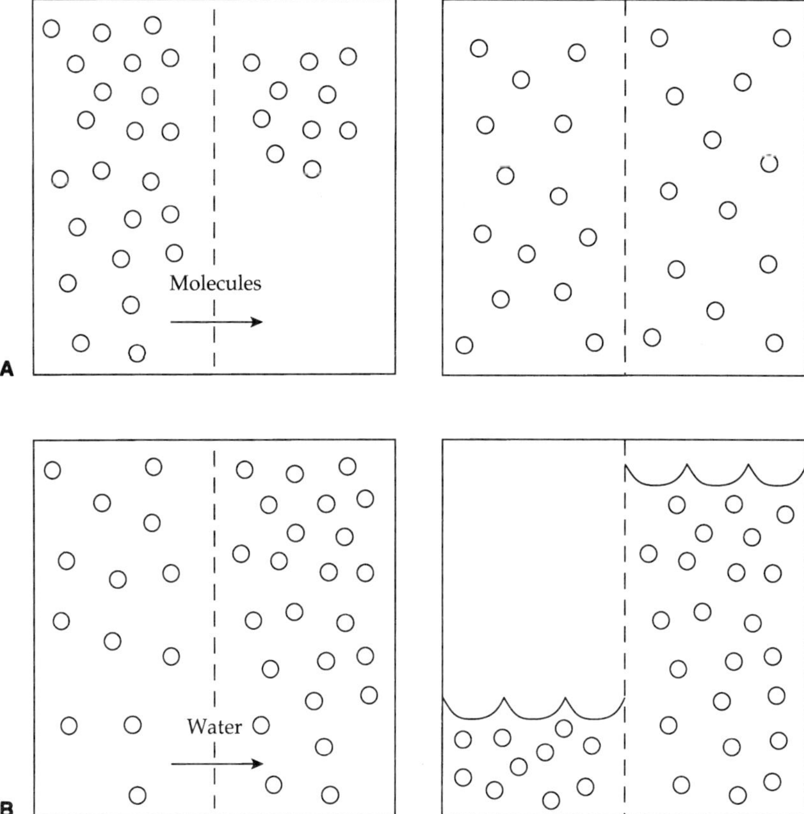


**FIGURE 13–1** **A,** Diffusion. **B,** Osmosis.

4. Hypotonic: extracellular concentration less than intracellular (water moves into cells)
   a. Osmolality less than 240 mOsm/L
   b. Example: half normal saline (0.45 NS) = 154 mOsm/L
5. Active transport: movement of molecules across cell membrane against concentration gradient
6. Filtration: transfer of water and dissolved substances across pressure gradient through permeable membrane from higher to lower pressure as with glomerular filtration in kidney

## REGULATION OF FLUID AND ELECTROLYTES

**I. Cerebral Regulation**

A. Hypothalamus: osmoreceptors affect antidiuretic hormone (ADH) synthesis, release, and storage
B. Pituitary regulation: ADH from posterior pituitary regulates water absorption in renal tubules and collecting ducts
   1. Increased ADH
      a. Increased plasma osmolality
      b. Decreased circulating blood volume
      c. Stimulated by
         (1) Stress: surgery, pain, trauma
         (2) Drugs: morphine, oxytocins, anesthetics
         (3) Mechanical ventilation

2. Decreased ADH (after hypophysectomy): diabetes insipidus
   a. Polydipsia
   b. Polyuria
   c. Dehydration
3. Right atrial baroreceptor
   a. Senses venous and arterial pressure changes
   b. Increases urinary output by decreasing ADH synthesis and release

**II. Adrenal Gland Regulation**

A. Secretion of aldosterone (principal mineralocorticoid)
   1. Influences renal tubules to increase sodium reabsorption
   2. Enhances potassium secretion into renal tubules

B. Increased aldosterone secretion promotes
   1. Sodium retention
   2. Potassium excretion
   3. Alkalosis
   4. Water retention

C. Decreased aldosterone secretion promotes
   1. Potassium retention
   2. Sodium excretion
   3. Metabolic acidosis
   4. Decreased cardiac output (weakness of contractions)

**III. Renal Regulation**

A. Concentration of electrolytes
   1. Aldosterone secretion in response to sodium and potassium concentrations, fluid volume status, and perfusion pressure of afferent renal arterioles
   2. ADH secretion in response to serum osmolality

B. Osmolality of body fluids: primarily through loop of Henle and proximal convoluted tubules

C. Blood volume: through response of renin-angiotensin-aldosterone system
   1. Preservation of blood pressure
   2. Retention of sodium and water

D. Blood pH: regulation of acid-base balance by retention and excretion of hydrogen and bicarbonate ions

E. Urine specific gravity: indicates relative portion of dissolved solutes in urine; reflects ability of kidneys to concentrate urine; normal is 1.010 to 1.025

**IV. Gastrointestinal Regulation (Bypassed in Operative Patient)**

**V. Insensible Water Loss**

A. Skin

B. Lungs

## FLUID AND ELECTROLYTE IMBALANCES

**I. Volume Imbalances**

A. ECF volume deficit (hypovolemia): plasma to interstitial fluid shift or total loss from body
   1. Causes
      a. Abrupt decrease in fluid intake: NPO status
      b. Acute loss of secretions and excretions
         (1) Diuretics
         (2) Ketoacidosis
         (3) Addison's disease
         (4) Third spacing

(5) Fistulous drainage
(6) Trauma or burns
(7) Vomiting
(8) Diarrhea
c. Hemorrhage
2. Diagnosis
a. Signs of dehydration
(1) Dry skin and mucous membranes
(2) Fatigue
(3) Decreased urinary output
(4) Decreased central venous pressure (CVP)
(5) Increased pulse and respirations
b. Hemoconcentration: increased osmolality, serum sodium, and urine specific gravity
3. Significance
a. Decreased cardiac output
b. Inadequate organ perfusion: kidney, brain, liver
c. Tubular necrosis, renal failure
4. Treatment
a. Fluid replacement with isotonic solutions
b. Treating underlying cause

B. ECF volume excess (hypervolemia): interstitial to plasma fluid shifts
1. Causes
a. Increased oral/parenteral fluid intake
b. Excess sodium retention
(1) Chronic kidney disease
(2) Chronic liver disease
(3) Congestive heart failure
c. Increased aldosterone level
(1) Hypotension in congestive heart failure (CHF)
(2) Hyperaldosteronism
d. Excess sodium intake intravenously or by seawater ingestion
e. Remobilization of third space fluid
2. Diagnosis
a. Signs of overhydration
(1) Peripheral edema
(2) Puffy eyelids
(3) Pleural effusion
(4) Pulmonary edema
(5) Increased CVP, pulmonary artery (PA) pressures
(6) Ascites
(7) Confusion
b. Laboratory data
3. Significance
a. Circulatory overload: CHF
b. Respiratory compromise (pulmonary edema)
4. Treatment
a. Goal: decrease excess fluid without altering electrolyte composition (unless hypernatremic)
b. Treat underlying cause
c. Diuretic therapy
d. Fluid restriction

## II. Fluid Spacing: Classification of Body Water Distribution

A. Definitions
  1. First spacing: normal distribution of body fluids
  2. Second spacing: excess accumulation of interstitial fluid (edema)
  3. Third spacing: fluid accumulation from vascular space into area normally having minimal or no fluid
     a. Localized to single area or organ (as in sprained ankle or blister)
     b. Multisystem involvement (after abdominal surgery, after severe burns, in intestinal obstruction)

B. Causes of third spacing
  1. Lowered plasma proteins
  2. Increased capillary permeability
     a. Sepsis
     b. Allergic reactions
     c. Radiation
     d. Direct trauma
  3. Lymphatic blockage (lymph system acts as accessory route whereby excess interstitial fluid and leaked proteins can flow back into vascular space)

C. Capillary and interstitial pressures (Fig. 13–2)
  1. Pressure within capillary exerting outward force against membrane
  2. Interstitial fluid pressure exerting inward pressure against membrane
  3. Plasma colloid osmotic pressure pulling fluid from interstitial space into capillaries
  4. Interstitial colloid osmotic pressure drawing fluid from capillary into interstitium (third space)

## III. Phases of Third Spacing

A. Phase I: fluid loss
  1. Occurs immediately after massive trauma or surgery
  2. Can last 48 to 72 hours
  3. Increased capillary permeability
     a. Allows protein leakage into areas of inflammation and trauma
     b. Fluid shifts from vascular to interstitial space
  4. Treatment (sometimes controversial)
     a. Colloids: colloid molecules preferentially retained in intravascular compartment
        (1) Albumin
        (2) Plasma

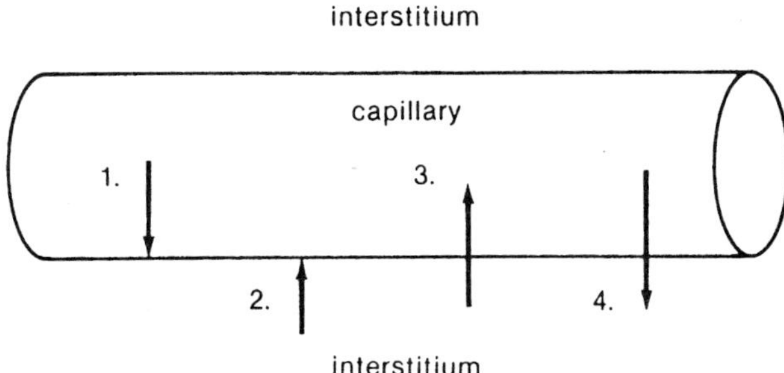


**FIGURE 13–2** Capillary and interstitial pressures. *1,* Capillary pressure; *2,* interstitial fluid pressure; *3,* plasma colloid osmotic pressure; *4,* interstitial colloid osmotic pressure.

(3) Dextran
(4) Hydroxyethyl starch (Hespan)
b. Crystalloids
(1) Hypertonic electrolyte solutions: $D_5NS$, $D_5LR$
(2) Saline
(3) Combined dextrose in saline
c. Colloids plus crystalloids in varying combinations
5. Intraoperative replacement
a. May require 1 to 2 L of Lactated Ringer's solution beyond blood replacement
b. May require 8 to 10 L in massive burns
6. Postanesthesia nursing concerns
a. Administer prescribed fluids; may require 200 to 1000 ml/hr for adequate replacement
b. Maintain renal perfusion
c. Monitor
(1) Vital signs
(2) Hemodynamic parameters: CVP, PA, pulmonary artery occlusion pressure (PAOP)
(3) Urinary output and specific gravity
(4) $K^+$, blood urea nitrogen (BUN), creatinine
(5) Chest auscultation for rales

B. Phase II: reabsorption
1. As injured tissues heal, capillaries repair and normal permeability returns
2. Lymph blockage clears
3. Plasma proteins return to normal
4. Capillary pressures, filtration, reabsorption restored
5. Fluid volume shifts to vascular compartment to be excreted by kidneys
6. Nursing care
a. Recognize reabsorption phase
(1) Increased urinary output
(2) Decreased specific gravity (urine)
(3) Fluid output exceeds intake
(4) Weight loss
b. Monitor signs of circulatory overload
(1) Distended neck veins
(2) Electrocardiogram (ECG) changes
(3) Shortness of breath
(4) Rales
(5) Increasing CVP
c. Electrolyte imbalances (Table 13–1)
(1) Sodium
(2) Potassium
(3) Chloride
(4) Phosphorus
(5) Magnesium

*Text continued on page 198*

**TABLE 13–1 Electrolyte Imbalances**

| | EXCESS | DEFICIT |
|---|---|---|
| **Sodium ($Na^+$)** *Normal:* serum sodium ($Na^+$) 135–145 mEq/L. Serum $Na^+$ reflects osmolality of blood. | | |
| Imbalance | **Hypernatremia**<br>Serum $Na^+$ >145 mEq/L<br>Blood contains excess salt relative to water<br>Hypernatremia indicates increased osmolality of blood<br>Imbalance may be called water depletion in cells | **Hyponatremia**<br>Serum $Na^+$ <130 mEq/L<br>Blood contains excess water relative to salt<br>Hyponatremia indicates decreased osmolality of blood<br>Imbalance may be called water intoxication in presence of hypervolemia but can be also found with hypovolemia |
| Causes of imbalance | Overall: factors that alter normal salt/water ratio | |
| | ***Conditions of increased water loss that raise salt/water ratio***<br>Severe vomiting ($H_2O$ loss vs. $Na^+$ loss)<br>Diabetes insipidus<br>Osmotic diuresis<br>Renal concentration disorders<br>Prolongs diarrhea without fluid replacement<br>Mechanical ventilation without humidification<br>Tracheobronchitis<br>Fever<br>Muscular exercise | ***Conditions of increased water intake that lower salt/water ratio***<br>Excessive infusion of 5% dextrose in water<br>Excessive tap water enemas<br>Stimulation of antidiuretic hormone (major surgery, trauma, volume depletion, inappropriate secretion of ADH)<br>Adrenal insufficiency<br>Overuse of ultrasonic nebulizers<br>Psychogenic polydipsia |
| | ***Conditions of decreased water intake or increased salt intake that raise salt/water ratio***<br>Inability to respond to thirst (confusion, weakness, coma, aphasia, paralysis)<br>No access to water<br>Difficulty swallowing fluids<br>High solute intake without adequate water (tube feedings, half-and-half for ulcer diet)<br>NaCl absorption<br>Excess administration of hypertonic NaCl or $NaHCO_3^-$<br>Hyperaldosteronism<br>Cushing's syndrome | ***Conditions of increased salt loss that lower salt/water ratio***<br>Nasogastric suction<br>Surgery: use of large amounts of hypotonic irrigating solutions (distilled water during prostatectomy resection)<br>Diuretic therapy<br>Salt-wasting renal disease (inability to retain $Na^+$)<br>Replacement of water but not lost electrolytes (burns, sweating, vomiting, diarrhea, nasogastric suction, fistula drainage)<br>Starvation<br>Dilutional hyponatremia, expansion of total body $H_2O$ (CHF, renal failure, cirrhosis)<br>Hyperlipidemia, hypoproteinemia, hyperglycemia (osmolality depends on total number of particles in solutions); with these conditions, osmolality of extracellular fluid is increased and $H_2O$ is pulled from intracellular compartments, thus diluting |

*Table continued on following page*

**TABLE 13–1 Electrolyte Imbalances** *(Continued)*

| | EXCESS | DEFICIT |
|---|---|---|
| Signs and symptoms | Basis: sodium imbalances affect osmotic pressure of extracellular fluid<br>Brain cells shrink with hypernatremia (desiccation)<br><br>***Manifestations of hypernatremia may include***<br>Thirst<br>Oliguria (unless mixed imbalance is present)<br>Confusion, lethargy<br>Muscle weakness, twitching<br>Convulsions, coma | Brain cells swell with hyponatremia (overhydration)<br><br>***Manifestations of hyponatremia may include***<br>Malaise<br>Nausea, vomiting<br>Headache<br>Confusion, lethargy<br>Convulsions, coma |
| Nursing interventions | ***To prevent hypernatremia***<br>Administer water between tube feedings<br>Keep humidifiers refilled<br><br>***To correct hypernatremia safely***<br>Monitor water loss replacement<br>Check specific gravity of urine | ***To prevent hyponatremia***<br>Use NS instead of distilled water for irrigations<br>Give isotonic ice chips to those on nasogastric suction<br><br>***To correct hyponatremia safely***<br>Restrict fluids if hypervolemic<br>Administer diuretics as ordered<br>Administer 3% NaCl carefully if ordered (used only in extremely rare cases of symptomatic hyponatremia; may cause circulatory overload)<br>Monitor intake and output, CNS status, laboratory data. |

**Potassium ($K^+$)** *Normal:* serum potassium ($K^+$) 3.5–5.0 mEq/L. $K^+$ is primarily intracellular: serum values do not necessarily reflect body stores. Insulin promotes entry of $K^+$ into cells.

| | | |
|---|---|---|
| Imbalance | **Hyperkalemia**<br>Serum $K^+$ >5.0 mEq/L | **Hypokalemia**<br>Serum $K^+$ <3.5 mEq/L |
| Causes of imbalance | Overall: conditions that affect intake or excretion, abnormal routes of potassium loss or gain, and factors that affect potassium movement in and out of cells<br><br>***Increased $K^+$ intake***<br>Excess or too rapid IV administration<br>Administration of large amounts of blood in which hemolysis of RBCs has occurred<br>Increased oral intake causes hyperkalemia only if accompanied by decreased $K^+$ excretion | <br><br>***Decreased $K^+$ intake***<br>Trauma, injury, surgery, burns<br>Gastrointestinal $K^+$ loss<br>Vomiting<br>Nasogastric suction<br>Diarrhea<br>Laxative abuse<br>Dehydration, starvation<br>Large sweat loss without $K^+$ replacement |

**TABLE 13–1 Electrolyte Imbalances** *(Continued)*

| | EXCESS | DEFICIT |
|---|---|---|
| | ***Decreased urinary excretion of $K^+$***<br>Oliguric renal failure<br>Volume depletion<br>$K^+$-sparing diuretics<br>Decreased effect of aldosterone (Addison's disease, chronic heparin administration, lead poisoning, hyporeninemia) | ***Increased urinary excretion of $K^+$***<br>Stress<br>Increased effect of aldosterone (hyperaldosteronism, excessive licorice ingestion, large doses of steroids)<br>Renal salt wasting<br>Hypomagnesemia<br>Diuretics (mercurials, thiazides, furosemide, ethacrynic acid, acetazolamide) |
| | ***Movement of $K^+$ into extracellular fluid***<br>Exercise (during)<br>Acidosis: pH, serum $K^+$<br>Tissue injury: burns or crush injuries<br>Massive digitalis overdose<br>Familial periodic paralysis | ***Entry of $K^+$ into cells***<br>Alkalosis: pH, $K^+$<br>Hypersecretion of insulin<br>Familial periodic paralysis |
| Signs and symptoms | Basis: potassium imbalances alter resting potential of muscle cells; muscle cells less sensitive to stimuli; circulating extracellular potassium is essential component in neuromuscular and cardiac function | |
| | ***Manifestations of hyperkalemia may include***<br>Abdominal distention, paralytic ileus, and muscle weakness starting in lower extremities and ascending upward, affecting respiratory muscles<br>Flaccid paralysis<br>Polyuria<br>Cardiac abnormalities: complete heart block, ectopy, ventricular fibrillation, standstill | ***Manifestations of hypokalemia may include***<br>Intestinal colic, diarrhea<br>Muscle weakness ascending from lower extremities but sparing respiratory muscles<br>Flaccid paralysis<br>Cardiac dysrhythmias: bradycardia, first- and second-degree blocks, atrial dysrhythmias, premature ventricular contraction (especially if taking digitalis), and cardiac arrest |
| | ECG changes: peaked T waves, disappearance of P wave progressing to idioventricular rhythm and asystole, prolonged PR, widened QRS | ECG changes: ST depression, flattened T waves, U wave |
| Nursing interventions | ***To correct hyperkalemia safely***<br>Encourage fluids to increase urinary output<br>Provide adequate carbohydrate (to prevent tissue breakdown and further $K^+$ release)<br>Withhold drugs containing $K^+$ (e.g., penicillin G)<br>Infuse IV glucose and insulin if ordered; $K^+$ moves to ICF when glucose and insulin are metabolized | ***To prevent complications and correct hypokalemia safely***<br>Observe ECG for signs of digitalis toxicity: hypokalemia potentiates digitalis<br>Administer IV potassium slowly (never more than 80 mEq/L or 30 mEq/hr)<br>Make sure patient is voiding and not oliguric when administering $K^+$ |

*Table continued on following page*

**TABLE 13–1 Electrolyte Imbalances** *(Continued)*

| | EXCESS | DEFICIT |
|---|---|---|
| Nursing interventions *(Continued)* | Administer sodium bicarbonate: facilitates $K^+$ movement back into cells<br>Administer calcium gluconate: antagonizes $K^+$ effect on myocardial irritability<br>Hemodialysis<br>Kaexylate enema | |
| **Chloride ($Cl^-$)** *Normal:* 95–109 mEq/L. | | |
| Imbalance | **Hyperchloremia** | **Hypochloremia** |
| Causes of imbalance | Overall: chloride competes with bicarbonate for combination with sodium ions; when $Cl^-$ decreases, bicarbonate rises in compensation (extra bicarbonate retained to balance $Na^+$ ions)<br>Excessive adrenal cortical hormone<br>Dehydration: $Cl^-$ retention<br>Head injury (neurogenic hyperventilation)<br>Hyperparathyroidism (kidneys waste phosphates so $Cl^-$ level rises)<br>Metabolic acidosis (excreted bicarbonate ions replaced by $Cl^-$)<br>Respiratory alkalosis (low carbonic acid because hyperventilation blows off $CO_2$)<br>Drugs: ammonium chloride, boric acid, ion exchange resins (Questran), Tandearil, phenylbutazone (Butazolidin), IV NaCl | Loss of $K^+$ accompanied by loss of $Cl^-$<br>Hyperhidrosis: sweating<br>Gastrointestinal disease (prolonged suctioning, vomiting, diarrhea)<br>Diabetic ketoacidosis (ketone anions replace $Cl^-$ in serum)<br>CHF (ECF excess)<br>Chronic renal failure<br>Low-salt diets<br>Metabolic alkalosis<br>Ingestion of excess bicarbonate<br>Ethacrynic acid (Edecrin) and furosemide (Lasix)<br>Thiazide and mercurial diuretics<br>Prolonged IV use of $D_5W$ |
| Signs and symptoms | Overall: usually when $Cl^-$ levels are abnormally high or low, there is a corresponding increase or decrease in $K^+$ and $Na^+$ levels; clinical signs and symptoms are those expected with $K^+$ and $Na^+$ | |
| Nursing interventions | ***To prevent hyperchloremia***<br>Assure adequate hydration in PACU and instruct patient regarding fluid intake<br>Decrease hyperventilation caused by anxiety by coaching, emotional support, and encouragement of verbalization<br>Assess patient for signs and symptoms of drug toxicity<br>***To correct safely***<br>Correct metabolic acidosis with sodium bicarbonate, $O_2$ as ordered<br>Monitor replacement of gastrointestinal losses | ***To prevent hypochloremia***<br>Monitor urine and blood glucose in diabetic patients<br>Accurate recording of gastrointestinal and IV intake and output (I & O)<br>Assess for signs and symptoms of drug toxicity<br>Monitor $Cl^-$ replacements carefully (if given)<br>***To correct safely***<br>Monitor fluid replacement and loss<br>Monitor urine and blood glucose in diabetic patient |

**TABLE 13–1 Electrolyte Imbalances** *(Continued)*

| | EXCESS | DEFICIT |
|---|---|---|
| **Calcium ($Ca^{++}$)** *Normal:* 8.5–10.5 mg/100 ml (slightly higher in children). Serum $Ca^{++}$ and $PO^{-}_4$ have reciprocal relationships when $Ca^{++}$ is increased and $PO^{-}_4$ is decreased and vice versa. | | |
| Imbalance | **Hypercalcemia**<br>Serum $Ca^{++}$ >11 mg/100 ml | **Hypocalcemia**<br>Serum $Ca^{++}$ <8 mg/100 ml |
| Causes of imbalance | Overall: conditions that affect intake, gastrointestinal absorption, excretion, bone homeostasis, physiologic availability of calcium, and abnormal routes of calcium loss | |
| | ***Increased gastrointestinal absorption of $Ca^{++}$***<br>Hypervitaminosis D<br>Milk-alkali syndrome<br>Sarcoidosis<br>***$Ca^{++}$ release from bone***<br>Hyperparathyroidism<br>Malignancy (bronchogenic carcinoma, hypernephroma, breast cancer, others)<br>Bone tumors<br>Multiple myeloma<br>Leukemia<br>Prolonged immobilization | ***Decreased gastrointestinal absorption of $Ca^{++}$***<br>Steatorrhea<br>Sprue<br>Diarrhea<br>Overuse of antacids<br>Chronic laxative abuse<br>Pancreatitis<br>Dietary lack of milk and vitamin D<br>Chronic uremia |
| | ***Increase in physiologically available $Ca^{++}$***<br>Acidosis (pH decreased, $Ca^{++}$ increased) | ***Decrease in physiologically available $Ca^{++}$***<br>Alkalosis (pH increased, $Ca^{++}$ decreased)<br>Massive transfusion of blood preserved with citrate phosphate dextrose (CPD), a $Ca^{++}$-binding agent<br>Rapid infusion of Plasmanate<br>Hypoparathyroidism<br>Surgical removal of parathyroid glands during thyroidectomy<br>Hypomagnesemia<br>Overuse of phosphate-containing laxatives and enemas<br>***Increased urinary excretion of $Ca^{++}$***<br>Chronic renal insufficiency<br>***$Ca^{++}$ loss in exudates***<br>Massive subcutaneous infection, burns, peritonitis |
| Signs and symptoms | Basis: calcium imbalances alter cell membrane permeability, which in turn alters neuromuscular excitability<br>Hypercalcemia decreases cell membrane permeability, producing decreased neuromuscular excitability | Hypocalcemia increases cell membrane permeability, producing increased neuromuscular excitability |

*Table continued on following page*

**TABLE 13–1 Electrolyte Imbalances** *(Continued)*

| | EXCESS | DEFICIT |
|---|---|---|
| | ***Manifestations of hypercalcemia may include***<br>Anorexia<br>Nausea and vomiting<br>Abdominal pain<br>Constipation<br>Headache<br>Muscle weakness, fatigue<br>Confusion, lethargy, CNS depression<br>Polyuria<br>Renal failure<br>Pathologic fractures<br>Cardiac arrest | ***Manifestations of hypocalcemia may include***<br>Muscle twitching and cramping<br>Positive Chvostek's sign*<br>Grimacing<br>Perioral and digital paresthesias<br>Positive Trousseau's sign†<br>Carpopedal spasm, tetany<br>Laryngospasm<br>Convulsions<br>Cardiac dysrhythmias<br>Cardiac arrest |
| Nursing interventions | ***To prevent hypercalcemia***<br>Increase patient mobility<br>Teach patients to avoid massive vitamin D supplementation<br>IV administration of loop diuretics (Lasix) and hydration | ***To prevent hypocalcemia***<br>Teach patients careful management of antacids and laxatives<br>Teach adults importance of drinking milk as tolerated |
| | ***To prevent complications while correcting hypercalcemia***<br>Ensure adequate hydration to prevent kidney damage<br>Maintain acid urine (increases solubility of $Ca^{++}$)<br>Prevent urinary tract infections (cause alkaline urine, which allows $Ca^{++}$ precipitation)<br>Handle patients gently when transferring or turning to prevent pathologic fractures<br>Watch for signs of toxicity in patients taking digitalis (hypercalcemia potentiates digitalis) | ***To prevent complications of hypocalcemia***<br>Teach patients that tetany may be exacerbated by hyperventilation or pressure on efferent nerve (e.g., by crossing legs)<br>Keep 10% calcium gluconate available for emergency use after parathyroid surgery |

**Phosphorus (phosphate, $PO^{-}_{4}$)** *Normal:* 2.5–4.5 mg/100 ml. Phosphorus (in the form of phosphate) is an essential part of energy storage compounds, nucleic acids, intermediary metabolites of carbohydrates, lipids, the enzyme 2,3-DPG (which controls release of oxygen from hemoglobin), and phospholipids of cell membranes.

| | | |
|---|---|---|
| Imbalance | **Hyperphosphoremia**<br>>4.5 mg/100 ml | **Hypophosphoremia**<br><2.5 mg/100 ml |
| Causes of imbalance | Overall: Conditions that affect parathyroid<br>Parathormone promotes phosphate excretion and maintains serum $Ca^{++}$<br>Serum $Ca^{++}$ and phosphorus levels very reciprocal<br>Damaged renal tubules (renal failure)<br>Vitamin D excess<br>Hypoparathyroidism | Vitamin D deficiency<br>Excessive alkalinity of intestinal contents<br>Malabsorption syndromes, steatorrhea, prolonged diarrhea<br>Hyperparathryoidism<br>Increased plasma insulin levels<br>Osteomalacia<br>Alcoholism<br>Vitamin D deficiency: rickets, soft bones, bowed legs, poor teeth, skeletal deformities |

**TABLE 13–1 Electrolyte Imbalances** *(Continued)*

| | EXCESS | DEFICIT |
|---|---|---|
| Signs and symptoms | Renal failure | |
| Nursing interventions | ***Prevention***<br>Discontinue exogenous vitamin D<br>Accurate I & O<br>Monitor electrolytes (especially $Ca^{++}$) | ***Prevention***<br>Discontinue or decrease amounts of alkalizers<br>Alcoholic counseling<br>Monitor diabetic carefully and correct imbalances as they occur<br>Accurate I & O<br>Monitor electrolytes<br>***Correction***<br>Vitamin D supplements |
| **Magnesium ($Mg^{++}$)** *Normal:* serum magnesium ($Mg^{++}$) 1.5–2.5 mEq/L. Serum levels may not reflect body stores. $Mg^{++}$ is absorbed primarily through small intestine. | | |
| Imbalance | Overall: conditions that affect magnesium intake, gastrointestinal absorption or excretion, and abnormal routes of magnesium loss or gain (found in green vegetables) | |
| Causes of imbalance | **Hypermagnesemia**<br>(excessive intake or absorption of $Mg^{++}$)<br>Overuse of $Mg^{++}$-containing antacids<br>Overuse of $Mg^{++}$-containing cathartics<br>Excess $Mg^{++}$ in renal dialysis fluid<br>Aspiration of seawater<br>$Mg^{++}$ overdose during replacement therapy<br>$Mg^{++}$ therapy in toxemia of pregnancy<br>***Impaired $Mg^{++}$ excretion***<br>Chronic renal failure: $Mg^{++}$ retention<br>Adrenal insufficiency<br>Epsom salt laxatives ($MgSO^{-}_4$ epsom salts)<br>Milk of magnesia: MgOH | **Hypomagnesemia**<br>Chronic malnutrition<br>Prolonged IV administration without $Mg^{++}$ supplementation<br>Chronic diarrhea<br>Malabsorption syndrome<br>Bowel resection (massive)<br>Inherited $Mg^{++}$ absorption defect<br>Chronic alcoholism<br>Prolonged diuresis<br>Severe dehydration loss from ICF<br>***Gastrointestinal $Mg^{++}$ loss***<br>Prolonged nasogastric suction<br>Steatorrhea<br>Acute pancreatitis<br>Biliary or intestinal fistula<br>***Increased urinary excretion of $Mg^{++}$***<br>Diuretic therapy<br>Diabetic ketoacidosis<br>Primary aldosteronism<br>Renal $Mg^{++}$ reabsorption defect<br>Chronic alcoholism |
| Signs and symptoms | Basis: magnesium imbalances alter release of acetylcholine at neuromuscular junction, which alters neuromuscular function<br>Hypermagnesemia decreases release of acetylcholine at neuromuscular junctions, which decreases neuromuscular excitability | Hypomagnesemia increases release of acetylcholine at neuromuscular junctions, which increases neuromuscular irritability |

*Table continued on following page*

**TABLE 13–1 Electrolyte Imbalances** *(Continued)*

| | EXCESS | DEFICIT |
|---|---|---|
| | ***Manifestations of hypermagnesemia may include***<br>Somnolence<br>Hypotension<br>Flushing, sweating<br>Drowsiness, lethargy, CNS depression<br>Slow, weak pulse<br>Weak or absent deep tendon reflexes<br>Flaccid paralysis<br>Respiratory depression<br>Cardiac dysrhythmias<br>Cardiac arrest | ***Manifestations of hypomagnesemia may include***<br>Insomnia<br>Hyperactive reflexes<br>Positive Chvostek's sign*<br>Leg and foot cramps, twitching, tremors<br>Positive Trousseau's sign†<br>Tetany<br>Convulsions<br>Extreme confusion, CNS stimulation<br>Cardiac dysrhythmias |
| Nursing interventions | ***To prevent hypermagnesemia***<br>Teach patients careful management of antacids and cathartics<br>Teach patients with renal problems to avoid $Mg^{++}$-containing preparations | ***To prevent hypomagnesemia***<br>Provide diet counseling for persons at risk |
| | ***To prevent complications and correct hypermagnesemia safely***<br>Give fluids to increase urinary output<br>Withhold preparations containing large amounts of $Mg^{++}$<br>Keep 10% calcium gluconate available for emergency use | ***To correct hypomagnesemia safely***<br>Administer intravenous $Mg^{++}$ slowly to prevent patients from feeling hot or flushed (150 mg/min)<br>Check renal function before administering $Mg^{++}$ replacement<br>$Mg^{++}$ inhibits absorption of tetracycline<br>Keep IV calcium gluconate ready to reverse $Mg^{++}$ excess |

*Positive Chvostek's sign: spasm of the cheek and corner of the mouth after a tap on cranial nerve VII in front of the ear.
†Positive Trousseau's sign: carpal spasm after occlusion of blood flow to the hand for 3 minutes.

## POSTANESTHESIA ASSESSMENT OF FLUID BALANCE

### NURSING DIAGNOSIS

Examples of related nursing diagnostic categories include:

- Fluid volume deficit
- Fluid volume excess
- Altered thought processes
- Decreased cardiac output
- Metabolic acidosis

**I. Assessing Fluid Balance in PACU** (Table 13–2)

A. Mental status

B. Cardiovascular function

1. Blood pressure: fluid volume excess and deficit may be masked by effects of anesthetic agents, adjuncts, depth of anesthesia, and septic shock or fever
2. Central venous pressure: useful when properly placed and no discrepancy exists between left and right ventricular function
3. PAOP: more accurate in assessing left-sided heart function and impending shock
4. Heart sounds, neck veins, pulses

C. Pulmonary function
  1. Lung sounds
  2. Respirations
  3. Arterial blood gases
  4. X-ray
D. Renal: urine output (normal range 30 to 50 ml/hr)
  1. Oliguria (less than 15 ml/hr)
    a. Fluid volume deficit
    b. Renal failure
    c. Mechanical obstruction
    d. Drug reaction
  2. Polyuria (more than 150 ml/hr)
    a. Fluid volume excess
    b. High output renal failure
    c. Release of urinary tract obstruction
    d. Diuretic therapy
    e. Diabetes insipidus
    f. Diabetes mellitus: ketoacidosis
E. Laboratory values
  1. Hyponatremia
    a. Addison's disease

**TABLE 13–2 Fluid Volume Status Summary**

| | EXCESS | DEFICIT |
|---|---|---|
| **Preexisting Conditions** | Congestive heart failure<br>Renal failure<br>Liver disease<br>Intraoperative overhydration<br>Excess sodium intake | Burns, trauma<br>Diuretic therapy<br>Infection, fever<br>Vomiting, diarrhea<br>Acute blood loss<br>Diabetes (mellitus, insipidus)<br>Pancreatitis<br>Fistula |
| **Assessment** | | |
| Cardiovascular | Increased (may be decreased in failure) | Decreased, postural hypotension |
| BP | Increased | Decreased |
| CVP | Increased | Decreased |
| PAOP | Increased | Normal/rapid, weak pulse |
| Neck veins/pulses | Distended/bounding | Normal, enhanced |
| Heart sounds | Muffled, $S_3$ present | Concentrated |
| Serum hematology/chemistry | Dilutional | |
| Pulmonary | Compensatory respiratory acidosis with decreased $Pa_{O_2}$ (also possible in deficit status) | $\dot{V}/\dot{Q}$ mismatch |
| Arterial blood gases | | Respiratory acidosis |
| X-ray | Pulmonary congestion | Normal |
| Lung sounds | Rales | Normal |
| Renal | | |
| Urine | Decreased | Increased |
| Specific gravity | | |
| Output | Increased | Decreased |
| Skin | Peripheral edema | Poor turgor |
| Body temperature | Normal or decreased depending on intraoperative conditions | Increased |
| Mental status | Restlessness, stupor | Weakness, stupor |

b. Diuretic therapy
c. Dilutional hyponatremia (after prostatectomy)
d. CHF
2. Hypernatremia
a. Diabetes insipidus
b. Hypertonic saline administration
3. Hematocrit
4. Serum osmolality
5. Serum glucose

F. Skin condition
1. Color
2. Turgor
3. Dry vs. moist

G. Body temperature: may be affected by anesthetic medications, duration and type of surgery, and administration of unwarmed intravenous fluid

H. Body weight

I. Wound drainage

J. Intravenous fluid and blood product administration

## II. Fluid Replacement in PACU (Table 13–3)

A. Crystalloids
1. Isotonic fluids: NS, LR, $D_5W$, $D_5$.25 NS
a. Advantages
(1) Expand ECF volume
(2) Replace gastrointestinal losses

**TABLE 13–3 Adult Fluid Replacement**

**Three-Part Formula for Deriving Amount of Fluid to Be Replaced**

A. Deficit: The time the patient is NPO to the time surgery begins = Number of hours × 2 ml/kg/hr
B. Maintenance: Depends on type of surgical procedure
1. Eye surgery, extremity procedure .......... 5 ml/kg/hr
2. Mastectomy .......... 8 ml/kg/hr
3. Minor abdominal procedures (appendectomy, herniorrhaphy, etc.) .......... 8–10 ml/kg/hr
4. Laparotomy/resection, thoracotomy .......... 12 ml/kg/hr
5. Extensive procedures (Whipple, accompanying peritonitis) .......... 15–20 ml/kg/hr
C. Blood replacement: ml/ml for blood replacement + 3 ml/ml crystalloid to estimated blood loss (EBL)

**Schedule for Replacement During Surgical Procedure**

A. First hour: ½ the deficit + Maintenance + Blood replacement
Second hour: ¼ the deficit + Maintenance + Blood replacement
Third hour: ¼ the deficit + Maintenance + Blood replacement
B. Example: A 70-kg patient, NPO from midnight, is scheduled for a small bowel resection at 8 AM
1. Deficit: 8 (hr NPO) × 2 ml × 70 (kg) = 1120 ml (total deficit)
2. Maintenance: Bowel resection = 12 ml × 70 kg = 840 ml/hr (maintenance)
3. Blood replacement: EBL = 500 ml = 500 ml blood to replace
+
3 ml crystalloid/ml EBL = 1500 ml crystalloid
C. Schedule of administration for 3-hour bowel resection:
First hour: 560 ml (½ deficit) + 840 ml/hr (maintenance) + 100 WB/300 LR
Second hour: 280 ml (¼ deficit) + 840 ml/hr (maintenance) + 200 WB/600 LR
Third hour: 280 ml (¼ deficit) + 840 ml/hr (maintenance) + 200 WB/600 LR
1120 ml deficit    2520 ml/hr maintenance    500 WB + 1500 LR
TOTAL REPLACEMENT: 5140 ml crystalloid + 500 ml blood

   b. Disadvantages
      (1) Hypernatremia
      (2) Overexpansion of ECF volume
      (3) Hypokalemia
2. Hypotonic fluids: 0.45 NS, 0.2 NS
   a. Advantages
      (1) Shift plasma into interstitial fluid
      (2) Supply normal salt and water requirements
   b. Disadvantages: should be given cautiously to cardiac, renal, and edematous patients
3. Hypertonic fluids: $D_5$LR, $D_5$NS, $D_{10}$W
   a. Advantages
      (1) Replace electrolytes
      (2) If dextrose solution, shift ECF from interstitium to plasma (useful in treating third spacing)
   b. Disadvantages
      (1) Cause fluid overload
      (2) Hypertonic dextrose irritates veins
      (3) Solutions with $D_{10}$W cannot be administered with blood; cause hemolysis

B. Colloids
1. Types
   a. Whole blood
   b. Whole blood components
      (1) Packed cells (with decreased plasma volume)
      (2) Plasma
         (a) Liquid serum albumin (5% and 25%) or Plasmanate
         (b) Frozen
         (c) Platelet concentrates
2. Advantages
   a. Increase hemoglobin content of blood, thereby increasing oxygen-carrying capacity of blood
   b. Replace volume
   c. Provide protein
3. Disadvantages
   a. Expensive
   b. Risk of hepatitis and acquired immune deficiency syndrome (AIDS) transmission
   c. Increase $K^+$
   d. Impair clotting
   e. Cause varied reactions
      (1) Febrile
      (2) Hemolytic
      (3) Allergic (urticaria)
      (4) Anaphylactic
   f. Calcium deficit caused by citrate binding

C. Synthetic colloids: blood products
1. Types
   a. Dextran 70
   b. Dextran 40
   c. Hespan (hydroxyethyl starch)
2. Advantages
   a. Effective volume expanders (especially in blood losses of patients who refuse blood and blood products)
   b. Less expensive than blood products
   c. Interfere with clotting (useful after vascular obstruction procedures)
   d. Metabolize slowly and remain in vascular system (but not as long as colloids)

3. Disadvantages
   a. Interfere with clotting
   b. Cause fluid overload
   c. Allergic reaction possible with hydroxyethyl starch

## BIBLIOGRAPHY


Ganong W: *Review of Medical Physiology,* 17th Ed. Norwalk, Conn, Appleton & Lange, 1995.

Halperin M, Goldstein M: *Fluid, Electrolyte, and Acid-base Physiology.* Philadelphia, WB Saunders, 1994.

Jones D: Fluid therapy in the PACU. *Crit Care Nurs Clin North Am* 3(1):109–120, 1991.

Kirvela O, Soreide E, Askanazi J: Management of fluid and electrolyte problems. *Anesth Clin North Am* 8(2):267–286, 1990.

Kokko J, Tannen R: *Fluids and Electrolytes,* 3rd Ed. Philadelphia, WB Saunders, 1996.

Litwack K: Perioperative fluid administration: Colloid or crystalloid. *Anesthesia Today* 8(2):15–18, 1997.

Litwack K, Keithley J: Fluid, electrolyte and nutrition therapy. In Nagelhout J, Zaglaniczny KL (eds): *Nurse Anesthesia* (pp 675–682). Philadelphia, WB Saunders, 1997.

Rose D: *Clinical Physiology of Acid-base and Electrolyte Disorders,* 4th Ed. New York, McGraw-Hill, 1994.

Tuman K: Fluid and electrolyte abnormalities and management. In Vender J, Spiess B (eds): *Post Anesthesia Care.* Philadelphia, WB Saunders, 1992.


## REVIEW QUESTIONS

1. **The secretion of ADH is regulated by:**
   A. Adrenal gland
   B. Kidneys
   C. Hypothalamus
   D. Gastrointestinal system

2. **Which solution is hypertonic?**
   A. $D_5$.2 NS
   B. $D_5$LR
   C. NS
   D. LR

3. **Which of the following will result in extracellular fluid volume deficit?**
   A. Ketoacidosis
   B. Chronic kidney disease
   C. Congestive heart failure
   D. Hyperaldosteronism

4. **The signs of extracellular fluid volume excess include:**
   A. Decreased CVP, fatigue, confusion
   B. Decreased urinary output, dry skin, tachycardia
   C. Peripheral edema, ascites, increased CVP
   D. Poor skin turgor

5. **What is the definition of third spacing?**
   A. Excessive accumulation of interstitial fluid
   B. Normal distribution of body fluids
   C. Decreased capillary permeability preventing accumulation of extracellular fluid
   D. Fluid accumulation from vascular space into area normally having no fluid

6. **Administration of isotonic solutions is indicated in the treatment of which imbalance?**
   A. Extracellular fluid volume deficit
   B. Extracellular fluid volume excess
   C. Intracellular fluid volume deficit
   D. Intracellular fluid volume excess

**7. If a patient is third spacing, what assessment parameters should the PACU nurse monitor?**

A. Urine output
B. Breath sounds
C. Vital signs
D. All of the above

**8. You assess your patient to be confused and lethargic with nausea and vomiting. Which electrolyte imbalance would you suspect?**

A. Hypermagnesemia, hypokalemia
B. Hyponatremia, hypercalcemia
C. Hyperkalemia, hyperchloremia
D. Hypophosphoremia, hypochloremia

**9. What are the signs and symptoms of electrolyte imbalance caused by cancer?**

A. Renal failure, CNS depression, pathologic fractures
B. Insomnia, hypotension, sweating, respiratory depression
C. Headache, diarrhea, laryngospasm
D. Flushing, seizures, hypotension

**10. In assessing adult fluid replacement needs, how can the patient's fluid deficit be calculated?**

A. Number of hours in surgery × 8 ml/kg/hr
B. Number of hours NPO × 5 ml/kg/hr
C. Number of hours NPO × 2 ml/kg/hr
D. 3 ml of crystalloid/ml estimated blood loss

**ANSWERS:** 1. C, 2. B, 3. C, 4. C, 5. D, 6. A, 7. D, 8. B, 9. A, 10. C

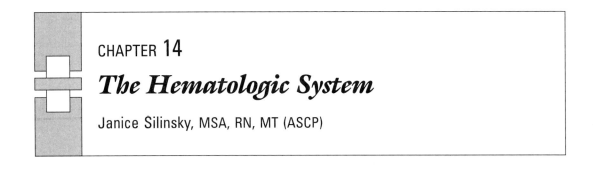

CHAPTER 14

# The Hematologic System

Janice Silinsky, MSA, RN, MT (ASCP)

## OBJECTIVES

**Study of the information represented by this outline will enable the learner to:**

1. Recognize and evaluate normal and abnormal laboratory values and initiate the appropriate nursing interventions as needed.
2. Describe the nursing care of a patient with a hematologic disorder.
3. Describe the nursing care of a patient with a disorder in hemostasis.
4. Discuss the nursing responsibilities associated with blood and blood component transfusions.
5. Identify the types of transfusion reactions and the appropriate nursing interventions.

This chapter covers the most common blood dyscrasias in the areas of hematology, hemostasis, and immunohematology. It is a broad presentation of the clinical signs, laboratory results, and nursing interventions for each area. For a detailed account of specific disease entities and syndromes not covered or for more in-depth information on disorders presented, refer to the bibliography at the end of this chapter.

## HEMATOLOGY

**I. Introduction to Hematology**

- A. Normal laboratory values*
  1. White blood cells (WBCs): 5000 to 10,000/μl
  2. Red blood cells (RBCs)
     - a. Male: 4.5 to 6.2 million per microliter
     - b. Female: 4 to 5.5 million per microliter
  3. Hemoglobin (Hb)
     - a. Male: 14 to 18 g/dl
     - b. Female: 12 to 16 g/dl
  4. Hematocrit (HCT)
     - a. Male: 40% to 52%
     - b. Female: 37% to 47%
- B. Differential
  1. Segmented neutrophils: 40% to 60%
  2. Band neutrophils: 0 to 3%
  3. Lymphocytes: 20% to 40%
  4. Monocytes: 4% to 8%
  5. Eosinophils: 1% to 3%

*The normal values listed are for guideline purposes only. Refer to the normal ranges established by your institution's clinical laboratory when evaluating test results.

6. Basophils: 0 to 1%
7. Nucleated red blood cells: 0

C. Platelet count: 150,000 to 400,000/µl
D. Reticulocyte count: 0.2% to 2%

**II. Anemias**

A. Acute blood loss
  1. Causes
    a. Surgery
    b. Trauma
    c. Gastrointestinal hemorrhage
  2. Laboratory results
    a. Hb, HCT may be normal*

B. Chronic blood loss
  1. Causes
    a. Menorrhagia
    b. Gastrointestinal hemorrhage
    c. Endocrine disorders
      (1) Addison's disease
      (2) Myxedema
      (3) Hypothyroidism
    d. Renal disease
      (1) Chronic renal failure
      (2) Malignant hypertension
    e. Hepatic disorders
      (1) Alcoholic cirrhosis
      (2) Drug-induced liver disease
    f. Cancer
      (1) Bone marrow infiltration by cancer cells
    g. Chronic infection
      (1) Subacute bacterial endocarditis
      (2) Tuberculosis
      (3) Osteomyelitis
    h. Inflammatory states
      (1) Collagen diseases
        (a) Rheumatoid arthritis
        (b) Lupus erythematosus
      (2) Inflammatory bowel disease

C. Aplastic, hypoplastic anemia
  1. Causes
    a. Radiation exposure (dose dependent)
    b. Infection
      (1) Viral: hepatitis
      (2) Bacterial: miliary tuberculosis
    c. Metabolic
      (1) Pancreatitis
      (2) Pregnancy
    d. Drugs/chemicals
      (1) Benzene
      (2) Chloramphenicol
      (3) Phenylbutazone

---

*Unreliable indicators of the extent of blood loss because of continued shifts of fluid from the extravascular space.

(4) Chemotherapy drugs
(5) Phenytoin
e. Systemic lupus erythematosus
f. Idiopathic
g. Cell-mediated immunologic disorders
h. Paroxysmal nocturnal hemoglobinuria
2. Laboratory results
a. WBCs decreased
b. Platelets decreased
c. RBCs decreased
d. Hb decreased
e. HCT decreased
f. Reticulocytes decreased
g. No immature cell forms seen on blood smear
3. Clinical signs
a. Occurs at any age
b. Gradual onset
c. Weakness, fatigue
d. Dyspnea on exertion
e. Abnormal skin and mucosal bleeding
f. Pallor of skin and mucous membranes

D. Vitamin $B_{12}$ deficiency anemia
1. Causes
a. Decreased production of intrinsic factor
(1) After gastrectomy
(2) Pernicious anemia
b. Decreased ileal absorption
(1) After extensive small bowel resection
(2) Crohn's disease
2. Laboratory results
a. Hb, HCT decreased
b. Hypersegmented neutrophils
c. $B_{12}$ level <100 pg/ml

E. Folic acid deficiency anemia
1. Causes
a. Dietary deficiency
(1) Alcoholism
(2) Anorectic cancer patients
b. After subtotal gastrectomy
c. Increased requirement
(1) Pregnancy
(2) Chronic hemolytic anemia
2. Laboratory results: same as $B_{12}$ except
a. $B_{12}$ level normal
b. Folic acid level decreased

F. Iron deficiency anemia
1. Causes
a. Chronic blood loss
(1) Gastrointestinal tract
(2) Menorrhagia
b. Deficient diet
c. Decreased absorption
d. Increased requirements
(1) Pregnancy

2. Laboratory results
   a. Hypochromic RBCs
   b. Serum iron decreased

## III. Hemolytic Anemias

A. Hereditary spherocytosis
   1. RBCs produced are spherical in shape instead of normal biconcave disk; cells are abnormal and removed from circulation by spleen; often diagnosed in childhood; when anemia is severe, splenectomy recommended
   2. Clinical signs
      a. Weakness
      b. Abdominal pain
      c. Loss of appetite
      d. Fever
      e. Jaundice
      f. Leg ulcers
      g. Hepatomegaly
   3. Laboratory results
      a. WBCs increased: 10,000 to 30,000/µl
      b. Hb decreased: 4 to 10 g/dl
      c. HCT decreased: 12% to 30%
      d. MCHC increased: >36%
      e. Reticulocyte count increased: 10% to 50%
      f. RBC survival decreased to 14 days
      g. Bilirubin increased: 0.8 to 5 mg/100 ml

B. Sickle cell anemia
   1. Hereditary condition, most commonly affecting 1% of African-Americans; person lacks normal Hb A and is homozygous for Hb S; becomes clinically apparent between 6 months and 1 year of age; low oxygen tension causes red cells to change shape to a sicklelike form; acidosis and fever also increase chance of sickling; sickle-shaped red cells get caught in capillaries, causing stasis, which leads to thrombosis and ischemic necrosis
   2. Clinical signs
      a. Diffuse pain in stomach, legs, arms, and joints
      b. Bone pain
      c. Ischemic necrosis of bone
      d. Ischemia and infarction in lungs, liver, spleen, kidney, eyes, and central nervous system (CNS)
      e. Lower leg ulcers
      f. Prone to infections, especially *Pneumococcus* and *Haemophilus influenzae*
      g. Cardiomegaly with systolic murmur
      h. Scleral jaundice
   3. Laboratory results
      a. WBCs increased: 10,000 to 30,000/µl
      b. Hb decreased: 3 to 12 g/dl
      c. HCT decreased: 10% to 30%
      d. Platelets increased
      e. Reticulocyte count increased: 10% to 40%
      f. RBC survival decreased to 1 to 19 days
      g. Positive sickle cell screen
      h. Positive Hb electrophoresis: Hb S, Hb F
      i. Bilirubin increased: 1 to 3 mg/100 ml
      j. RBC morphology
         (1) Sickle cells: 5% to 50%

(2) Target cells
(3) Nucleated red cells

C. Sickle cell trait
   1. Hereditary trait; occurs in about 10% of African-Americans; person is heterozygous for Hb A and Hb S; those affected are usually asymptomatic and have normal life expectancy
D. Thalassemia major (Cooley's anemia)
   1. Hereditary, homozygous form of β-thalassemia, affecting either sex of Italians, Greeks, Syrians, and Armenians; abnormal synthesis of Hb F; most affected die between 20 and 30 years of age
   2. Clinical signs
      a. Growth failure
      b. Moderate jaundice
      c. Slanted eyes
      d. Skeletal abnormalities
      e. Prominent facial bones
      f. Hepatomegaly
      g. Severe splenomegaly
   3. Laboratory results
      a. WBCs increased: 13,000 to 30,000/μl
      b. Hb decreased: 2 to 10 g/dl
      c. HCT decreased: 8% to 30%
      d. Reticulocyte count increased: 5% to 30%
      e. RBC survival decreased to 12 to 19 days
      f. Hb electrophoresis: Hb F 40% to 90%
      g. Bilirubin increased: 1.5 to 3 mg/100 ml
E. Thalassemia minor (Cooley's trait)
   1. Hereditary, heterozygous form of β-thalassemia, affecting either sex of Italians, Greeks, Syrians, and Armenians; abnormal synthesis of Hb F and $A_2$; normal life expectancy
   2. Clinical signs
      a. Mild to absent symptoms
   3. Laboratory results
      a. Hb: 9 to 11 g/dl
      b. Reticulocyte count increased: 2% to 5%
      c. RBC survival normal
      d. Hb electrophoresis: Hb F 5% to 10%
F. Physical trauma
   1. Prosthetic heart valves with crack or defect
   2. Extracorporeal circulation
   3. Long distance runners
   4. Karate activity
   5. Thermal damage from severe burns
G. Infections
   1. Malaria: most common cause of RBC hemolysis
   2. Clostridia
   3. *Streptococcus* species
   4. *Haemophilus influenzae*
   5. Black water fever
H. Drugs
   1. Methyldopa (Aldomet)
   2. Penicillin type
   3. Quinidine derivatives
   4. *p*-Aminosalicylic acid

5. Phenacetin
6. Sulfonamides

**Postanesthesia Nursing Care of the Anemic Patient**

1. Provide supplemental oxygen as ordered to maximize oxygen delivery to cells.
2. Elevate head of bed or stretcher (if not contraindicated) to promote adequate lung expansion.
3. Change patient position slowly to minimize orthostatic hypotension.
4. Monitor laboratory results carefully because anemia may alter:
   a. Oxygen saturation
   b. Acid-base balance
5. Minimize soft-tissue damage by using, soft-tipped, lubricated suction catheters, and decrease suction pressure.
6. Maintain adequate IV infusion rate to decrease blood viscosity.
7. Avoid hypothermia.
8. Administer RBCs per physician's order, observing all precautions.
9. Pad side rails to prevent potential bruising to patient.
10. Measure amount of all blood loss from dressings, surgical drains, and tubes.

**IV. Polycythemia, Leukemia, Lymphoma, and Multiple Myeloma**

A. Polycythemia vera
   1. Acquired myeloproliferative disorder characterized by excessive production of RBCs, WBCs, and platelets in bone marrow; cause unknown; both blood volume and blood viscosity increase several times over
   2. Clinical signs
      a. Affects males more often
      b. Occurs between 50 and 60 years of age
      c. Ruddy complexion
      d. Headache, visual disturbances
      e. Vertigo, dizziness
      f. Weakness, fatigue
      g. Irritability
      h. Angina, palpitations
      i. Peptic ulcer pain or bleeding
      j. Hypertension
      k. Splenomegaly
      l. Claudication, thrombophlebitis
   3. Laboratory results
      a. RBC: 7 to 12 million per microliter
      b. Hb: 18 to 24 g/dl
      c. HCT: 54% to 72%
      d. Reticulocyte count increased
      e. WBC increased
      f. Platelets increased
      g. Oxygen saturation of arterial blood normal

B. Secondary polycythemia
   1. Results from increased release of erythropoietin, which stimulates RBC production
   2. Clinical signs and laboratory results: see information on polycythemia vera above
   3. Contributing factors
      a. Living at high altitude for extended periods of time
      b. Chronic heart disease
         (1) Pulmonary stenosis

            (2) Septal defects
            (3) Rheumatic mitral disease
        c. Arteriovenous aneurysm
        d. Bronchial asthma
        e. Primary pulmonary hypertension
        f. Chronic pulmonary emboli
        g. Emphysema
        h. Renal disease
            (1) Hypernephroma
            (2) Hydronephrosis
        i. Pheochromocytoma
C. Acute lymphocytic leukemia
    1. Clinical signs
        a. Children more frequently affected before 10 years of age
        b. Fatigue, weakness
        c. Malaise
        d. Pain in extremities, bone pain
        e. Bleeding into skin, mucous membranes
        f. Easy bruisability
        g. Enlarged lymph nodes
        h. Splenomegaly
        i. Hepatomegaly
    2. Laboratory results
        a. WBCs increased: 20,000 to 100,000/μl
        b. Hb decreased: 2 to 6 g/dl
        c. Platelets decreased: 10,000 to 60,000/μl
        d. Differential
            (1) 15% to 75% lymphoblasts
            (2) 10% to 25% lymphocytes
        e. Reticulocyte count increased
        f. Serum lactic dehydrogenase (LDH) increased
D. Chronic lymphocytic leukemia
    1. Clinical signs
        a. In males older than 50 years most frequently
        b. Fatigue, weakness
        c. Swelling on either side of neck
        d. Lymph nodes enlarged
        e. Splenomegaly
    2. Laboratory results
        a. WBCs increased: 50,000 to 200,000/μl
        b. Hb decreased: 6 to 12 g/dl
        c. Platelets decreased: 50,000 to 200,000/μl
        d. Differential
            (1) 0 to 3% lymphoblasts
            (2) 75% to 95% lymphocytes
E. Acute myelocytic leukemia
    1. Clinical signs
        a. Accounts for about 80% of acute leukemia in adults
        b. Skin pallor
        c. Minor infections of skin and cuts
        d. Fever
        e. Petechiae, easy bruising
        f. Bone and joint tenderness

g. Fatigue, weakness
h. Anorexia, weight loss
i. Splenomegaly
j. Hepatomegaly
2. Laboratory results
a. WBCs increased: 20,000 to 100,000/μl
b. Hb decreased: 2 to 8 g/dl
c. Platelets: 50,000 to 150,000/μl
d. Differential: 20% to 90% myeloblasts
e. Reticulocyte increased 0.5% to 2%
f. Nucleated red cells

F. Chronic myelocytic leukemia
1. Clinical signs
a. Accounts for 20% of all leukemias
b. More often seen in adult men
c. Easily fatigued, weakness
d. Splenomegaly
e. Anorexia, weight loss
f. Excessive sweating
g. Sternal tenderness
2. Laboratory results
a. WBCs increased: 100,000 to 800,000/μl
b. Increase in WBC immaturity
c. Hb decreased: 4 to 8 g/dl
d. Platelets: 100,000 to 600,000/μl
e. Differential
(1) 2% to 10% myeloblasts
(2) 20% to 50% myelocytes
f. Philadelphia chromosome present in 85% of cases
g. Nucleated red cells
h. Hypersegmented neutrophils

G. Hodgkin's disease
1. Background information
a. Enlargement of lymphatic tissue
b. Usually begins in neck
c. Cause unknown
d. Incidence peaks late 20s
e. Gradual increase in incidence older than 45 years of age
2. Clinical signs
a. Chills, low-grade fever
b. Night sweats
c. Weight loss
d. Enlarged cervical and axillary lymph nodes
e. Fatigue
f. Splenomegaly, hepatomegaly
3. Laboratory results
a. WBCs increased: 10,000 to 20,000/μl
b. Hb decreased
c. Differential
(1) Lymphocytes decreased
(2) Neutrophils increased
(3) Monocytes increased
(4) Eosinophils increased

H. Lymphomas
   1. Types
      a. Reticulum cell sarcoma
      b. Lymphosarcoma
      c. Burkitt's lymphoma
   2. Clinical signs
      a. Enlarged lymph nodes
      b. Weight loss
      c. Fever
      d. Night sweats
      e. Splenomegaly
      f. Jaundice
   3. Laboratory results
      a. WBCs normal, decreased or increased
      b. Hb decreased
      c. HCT decreased
      d. Differential
         (1) Eosinophils increased
         (2) Monocytes increased
         (3) Neutrophils increased

I. Plasma cell myeloma, multiple myeloma
   1. Background information
      a. Uncontrolled proliferation of plasma cells in bone marrow
      b. Cells synthesize abnormal amounts of monoclonal immunoglobulins (G, A, D, E)
      c. Most frequently found in males older than 50 years of age; diagnosis at about 65 years of age
      d. Highest incidence is in men >80 years and women >70 years
   2. Clinical signs
      a. Weakness, fatigue
      b. Spontaneous fracture
      c. Bone pain
      d. Anorexia, weight loss
      e. Bruising
      f. Epistaxis
      g. Pallor
   3. Laboratory results
      a. Hb: 8 to 12 g/dl
      b. Differential
         (1) 0 to 10% plasmacytes
         (2) Rouleaux formation present
      c. Platelet count normal but platelet function abnormal
      d. Serum LDH increased
      e. Positive serum cryoglobulins
      f. Urinalysis
         (1) Positive albumin
         (2) Positive casts
         (3) Positive Bence Jones protein

**Postanesthesia Nursing Care of the Leukemic Patient**

1. Give supplemental oxygen as ordered to maximize oxygen delivery to the cells.
2. Elevate head of bed or stretcher (if not contraindicated) to promote lung expansion.
3. Change patient position slowly to minimize orthostatic hypotension.
4. Minimize soft-tissue damage by using soft-tip suction catheters, and decrease suction pressure.

5. Avoid hypothermia.
6. Avoid hypothermia. Maintain adequate IV infusion rate to decrease blood viscosity.
7. Monitor laboratory results carefully.
8. Administer blood components per physician's order, observing all precautions.
9. Administer antibiotics as ordered to maintain therapeutic blood levels.
10. Monitor temperature.
11. Maintain reverse isolation when indicated.
12. Avoid hematoma formation after venous or arterial punctures.
13. Pad side rails to prevent potential bruising.

## HEMOSTASIS

### I. Introduction to Hemostasis

A. Normal laboratory values*
   1. Prothrombin time (PT): 11 to 13 seconds (within 2 seconds of control). PT results may also be reported with an international normalized ratio (INR) value†
   2. Activated partial thromboplastin time (APTT): 25 to 37 seconds (within 5 seconds of control)
   3. Fibrin split products (FSP): 0 to 2 μg/ml (negative at >1:4 dilution)
   4. Platelets: 150,000 to 400,000/μl
   5. Fibrinogen: 200 to 400 mg/100 ml

B. Coagulation factor nomenclature (see Table 14–1)

C. Site of biosynthesis of coagulation factors‡
   1. Liver: I, II, V, VII, VIII, IX, X, XI, XII

---

*The normal values listed are for guidelines only. Refer to the normal ranges established by your institution's clinical laboratory.

†The INR concept was introduced by the World Health Organization to account for variations in thromboplastin reagents used by laboratories. Consult your clinical laboratory for normal INR values.

‡Each activated factor only activates the factor immediately following it in the cascade.

**TABLE 14–1 Coagulation Factor Nomenclature**

| FACTOR | NAME |
|---|---|
| I | Fibrinogen |
| II | Prothrombin, prethrombin |
| III | Tissue thromboplastin, tissue factor |
| IV | Calcium |
| V | Proaccelerin, labile factor |
| VI | Not assigned |
| VII | Proconvertin, SPCA, autoprothrombin I |
| VIII | Antihemophilic factor A, platelet cofactor I |
| VIII/vWF | von Willebrand's factor |
| VIII/C | Procoagulant activity |
| VIII/RCF | Ristocetin cofactor |
| IX | Christmas factor, antihemophilic factor B, autoprothrombin II, platelet cofactor II |
| X | Stuart-Prower factor, autoprothrombin III, Stuart factor |
| XI | Plasma thromboplastin antecedent, antihemophilic factor C |
| XII | Hageman factor |
| XIII | Fibrin-stabilizing factor, Laki-Lorand factor |
| High-molecular-weight kininogen | Fitzgerald factor |
| Prekallikrein | Fletcher factor |

2. All body fluids: III
3. Platelets: XIII
4. Vitamin K–dependent factors: II, VII, IX, X

D. Naturally occurring coagulation inhibitors
1. Protein C
2. Antithrombin 3
3. Complement (C1) inactivator
4. $\alpha_A$-macroglobulin
5. $\alpha_1$-antitrypsin

E. Coagulation tests
1. PT
   a. Measures factors I, II, V, VII, X
   b. Extrinsic and common pathway
   c. Monitors oral anticoagulant therapy
2. APTT
   a. Measures factors I, II, V, VIII, IX, X, XI, XII
   b. Intrinsic and common pathway
   c. Monitors heparin therapy
3. FSP
   a. Detects fibrinogen fibers
4. Fibrinogen
   a. Measures amount available

F. Basic scheme of coagulation: four components of hemostasis
1. Vascular system
   a. Normal vascular endothelium is very smooth and nonreactive to platelets, leukocytes, and coagulation factors; large breaks in vessel walls, especially in those under pressure, cannot be sealed by platelets or fibrin meshwork
2. Platelets
   a. Form initial plug at site of injury; surface membrane of platelet is required to initiate and support reactions of coagulation cascade
   b. Platelets localize clot formation; major function is to circulate until they locate a break in vascular integrity
   c. Platelets are disk shaped, about 3 to 4 μm in diameter
   d. Life span about 9 to 10 days
   e. Two thirds of platelets in systemic circulation
   f. One third kept in reserve in spleen
3. Coagulation cascade
   a. Because platelet plug is only temporary, it would fall apart without structural support of fibrin strands
   b. Goal is conversion of fibrinogen into fibrin, an insoluble gel
   c. Most coagulation factors circulate in inactive form in high concentrations in plasma
   d. Factors V and VIII circulate only in active form and are very labile
   e. Intrinsic pathway (Fig. 14–1)
      (1) Begins intravascularly with activation of factor XII
      (2) Factor XII activated by surface contact with vessel denuded of endothelium
      (3) Only factor not in intrinsic pathway is VII
   f. Extrinsic pathway (Fig. 14–1)
      (1) Begins extravascularly with release of tissue phospholipid from tissue damage
4. Fibrinolytic system
   a. Reestablishes normal blood flow by removing fibrin clot from vessel
   b. Limits coagulation to injury site, prevents uncontrolled coagulation
   c. Clot lysis is from "the inside out"; plasminogen activated locally within fibrin clot to plasmin
   d. Plasmin degrades fibrin or fibrinogen into FSP

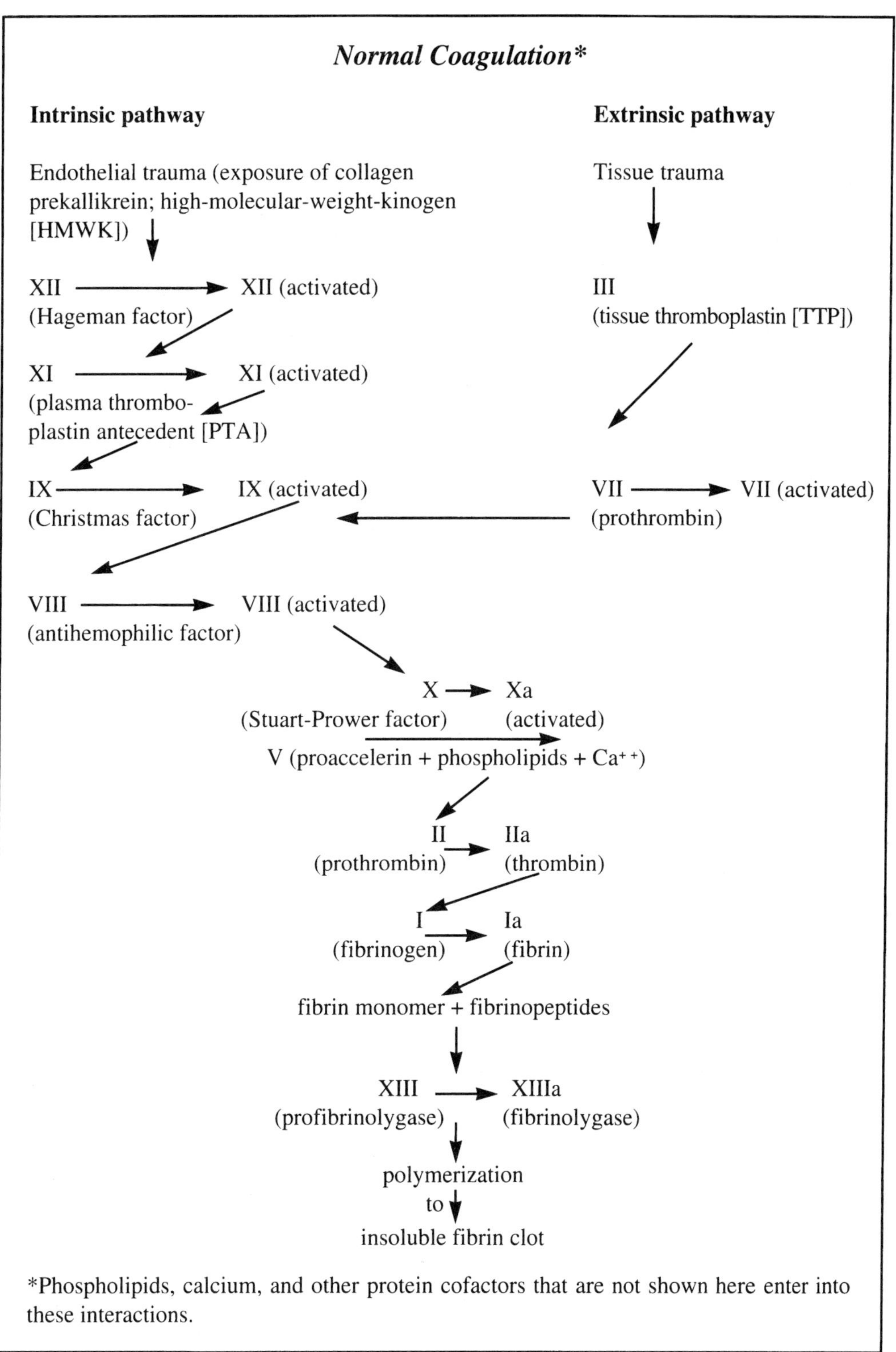


**FIGURE 14–1** Pathways for clot formation. (From Bailes BK: Disseminated intravascular coagulation. *AORN J* 55:519, 1992.)

## II. Inherited Disorders of Hemostasis

A. Hemophilia A: factor VIII deficiency
   1. Background information
      a. Inherited; primarily affects males
      b. Usually found in childhood
      c. Cause: factor VIII deficiency
   2. Clinical signs
      a. Epistaxis
      b. Bleeding into soft tissue or muscle
      c. Bleeding into joints (knees, elbows, ankles)
      d. Hematuria, melena
      e. Internal and external bleeding
      f. Intracranial bleeding
   3. Laboratory results
      a. Platelets normal
      b. Bleeding time increased
      c. Coagulation time increased
      d. PT normal
      e. Partial thromboplastin time (PTT) increased
      f. Factor VIII assay decreased

B. von Willebrand's disease
   1. Background information
      a. Inherited as autosomal dominant trait
      b. Affects both sexes
      c. Cause: low factor VIII level with platelet dysfunction
   2. Clinical signs
      a. Epistaxis
      b. Menorrhagia
      c. Mild bruising
      d. Mucous membrane bleeding
   3. Laboratory results
      a. Platelet count normal
      b. Bleeding time increased
      c. PT normal
      d. PTT increased
      e. Factor VIII assay decreased
      f. Platelet adhesion impaired

C. Hemophilia B (Christmas disease)
   1. Background information
      a. Sex-linked recessive trait
      b. Factor IX deficiency
   2. Clinical signs
      a. Epistaxis
      b. Bleeding into joints
      c. Spontaneous soft-tissue bleeding
   3. Laboratory results
      a. Platelet count normal
      b. Bleeding time normal to increased
      c. PT normal
      d. PTT increased
      e. Prothrombin consumption time increased

## III. Acquired Disorders of Hemostasis

A. Idiopathic immune thrombocytopenic purpura (ITP)

1. Background information
   a. Occurs in two forms
      (1) Chronic: seen most commonly in women 20 to 40 years old
      (2) Acute: seen in children; self-limiting
   b. Autoimmune disorder resulting from action of antiplatelet antibodies
2. Clinical signs
   a. Epistaxis
   b. Mucous membrane bleeding
   c. Prolonged menstrual periods
   d. Petechiae
3. Laboratory results
   a. Platelets decreased: 0 to 50,000/μl
   b. Bleeding time increased
   c. PT normal
   d. Prothrombin consumption test decreased
   e. Antiplatelet antibodies present

B. Disseminated intravascular coagulation (DIC)
1. Background information
   a. Acquired pathologic bleeding syndrome
   b. Spontaneous activation of coagulation cascade
   c. Is always a response to an underlying process
2. Causes
   a. Obstetric
      (1) Amniotic fluid embolism
      (2) Abruptio placentae
      (3) Toxemia
      (4) Missed abortion
   b. Surgery
      (1) Thoracic
      (2) Open heart
      (3) Leveen shunt
      (4) Abdominal aortic aneurysm, ruptured or dissecting
   c. Cancer
      (1) Prostate
      (2) Lung
      (3) Pancreas
   d. Disease states
      (1) Liver disease
      (2) Glomerulonephritis
      (3) Renal transplant rejection
      (4) Hemorrhagic pancreatitis
      (5) Acute promyelocytic leukemia
   e. Infection
      (1) Septicemia: viral, bacterial
      (2) Malaria
      (3) Protozoal
      (4) Rickettsial
   f. Shock states
      (1) Severe burns
      (2) Fat embolism
      (3) Cardiac arrest
      (4) Trauma with crush injury
      (5) Snake venom
      (6) Hypothermia

g. Transfusions
   (1) Hemolytic transfusion reaction
   (2) Acute antigen-antibody reactions
3. Clinical signs
   a. Diffuse bleeding from multiple sites
   b. Oozing from venipuncture, arterial puncture sites
   c. Mucosal bleeding: nose, gums
   d. Petechiae
   e. Hematuria
4. Laboratory results
   a. Platelet count decreased: <100,000/μl
   b. Bleeding time normal to increased
   c. PT increased
   d. PTT increased
   e. Fibrinogen decreased: <100 mg/dl
   f. Fibrinopeptide A increased
   g. FSP >2 μg/ml

**Postanesthesia Care of Patients with Hemostasis Disorders**

1. Maintain patent intravenous (IV) line for administration of blood, blood components, or factor replacement.
2. Observe all precautions when administering replacement factors or blood components.
3. Administer all medications by IV route if possible.
4. Provide support to affected extremities.
5. Avoid unnecessary repeated venipunctures by organizing blood sampling to be completed at designated collection times.
6. Provide adequate pressure to venous, arterial, or intramuscular (IM) puncture sites to decrease chance of hematoma formation.
7. Pad side rails to prevent potential bruising.
8. Monitor laboratory results carefully.
9. Minimize soft-tissue damage by using soft-tipped, lubricated suction catheters, and decrease suction pressure.

## IMMUNOHEMATOLOGY

**I. Immunohematology (Blood Transfusion Therapy)**
A. Basic concepts of ABO group and Rh type
   1. Four major blood groups: A, B, AB, O
      a. Red cells carry the A or B antigens or both on their surface and are group A, B, or AB
      b. Red cells without the A or B antigen are group O
      c. Plasma carries naturally occurring antibodies to antigens not present on the red cell

| *Group* | *Antigen* | *Antibody* |
|---|---|---|
| A | A | B |
| B | B | A |
| AB | A and B | None |
| O | None | A and B |

   2. Two Rh types: $Rh^+$ and $Rh^-$
      a. Rh antigen carried on red cell surface
      b. Rh system contains more than 30 antigens, but for practical purposes, the D antigen will be the determining factor

c. If D antigen is present: $Rh^+$ (85% of people)
d. If D antigen is lacking: $Rh^-$ (15% of people)
e. No naturally occurring antibodies present in Rh system

3. ABO recipient and ABO compatible donor
   a. A: A or O packed cells
   b. B: B or O packed cells
   c. AB: AB or A, B, O packed cells
   d. O: O only
4. Most common transfusion errors
   a. Improper identification of recipient blood sample
      (1) Right sample but wrong patient name
      (2) Wrong sample but right patient name
   b. Transfusion of blood into wrong recipient

B. Indications for transfusion therapy
   1. Restore circulating volume
   2. Increase oxygen transport to tissues
   3. Replace coagulation factors
   4. Replace platelets to correct bleeding
   5. Replace granulocytes or treat sepsis

## II. Blood and Blood Components

A. Whole blood
   1. Volume: 500 ml; HCT: 36% to 40%
   2. Composition
      a. Red blood cells
      b. Plasma
      c. White blood cells
      d. Platelets
   3. Storage
      a. 21 to 42 days at 1° to 6° C
      b. After 24 hours WBCs lose viability and platelet function greatly decreases
      c. As storage time increases
         (1) pH decreases
         (2) 2,3-DPG levels decrease*
         (3) Cell $K^+$ decreases
         (4) Plasma $K^+$ increases
         (5) Plasma ammonia and lactic acid levels increase
   4. Uses
      a. Actively bleeding patient with >2000 ml loss of total blood volume
      b. Exchange transfusion of neonate (use blood <24 hours old)

B. Packed red blood cells (PC, PRBC)
   1. Volume: 250 ml; HCT: 70% to 80%
   2. Composition
      a. Red blood cells
      b. Minimal plasma
      c. Nonfunctional white cells and platelets
   3. Uses
      a. Chronic anemia
      b. Cardiac disease
      c. Renal disease

---

*When RBCs lose 2,3-DPG, they lose 50% of their ability to deliver oxygen to tissues. This becomes a concern when a patient receives a massive transfusion of stored blood with low 2,3-DPG levels, which may result in tissue hypoxia. RBCs are able to regenerate their stores of 2,3-DPG within hours to days.

d. Hepatic disease
e. Cancer, leukemias

C. Washed red blood cells
1. Volume: 200 to 300 ml; 20% RBCs lost during washing
2. Composition (shelf life of 24 hours after washing)
a. Red blood cells
b. Minimal plasma
c. 10% white cells and platelets
3. Uses
a. Anemia
b. To minimize febrile and allergic transfusion reactions from plasma or leukocyte antibodies, platelets, or proteins such as IgA
c. To decrease sensitization to HLA antigens
d. Renal patients with Na, K, or citrate restrictions

D. Frozen washed red blood cells (FWRBC, FWC)
1. Volume: 200 ml
2. Composition
a. RBCs
b. 2% of white cells and platelets
c. No plasma
3. Uses
a. Bone marrow transplant recipient
b. Rare blood storage
c. Autologous transfusion for elective surgery
d. Patients with clinically significant antibodies to IgA

E. Granulocyte concentrates (WBC)
1. Volume: 400 ml (200 to 600 ml)
2. Composition*
a. Granulocytes
b. Lymphocytes
c. Platelets
d. Some red cells
e. Plasma
3. Uses†
a. Granulocytopenia with sepsis
b. Neutropenia (<500 segmented neutrophils)
c. Bone marrow with myeloid hypoplasia

F. Platelet concentrates‡
1. Volume: 50 to 300 ml
2. Composition
a. Platelets
b. Some red cells
c. Some white cells
d. Plasma
3. Uses
a. Leukemia
b. DIC
c. Bleeding caused by thrombocytopenia

---

*Must be crossmatched and ABO compatible.

†Administer slowly over 2 to 4 hours. Concentrate may be irradiated to prevent graft vs. host reaction.

‡Single donor platelets are collected from an individual during a 2- to 3-hour apheresis procedure. Random donor platelets are collected from individual units of blood.

   d. Chemotherapy-treated patient
   e. Radiation-treated patient
   f. Bleeding caused by thrombocytopathy

G. Fresh frozen plasma (FFP)—must be ABO compatible
   1. Volume: 125 to 250 ml (printed on unit label)
   2. Composition
      a. Plasma
      b. All coagulation factors
      c. Complement
      d. No platelets
   3. Uses
      a. Coagulation deficiencies secondary to liver disease
      b. DIC
      c. Antithrombin 3 deficiency
      d. Dilutional coagulopathy resulting from massive blood replacement

H. Factor IX concentrate (Konyne, Proplex)
   1. Volume: 25 ml (assay level stated on label)
   2. Composition
      a. Factor II
      b. Factor VII
      c. Factor IX
      d. Factor X
   3. Preparation
      a. Lyophilized form of plasma
      b. Shelf life: 1 to 2 years
      c. After reconstitution with sterile diluent, concentrate is stable for 12 hours
      d. Increased hepatitis risk with this concentrate
   4. Use
      a. Factor IX deficiency (Christmas disease)

I. Normal serum albumin (NSA, SPA)
   1. Volume
      a. 5%: 50, 250, 500 ml
      b. 25%: 20, 50, 100 ml
   2. Composition
      a. 96% albumin
      b. 4% globulin and other proteins
   3. Preparation
      a. Obtained from pooled plasma
      b. Heat treated to inactivate hepatitis virus, then sterilized
   4. Uses
      a. Plasma volume expander
      b. Hypoproteinemia

J. Factor VIII concentrate: antihemophilic factor (AHF, Koate, Factorate)
   1. Volume: 25 ml (assay level stated on label)
   2. Composition
      a. Lyophilized concentrate of factor VIII
   3. Preparation
      a. Reconstitute with sterile diluent only
      b. Increased hepatitis risk
      c. After reconstitution administer concentrate within 20 minutes
   4. Uses
      a. Moderate to severe factor VIII deficiency, hemophilia A

K. Cryoprecipitate (Cryo): must be ABO compatible
   1. Volume: 15 to 20 ml

2. Composition
   a. Fibrinogen
   b. Factors VIII: C, VIII: vWF, XIII
   c. Fibronectin
3. Preparation
   a. Obtained from FFP
   b. Shelf life: 1 year frozen at −18° C; 6 hours after thawing
4. Uses
   a. Hemophilia A
   b. DIC
   c. von Willebrand's disease
   d. Obstetric complications
   e. Fibrinogen deficiency

L. Plasma protein fraction (Plasmanate, PPF)
1. Volume: 50, 250, 500 ml
2. Composition
   a. 88% albumin
   b. 12% globulins
   c. No coagulation factors
3. Preparation
   a. Obtained from pooled plasma
   b. Heat treated to inactivate hepatitis virus
4. Uses
   a. Volume expander
   b. Hypoproteinemia

## III. Complications of Transfusions

A. Hemolytic transfusion reaction
1. Causes
   a. ABO incompatibility: immediate hemolysis after first few milliliters of blood are infused
   b. Human clerical error: patient or blood sample not properly identified
2. Clinical signs of hemolysis
   a. Burning sensation along vein receiving transfusion
   b. Temperature increases (105° F or higher), facial flushing, chills
   c. Patient may be restless, anxious, dyspneic, tachypneic
   d. Blood pressure decreases, pulse increases, may complain of palpitations
   e. Substernal or flank pain
   f. Abnormal bleeding or DIC (from liberation of thromboplastic substances from damaged RBCs followed by DIC)
   g. Chances for kidney damage high because of
      (1) Onset of hypotension
      (2) Massive antigen-antibody reaction
      (3) Presence of free hemoglobin
   h. In anesthetized surgical patient
      (1) Unexplained onset of significant oozing should receive immediate attention
      (2) Patient cannot report feelings of pain
      (3) Decreased blood pressure caused by transfusion reaction is difficult to distinguish from decreased blood pressure of hypovolemic shock for which transfusion was given
3. Treatment (per physician order)
   a. Stop transfusion
   b. Aggressive fluid management
   c. IV furosemide (Lasix) for diuresis

d. Renal dose of dopamine to improve blood flow
e. Drugs for shock as indicated
f. Send institution transfusion investigation form properly filled out to blood bank
g. Send unit, tubing, and accompanying IV fluid hanging to blood bank
h. Send one red top tube and one lavender top tube to blood bank
i. Send urine sample for hemoglobin to laboratory

B. Delayed hemolytic transfusion reaction
1. Usually occurs several days after transfusion
2. Causative antibodies
a. Anti-E
b. Anti-C
c. Kidd system
3. Delayed hemolysis occurs when transfused cells possess antigen to which recipient has been sensitized to at some time in the past
4. Clinical signs
a. Unexplained fever
b. Defined drop in hemoglobin 2 to 10 days after transfusion
c. Positive direct Coombs' test
d. Bilirubin increased
5. Prevention
a. Good history from patient
b. Good communication with blood bank

C. Febrile transfusion reaction
1. Causes
a. WBC or platelet antibodies
b. Contaminating pyrogenic bacteria
c. Pregnancy or previous transfusion
2. Clinical signs
a. Chills, fever (2° F increase usually)
b. Flushing
c. Headache
d. Tachycardia
e. Reaction begins about 1 hour after start of transfusion and may last for 8 to 10 hours
3. Treatment
a. Because signs are indistinguishable from early signs of hemolytic reaction, stop transfusion and start transfusion reaction investigation
b. Antipyretics
c. Administer blood with microaggregate filter

D. Allergic transfusion reaction: 1% to 3% of all transfusions
1. Causes
a. Antibodies to donor blood foreign proteins
b. Patient often has allergy history
2. Clinical signs
a. Itching
b. Urticaria (hives)
3. Treatment
a. Stop transfusion; allergic reactions may progress unpredictably
b. Assess for glottal edema
c. Give IV antihistamine (Benadryl)

E. Anaphylactic type of allergic reaction
1. Associated with transfusion of IgA to IgA-deficient recipient
2. No RBC destruction
3. Occurs very rapidly after a few milliliters of blood or plasma
4. Massive histamine release

5. Clinical signs
   a. Dyspnea
   b. Hypotension after hypertension
   c. Laryngeal edema
   d. Chest pain
   e. Shock
   f. Flushing
   g. Widespread edema
   h. Bronchospasm
6. Treatment
   a. Stop transfusion
   b. Combat hypotension, laryngeal edema, and bronchiolar constriction
   c. Transfuse with washed cells
   d. Obtain a detailed transfusion history

F. Circulatory overload
1. Causes
   a. May result from giving too much blood or too rapid an infusion rate
   b. Patient's blood loss may be overestimated, and rapid replacement of loss is enough to push patient into congestive heart failure (CHF)
   c. Patients at risk
      (1) Elderly
      (2) Cardiac history
      (3) Chronic anemia
      (4) Infants
2. Clinical signs
   a. Dry cough
   b. Chest tightness
   c. Premature ventricular contractions (PVCs)
   d. Labored breathing, dyspnea
   e. Pulmonary edema
   f. Basilar rales
   g. Tachycardia
   h. Systolic hypertension
   i. Distended neck veins
3. Treatment
   a. Slow transfusion rate
   b. Elevate head of bed 30 degrees
   c. Furosemide may need to be given
   d. Transfuse with packed cells

G. Hypothermia
1. Increases affinity of hemoglobin for oxygen; thus hemoglobin will not release oxygen at cell level
2. Hypothermia promotes release of intracellular $K^+$, which may lead to hyperkalemia
3. As heart rate and body temperature falls, oxygen consumption rises sharply
4. Cardiac output and blood pH decrease
5. Prevention
   a. Use commercial blood warmer
   b. Blood warmer recommended for
      (1) Exchange transfusion of infant
      (2) Children receiving >50 ml of blood per kilogram of body weight
      (3) Patient receiving rapid and multiple transfusions at rate >50 ml/min
      (4) Patients with cold agglutinins active in vitro at 37° C
   c. Infusing blood through warmer
      (1) Decreases vasoconstriction

(2) Decreases metabolic acidosis
(3) Facilitates reentry of $K^+$ into transfused red cells

## IV. Transmission of Disease Through Transfusion

A. Hepatitis (three types)
1. Hepatitis A: infectious hepatitis
a. Transmission: fecal-oral route or injection
b. Incubation: 2 to 6 weeks
2. Hepatitis B: serum hepatitis
a. Transmission: injection, parenteral, enteric route
b. Incubation: 2 to 6 months
3. Non-A, non-B hepatitis: hepatitis C
a. Accounts for 90% of posttransfusion hepatitis
b. Incubation: 2 to 20 weeks

B. Bacteria
1. Usually gram-negative *Pseudomonas,* coliforms, and *Achromobacter* bacteria grow rapidly in blood at refrigerator temperature and produce deadly endotoxins
2. Symptoms appear about 30 minutes after infusion of 50 ml of blood
3. Hemolyzed plasma in blood unit may be seen in bacterial contamination
4. Clinical signs
a. Shaking fever
b. Severe hypotension
c. Dry, flushed skin
d. Pain in abdomen and extremities
e. Vomiting and bloody diarrhea
f. Hemoglobinuria
g. DIC
h. Renal failure

C. Syphilis
1. Spirochete *Treponema pallidum* cannot survive past 72 hours
2. Little threat of acquiring this disease through transfusion

D. Cytomegalovirus (CMV)
1. Occurs 3 to 6 weeks after transfusion of large amounts of fresh blood during cardiopulmonary bypass in about 3% to 11% of patients
2. Resembles mononucleosis and is called the postperfusion syndrome
3. Especially threatening to immunosuppressed patients

E. Malaria
1. Seldom occurs in United States
2. Considerations for transmission
a. Increased travel abroad
b. Return of military personnel from Southeast Asia
c. Massive influx of immigrants from Southeast Asia
3. Plasmodia live in red cells and in some cases may be found years after infection

F. AIDS (acquired immune deficiency syndrome)
1. New screening test for blood units available
2. Donor centers continue to screen prospective donors carefully
3. Patients are encouraged to donate their own blood for use in surgery
4. Strict universal precautions when initiating or completing blood transfusion

## V. Synthetic Solutions

A. Perfluorochemicals (Fluosol-DA)*
1. Synthetic compounds related to Teflon and the refrigerant freon

---

*Not FDA approved.

2. Has almost three times oxygen-carrying capacity of blood
3. Has many self-limiting factors

B. Dextran
1. Polysaccharide produced by *Leuconostoc mesenteroides*
2. Fractionated into different molecular weights: 40, 75, 200
3. Primarily used as plasma expander
4. Remains in circulation 2 to 6 hours
5. Decreases blood viscosity by
   a. Hemodilution
   b. Decreasing red cell aggregation
   c. Decreasing platelet adhesiveness
6. Complications
   a. Bleeding
   b. Overloading
   c. Anaphylaxis
7. Draw blood for cross-match before starting infusion; dextran interferes with cross-match procedure
8. Contraindications
   a. Thrombocytopenia
   b. Coagulopathies
   c. Dextran potentiates heparin action; if given together, heparin dose should be cut by 50%

C. Hydroxyethyl starch (HES, Volex, Hespan)
1. 6% solution of starch in normal saline
2. Expansion property lasts about 24 hours
3. Slowly metabolized and excreted in urine
4. Dilutes hematocrit value
5. Advantages over dextran
   a. Less bleeding tendency
   b. No anaphylactic reaction
   c. Does not interfere with cross-matching procedure for transfusion
6. Complications
   a. PT increased
   b. PTT increased
   c. Pruritus

**Postanesthesia Nursing Responsibilities in Administering Blood and Blood Products**

1. Patient and blood component identification and verification
   a. Most mistakes caused by improper identification of patient or component
   b. Donor number on compatibility slip must be identical to donor number on component
   c. Donor ABO group and Rh type on compatibility slip must be identical to component label
   d. Patient name and hospital identification number on compatibility slip must be identical to patient wrist identification band
   e. If any discrepancy occurs in identification process, delay transfusion and notify blood bank immediately
2. Patient comfort and safety
   a. Take the chill off the unit to be transfused by placing it under your arm for a few minutes or within a warm blanket
   b. Examine unit carefully for bubbles, plasma discoloration
   c. No kinks in tubing; use arm board to stabilize IV site prn
   d. Record baseline vital signs; then every hour of transfusion and at completion
   e. Remain with patient for first 20 minutes of infusion to observe for any signs indicating a reaction

f. Continually observe IV site during transfusion to allow for early detection and resolution of problems interfering with infusion
g. Minimize environmental and transfusional hypothermia with warm blankets and other warming devices
h. Provide reassurance to patient
(1) Explain transfusion procedure
(2) Assure patient that frequent checks of vital signs and transfusion are part of normal routine

3. Documentation
a. Record vital signs before starting transfusion and at completion
b. Repeat and record vital signs after transfusion is in progress 10 minutes
c. Observe and record condition of IV site
d. Document patient response to each unit of blood and/or component received
e. Complete compatibility slip with required information
f. If transfusion reaction occurs, notify blood bank, surgeon, and anesthesiologist and follow established protocols of institution

4. Technical aspects of component administration
a. Lay component bag on flat surface when inserting administration set to avoid accidental puncture of bag
b. Prime filter set properly; blood should not drip directly on filter
c. Mix cells frequently to prevent sedimenting at insertion port
d. Change filter every 2 units
e. Use stopcock when possible to ease administration of infusion
f. *Only normal saline* is to be administered with blood or blood components
g. $D_5W$ is hypotonic and causes hemolysis
h. Ringer's lactate has calcium content and can initiate coagulation
i. Never add medications to a unit of blood, including PCA pump
j. Keep patient as warm as possible
k. All blood and blood products are administered through filters to remove clots and coagulant debris
l. A No. 18 or No. 19 gauge catheter needed for transfusion of red cells
m. Red cells can be diluted with normal saline only for easier infusion
n. For rapid administration, unit(s) can be infused with pressure bag
o. FDA regulations require transfusions to be completed within 4 hours

## BIBLIOGRAPHY

Babior BM: *Hematology: A Pathophysiological Approach,* 2nd Ed. New York, Churchill Livingstone, 1990.
Beck WS (ed): *Hematology,* 5th Ed. Cambridge, Mass, MIT Press, 1991.
Besa EC: *Hematology.* Baltimore, Williams & Wilkins, 1992.
Hoffman R (ed): *Hematology: Basic Principles and Practice.* New York, Churchill Livingstone, 1991.
Kapff CT: *Blood: Atlas and Sourcebook of Hematology.* Boston, Little, Brown, 1991.
Mollison PL: *Blood Transfusion in Clinical Medicine.* Chicago, Blackwell Scientific Publications, 1993.
Petz LD, Swisher SN, Kleinman S, Strauss R, Spence R: *Clinical Practice of Transfusion Medicine,* 3rd Ed. New York, Churchill Livingstone, 1995.
Ratnoff OD, Forbes CD (eds): *Disorders of Hemostasis,* 2nd Ed. Philadelphia, WB Saunders, 1991.
Rossi EC et al: *Principles of Transfusion Medicine.* Baltimore, Williams & Wilkins, 1991.
Williams WJ: *Hematology,* 4th Ed. New York, McGraw-Hill, 1990.
Wintrobe MM: *Wintrobe's Clinical Hematology,* 9th Ed. Philadelphia, Lea & Febiger, 1993.

## REVIEW QUESTIONS

**1. What are the normal hemoglobin and hematocrit values for an adult male?**
A. 12 to 16 g/dl and 37% to 47%
B. 14 to 18 g/dl and 42% to 52%
C. 4.7 to 6.1 g/dl and 14% to 18%
D. 12 to 16 g/dl and 42% to 52%

**2. Which of the following is not a hemolytic anemia?**
A. Sickle cell
B. Thalassemia minor
C. Hereditary spherocytosis
D. Polycythemia vera

**3. What percentage of African-Americans are affected by sickle-cell anemia?**
A. 5%
B. 20%
C. 1%
D. 40%

**4. What are the appropriate interventions in the nursing care of patients with anemias in the PACU?**
A. Provide supplemental oxygen
B. Minimize soft tissue damage
C. Avoid hypothermia
D. All of the above

**5. Which of the following is true of acute lymphocytic leukemia?**
A. Males older than 50 years of age are most frequently affected
B. No specific age or sex is affected
C. Children are more frequently affected
D. None of the above

**6. What are the clinical signs of Hodgkin's disease?**
A. Splenomegaly, hepatomegaly, enlarged lymph nodes
B. Skin pallor, fetid body odor, bone and joint tenderness
C. Weakness, neck swelling, enlarged lymph nodes
D. Angina, palpitations, hypertension, ankle edema

**7. What interventions are different for the patient with leukemia vs. the patient with anemia?**
A. Maintain adequate IV infusion rate, avoid hypothermia
B. Maintain reverse isolation, administer antibiotics
C. Monitor laboratory results, administer blood products as ordered
D. Minimize soft tissue damage, promote adequate lung expansion

**8. Which coagulation test monitors heparin therapy?**
A. Fibrin split products
B. PT
C. Fibrinogen
D. APTT

**9. What are the causes of DIC?**
A. Septicemia
B. Trauma
C. Major surgery
D. All of the above

**10. What is the cause of a hemolytic transfusion reaction?**
A. ABO incompatibility
B. Contaminating pyrogenic bacteria
C. Pregnancy
D. Antibodies to donor's foreign proteins

**11. The most common type of transfusion reaction is:**

A. Febrile
B. Hemolytic
C. Allergic
D. Anaphylactic

**12. To minimize allergic transfusion reactions, which type of cells should be used?**

A. Washed
B. Frozen
C. Leukocyte-free
D. White blood cells

**ANSWERS:** 1. B, 2. D, 3. C, 4. D, 5. C, 6. A, 7. B, 8. D, 9. D, 10. A, 11. C, 12. A

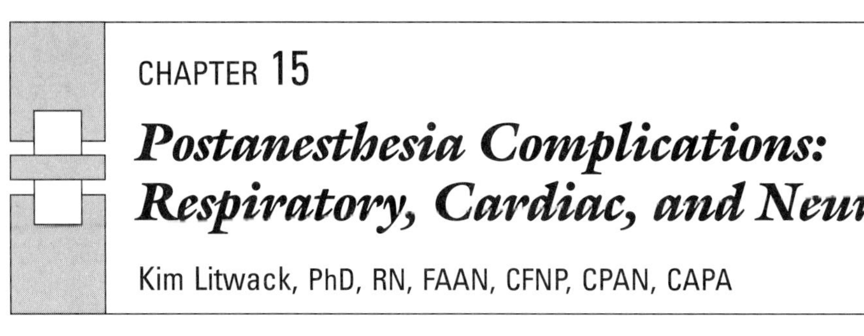

CHAPTER 15

# *Postanesthesia Complications: Respiratory, Cardiac, and Neurologic*

Kim Litwack, PhD, RN, FAAN, CFNP, CPAN, CAPA

## OBJECTIVES

**Study of the information represented by this outline will enable the learner to:**

1. Describe the common respiratory, cardiac, and neurologic emergencies seen in the postanesthesia care unit (PACU), including the following:
   a. A description of the emergency
   b. Signs and symptoms
   c. Risk factors
   d. Treatment
   e. Prevention

## RESPIRATORY COMPLICATIONS

### I. Airway Obstruction

A. Description: tongue, foreign body, or improperly placed airway falls into position that occludes pharynx, blocking flow of air in and out of lungs
B. Signs and symptoms
   1. Snoring
   2. Activation of accessory muscles
      a. Intercostal and suprasternal retractions
      b. Nasal flaring, especially in children
   3. Somnolence
C. Risk factors
   1. Anatomy: obesity, large neck, short neck, no jaw
   2. Poor muscle tone: narcotics, muscle relaxants, neuromuscular disease
   3. Swelling: anaphylaxis, surgical manipulation, edema
D. Treatment: Achieve a patent airway
   1. Stimulate patient
   2. Jaw thrust or chin lift
   3. Oral or nasal airway (correct placement if necessary)
   4. Reintubation with or without mechanical ventilation
   5. Pharmacologic reversal if indicated
E. Prevention
   1. Good intraoperative anesthetic and surgical management
   2. Ongoing assessment
   3. Judicious administration of narcotics
   4. Postoperative positioning in lateral position if patient is not awake

### II. Laryngospasm

A. Description: partial or complete spasm of laryngeal muscles blocking flow of air in and out of lungs

B. Signs and symptoms
   1. Agitation
   2. Decreased oxygen saturation
   3. If complete obstruction: absent breath sounds
   4. If partial obstruction: crowing sounds
   5. Stridor

C. Risk factors for airway irritation: may occur preoperatively, intraoperatively, or postoperatively
   1. Secretions
   2. Vomitus
   3. Blood
   4. Artificial airway placement
   5. Coughing
   6. Bronchospasm (asthma)
   7. Frequent suctioning
   8. Laryngoscopy
   9. Smoking history
   10. Traumatic or difficult intubation
   11. Exposure to pungent inhalational anesthetics
   12. Upper respiratory infection

D. Treatment
   1. Notify anesthesia provider
   2. Positive pressure ventilation with 100% oxygen
   3. Succinylcholine (subparalytic dose to relax laryngeal muscles)
   4. Steroids or lidocaine or both intravenously to decrease airway irritation and swelling

E. Prevention
   1. Hemostasis during surgery
   2. Suction oropharynx before extubation
   3. Minimize stimulation of extubation: extubate deep or when patient is awake
   4. Steroids and/or lidocaine to prevent or reduce airway irritation and swelling

## III. Hypoxemia

A. Description: $Pao_2$ <60 mm Hg

B. Signs and symptoms (all are nonspecific to hypoxemia and may be signs of other events)
   1. Agitation to somnolence
   2. Hypotension to hypertension
   3. Bradycardia to tachycardia and/or ventricular ectopy
   4. Oxyhemoglobin saturation <90%
   5. $Pao_2$ <60 mm Hg (blood gas)

C. Risk factors
   1. Inadequate oxygen concentration or delivery system
   2. Hypoventilation (decreased alveolar ventilation, increased $CO_2$)
      a. Risk factors
         (1) Decrease in central drive
            (a) Residual anesthetics
            (b) Loss of stimulation
            (c) Somnolence
         (2) Poor muscle tone
            (a) Abdominal surgery
            (b) Obesity
            (c) Neuromuscular disease
            (d) Residual anesthetics

b. Signs and symptoms
   (1) Low respiratory rate for age
   (2) Retention of $CO_2$
   (3) Hypoxemia
c. Treatment
   (1) Improve ventilation with stimulation to arouse
   (2) Remove cause if possible
   (3) Intubation and mechanical ventilation

3. Increased intrapulmonary shunting: atelectasis—*most common cause of postoperative hypoxemia* (causes right to left shunt)
   a. Risk factors
      (1) Bronchial obstructions
      (2) Secretions
      (3) Decreased lung volumes
      (4) Hypotension
      (5) Low cardiac output
   b. Signs and symptoms
      (1) Nonspecific signs of hypoxemia
      (2) Decreased breath sounds
      (3) Consolidation on chest x-ray
   c. Treatment
      (1) Humidified oxygen
      (2) Deep breathing
      (3) Increased mobility
      (4) Intermittent positive pressure ventilation (IPPV)
      (5) Incentive spirometry

## IV. Ventilation/Perfusion Mismatch

A. *Pulmonary edema:* increase in total lung water within interstitial spaces or in the alveoli. May occur as a result of an increase in hydrostatic pressure, decrease in interstitial pressure, or an increase in capillary permeability
   1. Risk factors
      a. Fluid overload
      b. Left-sided ventricular failure
      c. Mitral valve dysfunction
      d. Ischemic heart disease
      e. Sepsis
      f. Disseminated intravascular coagulation (DIC)
      g. Aspiration
      h. Anaphylaxis
      i. Transfusion reaction
      j. Naloxone administration in young adults (rare)
   2. Signs and symptoms
      a. Hypoxemia
      b. Rales on auscultation
      c. Decreased compliance
      d. Pulmonary infiltrates on chest x-ray film
   3. Treatment
      a. Remove or treat cause
      b. Maintain oxygenation
      c. Administer diuretics
      d. Maintain fluid restriction and intake/output records
      e. Consider afterload reduction

B. *Pulmonary embolism:* obstruction of pulmonary blood flow
  1. Risk factors
    a. Venous stasis
      (1) Immobility
      (2) Congestive heart failure (CHF)
    b. Hypercoagulability
    c. Abnormal blood vessel wall
      (1) Obesity
      (2) Elderly
      (3) Varicose veins
    d. Fat embolism
      (1) Pelvic or long bone fracture/surgery
      (2) Malignancy
  2. Signs and symptoms
    a. Acute onset of tachypnea
    b. Tachycardia
    c. Hypotension
    d. Hemoptysis
    e. Dysrhythmias
    f. Chest pain
    g. CHF
  3. Treatment
    a. Correct hypoxemia and hemodynamic instability
    b. IV heparin to achieve activated partial thromboplastin time (APTT) 1.5 to 2 times greater than control

C. *Aspiration* of foreign body, blood, or gastric contents
  1. Risk factors
    a. Loose teeth
    b. Surgical manipulation of oropharynx
    c. Obesity
    d. Pregnancy
    e. Hiatal hernia
    f. Peptic ulcer
    g. Trauma
  2. Signs and symptoms (depend on type of aspiration)
    a. Foreign body: cough, atelectasis, obstruction, bronchospasm
    b. Blood: minor airway obstruction, hypoxemia, hypercarbia
    c. Gastric contents: bronchospasm, hypoxemia, atelectasis, pulmonary edema
  3. Treatment (based on cause)
    a. Foreign body: removal
    b. Blood
      (1) Correct hypoxemia
      (2) Stop bleeding and restore airway patency
      (3) Possibly antibiotics if blood contained infected tissue
    c. Gastric contents
      (1) Correct hypoxemia
      (2) Maintain hemodynamic stability
      (3) Antibiotics if signs of infection develop
      (4) Steroid use is controversial
    d. NOTE: best treatment is prevention

D. *Bronchospasm:* increased bronchial smooth muscle tone resulting in airway closure
  1. Risk factors
    a. Aspiration

b. Tracheal and pharyngeal suctioning
c. Intubation
d. Histamine release
e. Allergic response
f. Chronic obstructive pulmonary disease (COPD), asthma
2. Signs and symptoms
a. Wheezing
b. Dyspnea
c. Use of accessory muscles
d. Tachypnea
3. Treatment
a. Decrease airway irritability
b. Promote bronchodilation through pharmacotherapy with $\beta_2$-agonist
c. Humidified oxygen

E. *Pneumothorax:* air in pleural space
1. Risk factors
a. Rupture of pleural bleb (COPD)
b. Positive pressure ventilation
c. Surgical chest procedures
d. Complication of central line placement
e. Complication of brachial plexus or intercostal nerve block
2. Signs and symptoms
a. Complaints of chest pain
b. Dyspnea
c. Decreased breath sounds on affected side
d. Hyperresonance on affected side
3. Treatment
a. If small (<20%) and patient is healthy: oxygen and observation
b. If larger or patient is compromised: chest tube placement and oxygen

## CARDIOVASCULAR COMPLICATIONS

**I. Hypotension**

A. Description: blood pressure <20% of baseline: clinical signs and symptoms more helpful than actual number

B. Signs and symptoms (hypoperfusion)
1. Initial compensation
a. Cool, clammy skin
b. Tachycardia
c. Tachypnea
2. Progressive fall in cardiac output
a. Disorientation, nausea, loss of consciousness
b. Chest pain, dysrhythmias
c. Oliguria, anuria, lactic acidosis

C. Risk factors
1. Hypovolemia (most common cause)
2. Primary myocardial dysfunction: myocardial infarction (MI), tamponade, embolism, dysrhythmias
3. Secondary myocardial dysfunction: negative inotropic and chronotropic medications
4. Low systemic vascular resistance: vasodilators, sepsis, spinal anesthesia, anaphylaxis

D. Treatment
1. Oxygen therapy
2. Evaluate and replace volume with fluid boluses

3. If myocardial dysfunction: coronary vasodilators, inotropic therapy, afterload reduction
4. Discontinue medications causing vasodilation
5. Vasoconstrictive medications to increase vascular resistance

E. Prevention
1. Attention to preoperative, intraoperative, and postoperative volume status
2. Ongoing monitoring and assessment
3. Titrating medications with myocardial or vasoactive effects

## II. Hypertension

A. Description: 20% to 30% increase above baseline blood pressure

B. Signs and symptoms
1. See description
2. Signs of sympathetic stimulation (see risk factors below)

C. Risk factors
1. Pain
2. Hypoxemia and hypercarbia
3. Distension of bowel, bladder, stomach
4. Hypothermia
5. History of preexisting hypertension
6. After revascularization (coronary artery bypass graft, abdominal aortic aneurysm repair, carotid endarterectomy)
7. Fluid overload
8. Preeclampsia
9. Pheochromocytoma
10. Autonomic hyperreflexia

D. Treatment
1. Alleviate cause
   a. Pain medication
   b. Correct respiratory compromise
   c. Catheter or nasogastric (NG) tube placement
   d. Rewarming
   e. Restart antihypertensive medications
   f. Fluid restriction and diuretics
2. Pharmacotherapy to directly reduce blood pressure
   a. Labetalol hydrochloride: peripheral vasodilator; slows heart rate
   b. Enalapril maleate: suppresses renin-angiotensin-aldosterone system
   c. Sodium nitroprusside: afterload reduction; vasodilator
   d. Hydralazine: relaxation of arterioles

E. Prevention
1. Address potential causes with prompt intervention
2. Patients to take routine antihypertensives on day of surgery with sip of water

## III. Dysrhythmias

A. Description: see rhythm strips in Chapter 16

B. Signs and symptoms: see rhythm strips in Chapter 16

C. Risk factors
1. Hypokalemia: wide QRS, premature ventricular contractions (PVCs), ventricular tachycardia, ventricular fibrillation
2. Hypoxia: atrioventricular dysrhythmias, conduction blocks
3. Hypercapnia: tachycardia, ventricular ectopy
4. Altered acid-base status: ventricular irritability
5. Circulatory instability: ventricular ectopy
6. Preexisting heart disease: myocardial ischemia
7. Hypothermia: AV block; sinus bradycardia, atrial or ventricular fibrillation
8. Vagal reflexes: severe sinus bradycardia

9. Anesthetic agents: junctional rhythm; bradydysrhythmias
10. Surgical stress: tachycardia
11. Pain: tachycardia
12. Hyperthermia: tachycardia
13. Hypovolemia: tachycardia

D. Treatment
1. Intervention directed toward underlying cause
2. See Chapter 16 for intervention according to ACLS protocols

E. Prevention
1. Avoid causes
2. Intervene to treat potential causes promptly

## IV. Bleeding

A. Description: loss of intravascular volume

B. Signs and symptoms
1. Presence of blood in drains, dressings, wounds, emesis
2. Hypotension resulting from hypovolemia
3. Compensatory tachycardia
4. Pain
5. Tight casts or dressings

C. Risk factors
1. Loss of vascular integrity
2. Alterations in coagulation
3. Surgical procedure associated with high blood loss

D. Treatment
1. Repair of bleeding vessels (return to operating room)
2. Volume replacement: usually not indicated to transfuse until hemoglobin <7 g or hematocrit <21% unless autologous blood is available or patient is symptomatic from blood loss
3. For alterations in coagulation, consider vitamin K, FFP, platelets

E. Prevention
1. Meticulous surgical care
2. Evaluation of coagulation profile before surgery
3. Discontinue anticoagulant therapy before surgery: aspirin, nonsteroidal anti-inflammatory drugs (NSAIDs), coumadin

## V. Chest Pain

A. Description: subjective complaint by patient of chest discomfort

B. Signs and symptoms
1. Subjective report of chest pain
2. Tachypnea
3. Tachycardia or other dysrhythmias
4. Hypotension

C. Risk factors (possible site of origin)
1. Cardiac: myocardial infarction, angina
2. Pulmonary: pneumothorax, pulmonary embolism, pneumonia
3. Gastrointestinal: reflux esophagitis, pancreatitis, cholecystitis, peptic ulcer
4. Musculoskeletal: rib fracture, costrochondritis
5. Miscellaneous: herpes zoster, anxiety

D. Treatment
1. *Always assume origin is cardiac until proven otherwise!!!*
2. Identify if patient has preexisting heart disease
3. Hemodynamic support
4. Obtain 12-lead electrocardiogram (ECG); compare with baseline ECG if available

5. Consider IV morphine titrated for pain
6. Continuous ECG monitoring
7. Administer antianginal or antidysrhythmic agents or both as indicated
8. Rule out pulmonary causes of pain

E. Prevention
1. Identify patients with preexisting heart disease
2. Maintain adequate oxygenation and hydration
3. Decrease myocardial work

## NEUROLOGIC COMPLICATIONS

**I. Emergence Delirium**

A. Description: responsive or unresponsive agitation

B. Signs and symptoms
1. Agitation
2. Disturbances in thought, orientation, attention, cognition

C. Risk factors
1. Hypoxemia or hypercapnia
2. Drug or alcohol withdrawal
3. Anesthetic agents: ketamine, droperidol
4. Adverse reactions to medications
5. Central anticholinergic syndrome: atropine, scopolamine
6. Metabolic disturbances: acid-base, electrolyte changes
7. Pain or anxiety
8. Visceral distension: bowel, bladder
9. Temperature alterations
10. Children more susceptible than adults

D. Treatment
1. *Always rule out hypoxemia as cause of agitation*
2. Patient and staff safety: restraints or sedation
3. Physostigmine for central anticholinergic syndrome

E. Prevention
1. Attention to oxygenation and ventilation
2. Inquire about alcohol or drug use preoperatively
3. Awareness of medications' side effects
4. Attention to potential causes

**II. Delayed Awakening or Failure to Awaken**

A. Description: lack of responsiveness or failure to return to baseline after administration of anesthetic

B. Signs and symptoms: lack of responsiveness, having allowed sufficient time for anesthetic metabolism and elimination

C. Risk factors
1. Prolonged drug effects (most common cause)
2. Neurologic injury: cerebrovascular accident (CVA), hypoxia
3. Hyperglycemia or hypoglycemia
4. Hypothermia: cold narcosis
5. Adrenal excess: Cushing's disease
6. Hypothyroidism
7. Organ failure

D. Treatment
1. Directed toward cause

2. Correction of acid-base and electrolyte disturbances
3. Evaluation of potential causes if specific cause is not identified, with review of anesthetic technique, patient history, laboratory values, intraoperative events
4. Supportive care

E. Prevention
1. Knowledge of patient baseline: neurologic status, laboratory results, history
2. Meticulous anesthetic delivery and care
3. Attention to drug and oxygen administration

## BIBLIOGRAPHY


Bines A, Landron S: Cardiovascular emergencies in the post anesthesia care unit. *Nurs Clin North Am* 28: 493–506, 1993.

Caplan R, Posner K, Ward R, et al: Adverse respiratory events in anesthesia: A closed claims analysis. *Anesthesiology* 72:828–833, 1990.

Drain C: *The Post Anesthesia Care Unit: A Critical Care Approach to Post Anesthesia Nursing*, 3rd Ed. Philadelphia, WB Saunders, 1994.

Fruth R: Differential diagnosis of chest pain. *Crit Care Nurs Clin North Am* 3:59–67, 1991.

Greenfield H: *Complications in Surgery and Trauma*. Philadelphia, JB Lippincott, 1990.

Herrick I, Mahendran B, Penny F: Postobstructive pulmonary edema following anesthesia. *J Clin Anesth* 2:116–120, 1990.

Leya C, Bandala, L: Respiratory complications. In Vender J, Spiess B (eds): *Post Anesthesia Care*. Philadelphia, WB Saunders, 1992.

Lipov E: Emergence delirium in the PACU. *Crit Care Nurs Clin North Am* 3:145–149, 1991.

Litwack K: Bleeding and coagulation in the PACU. *Crit Care Nurs Clin North Am* 3:121–127, 1991.

Litwack K: *Post Anesthesia Emergencies*. Philadelphia, RTN Healthcare Group, 1997.

Litwack K: *Postoperative Pulmonary Complications*. Sacramento, CME Resource, 1995.

Litwack K: *Post Anesthesia Care Nursing*, 2nd Ed. St. Louis, Mosby–Year Book, 1995.

Litwack K, Saleh D, Schultz P: Postoperative pulmonary complications. *Crit Care Nurs Clin North Am* 3:77–82, 1991.

Moser K: Venous thromboembolism: State of the art. *Am Rev Respir Dis* 141:235–249, 1990.

Pesola G, Kvetan V: Ventilatory and pulmonary problem management. *Anesthesiol Clin North Am* 8: 287–310, 1990.

Shub C: Stable angina pectoris: Clinical patterns. *Mayo Clin Proc* 64:234, 1990.

Sloan T: Postoperative central nervous system dysfunction. In Vender J, Spiess B (eds): *Post Anesthesia Care*. Philadelphia, WB Saunders, 1992.

Spiess B: Hemorrhagic disorders. *Anesthesiol Clin North Am* 8:441–492, 1990.

Spiess B: Hemorrhagic problems during the immediate postoperative period. In Vender J, Spiess B (eds): *Post Anesthesia Care*. Philadelphia, WB Saunders, 1992.

Tremblay D, Fischer R, Caouette C, et al: Arrhythmias in the PACU: A review. *Crit Care Nurs Clin North Am* 3:59–67, 1991.

Vender J, Spiess B: *Post Anesthesia Care*. Philadelphia, WB Saunders, 1992.


## REVIEW QUESTIONS

**1. The initial intervention for the patient presenting with laryngospasm is:**

A. 100 mg lidocaine intravenously
B. Positive pressure ventilation with 100% oxygen
C. 40 mg succinylcholine intravenously
D. 10 mg dexamethasone intravenously

**2. The patient at greatest risk for pulmonary embolism is:**

A. 45 years old, history of smoking and COPD, admitted for a cholecystectomy
B. 18 years old, 100 kg, admitted for a diagnostic laparoscopy
C. 70 years old, 50 kg, history of hiatal hernia, admitted for a cataract extraction
D. 80 years old, history of congestive heart failure, admitted for a hip pinning

**3. Aspiration of blood is characterized by:**
- A. Minor airway obstruction, hypoxemia, hypercarbia
- B. Cough, atelectasis, obstruction
- C. Bronchospasm, atelectasis, interstitial edema
- D. Tachypnea, dysrhythmias, chest pain

**4. Bronchospasm results from:**
- A. Pulmonary vasoconstriction
- B. Bronchodilation
- C. Increased bronchial smooth muscle tone
- D. Airway obstruction

**5. The most common cause of postoperative hypoxemia is:**
- A. Pulmonary edema
- B. Pulmonary embolism
- C. Atelectasis
- D. Excessive narcotic administration

**6. The most common cause of postoperative hypotension is:**
- A. Myocardial dysfunction
- B. Medication intolerance
- C. Hypovolemia
- D. Dysrhythmias

**7. Treatment of hypertension:**
- A. Requires intravenous antihypertensive medications
- B. Often depends on removal of the offending stimulus
- C. Requires suppression of parasympathetic stimulation
- D. Is not necessary because this is a normal postoperative finding

**8. Labetalol hydrochloride:**
- A. Relaxes arterial smooth muscle
- B. Is a peripheral vasodilator and slows heart rate
- C. Suppresses renin-angiotensin-aldosterone system
- D. Relaxes coronary artery smooth muscle

**9. Chest pain should always be considered:**
- A. To be of cardiac origin until proven otherwise
- B. To be a medical emergency
- C. To be a reaction to having been intubated
- D. To require transfer of patient to the intensive care unit

**10. The cause of emergence delirium should always be considered to be ______ until proven otherwise.**
- A. Increased intracranial pressure
- B. Medication intolerance
- C. A metabolic disturbance
- D. Hypoxemia

**11. The most common cause of delayed awakening in the PACU is:**
- A. Acute neurologic injury
- B. Prolonged drug effects
- C. Hypothermia
- D. Hypoglycemia

**ANSWERS:** 1. B, 2. D, 3. A, 4. C, 5. C, 6. C, 7. B, 8. B, 9. A, 10. D, 11. B

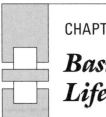

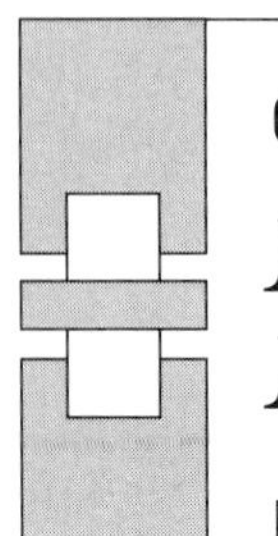

CHAPTER 16

# *Basic and Advanced Cardiac Life Support*

D. George Dresden, MSN, RN, CCRN

## OBJECTIVES

**Study of the information represented by this outline will enable the learner to:**

1. Understand basic life support (BLS) and airway management in emergency situations.
2. Identify life-threatening dysrhythmias.
3. Understand the pharmacotherapy of drugs used in emergency situations.
4. Identify the indications, precautions, and technique for defibrillation and cardioversion.
5. Be familiar with the American Society of Perianesthesia Nurses' (ASPAN's) *Standards of Nursing Practice* specific to advanced cardiac life support (ACLS) (see chapter appendixes).
6. Identify appropriate emergency drugs and equipment necessary in the postanesthesia care unit (PACU) for emergency care as identified by ASPAN.

I. **Basic Life Support—Airway Management and Cardiopulmonary Resuscitation (CPR)**
   A. Establish unresponsiveness
   B. Call for assistance; activate emergency system in your PACU
   C. Assess for breathing: look, listen, and feel
      1. If patient is not breathing, give two breaths over 2 seconds each (two puffs if an infant <1 year); child 1 to 8 years, use appropriately smaller volumes
         a. Bag-valve-mask (AMBU bag)
         b. Mouth to mask
         c. May be done mouth to mouth (not recommended)
         d. If an infant, both nose and mouth are covered
   D. Determine that airway is patent by observing chest movement
      1. If no movement noted, reposition airway and attempt to ventilate again; if unable to ventilate, suspect obstruction; attempt to remove obstruction by finger sweep of mouth, suctioning, and abdominal thrusts (For an infant, no finger sweep is used, and chest compressions replace abdominal compressions to relieve obstruction.)
   E. Once it is confirmed that patient is being ventilated, check for pulse (location: carotid artery in adults and children; brachial artery in infants); if pulse is present, ventilate patient once every 3 to 5 minutes; if pulse is not present, initiate CPR
   F. CPR: process of combining ventilation and external chest compression as means to reverse or prevent cardiac and/or respiratory arrest
      1. Ventilations are one breath every 3 to 5 minutes
      2. Chest compressions for one rescuer are given as 15 compressions to every 2 breaths at a rate of 100 compressions per minute
      3. Chest compressions for two rescuers (adult and child only) are given as 5 compressions to every 1 breath at a rate of 100 compressions per minute

## II. Arrhythmia Recognition*

A. Sinus bradycardia (Fig. 16–1)
   1. Description: characterized by decrease in heart rate caused by slowing of sinus node; may be a result of sinus node disease, increased parasympathetic tone, or drug effects (β-blockers, digitalis)
   2. ECG criteria
      a. Rate: <60 beats per minute (bpm)
      b. Rhythm: regular
      c. P waves: upright
   3. Treatment: if symptomatic, atropine, 0.5 to 1 mg intravenously (IV)

B. Pulseless electrical activity (PEA; electromechanical dissociation)
   1. Description: can be any rhythm on ECG (except VT/VF); however, no pulse and no blood pressure can be detected
   2. Frequent causes: remember the acronym MATCHED
      a. M: acute Myocardial infarction
      b. A: Acidosis
      c. T: Tension pneumothorax
      d. C: Cardiac tamponade
      e. H (×4): Hyperkalemia, or Hypoxemia, or Hypovolemia, or Hypothermia
      f. E: pulmonary Embolism
      g. D: Drug overdose
   3. Treatment
      a. CPR, 100% oxygen with immediate intubation
      b. Epinephrine, 1 mg IV every 3 to 5 minutes (may escalate)
      c. Consider and treat all possible causes
      d. Atropine 1 mg IV (only for bradycardic rhythms)

C. Ventricular tachycardia (Fig. 16–2)
   1. Description: three or more beats of ventricular origin in a row with a rate of greater than 100 bpm
   2. ECG criteria
      a. Rate: 100 to 220 bpm
      b. Rhythm: usually regular
      c. P waves: difficult to detect
      d. QRS complex: wide and bizarre

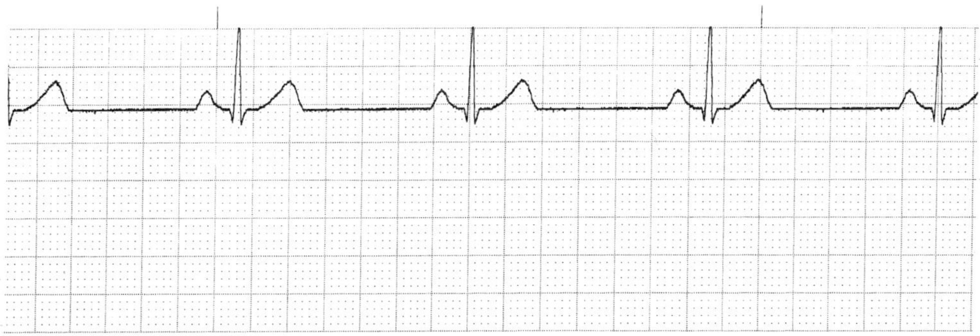

**FIGURE 16–1** Sinus bradycardia. (From Davis D: *Differential Diagnosis of Arrhythmias.* Philadelphia, WB Saunders, 1992.)

---

*NOTE: The electrocardiogram (ECG) treatment information given here summarizes accepted treatment as defined by the American Heart Association in current ACLS standards. The information given here is not intended to replace the ACLS manual, and therefore information is not given in algorithm format. The reader is encouraged to seek out the current American Heart Association manual or to become an ACLS provider.

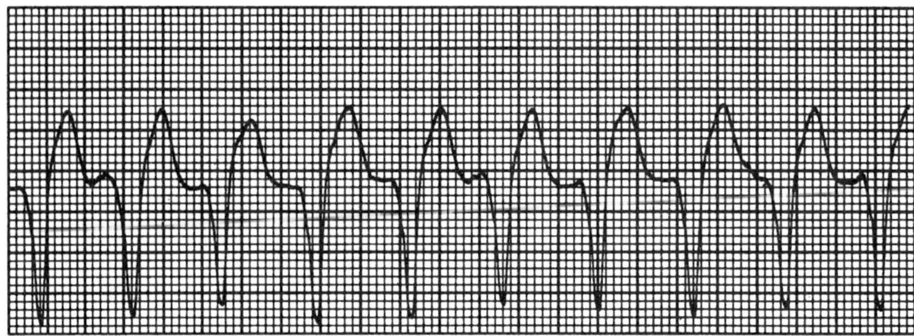

**FIGURE 16–2** Ventricular tachycardia. (From Davis D: *Differential Diagnosis of Arrhythmias.* Philadelphia, WB Saunders, 1992.)

3. Treatment
   a. Stable
      (1) Lidocaine, 1 mg/kg IV or by endotracheal (ET) tube
      (2) Procainamide if unsuccessful at 20 mg/min until ventricular tachycardia resolves, a total dose of 1 g has been given, the QRS widens by ≥50%, or hypotension occurs
      (3) Cardiovert if unstable
   b. Unstable: cardioversion—50, 100, 200 joules
   c. Pulseless: defibrillation—200, 300, 360 joules (treat as VF)

D. Ventricular fibrillation (Fig. 16–3)
   1. Description
      a. ECG with no organized rhythm

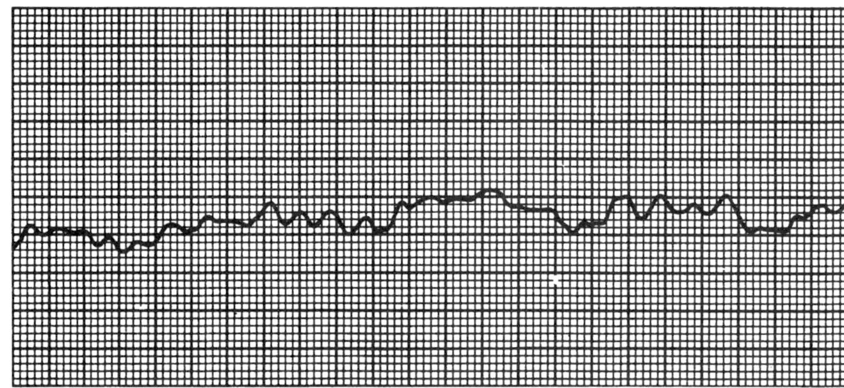



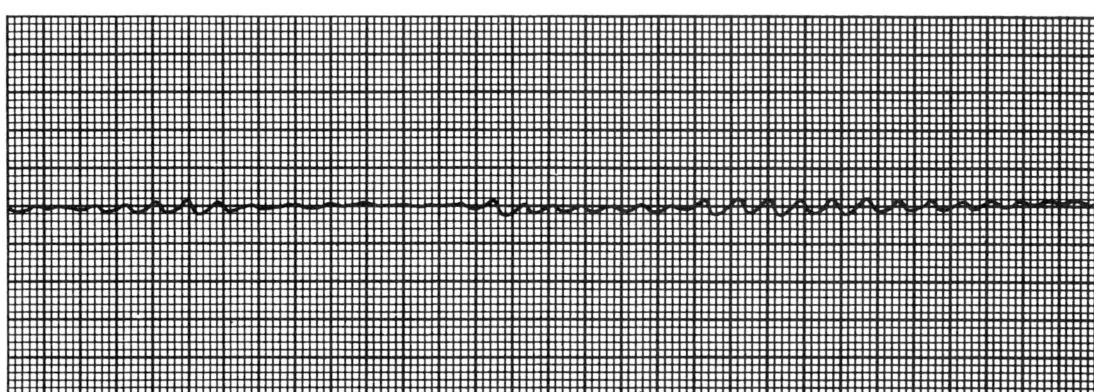



**FIGURE 16–3** **A,** Coarse ventricular fibrillation. **B,** Fine ventricular fibrillation. (From Davis D: *Differential Diagnosis of Arrhythmias.* Philadelphia, WB Saunders, 1992.)

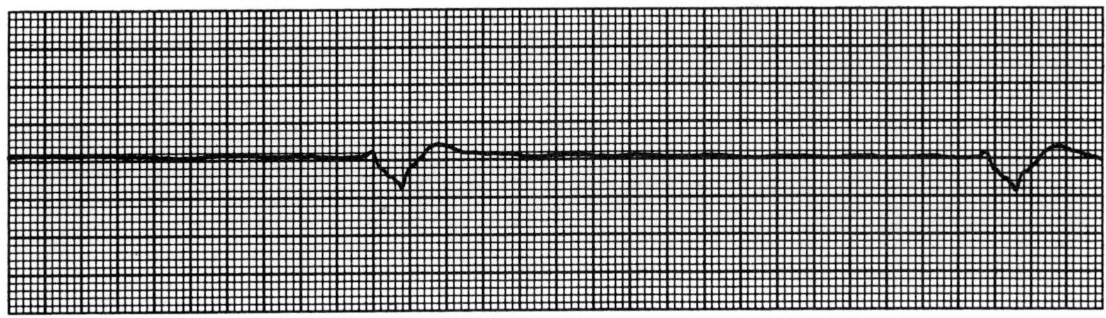

**FIGURE 16–4** Asystole. (From Davis D: *Differential Diagnosis of Arrhythmias.* Philadelphia, WB Saunders, 1992.)

   b. No cardiac output
   c. Coarse or fine refers to amplitude
2. ECG criteria
   a. Rate: rapid and too disorganized to count
   b. Rhythm: irregularly irregular
   c. No P wave, QRS complex, ST segment, or T wave
3. Treatment
   a. Immediate defibrillation: 200, 300, 360 joules
   b. Epinephrine, 1 mg IV or by ET tube (twice the IV dose)
   c. Intubate
   d. Defibrillate with 360 joules
   e. Lidocaine, 1 to 1.5 mg/kg IV or by ET tube (twice the IV dose)
   f. Defibrillate with 360 joules
   g. Epinephrine 1 mg IV (may escalate and repeat every 3 to 5 minutes)
   h. Defibrillate with 360 joules
   i. Bretylium, 5 mg/kg IV
   j. Defibrillate with 360 joules
   k. Repeat lidocaine (one half of initial dose) or bretylium (10 mg/kg)
   l. Defibrillate with 360 joules

E. Asystole (Fig. 16–4)
1. Description
   a. Total absence of ventricular electrical activity
   b. No pulse or blood pressure
2. ECG criteria: complete absence of activity; "flat line"
3. Treatment
   a. Rule out fine ventricular fibrillation by increasing gain on ECG monitor and checking in another lead
   b. Consider pacing
   c. Epinephrine, 1 mg IV or by ET tube (twice the IV dose)
   d. Intubate
   e. Atropine, 1 mg IV push or by ET tube (twice the IV dose)

F. Heart block (Fig. 16–5)
1. Description: delay in conduction
2. ECG criteria
   a. First-degree block
      (1) Regular rhythm
      (2) P wave followed by QRS
      (3) Prolonged PR interval (>0.20 sec)
      (4) QRS normal

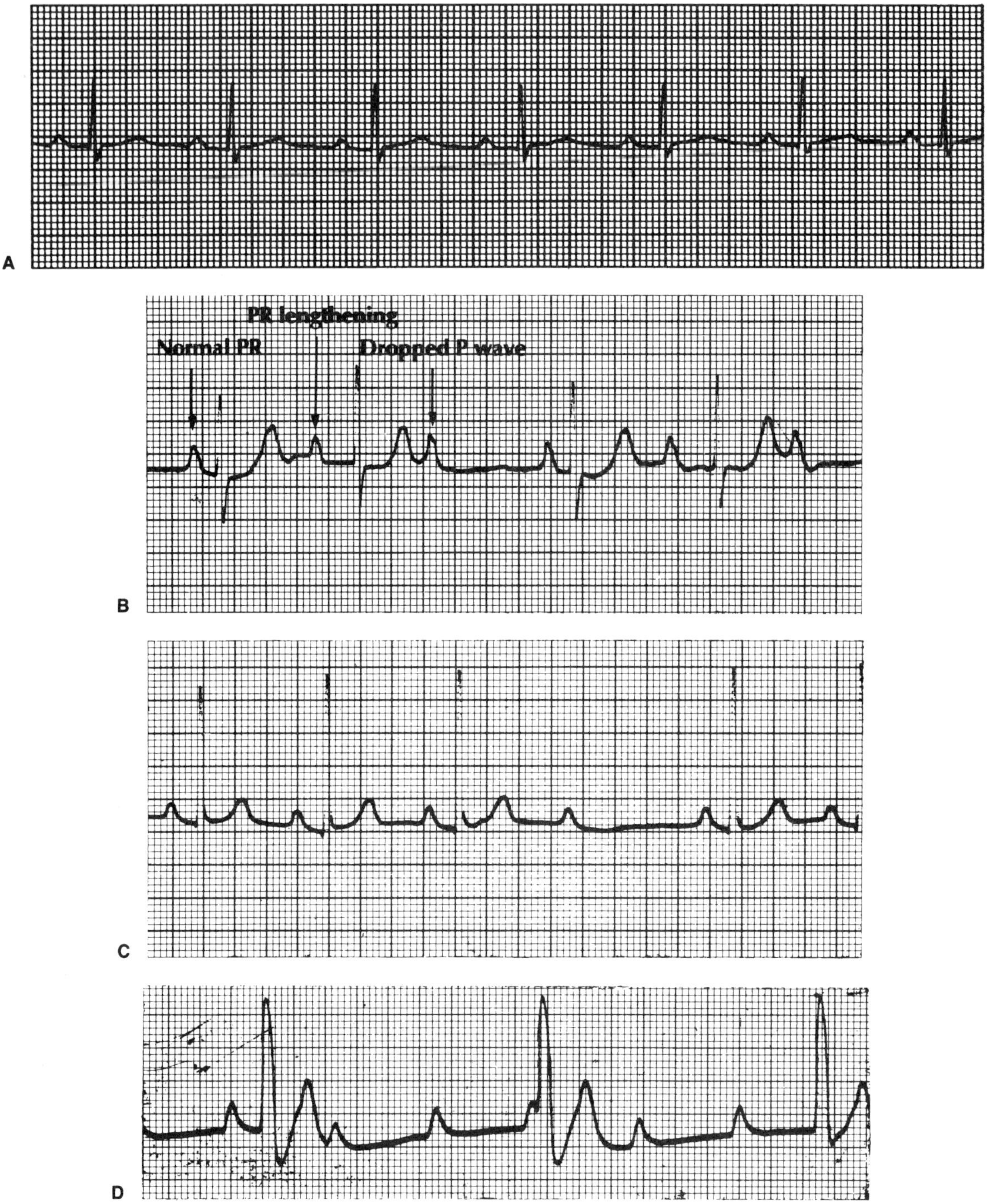

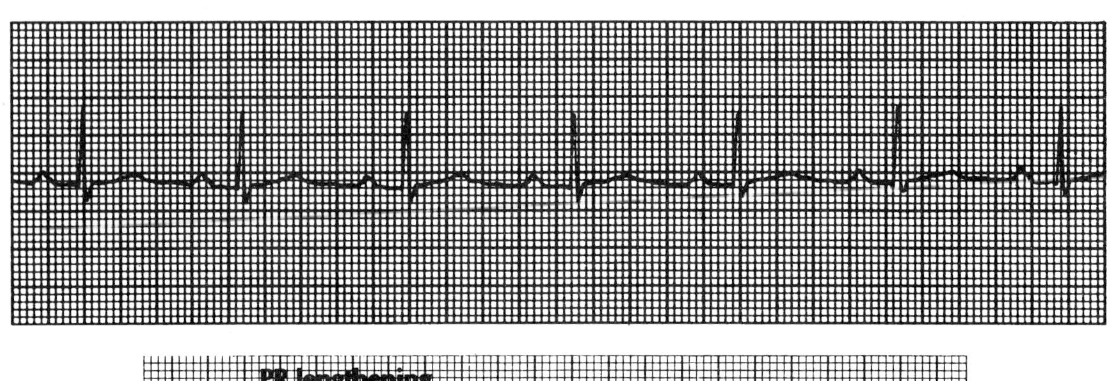


**FIGURE 16–5** **A,** First-degree AV block. **B,** Second-degree AV block, type I (Wenckebach). **C,** Second-degree AV block, type II (Mobitz). **D,** Third-degree AV block.

b. Second-degree type I Wenckebach block
   (1) Ventricular rate less than atrial rate
   (2) Rhythm usually irregular
   (3) P waves normal and followed by QRS except for dropped beat
   (4) PR interval gets progressively longer until beat is dropped
   (5) QRS normal

c. Second-degree type II Mobitz block
   (1) Ventricular rate less than atrial rate
   (2) Rhythm usually regular
   (3) P waves normal and PR interval consistent for conducted beats
   (4) Intermittent P wave not followed by a QRS: "march out" with those that are conducted
   (5) QRS normal
d. Third-degree block
   (1) Ventricular rate 40 to 60 bpm, atrial rate 60 to 100 bpm
   (2) P waves normal, QRS may be normal or widened
   (3) P waves and QRS unrelated to each other

3. Treatment
   a. First-degree: no intervention
   b. Second-degree type I
      (1) Stable: no intervention
      (2) Unstable: atropine, 0.5 to 1 mg IV or 1 to 2 by ET tube every 5 minutes to total of 2 mg (4 mg by ET tube)
   c. Second-degree type II
      (1) Stable: atropine, 0.5 to 1 mg IV or 1 to 2 by ET tube every 5 minutes to total of 2 mg (4 mg by ET tube)
      (2) Unstable: pacemaker (transcutaneous or transvenous)
   d. Third degree
      (1) Atropine, 0.5 to 1 mg IV or 1 to 2 by ET tube every 5 minutes to total of 2 mg (4 mg by ET tube)
      (2) Pacemaker (transcutaneous or transvenous)
      (3) Dopamine 5 to 20 μg/kg/min
      (4) Epinephrine 2 to 10 μg/min
      (5) Isoproterenol *(used very cautiously)*

## III. Defibrillation and Cardioversion

A. Defibrillation
   1. Indications
      a. Ventricular fibrillation—initial intervention
      b. Pulseless ventricular tachycardia—initial intervention
   2. Technique
      a. Confirm dysrhythmia
      b. Apply conductive gel to electrodes if necessary or use saline or gelled pads
      c. Turn on defibrillator
      d. Select energy level
         (1) Initial level is 200 joules for adult
         (2) Pediatric level, 1 to 2 joules per kilogram of body weight
      e. Charge defibrillator
      f. Apply paddles to chest
         (1) One paddle just below right clavicle on chest
         (2) One paddle to left of nipple in midaxillary line
         (3) Use 25 lb paddle pressure on both paddles
      g. Clear personal contact with patient—look!!
      h. Deliver countershock
      i. Evaluate rhythm
      j. Repeat as necessary; select energy level
         (1) If initial defibrillation was ineffective, increase to 300 joules
         (2) If second defibrillation was ineffective, increase to 360 joules (maximum)
   3. Precautions
      a. Know how defibrillator works in advance of need

b. Defibrillation most effective when done promptly
c. Clear area to avoid delivering shock to others
d. *Always confirm rhythm before and after shock*

B. Cardioversion
1. Indications
a. Treatment of choice for hemodynamically unstable tachydysrhythmias
(1) Ventricular tachycardia
(2) Supraventricular tachycardias
2. Technique
a. If patient is conscious, consider sedation or analgesia; provide explanation
b. Procedure is same as with defibrillation *except*
(1) Unit is set on synchronous mode
(2) Initial setting is 50 joules
(3) If unsuccessful, increase to 100 joules
(4) If unsuccessful, then increase to 200, then 300, and then 360 joules
c. If ventricular fibrillation occurs:
(1) Turn off synchronous mode
(2) Charge unit to 200 joules
(3) Defibrillate
3. Precautions
a. Same as with defibrillation
b. Recognition that ventricular fibrillation may occur
c. Confirm that mode of unit is synchronous

**IV. Pharmacologic Therapy for Life-Threatening Dysrhythmias***

A. Drug administration in emergency situation†
1. Know the drugs to be given; this is the principle of continuing education and ACLS repeat evaluation
2. IV drugs require circulation, either CPR or an effective, independent rhythm, and blood pressure of greater than 60 mm Hg systolic
3. IV drugs require an IV line; some require a central line; get IV access early in emergency situation in the largest vein possible
4. In absence of IV line, certain medications may be given by an ET tube, including naloxone, atropine, valium, epinephrine, and lidocaine (Some people remember these drugs with the acronym *NAVEL,* because this word is spelled by the first letters.)
5. If medications are given by an ET tube, they should be diluted into 10 ml of saline or distilled water, given as distally as possible, and followed with immediate AMBU bagging to force medications into lungs; double the IV dose when administering per ET tube
6. IV infusions of vasoactive medications recommend arterial line placement to monitor blood pressure changes
7. Route, dosage, and time of all medications given should be documented along with patient response and associated rhythm; use of an arrest record can facilitate documentation

---

*NOTE: The drugs selected for inclusion have been identified as being critical drugs by ASPAN in the *Standards of Perianesthesia Nursing Practice, 1998* (Resource 16). The drug information included is recommended by the American Heart Association.

†SPECIAL NOTE: The information provided in this section is not a substitute for ACLS course completion. It is provided as a reference only and therefore does not provide use of the drugs in the ACLS protocols or algorithms. The reader is encouraged to refer to the current American Heart Association manual or to attend an ACLS provider course.

B. Adenosine
  1. Mechanism of action
    a. Depresses AV and sinus node activity (supraventricular)
    b. Terminates reentry dysrhythmias (tachydysrhythmias)
  2. Indication: first line for narrow-complex supraventricular tachycardia (SVT)
  3. Dosage and route (in the most central vein possible)
    a. 6 mg rapid bolus over 1 to 3 seconds followed by 20 ml saline flush
    b. Repeat a 12 mg dose in 1 to 2 minutes
  4. Precautions
    a. Short half-life may result in recurrent SVT
    b. Less effective in patients taking theophylline

C. Amrinone
  1. Mechanism of action
    a. Positive inotropic agent without increasing myocardial oxygen consumption
    b. Cardiac output
    c. Preload and afterload
  2. Indication: congestive heart failure
  3. Dosage and route: 5 to 20 mg/kg/min IV after loading dose of 0.75 mg/kg bolus
  4. Precautions
    a. Hypotension
    b. Tachydysrhythmias
    c. Monitoring with central line is advised

D. Atropine sulfate
  1. Mechanism of action
    a. Parasympatholytic
    b. Increased automaticity
    c. Increased AV conduction
    d. Vagolytic
  2. Indications
    a. Initial treatment for symptomatic bradycardia
    b. May be beneficial in asystole after epinephrine
    c. May be beneficial in symptomatic bradycardia and bradycardic PEA
  3. Dosage and route
    a. 0.5 to 1 mg every 3 to 5 minutes IV or 1 to 2 mg by ET tube
    b. 0.04 mg/kg maximum dose (3 mg in 70 kg adult)
  4. Precautions
    a. Tachycardia that may result in ischemia or infarction
    b. Excessive dosing, ventricular fibrillation, or ventricular tachycardia

E. β-Blockers
  1. Mechanism of action
    a. Block effect of catecholamines on β-receptors
    b. Decrease heart rate, blood pressure, contractility
    c. NOTE: propranolol is a $\beta_1$- and $\beta_2$-blocker; metoprolol and atenolol are $\beta_1$-blockers (more selective)
  2. Indications
    a. Hypertension
    b. Angina pectoris
    c. Rapid supraventricular dysrhythmias
  3. Dosage and route
    a. Propranolol, 0.5 to 3 mg IV every 5 minutes (not >1 mg/min); maximum dose, 0.1 mg/kg
    b. Metoprolol, three 5 mg doses every 5 minutes over 2 minutes each; maximum dose, 15 mg
    c. Atenolol, 5 mg IV every 5 minutes times two doses

4. Precautions
   a. Hypotension, congestive heart failure
   b. Bronchospasm

F. Bretylium
   1. Mechanism of action
      a. Ventricular antidysrhythmic
      b. Decreases ventricular fibrillation threshold
      c. Decreases reentry phenomena
   2. Indications: ventricular dysrhythmias not responsive to lidocaine (because of adverse hemodynamic effects—not first choice antidysrhythmic)
   3. Dosage and route
      a. Initially 5 mg/kg IV, then 10 mg/kg every 15 to 30 minutes; maximum dose: 30 mg/kg
      b. Infusion: 2 g in 500 ml NS at 1 to 4 mg/min
   4. Precautions
      a. Postural hypotension
      b. Hypotension unresponsive to epinephrine
      c. Nausea and vomiting

G. Calcium channel blockers: diltiazem and verapamil
   1. Mechanism of action
      a. Inhibit cardiac smooth muscle activity
      b. Negative inotrope
      c. Decrease systemic vascular resistance
      d. Coronary vasodilation
   2. Indication: supraventricular tachycardia
   3. Dosage and route
      a. Diltiazem
         (1) 0.25 mg/kg followed by 0.35 mg/kg every 3 minutes
      b. Verapamil
         (1) 0.075 to 0.15 mg/kg IV over 1 minute (maximum, 10 mg)
         (2) In elderly patients, give over 3 minutes
         (3) Maintenance infusion: 5 to 15 mg/hr
         (4) Causes less myocardial depression
   4. Precautions
      a. Transient hypotension
      b. Potentiate β-blockers

H. Digoxin/digitalis
   1. Mechanism of action
      a. Increase myocardial contraction
      b. Increase atrial conduction
   2. Indications
      a. Atrial fibrillation
      b. Paroxysmal supraventricular tachycardia
      c. Congestive heart failure
   3. Dosage and route
      a. Emergency situation, give IV
      b. Nonemergency situation, oral
      c. Loading dose, 10 to 15 mg/kg
   4. Precautions
      a. Toxicity
         (1) Arrhythmias—all types
         (2) Nausea, vomiting, diarrhea

(3) Visual disturbances—yellow halos
(4) More common with hypokalemia, hypomagnesemia, and hypocalcemia

b. Treatment may require temporary pacemaker

I. Dopamine
1. Mechanism of action
   a. $\beta_2$-, $\alpha_1$-, and $\alpha_2$-agonist
   b. In low doses (2 to 5 mg/kg/min) dopamine causes vasodilation of renal, mesenteric, and cerebral arteries; urine output increases while blood pressure remains unchanged; in doses of 5 to 10 mg/kg/min, dopamine results in increased cardiac output ($\beta_1$ effects), peripheral vasoconstriction ($\alpha$ effects)
2. Indications
   a. Hemodynamically significant hypotension; systolic less than 90 mm Hg with signs of poor tissue perfusion
   b. Treatment of choice for cardiogenic shock
3. Dosage and route
   a. Infusion 400 or 800 mg in 250 ml $D_5W$
   b. Begin at 2 to 5 mg/kg/min
   c. Titrate to blood pressure, urine output, and signs of organ perfusion
4. Precautions
   a. Tachycardia may result in dysrhythmias
   b. Increases myocardial oxygen consumption at high doses
   c. Nausea and vomiting common
   d. Tissue necrosis if extravasation occurs
   e. Incompatible with sodium bicarbonate

J. Dobutamine
1. Mechanism of action
   a. Potent $\beta_1$-agonist
   b. Mild $\alpha$-agonist
   c. Increases cardiac output
   d. Increases peripheral resistance
   e. NOTE: effects of dobutamine have been compared to combining dopamine with nitroprusside
2. Indications
   a. Pulmonary congestion and low cardiac output
   b. Useful for patients who cannot tolerate low blood pressure
3. Dosage and route
   a. Infusion, 500 mg in 250 ml $D_5W$
   b. Begin at 2.5 mg/kg/min; titrate to effect
4. Precautions
   a. May cause tachycardia, arrhythmias
   b. Myocardial ischemia at high doses

K. Epinephrine
1. Mechanism of action
   a. Catecholamine with $\alpha$ and $\beta$ activity
   b. Increases systemic vascular resistance
   c. Increases blood pressure
   d. Increases heart rate
   e. Increases coronary and cerebral blood flow
   f. Increases myocardial contraction
   g. Increases myocardial oxygen consumption
   h. Increases automaticity
   i. Increases peripheral vasoconstriction

2. Indications
   a. Drug of choice in asystole, PEA
   b. Circulatory shock
3. Dosage and route
   a. 1 mg of 1:10,000 solution IV every 3 to 5 minutes
   b. Double dose by ET tube
   c. Infusion 4 mg/250 ml $D_5W$; start at 1 μg/min and titrate to effect
4. Precautions
   a. Not compatible with sodium bicarbonate
   b. Excessive effects can produce ischemia
   c. Excessive doses can cause hypertension
   d. May exacerbate ventricular ectopy, especially in patients taking digitalis

L. Lidocaine
1. Mechanism of action
   a. Suppresses ventricular dysrhythmias
   b. Elevates fibrillation threshold
   c. Local anesthetic properties
2. Indications
   a. Drug of choice with ventricular ectopy
   b. Ventricular fibrillation
   c. Ventricular tachycardia
   d. NOTE: treatment of premature ventricular contractions (PVCs) indicated when greater than 6/min, close coupled (R on T), multiformed, or occurring in runs
3. Dosage and route
   a. Initial: 1 to 1.5 mg/kg IV or by ET tube every 3 to 5 minutes
   b. Repeat doses: 0.5 to 0.75 mg/kg every 5 to 10 minutes
   c. Maximum dose: 3 mg/kg
   d. Infusion: 2 g/500 ml NS at 1 to 4 mg/min
4. Precautions
   a. Excessive doses → myocardial and circulatory depression
   b. Toxicity: drowsiness/disorientation/twitching
   c. Extreme toxicity → seizures

M. Magnesium sulfate
1. Mechanism of action
   a. Reduces SA node impulse formation
   b. Prolongs myocardial conduction time
2. Indications
   a. Hypomagnesemia
   b. Ventricular dysrhythmias: V-fib and V-tach (drug of choice for torsades de pointes)
   c. Symptoms of cardiac insufficiency
3. Dosage and route
   a. 1 to 2 g diluted in 100 ml $D_5W$ over 5 to 60 minutes
   b. Follow with infusion of 0.5 to 1 g/hr for up to 24 hours
4. Precautions
   a. Hypotension
   b. Asystole

N. Milrinone lactate
1. Mechanism of action
   a. Dose-dependent positive inotrope and vasodilator with minimal chronotropic response
   b. Decreases PCWP and SVR and increases CO
2. Indications
   a. Short-term management of CHF

3. Dosage and route
   a. IV infusion: 20 mg/180 ml NS
   b. Loading dose of 50 μg/kg over 10 minutes, then drip of 0.375 to 0.75 μg/kg/min
   c. Titrate to effect
4. Precautions
   a. Ventricular dysrhythmias
   b. Hypotension: arterial monitoring recommended
   c. Thrombocytopenia and hypokalemia

O. Morphine
1. Mechanism of action
   a. Analgesic
   b. Peripheral vasodilation
   c. Decreased venous capacitance → decreased pulmonary congestion
2. Indications
   a. Drug of choice for chest pain
   b. Acute cardiogenic pulmonary edema
3. Dosage and route: 2 to 10 mg IV every 5 to 30 minutes
4. Precautions
   a. Respiratory depression; reverse with naloxone
   b. Hypotension

P. Nitroglycerin
1. Mechanism of action
   a. Relaxes vascular smooth muscle
   b. Dilates coronary arteries
   c. Decreases systemic vascular resistance
2. Indications
   a. Drug of choice with angina pectoris/acute myocardial infarction (MI)
   b. Drug of choice with congestive heart failure
3. Dosage/route
   a. Sublingual with angina: 0.3 to 0.4 mg; may repeat in 5 minutes to three-dose total
   b. IV infusion: 50 mg in 250 ml $D_5W$; start at 10 to 20 mg/min and titrate to effect
4. Precautions
   a. Hypotension → ischemia of vital organs
   b. Bradycardia
   c. Recommended arterial line for infusion therapy
   d. Must be given by infusion pump

Q. Norepinephrine
1. Mechanism of action
   a. Positive inotrope
   b. $\beta_1$-agonist
   c. Increases myocardial contractility
   d. $\alpha_1$- and $\alpha_2$-agonist → vasoconstriction
2. Indication: hemodynamically significant hypotension that does not respond to epinephrine or dopamine
3. Dosage and route
   a. IV infusion: 1 mg/250 ml $D_5W$
   b. Begin at 2 μg/min
   c. Titrate to desired effect
4. Precautions
   a. Requires use of arterial line
   b. Increases myocardial oxygen needs
   c. May precipitate dysrhythmias
   d. Ischemic necrosis if extravasation occurs

R. Oxygen
  1. Mechanism of action
    a. Increases hemoglobin saturation
    b. Increases arterial oxygen tension
    c. Increases arterial oxygen content
    d. Improves tissue oxygenation
    e. Reduces extent of ST segment changes with MI
  2. Indications
    a. Acute chest pain secondary to ischemia
    b. Suspected hypoxemia of any cause
    c. Cardiopulmonary arrest
  3. Dosage and route
    a. If breathing spontaneously, nasal cannula or mask
    b. If not breathing, AMBU bag to mask or endotracheal tube and ventilator
  4. Precautions
    a. Oxygen toxicity with prolonged exposure to high oxygen concentrations
    b. Can diminish hypoxic respiratory drive in patients with chronic obstructive pulmonary disease (COPD)

S. Procainamide
  1. Mechanism of action
    a. Suppresses ventricular ectopy (may also suppress atrial dysrhythmias)
    b. Second-line therapy after lidocaine
  2. Indication: Suppressing PVCs and ventricular tachycardia not controlled with lidocaine
  3. Dosage and route
    a. 100 mg IV every 5 minutes at rate of 20 to 30 mg/min
    b. Given until dysrhythmia is suppressed, QRS complex widens by 50% of original width, hypotension develops, or total of 1 g of drug is given
    c. Infusion: 2 g in 500 ml NS at 1 to 4 mg/min
  4. Precautions
    a. Ganglionic blocker → vasodilation → hypotension
    b. Negative inotrope
    c. AV conduction disturbances

T. Sodium bicarbonate
  1. Mechanism of action: reacts with hydrogen ions to form water and $CO_2$ to buffer metabolic acidosis
  2. Indications
    a. *Only indicated after defibrillation,* effective CPR, intubation, hyperventilation with 100% oxygen, epinephrine, and lidocaine
    b. *Only indicated in documented metabolic acidosis and/or hyperkalemia*
  3. Dosage and route
    a. 1 mEq/kg initial dose
    b. Wait 10 minutes
    c. Repeat dose: 0.5 mg/kg
  4. Precautions
    a. In the past, sodium bicarbonate was drug of choice in resuscitation situations; now, as a result, the drug is often overused and used improperly.
    b. Sodium bicarbonate produces $CO_2$ and will worsen respiratory acidosis; $CO_2$ is also a negative inotrope; sodium bicarbonate causes oxyhemoglobin saturation curve to shift to left, decreasing oxygen release

U. Sodium nitroprusside
  1. Mechanism of action
    a. Arteriolar and venous vasodilator
    b. Afterload reduction

2. Indications
   a. Emergency treatment of hypertension
   b. Emergency treatment of heart failure
   c. Treatment of pulmonary congestion
   d. NOTE: frequently combined with dopamine for maximal effectiveness
3. Dosage and route
   a. IV infusion: 50 mg/250 ml $D_5W$
   b. Begin at 0.5 mg/kg/min; titrate to effect
4. Precautions
   a. Requires arterial line monitoring
   b. Can cause profound hypotension
   c. Hypotension can cause ischemia/infarction
   d. Elderly patients more sensitive to effects
   e. Metabolized to thiocyanate → cyanide toxicity
   f. Keep infusion protected from light (foil wrap)
   g. Must be given by infusion pump

## BIBLIOGRAPHY

American Heart Association: Guidelines for cardiopulmonary resuscitation and emergency cardiac care. *JAMA* 268(16):2171–2302, 1992.

American Heart Association: *Textbook of Advanced Cardiac Life Support.* Dallas, The Association, 1997.

American Society of Perianesthesia Nurses: *Standards of Perianesthesia Nursing Practice.* Thorofare, NJ, The Society, 1998.

Lester RM, Dente-Cassidy AM: *IV Medications for Critical Care,* 2nd Ed. Philadelphia, WB Saunders, 1996.

Taffet G, Teasdale T, Luchi R: In-hospital cardiopulmonary resuscitation. *JAMA* 260(14):2069–2072, 1990.

Vender J, Spiess B (eds): *Post Anesthesia Care.* Philadelphia, WB Saunders, 1992.

## REVIEW QUESTIONS

**1. You have arrived at the bedside 4 minutes after the cardiac arrest of a 100-pound man. Two other nurses are performing effective CPR and an IV is in place. The ECG monitor shows ventricular fibrillation. Your first priority should be to:**

A. Administer epinephrine, 0.5 mg by IV bolus
B. Administer lidocaine, 50 mg by IV bolus
C. Defibrillate with 200 joules
D. Intubate the patient

**2. Which of the following drugs when used in therapeutic doses directly depresses the contractility of the myocardium?**

A. Atropine
B. Isoproterenol
C. Lidocaine
D. Propranolol

**3. A 55-year-old man with a history of angina complains of chest pain. He is drowsy, his skin is cool and moist, and his heart rate is 45 bpm. His blood pressure is 86/60, and his ECG shows a high-grade AV block. The first drug to administer is:**

A. Atropine, 0.5 mg IV
B. Dopamine infusion, 5 mg/kg/min
C. Epinephrine, 0.5 mg IV
D. Isoproterenol, IV infusion at 2 mg/min

4. **You have been unsuccessful in the initial attempt to defibrillate a 70 kg adult. The recommended energy for the second attempt is:**
   A. 50 joules
   B. 100 joules
   C. 300 joules
   D. 360 joules

5. **During cardiac arrest the dose of epinephrine injected by the ET tube should be:**
   A. 0.5 ml of 1:1000 solution (0.5 mg)
   B. 1 mg of 1:1000 solution (1 mg)
   C. 10 ml of 1:10,000 solution (1 mg)
   D. 2 ml of 1:1000 solution (2 mg)

6. **Adenosine**
   A. Is capable of converting atrial fibrillation to normal sinus rhythm
   B. Decreases conduction time through the AV node
   C. Is given as a 1 mg IV bolus
   D. Is a long-acting choice for rate control of atrial flutter

7. **A bolus of sodium bicarbonate may be useful in the treatment of:**
   A. Hypoxic lactic acidosis
   B. PEA
   C. Hyperkalemia
   D. Asystole

8. **In stable ventricular tachycardia in a 70 kg patient, all of the following are end points for the administration of a procainamide loading infusion except:**
   A. A total of 1 g has been given
   B. Patient becomes hypotensive
   C. PR interval lengthens by more than 50%
   D. Rhythm converts to normal sinus

9. **Underlying causes of pulseless electrical activity include:**
   A. Tension pneumothorax
   B. Metabolic acidosis
   C. Massive pulmonary embolism
   D. All of the above

10. **Common adverse reactions to bretylium given IV include:**
   A. Respiratory depression and IV site pain
   B. Postural hypotension and vomiting
   C. Myocardial ischemia and chest pain
   D. Profound hypertension and tachycardia

**ANSWERS:** 1. C, 2. D, 3. A, 4. C, 5. D, 6. B, 7. C, 8. C, 9. D, 10. B

APPENDIX 16–1

# *Standard X Advanced Cardiac Life Support/ Pediatric Advanced Life Support (ACLS/PALS)*

**Standard:** Perianesthesia nursing practice involves autonomous decision-making and implementation of interventions in a crisis situation. Successful completion of an ACLS and/or PALS course or the equivalent is a necessary component to support this aspect of practice in Phase I.

**Rationale:** Postanesthesia care units are, by their nature, critical care units. The patient is in a very vulnerable stage of the perioperative course during the immediate postanesthesia period. Professional nurses with specific education, experience, and knowledge about the postoperative period can recognize and help manage anesthesia, surgery, and medically related complications. The competencies required are dictated by the patient population.

| *Structure Criteria* | *Process Criteria* | *Outcome Criteria* |
|---|---|---|
| 1. A job description for the professional nurse in Phase I includes a requirement for successful completion of an ACLS and/or PALS course or the equivalent educational process. | 1. Professional nursing staff successfully complete an ACLS and/or PALS course or the equivalent within six months of employment. | 1. Staff demonstrates competent management of emergency or critical situations. |
| 2. A mechanism exists for the provision of the educational requirements for an ACLS and/or PALS course or the equivalent educational process. | 2. Professional nursing staff participate, on a biannual basis, in the successful completion of an ACLS and/or PALS course or the equivalent educational process (see Resource 6).* | 2. Adequate opportunity for education exists. |
| 3. Policies and procedures, standing orders, and protocols direct the professional nurses' practice to respond to crisis situations. | 3. Professional nursing practice in Phase I reflects competency in ACLS and/or PALS or the equivalent educational process. | 3. Policies and procedures are congruent with competency levels. |

From American Society of Perianesthesia Nurses: *Standards of Perianesthesia Nursing Practice.* Thorofare, NJ, The Society, 1998.

*Excludes hands-on intubation experience.

APPENDIX 16–2

# Resource 6
# ACLS/PALS and Equivalent

In accordance to Standard X, an ACLS/PALS course and/or the equivalent is a necessary component to support PACU nursing practice in Phase I. Participation and completion should occur on a biannual basis.

The guideline that follows should be used in developing a program for your institution should they choose not to use the defined ACLS/PALS courses. Competence in this area must be documented and verified by the use of written tests and return demonstration with use of algorithms.

## GUIDELINES FOR ACLS EQUIVALENT PROGRAM

1. Advanced airway management
   a. Adult
   b. Pediatric
2. Identification and management of life threatening dysrhythmias
   a. Symptomatic bradycardia/heart blocks
   b. Pulseless electrical activity (PEA)
   c. Stable ventricular tachycardia
   d. Ventricular fibrillation/pulseless ventricular tachycardia
   e. Asystole
   f. Tachycardias including unstable ventricular tachycardia
   g. Hypotension, shock and pulmonary edema
   h. Acute MI
3. Pharmacologic therapy of life-threatening dysrhythmias
   a. Mechanism of action
   b. Indications
   c. Recommended dosage
   d. Route of administration
   e. Complications
   f. Drugs to be included
      (1) Adenosine
      (2) Atropine sulfate
      (3) Beta-blockers
      (4) Bretylium tosylate
      (5) Procainamide hydrochloride
      (6) Calcium chloride
      (7) Digoxin
      (8) Diltiazem hydrochloride
      (9) Dobutamine hydrochloride
      (10) Dopamine hydrochloride
      (11) Epinephrine hydrochloride
      (12) Lidocaine hydrochloride
      (13) Magnesium sulfate

(14) Morphine sulfate
(15) Nitroglycerin
(16) Norepinephrine bitartrate
(17) Oxygen
(18) Sodium bicarbonate
(19) Sodium nitroprusside
(20) Verapamil hydrochloride

4. Defibrillation and cardioversion, and external cardiac pacing
   a. Indications
   b. Precautions
   c. Technique

## GUIDELINES FOR PALS EQUIVALENT PROGRAM

Based on American Heart Association PALS Revision 8/97:

1. Advanced airway management
   a. Pediatric
2. Identification and management of life threatening dysrhythmias
   a. Symptomatic bradycardia
   b. Asystole and pulseless arrest
   c. Tachycardia with poor perfusion
3. Pharmacologic therapy of life threatening dysrhythmias
   a. Mechanism of action
   b. Indications
   c. Recommended dosage
   d. Route of administration
   e. Complications
   f. Drugs to be included
      (1) Adenosine
      (2) Atropine sulfate
      (3) Beta-blockers
      (4) Bretylium tosylate
      (5) Calcium chloride 10%
      (6) Digoxin
      (7) Dobutamine HCl
      (8) Dopamine HCl
      (9) Epinephrine HCl
      (10) Isoproterenol
      (11) Lidocaine HCl
      (12) Oxygen
      (13) Procainamide HCl (Pronestyl)
      (14) Sodium bicarbonate
4. Defibrillation, cardioversion and external cardiac pacing
   a. Indications
   b. Precautions
   c. Technique

---

From American Society of Perianesthesia Nurses: *Standards of Perianesthesia Nursing Practice.* Thorofare, NJ, The Society, 1998.

APPENDIX 16–3

# *Resource 7*
# *Emergency Drugs and Equipment*

**This list is not meant to be all-inclusive.**
**Refer to current ACLS and PALS protocols for dosing requirements.**

A. Adult
  1. Adenosine (Adenocard)
  2. Aminophylline
  3. Atropine sulfate
  4. Bretylium tosylate
  5. Calcium chloride
  6. Calcium gluconate
  7. Dextrose
  8. Diltiazem hydrochloride (Cardizem)
  9. Dopamine hydrochloride
  10. Epinephrine hydrochloride (Adrenalin chloride)
  11. Flumazenil (Romazicon)
  12. Furosemide (Lasix)
  13. Lidocaine hydrochloride
  14. Methylprednisolone sodium succinate (Solu-Medrol)
  15. Magnesium sulfate
  16. Naloxone hydrochloride (Narcan)
  17. Norepinephrine bitartrate (Levophed)
  18. Procainamide hydrochloride (Pronestyl)
  19. Propranolol hydrochloride (Inderal)
  20. Sodium bicarbonate
  21. Verapamil hydrochloride (Calan, Isoptin)

B. PALS Emergency Drugs
  Refer to current ACLS and PALS protocols for dosing requirements.
  AHA Guidelines 8/97
  1. Adenosine (Adenocard), 6 mg/2 ml vials/syringes
  2. Atropine sulfate: prefilled syringes 0.1 mg/ml (5 ml, 10 ml) or 1 mg/ml (1 ml)
  3. Bretylium 50 mg/ml (10 ml vial)
  4. Calcium chloride 10%: prefilled syringes 100 mg/ml (10 ml)
  5. Epinephrine HCl (Adrenalin): prefilled syringes 1:10.000 (0.1 mg/ml) 10 ml
  6. Epinephrine HCl (1:1000) should be available for ET and high dose IV infusion (1 mg/ml) syringes 1 ml, or vial 30 ml
  7. Dextrose 25% or 50 ml vial of $D_{50}$ and dilute
  8. Dopamine HCl 40 mg/ml (5 ml)
  9. Dobutamine HCl 25 mg/ml (10 ml) or 12.5 mg.ml (20 ml)
  10. Isoproterenol HCl: 0.2 mg/ml (5 ml)
  11. Lidocaine HCl 1%: prefilled syringes 10 mg/ml (5 ml), 20 mg/ml and vials 40 mg/ml, 100 mg/ml, 200 mg/ml
  12. Naloxone: vials 0.4 mg/ml (1 ml, 10 ml) or 1 mg/ml (2 ml)
  13. Norepineprine: for IV infusion only
  14. Sodium bicarbonate: prefilled syringes of 8.4% solution 1 mEq/ml (50 ml or 10 ml) or 0.5 mEq/ml of 4.2% (10 ml)

15. Sterile normal saline 10 ml vials (preservative free)
16. Sterile water 10 ml vials (preservative free)
17. TB or 1 cc syringes are necessary to mix meds

C. Emergency supplies
1. Portable defibrillator (adult and pediatric paddles)
2. External cardiac pacing
3. Defibrillator pads or gel
4. Electrodes (include pediatric and diaphoretic)
5. Gloves (sterile and nonsterile)
6. Personal protective equipment
7. Oral airways: assorted sizes including pediatric
8. Nasal airways: assorted sizes including pediatric
9. Laryngoscope
10. Extra bulb
11. Blades: straight and curved (include size appropriate for pediatrics)
12. Endotracheal tubes (various sizes including pediatric)
13. Stylet (adult and pediatric)
14. Magill forceps
15. Yankauer suction handle
16. Syringes: assorted sizes
17. Assorted needles
18. IV catheters
19. IV solutions: $D_5W$, NS/100 ml, 250 ml, & 500 ml
20. IV tubings: standard and infusion regulator
21. Central venous catheter (CVC) kit
22. Alcohol swabs
23. Betadine swabs
24. Tincture of benzoin
25. Sponges: sterile 4×4, 2×2
26. Medication labels
27. Cardiac arrest documentation forms
28. Arterial blood gas (ABG) kit
29. Tape

D. Additional pediatric needs
1. Assorted needles: 18-, 20-, 22-, and 25-gauge
2. Butterfly 25-gauge × 5/8 inch (winged infusion needle)
3. LP needles: 3 inch fine 19-, 20-, and 22-gauge
4. Minidrip tubing
5. Volume control chamber
6. Syringes: add TB & 50 ml
7. Arm restraints
8. Wrist restraints
9. Interosseous needles: 18-gauge

E. Sterile packs
1. Cutdown
2. Tracheostomy
3. Suture set
4. Emergency tonsil set
5. Pediatric: infant gauge tray with assorted feeding tubes
6. Central line

---

From American Society of Perianesthesia Nurses. *Standards of Perianesthesia Nursing Practice.* Thorofare, NJ, The Society, 1998.

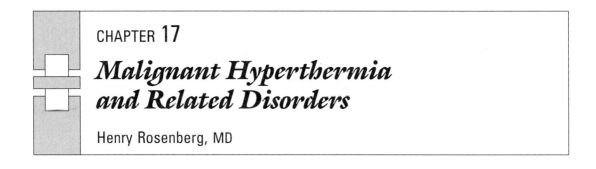

CHAPTER 17

# *Malignant Hyperthermia and Related Disorders*

Henry Rosenberg, MD

## OBJECTIVES

**Study of the information represented by this outline will enable the learner to:**

1. Describe the pathophysiology of malignant hyperthermia (MH).
2. Describe the drugs and situations that may trigger MH.
3. Identify patients at risk for MH.
4. Describe the signs of MH.
5. Describe the treatment of MH.
6. Be aware of available resources regarding MH.
7. Describe similarities and differences between MH and other potentially fatal disorders that may occur in the perioperative period

MH is a potentially fatal syndrome that can affect patients of all races and both sexes, particularly the young. It can occur in the operating room and later in the patient's postoperative course in the postanesthesia care unit (PACU). Particular vigilance is required by the postanesthesia nurse in detecting signs and symptoms of MH because serious morbidity and mortality can result from tardy or inadequate intervention. With prompt diagnosis and treatment, mortality from MH can be avoided in almost all cases.

## OVERVIEW

**I. Definition of MH**

- A. Pharmacogenetic disease of skeletal muscle
  - 1. Requires a drug to trigger syndrome
    - a. Potent inhalation anesthetic agents, such as halothane, enflurane, isoflurane, desflurane, or sevoflurane; nitrous oxide is not an MH trigger
    - b. Depolarizing muscle relaxants, such as succinylcholine
  - 2. Patient must have specific genes for MH to occur
    - a. Relatives of patient who has MH crisis are at risk (siblings, parents, children)
    - b. Inheritance by autosomal dominant pathway; risk diminishes as relationship to MH-susceptible person becomes further removed

**II. Manifestations of MH Syndrome**

- A. Hypermetabolism
  - 1. Increase in end tidal $CO_2$, typically doubled or tripled
  - 2. Tachycardia
  - 3. Tachypnea
  - 4. Cyanosis, mottling
  - 5. Respiratory and metabolic acidosis
  - 6. Muscle rigidity

7. High fever
8. Rhabdomyolysis
9. Coagulopathy a late sign

B. Increased level of intracellular calcium in skeletal muscle
1. Results from enhanced release of calcium from sarcoplasmic reticulum or other storage organelles within muscle cell
2. Sustained, elevated level of ionized calcium
   a. Causes continued muscle contraction
   b. Series of hypermetabolic reactions
      (1) Increases heat production
      (2) Increases membrane permeability

**III. Agents and Conditions That May Trigger or Sustain Episode of MH**

A. Inhalation anesthetic agents
1. Halothane
2. Enflurane
3. Isoflurane
4. Desflurane
5. Sevoflurane

B. Depolarizing muscle relaxant: succinylcholine

C. Environmental factor: increased environmental heat (?)

**IV. Incidence**

A. More common in children
1. Children: 1:15,000 anesthetics administered
2. Adults: 1:20,000 to 1:50,000 anesthetics administered

B. Many cases undetected
1. Never anesthetized
2. Short anesthetic period
3. Effects of triggering agent may be modified by preceding it with use of nontriggering agents, such as thiobarbiturates, nondepolarizing muscle relaxants, or hypothermia
4. Many cases mild, not diagnosed

**V. Prognosis**

A. Chances of successful treatment are good if early signs are recognized

B. Prognosis poorer if late signs appear

**VI. Mortality Significantly Reduced Since Availability of Dantrolene in Late 1970s**

A. Before 1970: 70%

B. 1976: 28%

C. 1987: 6% to 7%

D. Most deaths still occur in otherwise healthy children and adults

## PREOPERATIVE DETECTION

**I. History**

A. Patient with previous MH episode obviously at risk
1. 50% of patients with MH have had previous anesthesia without a problem

B. Family member who has had MH crisis provides warning of possibility

C. History of any family member who died during surgery and anesthesia should be a red flag

**II. Examination**

A. Usually reveals nothing
1. Patients with muscular dystrophy at special risk for anesthetic complications, i.e., hyperkalemic cardiac arrest

B. Muscle weakness and myopathies associated with MH-like syndromes
   1. Duchenne muscular dystrophy
   2. Central core disease
   3. Myotonia
   4. Other unusual myopathies

**III. Laboratory Tests**

A. Caffeine-halothane contracture test
   1. Most reliable test for preoperative diagnosis
   2. Few (about 10) hospitals in United States can perform this test
   3. Requires muscle biopsy
      a. Must be performed at one of the testing hospitals
      b. Cannot be mailed to testing center

B. No simple screening tests
   1. Creatinine phosphokinase (CK)
      a. Muscle enzyme
      b. Unreliable diagnostic test for MH
      c. 40% of MH patients have elevated CK
      d. 10% of normal people have elevated CK
      e. Other diseases produce elevated CK

## SIGNS AND SYMPTOMS

**I. Early Signs**

A. Muscle rigidity
   1. Masseter muscle spasm after administration of succinylcholine
      a. Intubation difficult
      b. Indication to cancel anesthesia immediately in elective cases
      c. Emergent cases may be carried out with nontriggering agents
   2. Generalized rigidity
      a. Definitive sign of MH
      b. Begin MH treatment immediately

B. Tachycardia and dysrhythmia
   1. Very consistent and early sign of MH crisis
   2. Premature ventricular contractions, bigeminy common
   3. Sudden cardiac arrest resulting from hyperkalemia after succinylcholine in patients with muscle diseases
   4. Very nonspecific sign

C. Cutaneous changes (inconsistent)
   1. Early generalized erythematous flush
      a. Skin feels warm
      b. Core temperature may be normal
   2. Later, skin becomes mottled followed by cyanosis

D. Tachypnea
   1. Results from increased $CO_2$ production
      a. If ventilation is controlled, increasing minute ventilation may mask rise of end tidal $CO_2$

E. Hyperkalemia
   1. Increased $PCO_2$
   2. Acidosis
   3. Cardiac changes noted above
   4. Results from muscle membrane breakdown

## II. Late Signs

A. Pyrexia
   1. Temperature elevation
      a. Hallmark of disease but often a late sign
      b. Develops early if succinylcholine and volatile anesthetics used
   2. Rate of increase may be 1° F/3 min
   3. Best measured by core temperature rise (e.g., nasopharyngeal, tympanic, bladder, rectal, axillary)
   4. Excessive heat production centered in skeletal muscle hypermetabolism

B. Coagulopathy
   1. Disseminated intravascular coagulation (DIC)
   2. Venipuncture sites begin to bleed
   3. Generally occurs after massive acidosis, marked hyperthermia a nonspecific sign

C. Rhabdomyolysis
   1. Result of muscle membrane breakdown
   2. Manifested first by brown or cola-colored urine
   3. Elevated levels of myoglobin in urine and serum
   4. Elevated CK levels (peak at 20 hours after event)

D. Left ventricular failure (usually terminal event)
   1. Pulmonary edema
   2. Rales
   3. Frothy sputum

E. Biochemical changes during MH
   1. Decreased pH secondary to $CO_2$ and lactic acidosis
   2. Increased $P_{CO_2}$ (marked increase in $CO_2$ production)
   3. Decreased $Pa_{O_2}$ (despite administration of 100% oxygen)
   4. Increased CK
   5. Increase in myoglobin in urine; hypercalcemia or hypocalcemia

## III. Sequelae to MH Crisis

A. Late diagnosis or unsuccessful treatment leads to death or permanent disability
   1. Central nervous system (CNS) damage
      a. Coma
      b. Convulsions
      c. Permanent CNS damage
         (1) Paralysis
         (2) Blindness
   2. Renal failure
      a. Myoglobinuria
         (1) Caused by breakdown of skeletal muscle
         (2) Clogs renal tubules, producing oliguria
   3. Recurrence of syndrome
      a. May recur several hours after initial successful treatment in as many as 25% of cases
      b. Patients must be monitored in an ICU and treated for at least 36 hours postoperatively
   4. Muscle edema/weakness
      a. Development of compartment syndrome

## TREATMENT AND PACU NURSING CONCERNS

**NURSING DIAGNOSIS**

Examples of related nursing diagnostic categories include:
- Altered thermoregulation
- Impaired gas exchange
- Decreased cardiac output
- Potential for altered tissue perfusion

**I. Initiate Immediate Treatment**

A. Discontinue anesthesia and surgery immediately
B. Administer 100% oxygen
C. Administer dantrolene (Dantrium) as soon as possible
  1. Dantrolene supplied in 20 mg vials and reconstituted with 60 ml preservative-free sterile water and shaking vigorously; warming bottle of solution may hasten mixing
  2. Recommended dose of dantrolene is 2.5 mg/kg body weight up to a total of 10 mg/kg; if syndrome not under control, even this limit may be exceeded. Administer by push initially. May be infused more slowly once syndrome under control
  3. Side effects of dantrolene include difficulty in walking, fatigue, muscle weakness, dizziness, blurred vision, nausea, and thrombophlebitis (late problems)

**II. Initiate Patient Cooling**

A. Intravenous (IV) infusion of iced sodium chloride (NaCl)
B. Surface cooling for all patients
  1. Ice packs to groin, axillae, head
  2. Cooling blankets
  3. Immersion in container of ice
C. Lavage stomach, bladder, and rectum with cold saline
D. Lavage peritoneal cavity with cold saline if open
E. Extracorporeal cooling by heart-lung machine in exceptional cases
F. Discontinue cooling interventions when body temperature decreases to 38° C
G. In almost all situations, treatment with dantrolene, discontinuation of anesthetic combined with surface, stomach, and bladder lavage will be effective

**III. Maintain Fluid and Electrolyte Balance**

A. Monitor arterial blood gases frequently
B. Monitor central venous pressure (CVP) or pulmonary artery catheter to guide fluid therapy as needed
C. Administer sodium bicarbonate as ordered to treat metabolic acidosis, 1 to 4 mEq/kg, on the basis of blood gas analysis
D. Use indwelling urinary catheter to monitor urine output
E. Administer IV fluids as ordered
F. Administer furosemide and mannitol as ordered
G. Administer glucose (or dextrose) and insulin as ordered for hyperkalemia

**IV. Monitor Cardiac Output**

A. Maintain continuous cardiac monitoring
B. Treat ventricular dysrhythmias with procainamide or lidocaine (do not use calcium channel blockers)

## V. Monitor Patient Status Continuously After MH Treatment

A. Repeat dantrolene every 4 to 6 hours either IV or orally for up to 48 hours
B. Monitor patient for 36 hours postoperatively in an ICU to detect possible recurrence of MH
C. Follow CK for several days until normalized

## VI. Preparation of PACU for MH Treatment

A. Maintain MH cart of all drugs and fluids required to treat acute MH episode (may share with operating room)
B. Keep clear instructions with MH cart at all times
C. Make sure MH treatment protocol is posted in highly visible place
D. Monitor and update education of every PACU nurse
E. Have dantrolene immediately available (not in locked cabinet or stored in pharmacy)
F. Have arterial blood gas (ABG) laboratory immediately available
G. Monitor temperatures of all PACU patients

## VII. Miscellaneous

A. Ambulatory patients who are MH susceptible and have undergone uneventful surgery may be discharged after 4 hours in PACU
B. Low levels of inhalation agents in the PACU (or OR) atmosphere do not trigger MH
C. For inpatients, prominently label the patients chart as *"MH risk—do not use succinylcholine"* because some MH patients who have required resuscitation have been given succinylcholine

## VIII. Syndromes Resembling or Mimicking MH

MH is one of several syndromes that are marked by muscle breakdown or other abnormalities on exposure to succinylcholine and/or inhalation agents. Although these syndromes share clinical features with MH, they are fundamentally different from MH and may require different treatment.

*Hyperkalemic Cardiac Arrest in Patients with Occult Myopathy*

A. Duchenne muscular dystrophy: X-linked disorder, therefore a syndrome of males. Onset is between age 2 and 8 years with muscle weakness progressing to death by late teens
   1. Patients with muscular dystrophy who are too young to manifest signs of the disease may develop sudden, catastrophic hyperkalemia if given succinylcholine and/or a potent inhalation agent, which manifests as ventricular tachycardia and ventricular fibrillation; mild muscle rigidity and fever may also occur
   2. Sometimes patients with muscular dystrophy may have catastrophic hyperkalemia develop after anesthesia with inhalation agents only, without succinylcholine
      a. The first manifestation may be cardiac arrest in PACU
   3. Diagnosis
      a. Sudden cardiac arrest in a child or young adult with no cardiac or pulmonary risk factors after anesthesia with succinylcholine and/or potent inhalation agents strongly suggests hyperkalemic arrest
      b. Draw specimens for blood gas and potassium
   4. Treatment
      a. Glucose and insulin, plus bicarbonate given intravenously
      b. For acute situations with ventricular tachycardia, calcium chloride or gluconate may be needed to prevent progression to ventricular fibrillation
   5. Follow-up
      a. Evaluation by neurologist; muscle biopsy
B. Neuroleptic malignant syndrome: A disorder occurring in as many as 1.5% of patients receiving antipsychotic medications (e.g., clonazepine); *not* inherited; syndrome may occur during any time of therapy; usually occurs in hospital ward or as an outpatient
   1. Signs and symptoms; signs similar to MH:
      a. Fever

b. Muscle tone increased
c. Acidosis
d. Rhabdomyolysis
e. Mental status changes
f. Tachycardia, hyper/hypotension
2. Treatment:
a. Cooling
b. Dantrolene
c. Bromocriptine (a dopamine agonist)
d. Symptomatic therapy
3. Testing
a. No diagnostic test available
4. Miscellaneous
a. Electroshock therapy sometimes used for patients who cannot take phenothiazines

C. Endocrine disturbances
1. Thyrotoxicosis
a. Fever, tachycardia, hypertension, agitation, sometimes acidosis are cardinal signs
b. When occurring after anesthesia, may be confused with MH. However, no rigidity, little to no acidosis, no myoglobinuria
2. Pheochromocytoma (the great mimicker)
a. Hypertension, tachycardia, fever may be presenting signs. Crisis may be precipitated by anesthesia and surgery for unknown reasons
b. Some patients may present with unexpected pulmonary edema after anesthesia
c. Dantrolene is of little or no value
d. Do not treat with beta blockers only
e. Diagnosis very difficult acutely, requires urinary metanephrine levels, plasma catecholamine assays, and MRI

D. Hypoxic brain damage
1. Periods of hypoxia, such as after cardiac arrest, can lead to hyperthermia in PACU because of hypothalamic dysfunction
2. Opisthotonic posturing and/or seizures occur
3. Patient usually fails to awaken
4. Dantrolene may help with treatment of fever, but not specific
5. Muscle enzymes (CK) may be elevated because of seizures, posturing
Diagnosis requires high suspicion, CT scan
6. Treatment: mannitol, steroids

E. Ascending tonic/clonic syndrome: A rare syndrome occurring after radiologic contrast agent injected into CSF for myelogram. Occurs usually with water-soluble contrast agent
1. Signs:
a. Jerking movements of muscles in legs progress to whole body tonic activity
b. Patient loses consciousness and seizures develop. Seizures lead to hyperthermia.
c. Signs usually begin within 1 to 2 hours of myelogram
2. Treatment is support of ventilation and vital signs. Dantrolene may help keep temperature normalized, but not a specific treatment
a. High mortality if not recognized and treated aggressively

## IX. Make Use of Available Support Services

A. Malignant Hyperthermia Association of the United States (MHAUS), 32 South Main Street, Sherburne, New York (phone: 607-674-7901 or 1-800-98-MHAUS), Fax: 607-674-7910
E mail: *mhaus@Norwich.net*
Web site: *http://www.mhaus.org*
NMS web site: *http://www.nmsis.org*

1. A note to this organization will get a large treatment protocol poster for your PACU
2. Telephone hotline: 1-800-MH HYPER; call any time day or night for treatment advice

B. Report MH event to the North American MH Registry, division of MHAUS (same address)

## BIBLIOGRAPHY


Drain C, Christoph S: *The Recovery Room: A Critical Care Approach to Post Anesthesia Nursing*, 2nd Ed. Philadelphia, WB Saunders, 1987.

Frederick C, Rosemann D, Austin M: Malignant hyperthermia: Nursing diagnosis and care. *JOPAN* 5:29–32, 1990.

Greenberg C: Diagnosis and treatment of hyperthermia in the postanesthesia care unit. *Anesth Clin North Am* 8:377–397, 1990.

Larach MG, Localio AR, Allen GA, et al. A clinical grading scale to predict malignant hyperthermia susceptibility. *Anesthesiology* 80:771–779, 1994

Larach MG, Rosenberg H, Gronert GA, Allen GC: Hyperkalemic cardiac arrest during anesthetics in infants and children with occult myopathies. *Clin Pediatr* January: 9–18, 1997.

Litwack-Saleh K: Practical points in the management of malignant hyperthermia. *JOPAN* 7:327–329, 1992.

Newberry J: Malignant hyperthermia in the postanesthesia care unit: A review of current etiology, diagnosis, and treatment. *JOPAN* 5:25–28, 1990.

Pessah IN, Lynch C, Gronert GA: Complex pharmacology of malignant hyperthermia. *Anesthesiology* 84: 1275–1279, 1996.

Rosenberg H, Fletcher JE, Seitman, D: Pharmacogenetics. In Barash P, Cullen B, Stoelting R (eds): *Clinical Anesthesia,* 3rd Ed. Philadelphia, JB Lippincott, 443–460, 1992.


## REVIEW QUESTIONS

**1. Malignant hyperthermia may be triggered by what drug?**

A. Pancuronium (Pavulon)
B. Succinylcholine
C. Fentanyl
D. Sodium pentothal

**2. Excessive levels of what intracellular electrolyte begin malignant hyperthermia?**

A. Potassium
B. Sodium
C. Glucose
D. Calcium

**3. If when interviewing a patient preoperatively you discover the patient's brother died in surgery of unknown causes, should you consider this patient a potential candidate for malignant hyperthermia?**

A. Yes
B. No

**4. The most reliable laboratory test for detecting malignant hyperthermia is:**

A. Creatinine phosphokinase
B. Caffeine/halothane contracture test
C. Cardiac enzymes
D. Serum electrolytes

**5. What signs and symptoms are an early indication of a malignant hyperthermia crisis?**

A. Increased end tidal $CO_2$, tachycardia
B. Cyanosis, muscle rigidity
C. Mottled skin, fever
D. Pulmonary edema, seizures

**6. The drug of choice for treatment of malignant hyperthermia is:**

A. Pancuronium (Pavulon)
B. Lidocaine
C. Dantrolene
D. Sodium bicarbonate

**7. The recommended initial dose of dantrolene is:**

A. 1 mg/kg
B. 10 mg/kg
C. 2.5 mg/kg
D. 25 mg/kg

**8. The first intervention in the PACU for the patient with suspected malignant hyperthermia is:**

A. 100% oxygen
B. Decrease IV fluid rates
C. Draw serum electrolytes
D. Apply ice packs

**9. How long should malignant hyperthermia candidates be intensively monitored after successful treatment of an MH episode?**

A. 2 to 3 days
B. 12 hours
C. 36 hours
D. 3 to 4 hours

**10. A young male has a cardiac arrest after being admitted to the PACU after an uneventful halothane anesthetic. The initial temperature is 38° C and the patient is breathing satisfactorily before the arrest. What diagnosis should is most likely?**

A. Myotonic dystrophy
B. Malignant hyperthermia
C. Anaphylaxis
D. Muscular dystrophy

**11. Which is true regarding MH and ambulatory surgery?**

A. Ambulatory surgery is contraindicated
B. Dantrolene pretreatment is necessary for all ambulatory MH patients
C. May only be conducted where there is a 24-hour recovery room
D. There is no contraindication on the basis of MH susceptibility only

**ANSWERS:** 1. B, 2. D, 3. A, 4. B, 5. A, 6. C, 7. C, 8. A, 9. C, 10. D, 11. D

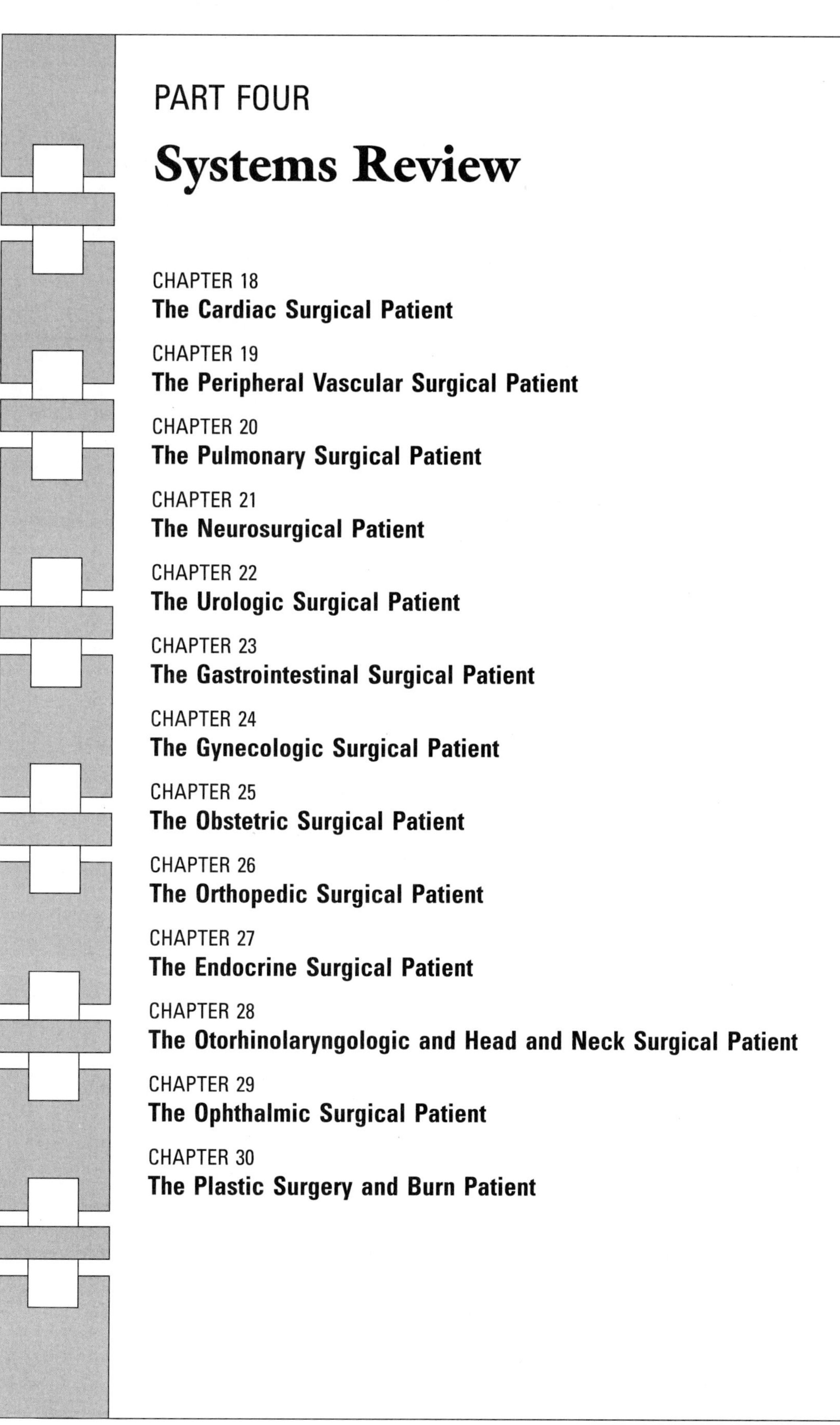

PART FOUR

# Systems Review

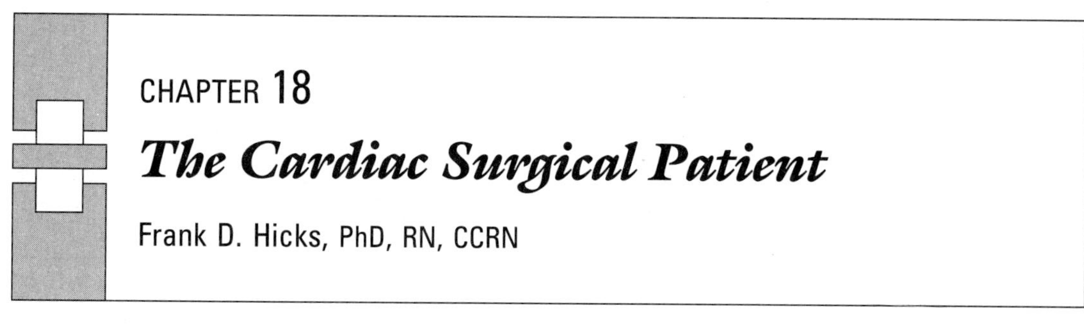

CHAPTER 18

# The Cardiac Surgical Patient

Frank D. Hicks, PhD, RN, CCRN

## OBJECTIVES

**Study of the information represented by this outline will enable the learner to:**

1. Explain the interrelationship of preload, afterload, contractility, and heart rate in the determination of cardiac output.
2. Identify and explain the effects of congenital heart defects on the hemodynamics of the cardiovascular system.
3. Explain the effects of atherosclerosis on the coronary arteries.
4. Identify risk factors associated with coronary artery disease.
5. Identify complications that may result from coronary artery disease.
6. Explain the diagnostic studies used to examine the cardiovascular system.
7. Describe and interpret hemodynamic monitoring and values.
8. Identify psychosocial concepts that are applied to the nursing care plan for the cardiovascular surgical patient.
9. Explain the goals of preoperative teaching for the cardiovascular surgical patient.
10. Identify the operative procedures for each of the following: congenital heart defects, coronary artery disease, valvular heart disease.
11. Describe the preoperative assessment of the cardiovascular surgical patient.
12. Relate assessment findings to the selection of anesthetics to be used during the surgical procedure.
13. Compare and contrast the intraoperative management of the adult cardiac patient vs. the pediatric cardiac patient.
14. Implement the nursing process for a postoperative cardiovascular patient in the postanesthesia care unit (PACU).
15. Identify basic cardiac dysrhythmias that may occur after cardiac surgery and identify possible causes and treatments.
16. Identify the use of and management of a patient with a pacemaker in the PACU after cardiac surgery.
17. Identify the use of and management of a patient with an intraaortic balloon pump (IABP).

Intelligent care of the postoperative cardiovascular patient depends on a thorough understanding of the concept of oxygenation. The primary concern when caring for a patient in the early postoperative phase is to maximize oxygen delivery to body tissues and to minimize the oxygen consumption (i.e., work load) of the heart. This requires a sound understanding of normal cardiac physiology (Figs. 18–1 to 18–3), pathophysiology, pharmacology, and psychosocial aspects of postoperative nursing care. Although much progress has been made with respect to the care of these challenging patients in the past two decades, the knowledge base and assessment skills of the nurse are the primary determinants of positive outcomes after surgery.

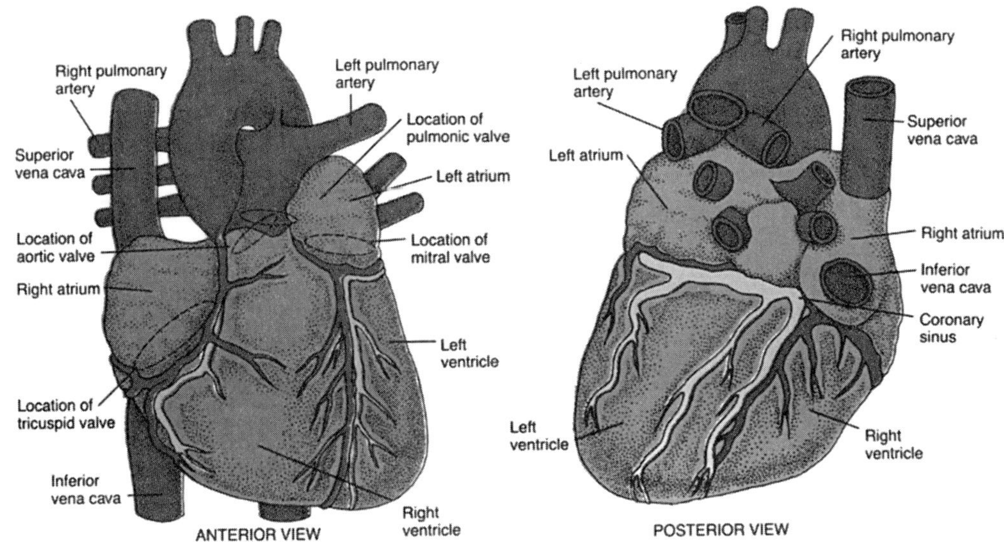


**FIGURE 18–1** Surface anatomy of heart. (From Ignatavicius DD, Bayne MV: *Medical-Surgical Nursing: A Nursing Process Approach* [p 2068]. Philadelphia, WB Saunders, 1991.)

## REVIEW OF CARDIAC PHYSIOLOGY: FOUNDATIONS OF ADEQUATE OXYGEN DELIVERY

### I. Cardiac Determinants of Oxygen Delivery

A. Cardiac cycle consists of two major periods

1. Systole (ventricular contraction): occurs when ventricular pressure exceeds vascular pressure (pulmonic and aortic) and respective valves open, tricuspid and mitral valves close
   a. Results in ejection of blood out of ventricles into vasculature

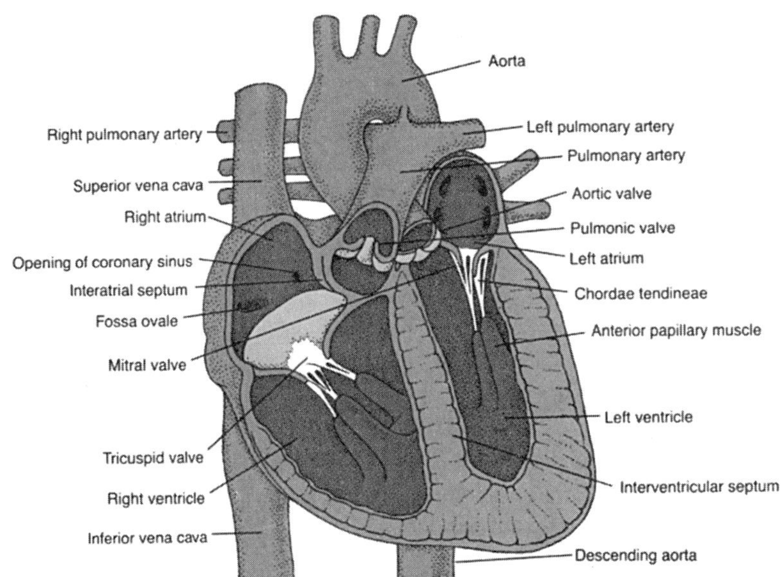


**FIGURE 18–2** Cross-section of heart. (From Ignatavicius DD, Bayne MV: *Medical-Surgical Nursing: A Nursing Process Approach* [p 2068]. Philadelphia, WB Saunders, 1991.)

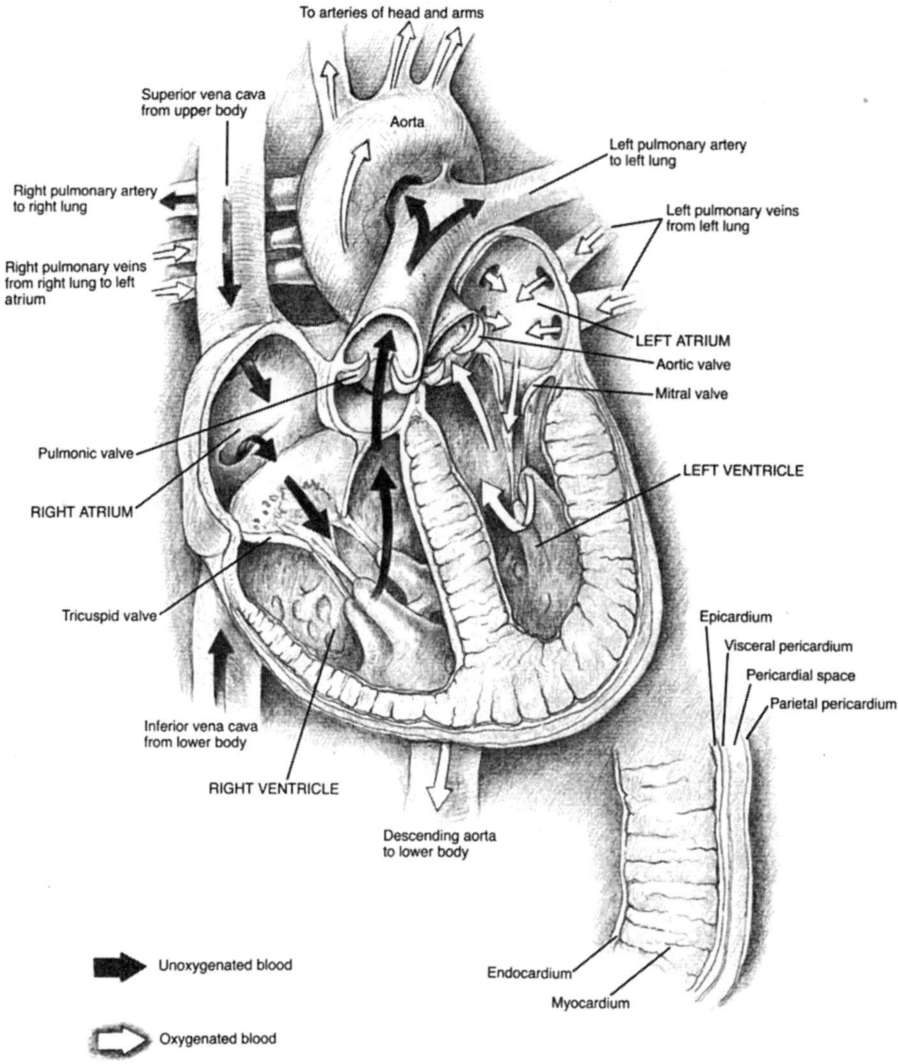


**FIGURE 18–3** Blood flow through heart. (From Ignatavicius DD, Bayne MV: *Medical-Surgical Nursing: A Nursing Process Approach* [p 2071]. Philadelphia, WB Saunders, 1991.)

b. Comprises approximately one third of cardiac cycle
c. Is assisted through atrial contractions just before beginning of systole; atrial kick can add as much as 30% to cardiac output

2. Diastole (ventricular relaxation): occurs when ventricular pressure is less than vascular pressure; tricuspid and mitral valves open so ventricles fill, pulmonic and aortic valves close
   a. Blood flows passively into ventricles until last third of diastole, when atrial kick occurs
   b. Comprises about two thirds of cardiac cycle
   c. Allows for ventricular filling and myocardial tissue perfusion

B. Determination of cardiac output (hemodynamics)
   1. Stroke rate; under control of
      a. Sympathetic nervous system (epinephrine): increases rate
      b. Parasympathetic nervous system (acetylcholine): decreases rate
      c. Increased heart rate (>130) decreases diastolic filling time and myocardial perfusion
      d. Decreased heart rate (<50 but can vary) decreases cardiac output

2. Stroke volume; determined by
   a. Preload: end-diastolic ventricular pressure; related to venous return; controls "stretch" of myocardial fibers
      (1) As preload increases, stretch increases and contractility improves to a point
      (2) High preload (i.e., increased volume) can lead to overstretch and result in decreased contractility (Starling's law)
   b. Afterload: resistance to ejection of blood from heart; increased from
      (1) Peripheral: constriction of arterioles
      (2) Ventricular outflow: valve stenosis
      (3) Ventricular diameter: congestive heart failure (CHF)
      (4) Blood viscosity: increased hematocrit (higher concentrations of red blood cells increase resistance along blood vessels)
   c. Contractility: physiologic parameters needed for actin/myosin coupling; affected by
      (1) Temperature: decreased with hypothermia
      (2) Calcium: decreased with hypocalcemia
      (3) pH: decreased with acidosis
      (4) Cellular changes: decreased with CHF, cardiomyopathy

## PATHOPHYSIOLOGY

**I. Congenital Heart Disease**

A. Malformation of heart or its associated blood vessels during fetal life
   1. Incidence: about 1% of live births
   2. Three major types
      a. Stenosis: obstruction to blood flow
      b. Left-to-right shunt: blood flows directly from left side of heart, or aorta, to right side of heart, or pulmonary artery, bypassing systemic circulation
      c. Right-to-left shunt: blood flows from right side of heart, or pulmonary artery, directly into left side of heart, or aorta, bypassing lungs

B. Left-to-right shunts
   1. Patent ductus arteriosus (PDA)
      a. Accounts for about 10% of all types of congenital heart disease; 1/2000 full-term live births
      b. Backward flow of blood from aorta (high pressure) to pulmonary artery (low pressure) through open ductus arteriosus
         (1) Failure of ductus arteriosus to close during early months of life
      c. High pulmonary pressures caused by pulmonary congestion lead to increased right ventricular afterload, resulting in right ventricular hypertrophy
      d. Left ventricular hypertrophy results from increased pumping requirements of left ventricle (two or more times cardiac output)
      e. Diastolic murmur present (machinery murmur)
         (1) Best heard over pulmonic area (left second intercostal space close to sternum)
      f. Corrective surgical procedure: ligation or ligation and division of ductus arteriosus
   2. Ventricular septal defect (VSD)
      a. Accounts for about 29% of congenital heart defects
      b. Hole in ventricular septum
         (1) May vary in size
         (2) Results in blood flow from left to right ventricle
      c. Increase in right ventricular volume (increased preload) and pressure results in hypertrophy
      d. Physical examination
         (1) Right ventricular hypertrophy

        (2) Systolic murmur of VSD shunt
        (3) Presternal thrill
    e. Chest film
        (1) Right ventricular hypertrophy
        (2) Pulmonary artery enlargement
        (3) Left atrial and left ventricular enlargement
    f. Corrective surgical procedure: patch closure of defect
3. Atrial septal defect (ASD)
    a. Constitutes 7% of congenital heart defects
    b. Communicating defect
        (1) Between left and right atria
        (2) Results in blood flow from left to right atrium
    c. Three types of defects classified by location
        (1) Ostium primum ASD: located at base of interatrial septum
        (2) Ostium secundum ASD: large interarterial communication (most common type)
        (3) Sinus venosus ASD: located high on developing interatrial septum (least common type)
    d. Patients usually asymptomatic; surgery done to prevent development of pulmonary hypertension that could lead to right ventricular failure
    e. Clinical findings
        (1) Cardiac catheterization demonstrates increased oxygen content in right atrium
        (2) Chest film reveals right ventricular enlargement and prominent main pulmonary artery
    f. Corrective surgical procedure: suture or patch closure of defect

C. Right-to-left shunts
1. Tetralogy of Fallot
    a. Accounts for about 10% of congenital heart defects
    b. Composed of four anatomic defects
        (1) VSD
        (2) Aorta overriding VSD
        (3) Right ventricular outflow obstruction: pulmonic stenosis
        (4) Right ventricular hypertrophy
    c. Presence of cyanosis depends on amount of right ventricular outflow obstruction and degree of right-to-left shunting caused by obstruction
    d. Corrective surgical procedure
        (1) Aortopulmonary shunt for palliation
        (2) Patch closure of VSD
        (3) Right ventricular outflow reconstruction
2. Other right-to-left shunts
    a. Complete transposition of great vessels
        (1) Aorta arises from right ventricle
        (2) Pulmonary artery arises from left ventricle
    b. Total anomalous pulmonary venous return
        (1) No pulmonary veins enter left atrium
        (2) Anomalous common pulmonary venous channel formed
        (3) ASD also present

D. Obstruction to blood flow
1. Valvular pulmonic stenosis
    a. Accounts for approximately 10% of patients with congenital heart disease
    b. Thickening of valve with fusion of leaflets at their commissures, narrowing pulmonary outflow tract
    c. Poststenotic dilatation of pulmonary artery
    d. Right ventricular hypertrophy (increased afterload of right ventricle)

e. VSD or ASD may also be present
f. Cardiac catheterization defines level of obstruction and identifies other lesions
g. Corrective surgical procedure: pulmonary valvotomy

2. Valvular aortic stenosis
a. Accounts for 5% to 10% of congenital heart disease
b. May be present with PDA, coarctation of aorta, or both
c. Normal aortic valve is tricuspid, whereas stenotic valve is most commonly bicuspid with narrowing of aortic outflow
d. Increase in left ventricular volume (preload) and pressure (afterload) results in hypertrophy
e. Physical examination
(1) Different blood pressure between two arms
(2) Systolic thrill
(3) Systolic ejection murmur
(4) Tachypnea
(5) Tachycardia
(6) Cyanosis with severe stenosis
f. Corrective surgical procedure: aortic valvotomy

3. Coarctation of aorta
a. Accounts for 5% to 8% of congenital heart disease, with male/female ratio of 2:1
b. May be present with PDA, valvular aortic stenosis, VSD, and other left-sided lesions
c. Localized narrowing of aortic lumen (usually at ligamentum arteriosum) presents as two types of coarctations
(1) Preductal (infantile): upper body supplied by left ventricle and lower body supplied by right ventricle through ductus arteriosus
(2) Postductal (adult): left ventricle supplies upper body and collaterals develop in utero through intercostal and internal mammary arteries to supply lower body
d. CHF may occur in early infancy because of increased left ventricular afterload and increased arteriolar resistance (peripheral resistance)
e. Physical examination
(1) Preductal coarctation: CHF, cyanosis, diminished pulses in lower body
(2) Postductal coarctation: acyanotic, upper extremity hypertension, diminished pulses in lower body, midsystolic ejection murmur, leg pain with exercise, fatigability, and headaches
f. Corrective surgical procedure: patch angioplasty or resection with end-to-end anastomosis

E. Effects on hemodynamics
1. Elevated preload (volume overload) from ASD or VSD
2. Elevated afterload (pressure overload) from obstruction to outflow of blood from heart; results in increased oxygen demand for ventricle
3. Desaturation decreases blood oxygen content

F. Signs and symptoms
1. Cyanosis
a. Shunting of unoxygenated blood into left side of heart: tetralogy of Fallot
b. Poor oxygen uptake: CHF, pulmonary edema
2. Tachypnea
a. Physiologic response to low oxygen content in blood
b. Precipitated by mild exercise
3. Effort intolerance
a. Inability of infant to tolerate feedings; respiratory distress
b. Fatigue with activity, inability to keep up with other children
4. Failure to thrive
a. Usually indicates left-to-right shunt or CHF
b. Growth retardation, inability to gain weight

5. Miscellaneous findings
   a. Frequent upper respiratory infections with ASD or PDA
   b. Headaches and leg pains with activity: coarctation of aorta
   c. Chest pain on exertion, fainting: aortic stenosis
   d. Clubbing of fingers, hypoxic episodes: tetralogy of Fallot

**II. Coronary Artery Disease (CAD)**

A. Definition: narrowing or total occlusion of arterial lumen characterized by accumulation of lipids, fibrous tissue, and calcium deposits in arterial wall

B. Risk factors
1. Nonmodifiable
   a. Age: increased incidence in those over 50 years
   b. Sex: higher incidence in males than premenopausal females (risk equalizes after menopause)
   c. Heredity: family history of premature atherosclerosis
   d. Diabetes mellitus
2. Modifiable
   a. Hyperlipidemia: elevated serum cholesterol and triglycerides
   b. Dietary habits: diet high in calories, fats, salt
   c. Obesity
   d. Hypertension
   e. Cigarette smoking
   f. Stressful environments/lifestyles
   g. Sedentary lifestyle
   h. Oral contraceptives
   i. High levels of homocysteine from increased intake of folate

C. Angina pectoris: chest pain associated with myocardial ischemia
1. Results from imbalance between oxygen supply and oxygen demand to myocardium
   a. Oxygen supply limited with reduction of coronary blood flow as in narrowing of coronary arteries by plaque (CAD) or with coronary artery spasm
2. Factors affecting myocardial oxygen delivery
   a. Factors increasing demand
      (1) Hypertension (increased afterload)
      (2) Increased blood volume (increased preload)
      (3) Dysrhythmias: tachydysrhythmias, including tachycardia
      (4) Increased contractility
      (5) Increased metabolism (fever, thyrotoxicosis)
   b. Factors decreasing oxygen supply
      (1) Decreased blood pressure (hypovolemia)
      (2) Peripheral vasodilation
      (3) Increased left ventricular diastolic pressure (CHF)
3. Precipitants
   a. Physical activity and exercise (most common)
   b. Emotional excitement and stress
   c. Eating heavy meals
   d. Exposure to cold
   e. Sleep (nocturnal angina)
   f. Chemical irritants and smoking
   g. Pain (postoperative)
   h. Stress of surgery
4. Characteristics
   a. Duration: lasts 1 to 5 minutes and subsides when precipitating factor removed
   b. Described as heaviness in chest, squeezing, burning, aching, or tightness

c. Location: usually precordial, middle, or lower sternum; may radiate to jaw, neck, shoulder, arm, or hand, usually on left side
d. May be accompanied by dyspnea, diaphoresis, nausea, vomiting, general fatigue
e. Subsides with rest
f. Usually relieved with nitroglycerin within 30 to 90 seconds; no relief may indicate that pain is not cardiac in origin or infarct pain

5. Classification
   a. Stable angina
      (1) Associated with characteristic onset, duration, location, radiation, and quality of pain
   b. Vasospastic (Prinzmetal's)
      (1) Associated with anginal pain at rest that is cyclic and unrelated to effort
      (2) Discomfort longer in duration than stable angina
      (3) Results from coronary artery spasm
      (4) Usually does not result in myocardial ischemia
   c. Unstable angina (Preinfarction)
      (1) Increased frequency, intensity, duration of pain, and/or change in character of pain from previous experiences with angina
      (2) May signify impending infarction
6. Noninvasive management
   a. Identify and reduce modifiable risk factors
   b. Reduce myocardial oxygen demand
      (1) Preload reduction
      (2) Afterload reduction
      (3) Reduction of contractility (only if left ventricular function is adequate)
   c. Improve oxygen delivery with calcium channel blockers
   d. Diagnostic studies to evaluate and confirm cardiac disease
7. Invasive management
   a. Percutaneous coronary transluminal angioplasty (PTCA)
   b. Laser angioplasty
   c. Coronary artery bypass grafting (CABG)
   d. Intraaortic balloon counterpulsation (IABP)
   e. Atherectomy
   f. Stent placement

## III. Myocardial Infarction (MI)

A. Definition: sustained myocardial ischemia resulting in death of myocardial tissue because of oxygen deprivation
B. Causes
   1. Atherosclerosis of coronary arteries (most common cause)
   2. Coronary artery embolism (thrombi, fat, air, calcium deposits)
   3. Coronary artery spasm
   4. Imbalance of myocardial oxygen demand vs. supply such as seen in cocaine abuse, thyrotoxicosis
C. Location described by affected wall of heart
D. Types
   1. Nontransmural infarction (subendocardial): affects heart's inner lining (endocardium)
   2. Transmural infarction: full-thickness myocardial necrosis extending through entire ventricular wall (from endocardium to pericardium)
E. Symptoms
   1. Chest pain
      a. Occurs suddenly
      b. Severe crushing quality
      c. Usually substernal, radiating across chest to arms

   d. More intense than anginal pain
   e. Constant pain unrelieved by nitroglycerin or rest
   f. Duration usually 20 to 30 minutes or longer
2. Nausea and vomiting
3. Dyspnea and weakness
4. Diaphoresis
5. Anxiety, apprehension, feeling of doom
6. Dysrhythmias
7. Noncardiac chest pain characterized by
   a. Location generally not substernal
   b. Radiation may differ
   c. Generally less intense
   d. May be relieved by antacids
   e. Generally not described as pressure-like
   f. Precipitating factors not consistent with cardiac presentation

F. Diagnostic findings
1. History reflective of MI
   a. Type, location, duration of pain and associated symptoms
   b. History of angina
   c. Family history of CAD
   d. History positive for other risk factors
2. Electrocardiogram (ECG) changes: pattern of ischemia progressing to infarction
   a. ST segment depression and T-wave inversion indicate possible ischemia
   b. ST segment elevation indicates pattern of injury
   c. Q-wave appearance (more than 0.03 second in width) indicates pattern of necrosis and becomes definitive diagnosis of infarction
3. Physical assessment reveals one or more of following
   a. Inspection
      (1) Dyspnea or shortness of breath
      (2) Anxiousness, feeling of doom
      (3) Cyanosis
      (4) Diaphoresis
      (5) Cool skin
   b. Palpation
      (1) Thrills: turbulent blood flow produces vibrations
      (2) Heaves: pronounced lifting sensation when palpating chest wall
      (3) Point of maximal impulse (PMI) may shift caudally and laterally
   c. Auscultation
      (1) Crackles
      (2) Gallop rhythms ($S_4$, maybe $S_3$)
      (3) Murmurs
      (4) Precordial friction rubs (Usually late; related to postinfarction pericarditis [Dressler's syndrome])

G. Laboratory findings: elevated cardiac enzymes (Table 18–1)

H. Complications
1. Dysrhythmias: number one complication within first 2 hours after infarction
2. CHF, pulmonary edema
3. Cardiogenic shock
4. Conduction defects
5. Thromboembolism
6. Pericarditis
7. Ventricular aneurysm
8. Myocardial rupture
9. Papillary muscle rupture, mitral insufficiency

**TABLE 18–1 Cardiac Enzyme Activity after Myocardial Infarction**

| ENZYME | ONSET OF ELEVATION (HR) | PEAK ELEVATION (HR) | RETURN TO NORMAL (DAYS) |
|---|---|---|---|
| Troponin I (cTnI)* normal <3.1 ng/ml | Within minutes | 1 | 7–10 |
| CK 12–80 u/L males; 10–70 u/L females | 3–6 | 12–24 | 24–48 |
| CK-MB (cardiac specific) 0%–3% total CK | 4–8 | 18–24 | 3 |
| LDH 45–90 u/l | 24–72 | 72–96 | 10–14 |
| $LDH_1$ (cardiac specific) 20%–30% total LDH | 12–24 | 48 | 10–14 |
| LDH1:LDH2 ratio <1 (i.e., LDH2 > LDH1) | 12–24 | 48 | 10–14 |

*Considered most diagnostic of myocardial injury.

10. VSD
11. Sudden cardiac death, usually from ventricular fibrillation

I. Management
1. ECG and hemodynamic monitoring: most important for reduction of mortality by improving ability to detect and prevent complications
2. Oxygen therapy
3. Bedrest in acute stage
4. Pain relief: morphine reduces anxiety and preload
5. Antiarrhythmics for documented dysrhythmias: lidocaine, procainamide (Pronestyl), bretylium
6. Calcium channel blockers and ACE inhibitors
7. β-blockers if contractility sufficient
8. Positive inotropes if necessary: dobutamine, digoxin
9. Tranquilizers and sedatives
10. Magnesium (1 to 2 g over an hour, followed by 0.5 to 1 g/hr over 24 hours) regardless of serum level.
11. Emergency drugs and equipment close at hand
12. Low-sodium diet
13. Prevention of complication of immobility (i.e., thrombophlebitis)
14. Tissue plasminogen activator (tPA) or streptokinase infusion in early stages of MI
15. Aspirin and anticoagulation (Heparin)
16. Nitrates (especially nitroglycerin); if administering IV nitroglycerin, higher doses of heparin may be required.

## IV. Valvular Heart Disease

A. Rheumatic heart disease (RHD)
1. Characterized by scarring and deformity of heart valves resulting from rheumatic fever
2. Rheumatic fever: diffuse inflammatory disease affecting joints, heart, skin, nervous system
3. Probably result of autoimmune process induced by streptococcal antigens
4. Valves commonly involved
   a. Mitral and aortic (most common)
   b. Tricuspid
   c. Pulmonary (almost never)
5. Extent of resulting cardiac disease depends on following factors
   a. Variability in duration and severity of rheumatic inflammation

b. Location and severity of hemodynamic lesion caused by valvular insufficiency and stenosis
c. Frequent recurrences of carditis
d. Degree of valvular and myocardial scarring after resolution of inflammation
e. Advancement of valvular sclerosis and calcification unrelated to underlying rheumatic inflammation

6. Management
    a. Antibiotic therapy: penicillin (vancomycin if patient is allergic to penicillin)
    b. Antiinflammatory agents: salicylates, corticosteroids
    c. Prevention of recurrence of streptococcal infections with prophylactic penicillin
    d. Valve surgery if hemodynamics significantly affected

B. Other causes
1. Atherosclerotic heart disease
2. Congenital abnormalities
3. Cardiothoracic trauma
4. Calcification caused by age
5. Systemic infections
6. Tumors
7. Syphilis
8. Marfan's syndrome

C. Valvular pathologic findings
1. Stenosis: narrowing of valve orifice; obstructs blood flow
2. Insufficiency: incompetent valve results in regurgitation through valve orifice
3. Mixed lesion: stenosis and insufficiency

D. Valvular abnormalities
1. Mitral stenosis
    a. Principal cause is rheumatic fever
    b. Most common valvular defect
    c. Pathologic findings
        (1) Fusion of commissures
        (2) Scarring of anterior and posterior leaflets' free margins
        (3) Shortening, fusion, and nodularity of chordae tendineae
    d. Effects on hemodynamics (Table 18–2)
    e. Clinical manifestations
        (1) Exertional dyspnea
        (2) Decreased vital capacity
        (3) Atrial fibrillation
            (a) May decrease cardiac output (CO) by as much as 15% to 20%
            (b) Increased likelihood of clot formation caused by incomplete emptying of atria
        (4) Thromboembolism
            (a) 80% of patients in whom systemic emboli develop are in atrial fibrillation
        (5) Murmur is early to middiastolic, low-pitched rumbling sound heard best at apex

**TABLE 18–2 Summary of Mitral Valve Disease Effects**

| EFFECT | STENOSIS | INSUFFICIENCY |
|---|---|---|
| Decreased cardiac output | X | X |
| Increased left atrial pressure | X | X |
| Increased pulmonary pressure | X | X |
| Increased pulmonary capillary wedge pressure | X | |
| Increased right ventricular pressure | X | |
| Increased left ventricular pressure and volume | X | X |

f. Diagnostic studies
    (1) ECG
    (2) Vectorcardiogram
    (3) Cardiac radiography
    (4) Echocardiogram
g. Management
    (1) Restrict sodium intake
    (2) Administer diuretics
    (3) Treat dysrhythmias
    (4) Use anticoagulants
    (5) Right and left cardiac catheterization to determine size of valve orifice
h. Surgical intervention: considered when patient becomes symptomatic (atrial fibrillation, pulmonary edema, pulmonary hypertension, orthopnea, fatigue)
    (1) Closed mitral commissurotomy
    (2) Open mitral commissurotomy
    (3) Mitral valve replacement
    (4) Balloon mitral valvotomy

2. Mitral insufficiency
    a. Causes
        (1) Rheumatic fever
        (2) Bacterial endocarditis
        (3) Ruptured chordae tendineae
        (4) Annular dilatation
        (5) Ischemic degeneration of papillary muscle
        (6) Prolapse of valve
        (7) Cardiothoracic trauma
    b. Second most common valvular defect
    c. Pathologic findings
        (1) Scarring and calcification
        (2) Bacterial destruction of uninvolved tissue (bacterial endocarditis)
        (3) Dilatation of anulus of mitral valve
        (4) Regurgitation of blood back into left ventricle
    d. Effects on hemodynamics (see Table 18–2)
    e. Clinical manifestations
        (1) Blowing, high-pitched, pansystolic murmur heard best at PMI, with radiation to left axilla or infrascapular areas
        (2) Weakness and fatigue
        (3) Atrial fibrillation
        (4) Pulmonary edema
        (5) CHF
    f. Diagnostic studies: same as for mitral stenosis
    g. Management
        (1) Improve contractility with cardiac glycosides: digoxin
            (a) Positive inotrope (increases force), negative chronotrope (decreases rate)
            (b) Absorption, distribution, and excretion variable
            (c) Toxicity common; normal level, 1 to 2 ng/dl
            (d) Toxic symptoms include anorexia, nausea, vomiting, yellow-tinted vision, cardiac dysrhythmias; symptoms correlated with degree of toxicity
        (2) Reduce afterload with nitroprusside or other arteriodilators (calcium channel blockers, angiotensin converting enzyme [ACE] inhibitors)
        (3) Left side of heart catheterization to confirm and evaluate regurgitation
    h. Surgical intervention
        (1) Valve replacement
        (2) Annuloplasty

**TABLE 18–3 Summary of Aortic Valve Disease Effects**

| EFFECT | STENOSIS | ACUTE INSUFFICIENCY | CHRONIC INSUFFICIENCY |
|---|---|---|---|
| Left ventricular hypertrophy | X | X | X |
| Increased left ventricular end-diastolic pressure | X | X | |
| Increased left ventricular end-diastolic volume | | X | X |
| Decreased cardiac output | X | X | |
| Increased left atrial pressure | X | | |
| Increased systemic arterial pulse pressure | | | X |
| Pulmonary congestion | | X | |

3. Aortic stenosis
   a. Causes
      (1) Congenital abnormality (<30 years of age)
      (2) Rheumatic fever (30 to 70 years of age)
      (3) Calcification caused by aging (>70 years of age)
      (4) Idiopathic hypertrophic subaortic stenosis (IHSS)
   b. Combined aortic and mitral disease most likely caused by rheumatic fever
   c. Effects on hemodynamics (Table 18–3)
   d. Clinical manifestations
      (1) Chest pain (most frequent symptom)
      (2) Syncope after exertion
      (3) CHF
      (4) Dysrhythmias, conduction defects
      (5) Harsh, high-pitched systolic crescendo-decrescendo best heard at right sternal border at second intercostal space; may radiate to neck or apex
      (6) Systolic thrill over apex
      (7) Narrowed pulse pressure
   e. Diagnostic studies same as for mitral stenosis
   f. Management
      (1) Prophylactic antibiotics
      (2) Treat dysrhythmias
      (3) Treat CHF
   g. Surgical intervention
      (1) Valve replacement (most common procedure)
      (2) Commissurotomy
4. Aortic insufficiency
   a. Causes
      (1) Congenital abnormalities
      (2) Rheumatic fever
      (3) Syphilis
      (4) Bacterial endocarditis
      (5) Dissecting aneurysm
      (6) Trauma
   b. Effects on hemodynamics (see Table 18–3)
   c. Clinical manifestations
      (1) Chronic
         (a) CHF in early stages
         (b) High-pitched, blowing crescendo diastolic sound heard best at second right intercostal space while patient is sitting
         (c) Rapid up stroke and down stroke of carotid pulse (Corrigan's pulse)
         (d) Exertional dyspnea, orthopnea
         (e) Markedly enlarged heart on x-ray film

(2) Acute
   (a) CHF in early stages
   (b) Tachycardia
   (c) Dyspnea
   (d) Pulmonary edema
   (e) Peripheral vasoconstriction and cyanosis
   (f) Midpitched, short, diastolic murmur

d. Diagnostic studies: same as for mitral stenosis

e. Management
   (1) Acute
      (a) Valve replacement
      (b) Preoperative antibiotic therapy for 10 to 14 days if secondary to active infective endocarditis and patient remains hemodynamically stable
   (2) Chronic
      (a) Cardiac glycosides
      (b) Antihypertensives
      (c) Antidysrhythmics
      (d) Prophylactic antibiotics
      (e) Valve replacement as symptoms occur or evidence of left ventricular dysfunction at rest

5. Tricuspid valve disease (Table 18–4)
   a. Causes
      (1) Stenosis
         (a) Rheumatic fever
         (b) Right atrial tumors
         (c) Congenital abnormalities
      (2) Insufficiency
         (a) Dilatation of right ventricle
         (b) Right ventricular hypertrophy resulting from any form of cardiac or pulmonary vascular disease
         (c) Congenital abnormality
   b. Comparison of effects on hemodynamics
   c. Clinical manifestations
      (1) Jugular vein distension, ascites, edema
      (2) Low cardiac output; fatigue and weakness
      (3) Symptoms of mitral valve disease
      (4) Cardiomegaly
      (5) Hepatomegaly
      (6) Diastolic murmur with stenosis
      (7) Pansystolic murmur with insufficiency
   d. Diastolic studies: see mitral stenosis

**TABLE 18–4 Summary of Tricuspid Valve Disease Effects**

| EFFECT | STENOSIS | INSUFFICIENCY |
|---|---|---|
| Elevated mean right atrial pressure | X | X |
| Low cardiac output | X | X |
| Most commonly found with mitral valve disease | X | X |
| Diastolic pressure gradient between right atrium and ventricle | X | |
| Regurgitation usually present | X | |

e. Management for stenosis and insufficiency
   (1) Surgical intervention
      (a) Open commissurotomy
      (b) Valve replacement
   (2) Sodium restriction
   (3) Diuretic therapy

6. Pulmonary valve disease
   a. Most common cause of pulmonic stenosis is congenital abnormality
   b. Most common cause of pulmonic insufficiency is dilatation of valve ring resulting from pulmonary hypertension
   c. May be tolerated for years without difficulty unless it complicates, or is complicated by, pulmonary hypertension
   d. Physical findings
      (1) Hyperdynamic right ventricle
      (2) Palpable systolic pulsations
      (3) Enlarged pulmonary artery
      (4) Midsystolic ejection murmur
   e. Management
      (1) Cardiac glycosides
      (2) Treatment of primary condition responsible for pulmonary hypertension
      (3) Valve replacement
7. Multivalvular disease
   a. Common in patients with rheumatic heart disease
   b. Should undergo right- and left-sided heart catheterization if surgery required
   c. Types
      (1) Mitral stenosis and aortic insufficiency
      (2) Mitral stenosis and aortic stenosis
      (3) Aortic stenosis and mitral insufficiency
      (4) Aortic and mitral insufficiency
   d. Management
      (1) Double valve replacement
         (a) Operative mortality approximately 18.6%
         (b) 5-year survival rate is 47%
      (2) Triple-valve replacement
         (a) Presents with severe heart failure
         (b) Surgical correction imperative
         (c) 18% to 40% operative mortality

## V. Miscellaneous Acquired Lesions

A. Myocardial disease
   1. Unrelated to rheumatic or atherosclerotic heart disease
   2. Primary myocardial diseases
      a. Myocarditis caused by bacteria, viruses, fungi, or parasites
      b. Cardiomyopathy (usually idiopathic)
      c. Hypertrophic cardiomyopathy (IHSS): overgrowth of ventricular muscle mass, small ventricular cavities
   3. Pericardial disease (pericarditis)
      a. Causes: idiopathic origin infection, inflammation, postpericardiectomy syndrome, metabolic origin, trauma, tumor
      b. Physical findings
         (1) Pleuritic substernal chest pain
         (2) Dyspnea
         (3) Pericardial friction rub
      c. Complication: pericardial restriction resulting in cardiac tamponade

d. Management
(1) Antiinflammatory agents
(2) Pericardectomy

4. Traumatic heart disease
   a. Types of injuries
      (1) Penetrating
      (2) Blunt
   b. Treatment depends on location of injury and effect on hemodynamics
5. Cardiac tumors
   a. Primary or metastatic
   b. Complications
      (1) Pericardial effusions
      (2) Restrictive disease
      (3) Obstruction to blood flow
      (4) Impaired contractility
   c. Treatment depends on location of tumor and hemodynamic effects
6. Aneurysms
   a. Weakening of aortic walls
   b. Thoracic or abdominal
   c. Thoracic may involve aortic valve
   d. Danger of rupture; mortality >95%
   e. Treatment generally surgery

## ASSESSMENT

**I. Diagnostic Tests**

A. Laboratory values (serum)
   1. Electrolyte profile, including glucose and calcium
   2. Blood urea nitrogen (BUN) and creatinine
   3. Serum lipids: cholesterol, high-density lipoproteins (HDL), low-density lipoproteins (LDL), triglycerides
   4. Hematology profile
   5. Enzymes (see Table 18–1)
   6. Coagulation profile
   7. Blood gas analysis (arterial = ABG; venous = VBG)
   8. Rapid plasma reagin (RPR)

B. Laboratory values (urine)
   1. Routine urinalysis
   2. Culture and sensitivity
   3. Electrolytes

C. Noninvasive cardiac diagnostic studies
   1. Cardiac radiography
      a. Provides information on cardiac size, chamber configuration, pulmonary vasculature
   2. Electrocardiography
      a. 12-lead ECG to demonstrate or detect
         (1) Disturbances of rate, rhythm, conduction
         (2) Ischemia or infarction
         (3) Electrolyte abnormalities
         (4) Anatomic orientation of heart
         (5) Chamber enlargement
         (6) Drug toxicity

   b. Preoperative electrocardiogram necessary to establish baseline for all patients undergoing cardiac surgery
3. Echocardiography
   a. Ultrasonic method of cardiac examination
   b. Records existing abnormalities of anatomy and motion
   c. Transesophogeal echocardiogram (TEE) especially useful to assess for atrial clots before balloon mitral valvotomy
4. Radionuclide scans
   a. Perfusion imaging: evaluates myocardial blood flow
   b. Infarction scintigraphy: detects injured or necrotic myocardium
   c. Thallium imaging (cold spot)
   d. Technetium pyrophosphate imaging (Tc-PYP)
   e. Gated blood pool imaging (e.g., MUGA)
5. Exercise electrocardiography (stress testing): permits evaluation of cardiac response to exercise stress
6. Tomography
   a. Digital subtraction angiography (DSA)
   b. Computed tomography (CT)
   c. Positrom emission tomography (PET)
   d. Magnetic resonance imaging (MRI)

D. Invasive cardiac diagnostic studies
1. Purposes
   a. Visualize heart chambers and identify shunts
   b. Confirm and evaluate lesions in valves, arteries, muscle tissue
   c. Measure cardiac and pulmonary pressures
   d. Measure CO and blood gases
   e. Evaluate left ventricular function
2. Cardiac catheterization complications
   a. Cardiac dysrhythmias and conduction defects
   b. Embolism: systemic, coronary, and pulmonary
   c. Arterial thrombosis
   d. Perforation of heart or great vessels leading to cardiac tamponade, pneumothorax, pleural effusion
   e. Local or systemic infection
   f. Allergic reactions to contrast media
   g. Bleeding at site
3. Pulmonary artery catheter (see Chapter 33)
4. Ventriculography: left side of heart catheterization; standard technique for evaluating left ventricular performance
5. Selective coronary arteriography: left side of heart catheterization; definitive method for diagnosing and describing coronary artery abnormalities
6. Pulmonary angiography
   a. Purposes
      (1) Confirm suspected pulmonary thromboembolism
      (2) Identify congenital malformations
      (3) Visualize pulmonary artery and left atrium
7. Aortography
   a. Diagnostic for
      (1) Aortic valve disease
      (2) Aortic coarctation
      (3) Dissecting aortic aneurysm
   b. Radiopaque contrast fluid injected by catheter placed in aortic root

E. Blood pressure measurement
   1. Noninvasive: cuff, Doppler ultrasonography palpation
   2. Invasive: placement of intraarterial catheter (see Chapter 33)
F. Central venous pressure (CVP) measurement (see Chapter 33)
G. Pulmonary artery pressure (PAP) measurement (see Chapter 33)

**II. Psychosocial Factors**

A. Goals of nursing care
   1. Assessment of patient needs
   2. Planning and implementing of nursing strategies
   3. Evaluation of expected patient outcomes
   4. Provision of holistic nursing care
B. Psychosocial concepts to consider when planning care for critically ill patient
   1. Perception
   2. Self-concept
   3. Self-esteem
   4. Stress
   5. Fear and anxiety
   6. Body image
   7. Pain
   8. Death
   9. Sensory deprivation/overload
C. Structured preoperative family and patient teaching
   1. Reduce patient and family anxiety related to perioperative course
   2. Preoperative instruction
      a. Surgical procedure specific to patient
      b. Tour of postoperative unit and visiting hours
      c. Sequence of events of operative day: premedication, time of procedure, surgical waiting area for family
      d. Identification of equipment to be used postoperatively
      e. Procedure for coughing and deep breathing, stating rationale for their importance
      f. Review of expected postoperative course
      g. Adequate time for discussion to enable patient or family to ask questions and verbalize concerns

## OPERATIVE PROCEDURES

**I. Treatment of Congenital Heart Defects**

A. Left-to-right shunts
   1. PDA: ligation or ligation and division of PDA
   2. VSD: pulmonary artery banding for palliation or total correction with patch closure of defect; requires cardiopulmonary bypass (CPB)
   3. ASD: suture or patch closure; requires CPB
B. Right-to-left shunts
   1. Tetralogy of Fallot: aortopulmonary shunt for palliation, patch closure of VSD, right ventricular outflow reconstruction; requires CPB
   2. Complete transposition of great vessels: atrial septectomy for palliation, total correction of transposition to increase communication between pulmonary and systemic circulation; requires CPB
   3. Total anomalous pulmonary venous return: anastomosis of collecting vein and enlargement of left atrium; requires CPB and profound hypothermia

C. Obstruction to blood flow
 1. Pulmonic stenosis: pulmonary valvotomy; requires CPB
 2. Aortic stenosis: aortic valvotomy; requires CPB
 3. Coarctation of aorta: patch angioplasty or resection with end-to-end anastomosis

## II. Treatment of Coronary Artery Disease (CAD)

A. Indications for coronary artery bypass grafting (CABG): requires CPB
 1. Left main coronary artery disease, with or without angina
 2. Left anterior descending (LAD) coronary artery disease, with angina pectoris
 3. LAD, plus right coronary artery (RCA) or circumflex coronary artery disease, or both, with angina pectoris
 4. RCA (dominant) single-vessel disease, with angina pectoris despite medical therapy

B. Resection of left ventricular aneurysm (LVA): easier to manage CHF when caused by LVA; requires CPB

C. Repair of interventricular septal defect (rupture of interventricular septum as result of acute coronary occlusion); patch closure; requires CPB

D. Minimally invasive coronary artery bypass grafting
 1. For occluded anterior coronary arteries
 2. Uses pedicled form of the internal thoracic artery (ITA) as graft conduit by means of limited anterior thoracotomy incision; does *not* require CPB or aortic cross-clamping.
 3. Right ITA used for RCA; left ITA for descending LAD
 4. CPB used, chest tubes, pulmonary artery or CVP catheters placed
 5. Hospitalization time reduced by 2 to 3 days

E. Transmyocardial laser revascularization (TMLR)

F. Percutaneous transluminal coronary angioplasty (PTCA)

G. Arthrectomy

H. Coronary artery stents

## III. Treatment of Valvular Heart Disease

A. Aortic valve disease
 1. Indications for valve replacement
  a. Symptomatic angina, syncope
  b. Calculated aortic valve area index is less than 0.8 $cm^2/m^2$
  c. Stenosis significant enough to cause large pressure drop across valve

B. Mitral valve disease
 1. Indications for valve replacement
  a. Decrease in calculated cross-sectional area of mitral valve orifice
  b. Commissurotomy performed if valve is only stenotic with fusion of uncalcified commissures, chordae tendineae are not severely deformed, leaflets are mobile, and there is no associated insufficiency
  c. Valve replacement performed if preoperative catheterization, angiography, and echocardiography indicate valvular or subvalvular calcification and thickening
  d. Balloon valvuloplasty is an effective, safe alternative to commissurotomy and valve replacement; may be performed on outpatient basis with discharge in 7 to 8 hours after the procedure; most dangerous complication is damage to the MV that would require open heart surgery (OHS) and mitral valve replacement (MVR)

C. Tricuspid valve disease
 1. General information
  a. Associated with severe mitral or aortic valve lesions or both
  b. Implies far advanced left-sided structural and hemodynamic impairment
 2. Indications for surgery
  a. Replace or repair valve
  b. Treatment of left-sided valvular lesions

## INTRAOPERATIVE CONCERNS

**I. General Concerns**

A. Preoperative evaluation
   1. Type of disease: congenital, acquired, valvular, CAD
   2. Severity and stability of cardiac disease; stable vs. accelerating angina
   3. Other medical disorders: diabetes, renal, pulmonary
   4. Medications: types, doses
   5. Psychosocial: anxiety, depression, family support
   6. Perioperative monitoring: pulmonary artery or left atrial catheter (varies by surgeon), CVP, arterial line
   7. Consideration of anesthetic and surgical approach
   8. Goals of preoperative medication
      a. Reduce anxiety
      b. Decrease stress on cardiovascular system resulting from anxiety
      c. Reduce or prevent catecholamine-induced stress on cardiovascular system as a result of anxiety
      d. Prevent increase in afterload and heart rate as a result of stress-induced catecholamine release
      e. Provide maximum sedation possible without further depressing myocardium or respiratory system

B. Preparation for anesthesia induction
   1. Line placement: peripheral and central catheters
   2. ECG: five lead, baseline tracings recorded
   3. Positioning: supine, "frogleg" position
   4. Temperature control and monitoring
   5. Complete chart review for recent entries

C. Intraoperative concerns
   1. Insertion of urinary catheter for accurate output
   2. Label all drugs for ready and immediate use
   3. Goal of induction: maintain stable preoperative heart rate, blood pressure, and central pressures during stressful periods (intubation, sternotomy)
   4. Incision: usually median sternotomy, unless miniCAB
   5. Anticoagulation: heparin given before cannulation. of heart and during CPB to prevent blood clotting
   6. Purposes of CPB
      a. Maintain systemic perfusion
      b. Add oxygen to blood
      c. Remove $CO_2$ and debris from blood
      d. Allow heart and lungs to be bypassed and motionless during surgery
      e. Initiated after cannulation of aorta and vena cava, or right atrium
   7. Induced hypothermia: lowers oxygen demand of vital organs (brain, kidneys); protects from ischemic injury
   8. Cardioplegia solution
      a. 4° C saline solution with high potassium concentration injected into chambers and vessels of heart
      b. Stops all mechanical and electrical activity and retards metabolism of heart
      c. Used concomitantly with hypothermia to reduce oxygen demand
   9. Completion of surgical procedure: cardioplegia solution purged from heart; body and heart rewarmed, and air removed from heart
   10. After rewarming begins, heart usually restarts spontaneously but may require cardioversion or temporary or permanent pacing
   11. CPB support gradually withdrawn and controlled lung ventilation restarted
   12. Pharmacologic support added as needed (dobutamine, nitroglycerin)

13. CPB discontinued when patient is rewarmed and cardiac function adequate
14. Reversal of anticoagulation: heparin-induced anticoagulation reversed with protamine
15. Closure of median sternotomy incision: before closure of incision, chest tubes are inserted to drain mediastinum and sometimes lung cavities, temporary pacing wires are placed if needed, and sternum is closed with wire suture

D. Immediate postoperative concerns
1. Goal: prevent or minimize potential complications during this critical period
2. Notification of nursing unit: preadmission report of necessary equipment or drugs to be ready to receive patient
3. Transport from operating room to nursing unit
   a. Ventilatory support with an $F_{IO_2}$ of 100%
   b. Continuous physiologic monitoring
   c. Pharmacologic support if necessary
   d. Esophageal stethoscope for monitoring respiratory and cardiovascular sounds
   e. Availability of portable defibrillator

## II. Special Considerations in CHD

A. Overview
1. Surgery for congenital heart defects requires thorough understanding of unique physiology of each type of defect
2. CHD surgical patient usually pediatric with unique requirements

B. Preoperative concerns
1. Surgical and anesthetic planning requires knowledge of weight and body surface area, cardiac status, general health, and laboratory data, chest radiograph findings, ECG results
2. Awareness of other significant congenital defects that may influence surgical course (e.g., hypoplastic lungs)

C. Operative concerns
1. Body temperature: pediatric patient has larger body surface area per kilogram than adult and can rapidly lose heat; methods for intraoperative temperature control must be available (e.g., hyperthermia blanket, IV solution warmers, increase in room temperature)
2. Patients with severe CHF and little cardiac reserve require narcotic anesthetics
3. Patients with severe outflow obstruction may benefit from ketamine
4. At end of corrective procedure, heart must be carefully purged of air to prevent embolism
5. For optimal postoperative care, personnel trained in nursing of critically ill child should be used

## III. Special Considerations in Acquired Valvular Disease

A. Preoperative concerns
1. Evaluation of cardiac disease: exertional tolerance, history of CHF, response to drug therapy
2. Review of cardiac catheterization data, laboratory data, ECG, radiography reports
3. Decision on type of valve (mechanical vs. porcine) required by patient

B. Operative concerns
1. Considerations in aortic stenosis
   a. Most difficult to manage of all valvular diseases
   b. Adequate preload essential for maintenance of ventricular filling and cardiac output
   c. Dysrhythmias: atrial fibrillation and tachycardia can significantly reduce ventricular filling and should be avoided and minimized
2. Considerations in aortic insufficiency
   a. Left ventricular preload greatly increased (overload)
   b. Prevent bradycardia to prevent prolonged filling and volume overload
   c. Reduce afterload with vasodilators: nitroglycerin, nitroprusside

3. Considerations in mitral stenosis
    a. Pulmonary hypertension common because ventricular filling limited by lesion
    b. Maintain adequate cardiac output and avoid pulmonary edema through careful preload management
    c. Preventing and minimizing dysrhythmias while controlling ventricular rate are essential
4. Considerations in mitral insufficiency
    a. Both ventricle and atrium are usually volume overloaded and dilated
    b. Goal of anesthesia is to maintain heart rate at normal levels, reduce afterload with nitroglycerin or nitroprusside

## IV. Special Considerations in CAD

A. Preoperative concerns
1. Current condition of patient: left ventricular function, CHF, and others
2. Angina: severity (i.e., accelerating)
3. Review of cardiac catheterization data

B. Operative concerns
1. Goal of anesthesia is to maintain myocardial oxygen supply and keep oxygen demand as low as possible
2. Objective of anesthesia in patient with ischemic heart disease is to maintain heart rate, blood pressure, preload, and afterload at or near stable preoperative values
3. Use of pharmacologic support therapy: vasoactive drugs, antidysrhythmics, diuretics
4. Intraaortic balloon pump (IABP) support for persistently low cardiac output or refractory angina
5. Right ventricular, left ventricular, or biventricular assist devices may be used in severe cases of ventricular failure

## V. Classification of Patients with Cardiovascular Disease

A. New York Heart Association guidelines (Table 18–5)

B. American Society of Anesthesiologists' Physical Status Classification
1. Descriptive analysis of patient status
2. Often used to classify patient's status relative to risks of operative intervention
3. Classes
    a. Class 1: patient has no organic, physiologic, biochemical, or psychiatric disturbances; pathologic process for which operation is to be performed is localized and does not entail systemic disturbance
    b. Class 2: mild to moderate systemic disturbance caused by either condition to be treated surgically or other pathophysiologic process
    c. Class 3: severe systemic disturbance or disease from whatever cause, even though it may not be possible to define degree of disability with finality
    d. Class 4: patient with severe systemic disorders that are already life threatening, not always correctable by operation
    e. Class 5: moribund patient who has little chance of survival but has submitted to operation in desperation

**TABLE 18–5 Cardiovascular Disease Guidelines**

| CARDIAC STATUS | PROGNOSIS |
|---|---|
| I. Uncompromised | I. Good |
| II. Slightly compromised | II. Good with therapy |
| III. Moderately compromised | III. Fair with therapy |
| IV. Severely compromised | IV. Guarded with therapy |

From Criteria Committee of the New York Heart Association: *Nomenclature and Criteria for Diagnosis of Diseases of the Heart and Great Vessels,* 7th Ed. © Copyright 1973, published by Little, Brown and Company.

f. Emergency operation (E): any patient in one of the classes listed previously who is operated on as an emergency is considered to be in less than optimal physical condition; the E is placed after the numeric classification

## POSTANESTHESIA CARE

**I. Unit Admission**

A. Major goals of patient care
1. Maintain adequate cardiac function by minimizing oxygen demand of myocardium and maximizing oxygen delivery to all body tissues
   a. Ensure adequate tissue perfusion
   b. Ensure adequate tissue oxygenation
2. Maintain pulmonary function
3. Maintain fluid and electrolyte balance
4. Prevent and manage postoperative complications
5. Promote physical and mental well-being

B. Operative report
1. Type of surgical procedure
2. Type of anesthesia; combination of inhalation and narcotic, muscle relaxants, and reversal agents used
3. Hemodynamic problems: pulmonary artery and/or central venous pressure values
4. Ventilatory problems: ABG results
5. CPB time: the more time on CPB, the greater the likelihood of coagulation problems
6. Recent laboratory data: serum potassium, hemoglobin and hematocrit, serum glucose (often elevated immediately postoperatively because of stress response and CPB)
7. Types of IV fluids and blood products transfused
8. Reversal of anticoagulation: reverse heparin by protamine sulfate in ratio of 1.3 mg protamine to 1 mg heparin used in procedure, including priming of pump
9. Pertinent medical history—especially pulmonary and cardiovascular

C. Admission procedure
1. Respiratory support
   a. Record mechanical ventilator settings: rate, tidal volume, $FIO_2$, mode, positive end-expiratory pressure (PEEP), set alarms
   b. Administer high humidity and adjust $O_2$, flow rate as per order (T-piece, face mask)
   c. Record rate and quality of respirations
   d. Assess breath sounds: auscultate lung fields bilaterally for abnormal breath sounds, pneumothorax, right main-stem bronchus intubation
   e. Monitor ABGs at regular intervals: acidosis increases myocardial oxygen demand; reduces contractility
2. Cardiac support
   a. ECG monitor: select lead (usually $V_5$ or modified chest lead); record heart rate and rhythm; set alarm
   b. Pressure monitoring: pulmonary artery or left atrial catheter, arterial line, blood pressure, CVP; record baseline values
   c. Assess heart sounds: murmurs, gallops, rubs
   d. Obtain baseline rhythm strip
   e. Assess peripheral pulses, skin color, temperature
   f. Pacemaker (Tables 18-6 and 18-7); check for
      (1) Type: permanent (transvenous or epicardial) vs. temporary (external)
      (2) Mode: ventricular, atrial, AV sequential
      (3) Sensitivity: synchronous (senses intrinsic cardiac rhythm) vs. asynchronous (does not sense intrinsic cardiac rhythm)

**TABLE 18–6 Three-Position Pacemaker Code**

| CHAMBER PACED | CHAMBER SENSED | MODE OF RESPONSE* |
|---|---|---|
| V = Ventricle | V = Ventricle | I = Inhibited |
| A = Atrium | A = Atrium | T = Triggered |
| D = Atrium and ventricle | D = Atrium and ventricle | D = Atrial triggered and ventricle inhibited |
| O = None | O = None | O = None |

*Inhibited = Will not pace on sensing spontaneous cardiac activity. Triggered = Delivers stimulus just after spontaneous depolarization and resets timing immediately on sensing spontaneous cardiac activity.

(4) Monitor asynchronous carefully: may compete with patient's own rhythm; could cause ventricular fibrillation if R-on-T phenomenon occurs
(5) Milliamperage (mA): amount of current delivered to heart; helps determine capture
(6) Rate: frequency of pacing; depends on patient's cardiac output needs

3. Neurologic assessment
4. Renal assessment
5. Temperature monitoring and control
6. IV fluid support: crystalloids, colloids, blood
7. Miscellaneous
   a. Chest tube drainage system: gently strip tubes and connect to suction, record time and amount of drainage; drainage >100 ml/hr should be monitored closely; notify surgeon if this continues for more than 1 hour
   b. Routine laboratory studies
      (1) ABGs
      (2) Electrolytes: low potassium and magnesium cause ventricular irritability (PVCS); low $Ca^{2+}$ causes decreased contractility
      (3) Prothrombin time (PT) and partial thromboplastin time (PTT) to assess for potential bleeding
      (4) Complete blood count (CBC) and platelet count as indicator for blood replacement; CPB affects platelet production and hemodilution of intravascular volume
      (5) Serum glucose: CPB usually causes decline in insulin secretion leading to hyperglycemia; insulin secretion resumes on termination of CPB
      (6) BUN and creatinine: indicators of renal function
      (7) Cardiac enzymes: monitor for potential MI
   c. Serial 12-lead ECG studies to monitor for potential electrophysiologic disturbances, ischemia, drug toxicity
   d. Check surgical incisions for postoperative bleeding
   e. Review patient's records for baseline values

**TABLE 18–7 Troubleshooting Temporary Pacemakers**

| PROBLEM | ACTION |
|---|---|
| Failure to capture | 1. Check lead connections<br>2. Check lead placement by x-ray film if transvenous<br>3. mA may be too low<br>4. Battery is low<br>5. Significant scar tissue formation |
| Failure to sense | 1. Sensitivity may be too low<br>2. Battery low<br>3. In asynchronous mode |

**NURSING DIAGNOSIS**

Examples of related nursing diagnostic categories include:

- High risk for decreased cardiac output
- High risk for impaired tissue perfusion
- Ineffective breathing pattern
- High risk for impaired airway clearance
- High risk for fluid volume deficit/excess
- Hypothermia
- Altered urinary elimination
- Pain
- Anxiety
- Impaired verbal communication
- Self-esteem disturbance
- Disturbance in role performance
- Total self-care deficit (specify level)
- Activity intolerance

## II. Immediate Postoperative Patient Management

A. Dysrhythmias of sinus origin
  1. Sinus tachycardia
    a. Causes
      (1) Hypoxia
      (2) Shock
      (3) Fever
      (4) Pain
      (5) Anxiety
      (6) CHF
      (7) Hypovolemia
      (8) Drugs: epinephrine, atropine, isoproterenol, dobutamine
      (9) Anemia
      (10) Thyrotoxicosis
      (11) Exertion
    b. Treatment
      (1) Identify and treat underlying cause
      (2) Evaluate patient's ability to tolerate dysrhythmia
      (3) Drug therapy depends on cause
  2. Sinus bradycardia
    a. Causes
      (1) Acute MI
      (2) Drugs: propranolol, digitalis, neostigmine
      (3) Myxedema
      (4) Increased intracranial pressure
      (5) Valsalva's maneuver
      (6) Hypothermia
      (7) Reflex following vasopressors
      (8) Vagal influence
      (9) Carotid sinus pressure
      (10) Athletes with healthy cardiac tone
      (11) High spinal anesthetic level
    b. Treatment
      (1) Identify and treat underlying cause; evaluate patient's ability to tolerate dysrhythmia

(2) Drugs to increase heart rate such as atropine or isoproterenol if patient is symptomatic; use isoproterenol with caution because it significantly increases myocardial oxygen consumption
(3) Evaluate patient's ability to increase heart rate in response to volume change

3. Sinus dysrhythmia
   a. Causes
      (1) Common in young people
      (2) May indicate disease of sinoatrial node in elderly
   b. Treatment: usually none indicated
4. Sinus block/arrest
   a. Causes
      (1) Impulse formation defect
      (2) Impulse conduction defect
      (3) Vagal influence
      (4) Carotid sinus stimulation
      (5) Drugs: digitalis, propranolol, myocardial depressants such as anesthetic agents
      (6) Ischemic injury to sinoatrial node

B. Dysrhythmias of atrial origin
   1. Premature atrial contraction: may be precursor to atrial tachydysrhythmias
      a. Causes
         (1) Stress
         (2) Caffeine
         (3) Rheumatic heart disease
         (4) Atherosclerotic heart disease
         (5) Thyrotoxicosis
      b. Treatment
         (1) Usually none indicated; drug therapy for atrial dysrhythmias: propranolol, digitalis, quinidine, procainamide (Pronestyl)
   2. Wandering atrial pacemaker
      a. Causes
         (1) Increased vagal tone
         (2) Disease of sinus node
         (3) Digitalis toxicity
         (4) Rheumatic heart disease
      b. Treatment: usually none indicated
   3. Paroxysmal atrial tachycardia (PAT)
      a. Causes
         (1) MI
         (2) Rheumatic heart disease
         (3) Hypertensive heart disease
         (4) Stress
         (5) Hyperventilation
         (6) Pulmonary emboli
         (7) Caffeine
      b. Treatment
         (1) Identify and treat underlying cause; evaluate tolerance of dysrhythmia
         (2) Carotid massage may stimulate vagus nerve to decrease heart rate
         (3) Drug therapy: digitalis, propranolol, verapamil, adenosine
         (4) Valsalva's maneuver
         (5) Cardioversion if patient severely symptomatic and other therapies have failed
   4. Atrial flutter
      a. Causes
         (1) Atherosclerotic heart disease

(2) Rheumatic heart disease
(3) Congenital heart disease
(4) Hypertensive heart disease
(5) Hypoxia
(6) Stress
(7) Exercise
(8) MI
(9) Drug toxicity: digitalis, quinidine

b. Treatment
(1) Identify and treat underlying cause; evaluate tolerance
(2) For rapid ventricular rate, administer digitalis, adenosine

5. Atrial fibrillation
a. Causes
(1) Myocardial disease
(2) Stress and nausea
(3) Pain
(4) Electrolyte disturbance
(5) Infection
(6) Commonly occurs with mitral valve disease
(7) Sympathomimetic drugs: dobutamine, dopamine, epinephrine, terbutaline

b. Treatment goal: control ventricular response
(1) Identify and treat underlying cause
(2) Evaluate tolerance to dysrhythmia; may lead to decreased CO, clot formation, CHF, or angina
(3) Drug therapy: digitalis, propranolol, or verapamil to decrease ventricular rate; quinidine to convert to sinus
(4) Cardioversion

C. Dysrhythmias of AV junctional origin
1. Premature junctional (nodal) contraction (PJC or PNC); may be precursor to junctional tachycardia
a. Causes
(1) Irritation of AV node
(2) Carotid sinus pressure
(3) Rheumatic or atherosclerotic heart disease
(4) Ischemia
(5) Damage to conduction system during surgery

b. Treatment
(1) Usually none indicated
(2) Frequent PNCs (>6/min) may indicate myocardial irritability

2. Junctional (nodal) rhythm
a. Causes
(1) Sinus node disease
(2) Digitalis toxicity
(3) Increased vagal tone

b. Treatment
(1) Depends on underlying cause and clinical circumstances
(2) Transient episodes usually require no treatment
(3) Patients unable to tolerate dysrhythmia may require either drug therapy or pacemaker to increase heart rate

3. Junctional (nodal) tachycardia
a. Causes
(1) Paroxysmal: same as PAT
(2) Nonparoxysmal: inferior wall MI, after cardiac surgery, digitalis toxicity

b. Treatment
   (1) Identify and treat underlying cause; evaluate tolerance
   (2) Drug therapy: propranolol, esmolol, or verapamil

D. Dysrhythmias of ventricular origin
   1. Premature ventricular contraction (PVC): may be precursor to ventricular tachycardia or ventricular fibrillation
      a. Causes
         (1) Electrolyte imbalance: hypokalemia, hypomagnesemia
         (2) Irritation of ventricles by intracardiac catheters
         (3) Myocardial ischemia
         (4) Digitalis toxicity
         (5) Hypoxia
         (6) Drugs: epinephrine, isoproterenol
         (7) Acidosis
      b. Treatment
         (1) Identify and treat underlying cause; evaluate tolerance of dysrhythmia; drug therapy (lidocaine, procainamide, bretylium) indicated for frequent episodes of PVCs (>6/min, couplets, runs)
         (2) Provide supplementary oxygen; encourage deep breathing
   2. Ventricular escape beats and rhythms: may be preterminal rhythm
      a. Causes
         (1) MI
         (2) Cardiac disease
         (3) Electrolyte imbalance
         (4) Vagal influence
         (5) Complete heart block
      b. Treatment: identify underlying cause and treat accordingly
   3. Ventricular tachycardia (V-tach): life-threatening dysrhythmia requiring immediate treatment
      a. Causes
         (1) Electrolyte imbalance
         (2) Irritation caused by intracardiac catheters
         (3) Digitalis toxicity
         (4) Cardiac disease
         (5) MI
         (6) Acidosis
      b. Treatment: follow ACLS guidelines (see Chapter 16)
   4. Ventricular flutter: incompatible with life
      a. Causes
         (1) Ventricular tachycardia and its causative factors (listed above)
         (2) MI
      b. Treatment: follow ACLS guidelines (see Chapter 16)
   5. Ventricular fibrillation: incompatible with life
      a. Causes
         (1) MI
         (2) PVC on T wave (R-on-T phenomenon)
         (3) Cardiac disease
         (4) Ventricular tachycardia or flutter
      b. Treatment: follow ACLS guidelines (see Chapter 16)

E. Dysrhythmias: AV conduction defects
   1. First-degree AV block: may precede higher degree of heart block
      a. Causes
         (1) Drugs that prolong P-R interval: digitalis, quinidine, procainamide, propranolol, verapamil

(2) Atherosclerotic or rheumatic heart disease
(3) Acute MI
b. Treatment: see Chapter 16
2. Second-degree AV block (Mobitz type I, Wenckebach): may precede higher-degree heart block
a. Causes
(1) Atherosclerotic or rheumatic heart disease
(2) Drugs: digitalis, propranolol
(3) Acute inferior MI (dysrhythmia usually transient)
b. Treatment: see Chapter 16
3. Second-degree AV block (Mobitz type II): often precedes complete heart block
a. Causes
(1) Atherosclerotic or rheumatic heart disease
(2) Digitalis toxicity
(3) Acute anterior MI
b. Treatment: see Chapter 16
4. Third-degree (complete) heart block
a. Causes
(1) Atherosclerotic or rheumatic heart disease
(2) Acute MI
(3) Cardiac surgery
(4) Myocarditis
(5) Digitalis toxicity
(6) Hyperkalemia
b. Treatment: see Chapter 16

F. Intraventricular conduction defects
1. Right bundle branch block (RBBB)
a. Causes
(1) Cardiac disease
(2) Congenital lesion
(3) Trauma (especially after valve replacement)
b. Clinical significance
(1) Underlying heart disease determines treatment
(2) If chronic condition, patient may be asymptomatic
(3) If acute onset after cardiac event, may indicate deterioration of condition and may precede complete heart block or cardiac arrest
2. Left bundle branch block (LBBB)
a. Causes: same as RBBB, with most common cause being CAD
b. Clinical significance: same as RBBB

G. Low cardiac output: refer to beginning of chapter
1. Causes
a. Heart rate and rhythm disturbances: bradycardias, tachycardias, atrial fibrillation
b. Preload (most common): relating to inadequate intravascular volume
(1) Preoperative hypovolemic fluid status
(2) Post CPB fluid loss
(3) Fluid shifts caused by third-space loss
(4) Blood loss
(5) Tamponade
c. Afterload
(1) Effects of hypothermia: vasoconstriction increases peripheral resistance
(2) Effects of CPB
(3) Development of hypertension
d. Contractility
(1) Preoperative dysfunction: CHF, MI

(2) Intraoperative injury
(a) Mechanical: manipulation, cannulation, restrictive or misplaced suturing
(b) Ischemia: hypotension/hypertension, lengthy CPB period
(c) Coronary artery injury
(3) Postoperative dysfunction
(4) Residual defects
(a) Hypoxia: may produce acidosis and dysrhythmias
(b) Acidosis: metabolic, respiratory
(c) Electrolyte imbalance: hyperkalemia, hypocalcemia
(d) Hypoglycemia
(e) Drug induced

2. Nursing interventions
a. Frequent monitoring of vital signs
b. Close observation of fluid and electrolyte balance
c. Observe for clinical signs
(1) Hypotension
(2) Cold, clammy, mottled skin
(3) Diminished peripheral pulses
(4) Narrowing of pulse pressure
(5) Decreased urine output
(6) Crackles in lung fields
(7) Elevation of CVP and/or PCWP; or reduction of same in volume loss
(8) Metabolic or respiratory acidosis per ABGs

3. Treatment goal: maximize cardiac output by treating underlying causes of low cardiac output
a. Stabilize heart rate and rhythm
(1) Cardiac pacing
(2) Antidysrhythmics: lidocaine (PVCs), propranolol, verapamil
b. Optimize preload
(1) Fluid replacement as appropriate: blood or colloid
(2) Administer diuretics if necessary; restrict crystalloid intake
(3) Administer vasodilators if necessary (nitroglycerin, morphine)
(4) Monitor hematocrit and hemoglobin
c. Reduce afterload
(1) Administer vasodilators to reduce peripheral vascular resistance: nitroglycerin, nitroprusside; substituting labetolol has been shown to improve arterial oxygenation and allow earlier weaning in hypertensive cardiac surgery patients who require high $F_{IO_2}$
(2) Monitor and control body temperature: hypothermia causes vasoconstriction, resulting in increased peripheral resistance
d. Improve contractility with positive inotropic drugs: dopamine, epinephrine (use epinephrine cautiously because it has been shown to precipitate lactic acidosis in some patients)
e. Intraaortic balloon pump (IABP) may be indicated if above measures are not adequate or if myocardial ischemia is suspected (Table 18–8)

H. Cardiac tamponade
1. Definition: impaired ventricular diastolic filling resulting from increased intrapericardial pressure from accumulated fluid (blood or serum) or pericardial fibrosis
2. Patient management
a. Causes of tamponade
(1) Bleeding at graft suture site
(2) Small arterial bleeders
(3) Removal of cardiac pacing wires and left atrial lines

**TABLE 18–8 Care of Patient on an Intraaortic Balloon Pump (IABP)**

| | | |
|---|---|---|
| Rationale for use | The IABP is a counterpulsation device in which the balloon inflates when the heart is in diastole and deflates when the heart begins systole. Its two main functions are (1) to increase coronary artery perfusion (in diastole, balloon inflates) and (2) to decrease afterload (in systole, balloon deflates) | |
| Placement | Generally in the femoral artery; can use percutaneous or cutdown technique | |
| Timing | Balloon is set to inflate on or near the dicrotic notch of the arterial waveform and deflate slightly before systole; the goal is to reduce afterload | |
| Troubleshooting | Early/late inflation/deflation | Adjust timing |
| | Inadequate augmentation | Check trigger<br>Check actual gas volume in balloon<br>Cardiac status is improved |
| | Balloon not pumping | Check trigger<br>Check power source<br>Check connections |

The reader is referred to the articles in the Bibliography for a more in-depth discussion of this treatment modality and related nursing care.

(4) Anticoagulation problems
(5) Postpericardiotomy syndrome

b. Nursing intervention
   (1) Observe for clinical signs of tamponade
      (a) Cold, clammy skin
      (b) Narrowing pulse pressure
      (c) Rapidly rising CVP and/or PCWP
      (d) Equalization of CVP and PCWP (high pressures)
      (e) Decreasing blood pressure
      (f) Diminished peripheral pulses
      (g) Pulsus paradoxus: decrease in systolic pressure by more than 20 mm Hg during inspiration
      (h) Widening of mediastinal shadow on chest film
      (i) Distant heart sounds
      (j) Rapid, thready pulse
      (k) Chest tube drainage: profuse bleeding is suggestive of intramediastinal bleeding; decreased drainage suggests inadequate decompression of mediastinal bleeding
      (l) Decreased urine output
c. Treatment
   (1) Supportive fluid and drug therapy: blood transfusions, colloid
   (2) Surgical decompression and evacuation of hemopericardium or hemomediastinum, preferably done in operating room, but may be done on nursing unit in extreme emergencies

I. Bleeding
   1. Causes of postoperative bleeding
      a. Clotting abnormalities: preexisting, or after CPB
      b. Bleeding at graft suture lines
      c. Protamine rebound
   2. Nursing interventions
      a. Notify surgeon of chest tube drainage >100 ml/hr
      b. Obtain coagulation profile, hematocrit, and hemoglobin
      c. Monitor patient's vital signs and pressures
      d. Maintain adequate intake and output
      e. Maintain adequate cardiac pressures through fluid replacement as ordered

3. Treatment
   a. Correction of coagulopathy: replace appropriate clotting factors
      (1) Protamine to reverse effects of heparin
      (2) Fresh frozen plasma to provide clotting factors
      (3) Vitamin K to counter hypoprothrombinemia
      (4) Epsilon-aminocaproic acid (EACA) to counter hyperfibrinolysis
   b. Replace blood loss with blood products and colloid solutions as ordered
   c. Prepare patient for return to operating room as soon as possible

J. Hypertension (see Chapter 15)
K. Impaired oxygenation and ventilation (see Chapter 15)
L. Impaired renal function
1. Causes
   a. Preexisting renal disease
   b. Decreased renal perfusion resulting from low cardiac output. Be alert for hypotensive episode perioperatively, hypovolemia
2. Nursing interventions
   a. Hourly monitoring of urine output
   b. Serial BUN and creatinine levels
   c. Observe patient for clinical signs of renal failure
      (1) Decreased urinary output with adequate hydration
      (2) Elevation of BUN, creatinine, serum potassium
      (3) Persistent proteinuria and hematuria
      (4) Metabolic acidosis
3. Treatment goals: prevention and avoidance of renal failure
   a. Monitor continually for signs of failure throughout immediate postoperative recovery
   b. Maintain cardiac output
   c. Maintain fluid and electrolyte balance
   d. Initiate dialysis if indicated

M. Neurologic impairment
1. Causes
   a. Air embolism
   b. Preexisting cerebrovascular disease
   c. Hypoxemia/hypercapnea
2. Nursing interventions
   a. Assess patient's neurologic function
   b. Report significant changes to physician
3. Treatment
   a. Administer pharmacologic agents: narcotic antagonists, physostigmine for reversal
   b. Maintain adequate ventilation: if increased intracranial pressure (IICP) present, may adjust ventilator to produce mild to moderate hypocarbia (constricts cerebral vessels)
   c. Administer dexamethasone (Decadron) and/or mannitol to reduce IICP

N. Other nursing considerations
1. Assessment of patient for other potential complications
   a. Peripheral arterial embolization: pulse deficits and cool, pale skin in affected extremity; may require embolectomy
   b. Pericarditis: pericardial friction rub, ECG changes, complaint of pain; treated with antiinflammatory agents and analgesics
   c. Paralytic ileus: abdominal distension, expanding girth, diminished bowel sounds, vomiting
   d. Stress/pain: tachycardia, peripheral vasoconstriction, stress ulcers, hyperglycemia
   e. Postoperative psychosis
      (1) Symptoms
         (a) Sudden changes in behavioral patterns

(b) Disorientation

(c) Combativeness

(2) Goals of nursing care

(a) Reorientation

(b) Provide adequate sedation, analgesia

(c) Limit sensory overload from unit

2. Continuous observation, assessment, and ventilation of patient's status is mandatory during immediate postoperative period

## BIBLIOGRAPHY


Adams JE, Bodor GS, Davila-Roman VG, et al: Myocardial injury/infarction: Cardiac troponin I: A marker with high specificity for cardiac injury. *Circulation* 88(1):101–110, 1993.

Black JM, Matassarin-Jacobs E: *Medical-Surgical Nursing: Clinical Management for Continuity of Care,* 5th Ed. Philadelphia, WB Saunders, 1997.

Braunwald E: Pathophysiology of heart failure. In Braunwald E (ed): *Heart Disease: A Textbook of Cardiovascular Medicine,* 3rd Ed. Philadelphia, WB Saunders, 1988.

Braunwald E: Valvular heart disease. In Braunwald E (ed): *Heart Disease: A Textbook of Cardiovascular Medicine,* 3rd Ed. Philadelphia, WB Saunders, 1988.

Brody TM, Larner J, Minneman KP, Neu HC: *Human Pharmacology: Molecular to Clinical,* 2nd Ed. St Louis, Mosby, 1994.

Coleman B, Lavieri MC, Gross S: Patients undergoing cardiac surgery. In Clochesy JM, Breu C, Cardin S, et al (eds): *Critical Care Nursing.* Philadelphia, WB Saunders, 1993.

Fleury J, Murdaygh C: Patients with coronary artery disease. In Clochesy JM, Breu C, Cardin S, et al (eds): *Critical Care Nursing.* Philadelphia, WB Saunders, 1993.

Groth EJ, Lindahl B, Wallentin L: Early assessment of patients with acute myocardial infarction by biochemical monitoring and neural network analysis. *Clinical Chemistry* 43(10):1919–1925, 1997.

Guzzetta C, Dossey B: Nursing diagnosis: Framework, process and problems. *Heart Lung* 12:281–291, 1983.

Hall LT: Cardiovascular lasers, a look into the future. *Am J Nurs* 90:27–30, 1990.

Hicks FD, Klein DM: Pharmacokinetics in postanesthesia recovery: Implications for nurses. *J Post Anesth Nurs* 11(2):97–103, 1996.

Holloway S, Feldman T: An alternative to valvular surgery in the treatment of mitral stenosis: Balloon mitral valvotomy. *Crit Care Nurse* 17(3):27–36, 1997.

Hollenberg SM, Hoyt J: Pulmonary artery catheters in cardiovascular disease. *New Horizons: The Science and Practice of Acute Medicine* 5(3):207–213, 1997.

Kuhn M: *Pharmacotherapeutics: A Nursing Process Approach,* 4th Ed. Philadelphia, FA Davis, 1998.

LeMone P, Burke K: *Medical-Surgical Nursing: Critical Thinking in Client Care.* Menlo Park, California, Addison-Wesley, 1996.

Litwack K, Hicks F, Brooks D: Practical points in the care of the patient postcardiac surgery. *J Post Anesth Nurs* 5(2):106–111, 1990.

McCance KL, Huether SE: *Pathophysiology: The Biologic Basis for Disease in Adults and Children,* 3rd Ed. St Louis, Mosby, 1998.

Mizell JL, Maglish BL, Matheny RB: Minimally invasive direct coronary artery bypass graft surgery: Introduction for critical care nurses. *Crit Care Nurse* 17(3):46–55, 1997.

Owens MW, Daniel JL: IV magnesium sulfate in the treatment of ventricular tachycardia and acute myocardial infarction. *Crit Care Nurse* 13(6):83–85, 1993.

Perviaz S, Anderson FP, Lohmann TP, et al: Comparative analysis of cardiac troponin I and creatine kinase-MB as markers of acute myocardial infarction. *Clin Cardiol* 20(3):269–71, 1997.

Pill MW: Ibutilide: A new antiarrhythmic agent for the critical care environment. *Crit Care Nurse* 17(3): 19–22, 1997.

Porterfield LM, Porterfield JG: Digitalis toxicity: A common occurrence. *Crit Care Nurse* 13(6):40–43, 1993.

Purcell JA, Haynes L: Using the ECG to detect MI. *Am J Nurs* 84:627–642, 1984.

Purcell JA, Pippin L, Mitchell M: IABP therapy. *Am J Nurs* 83:775–790, 1983.

Pursley P: Acute cardiac tamponade. *Am J Nurs* 83: 1414–1418, 1983.

Rupert SD, Kernicki JG, Dolan JT: *Dolan's Critical Care Nursing: Clinical Management Through the Nursing Process,* 2nd Ed. Philadelphia, FA Davis, 1996.

Sanderson RG: Anatomy, embryology, and physiology. In Sanderson RG, Kurth CL (eds): *The Cardiac Patient: A Comprehensive Approach.* Philadelphia, WB Saunders, 1983.

Schakenbach LH: Patients with valvular disease. In Clochesy JM, Breu C, Cardin S, et al (eds): *Critical Care Nursing.* Philadelphia, WB Saunders, 1993.

Stephenson NL, Combs W: Artificial cardiac pacemakers and implantable cardioverter defibrillators. In Kinney MR, Packa DR, Andreoli KG, Zipes DP (eds): *Comprehensive Cardiac Care,* 7th Ed. St Louis, Mosby–Year Book, 1991.

Totaro RJ, Raper, RF: Epinephrine-induced lactic acidosis following cardiopulmonary bypass. *Crit Care Med* 25(10):1693–1699, 1997.

Tucker JF, Collins RA, Anderson AJ, et al: Early diagnostic efficiency of cardiac troponin I and troponin T for acute myocardial infarction. *Acad Emerg Med* 4(1):13–21, 1997.

Wood G: Effect of antihypertensive agents on the arterial partial pressure of oxygen and venous admixture after cardiac surgery. *Crit Care Med* 25(11):1807–1812, 1997.

## REVIEW QUESTIONS

**1. A client with a history of hypertension is received in the PACU after coronary artery bypass grafting. Which of the following best represents an increase in afterload?**

A. Increased PCWP and SVR
B. Increased PCWP, decreased SVR
C. Decreased PCWP and SVR
D. Decreased PCWP, increased SVR

**2. A postoperative coronary artery bypass patient begins to shiver. The nurse is concerned with this development because it:**

A. Increases myocardial oxygen consumption
B. Increases oxygen delivery to peripheral tissues
C. Decreases $CO_2$ levels in the blood
D. Promotes the development of hyperoxemia

**3. Four hours after a mitral valve replacement, the client's chest tube output is about 150 ml/hr. Which of the following would be the best intervention to implement at this time?**

A. Assess PCWP and CVP pressures
B. Elevate head of bed 45 degrees
C. Monitor BP and UO
D. Draw PTT and HCT

**4. A client is returned to the PACU after CABG. Two hours after admission, the client's chest tube output is 20 ml/hr, and the blood pressure is 86/68. Which of the following would be expected?**

A. Urine output in excess of 200 ml/hr
B. Equalization of PCWP and CVP pressures
C. Declining $Pao_2$ and $Paco_2$
D. Shift of PMI laterally and caudally

**5. Which of the following is most diagnostic of an MI?**

A. Troponin I
B. CK-BB
C. MB-CK
D. LDH

**6. The most frequently seen complication after an MI is:**

A. Papillary muscle rupture
B. CHF
C. Cardiogenic shock
D. Dysrhythmia

**7. All of the following are common to tricuspid valve disease except:**

A. Elevated right atrial pressures
B. Presence of regurgitation
C. Commonly seen with mitral valve disease
D. Low cardiac output

**8. The purposes of an intraaortic balloon pump (IABP) are to:**
   A. Increase preload, decrease afterload
   B. Increase coronary artery perfusion and preload
   C. Decrease coronary artery perfusion, increase preload
   D. Increase coronary artery perfusion, decrease afterload

**9. A patient returns from surgery with a DDI permanent pacemaker. This means that the:**
   A. Atrium and ventricles are sensed and paced
   B. Atrium alone is sensed, the ventricle is paced
   C. Ventricle is sensed, the atrium paced
   D. Atrium is inhibited, the ventricle triggered

**10. Temporary pacemakers should never be on "asynchronous" because this could lead to:**
   A. Overriding intrinsic rhythm
   B. Undersensing
   C. R-on-T phenomenon
   D. Loss of capture

**ANSWERS:** 1. A, 2. A, 3. D, 4. B, 5. A, 6. D, 7. C, 8. D, 9. A, 10. C

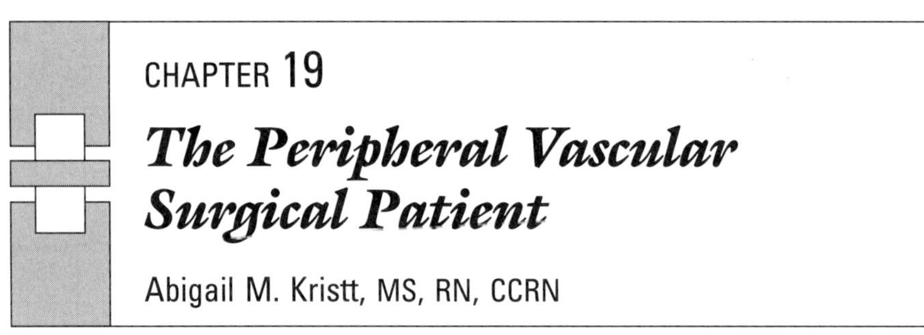

CHAPTER 19

# The Peripheral Vascular Surgical Patient

Abigail M. Kristt, MS, RN, CCRN

## OBJECTIVES

**Study of the information represented by this outline will enable the learner to:**

1. Explain three factors that affect peripheral circulation.
2. Describe three causes of arteriosclerosis.
3. Compare the signs and symptoms of arterial and venous vascular disease.
4. Identify the risk factors that contribute to the development of peripheral vascular disease.
5. Discuss three postarteriography assessment criteria.
6. Identify the most common sites of occurrence of peripheral vascular disease.
7. Describe the 19 operative procedures performed on patients with peripheral vascular disease as outlined in this chapter.
8. Describe the immediate postoperative nursing considerations for each operative procedure.
9. State at least six major postoperative complications of vascular surgery.
10. List at least two postanesthesia nursing interventions for each of the surgical procedures described.
11. By use of the nursing process, discuss how you would synthesize the preoperative assessment and intraoperative concerns of the surgical team into a rationale for postanesthesia care of the vascular patient.

The most common causative factor in the development of peripheral vascular disease (PVD) is atherosclerosis. The most common form of arteriosclerosis is obliterans. Atherosclerotic occlusive disease affects not only the peripheral vascular system but the coronary arterial circulation as well. The presence of vascular disease in the extremities may precipitate the development of acute or chronic disability with a diminished quality of life, whereas the coexisting cardiac problems may complicate the prognosis of the patient with PVD. Therefore cardiac monitoring is an integral part of the postoperative (postanesthesia) care of the patient with PVD.

PVD refers to any pathophysiologic process that interferes with the blood flow in the arteries or veins of the extremities, abdomen, thorax, and neck. This chapter discusses atherosclerosis in addition to the other common causes of PVD, related surgical interventions, and the appropriate nursing management criteria. A brief outline of the risk factors, pathophysiology, and assessment parameters is presented, along with a systems approach to nursing care in the postanesthesia setting. Surgical reconstructive procedures for the patient with PVD are outlined to facilitate comprehension and applicability to the postoperative population. Because individuals preparing for the CPAN or CAPA certification examination are employed in postanesthesia care units of varying sizes and acuity levels, it is important to remember that execution of certain of the recommendations depends on the policy of the specific unit and the expertise and clinical decision-making skills of the caregiver.

## ANATOMY AND PHYSIOLOGY

**I. Peripheral Vascular Anatomy: Includes Peripheral Arterial and Venous Systems and Excludes Cardiac, Pulmonary, and Cerebral Systems**

A. Arterial and venous wall structure: contains three layers
   1. Adventitia: thin outer layer containing collagen and lymphatics
   2. Media: thick middle layer containing smooth muscle cells arranged into strong, intertwining sheets of elastin that constrict or dilate. The medial layer is thinner in veins
   3. Intima: thin, inner, single endothelial layer; easily traumatized

B. Circulatory path (Fig. 19–1)
   1. Artery → arteriole → precapillary sphincter → capillary
      a. Artery: high pressure, low volume
      b. Arteriole (diameter <0.5 mm): offers resistance to blood flow, regulates blood flow into capillary bed
      c. Precapillary sphincters: rings of smooth muscle located at proximal end of a true capillary that regulate flow of blood and oxygen
      d. Capillary: site of gas and nutrient exchange
   2. Capillary → venule → vein
      a. Venule: as venules merge, the rate of blood flow increases
      b. Vein: low pressure, high volume; veins are capacitance vessels because they accommodate large volumes of blood; unidirectional valves direct venous flow from feet toward heart and prevent reflux; approximately 70% of blood volume contained in venous circulation

C. Arterial circulation (Fig. 19–2)
   1. Aorta: largest peripheral vessel, which includes four sections
      a. Ascending aorta: from aortic valve to arch
      b. Arch: where brachiocephalic and carotid vessels originate
      c. Descending thoracic aorta: from aortic arch to level of diaphragm
      d. Abdominal aorta: from thoracic to aortic bifurcation
   2. Aortic bifurcation: where aorta divides into right and left common iliac arteries
      a. Common iliac divides
         (1) Internal iliac (hypogastric)
         (2) External iliac: continuation of common iliac artery that becomes the common femoral artery in the thigh
      b. Common femoral (thigh)
         (1) Lateral and medial femoral circumflex
         (2) Profunda (deep) femoral
      c. Popliteal: continuation of common femoral located posterior to knee surface divides
         (1) Anterior tibial
            (a) Dorsalis pedis
         (2) Posterior tibial
            (a) Medial and lateral plantar
            (b) Peroneal

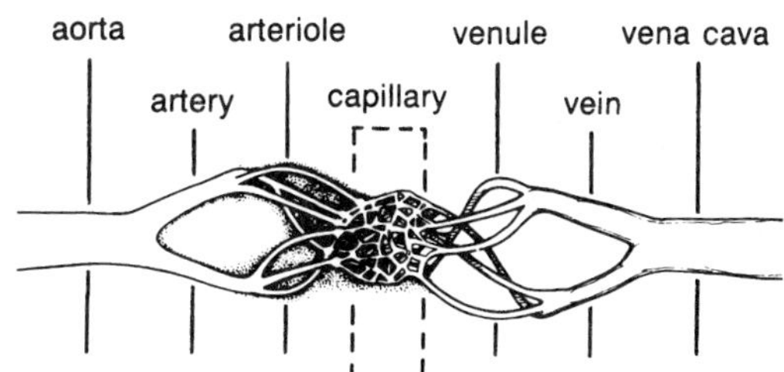


**FIGURE 19–1** Arterial and venous circulation. (From Ruppert SD, Kernicki JG, Dolan JT: *Dolan's Critical Care Nursing: Clinical Management Through the Nursing Process,* 2nd ed. Philadelphia, FA Davis, 1996.)

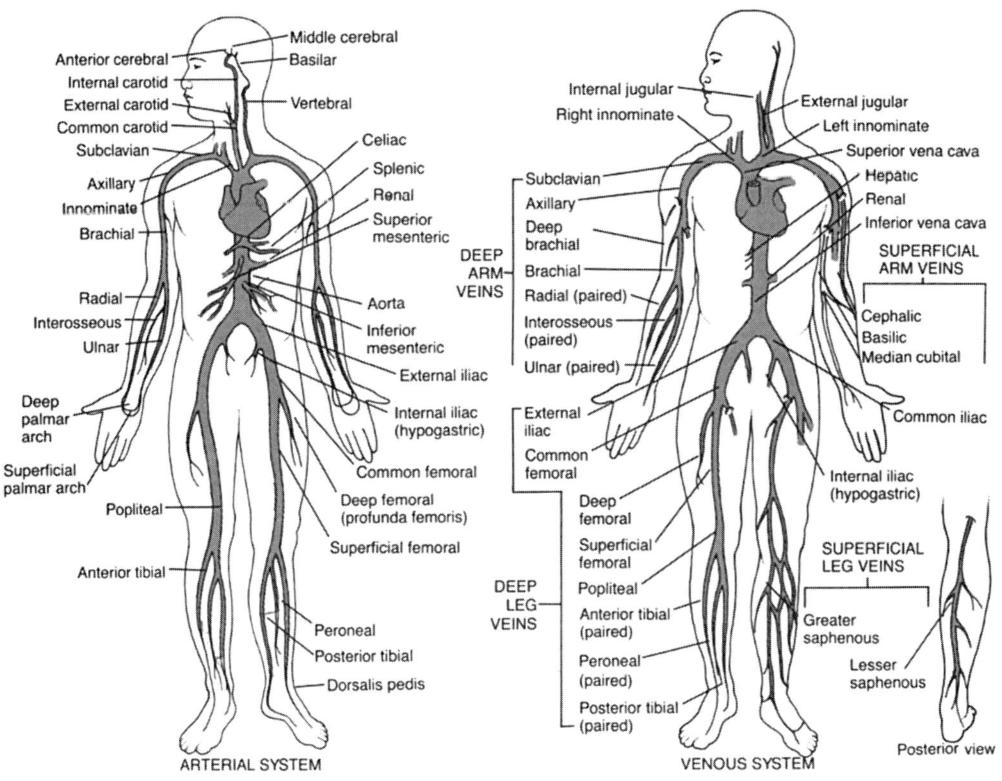


**FIGURE 19–2** Anatomy of arterial and venous systems. (From Ignatavicius DD, Bayne MV: *Medical-Surgical Nursing: A Nursing Process Approach* [p 2082]. Philadelphia, WB Saunders, 1991.)

D. Venous circulation
   1. Superficial system: in subcutaneous tissue
      a. Greater saphenous: longest vein in the body extending from malleolus of the ankle to the femoral vein (saphenous junction)
      b. Lesser saphenous: extends from the ankle to the popliteal vein in the knee (saphenopopliteal junction)
   2. Deep veins: in muscular layers
      a. Anterior and posterior tibial
      b. Peroneal
      c. Popliteal
      d. Femoral, profunda femoris
      e. Iliac
   3. Perforating (communicating): vascular channels (Fig. 19–3)
      a. Communicate between deep and superficial veins
      b. Flow is shunted from superficial to deep system with the help of unidirectional valves and finally to the inferior vena cava
      c. Muscle contraction promotes forward flow, valves prevent backflow during muscular relaxation

## II. Factors Affecting Circulation

A. Cardiac output (Cardiac output = Stroke volume × Heart rate): Venous capacity will determine venous return that will affect stroke volume of the heart

B. Arteriolar resistance: systemic vascular resistance (SVR) depends on the degree of arteriolar constriction, resistance increases as vessels constrict and decreases as vessels dilate, high SVR will decrease blood flow and increase myocardial workload

C. Vessel wall elasticity: with low compliance, the pressure is greater; increased pressure will increase myocardial oxygen consumption
D. Fluid volume status: low fluid volume will reduce peripheral resistance
E. Diameter of vessel (arteriole diameter <0.5 mm)
    1. Vasoconstriction: exposure to cold, vasoconstrictive agents
    2. Vasodilation: exposure to heat, vasodilator agents
F. Sympathetic nervous system: regulates amount of vasoconstriction

**III. Common Sites of Vascular Disease** (Fig. 19–4)
A. Internal carotid arteries
B. Aorta
C. Aortoiliac: bifurcation of aorta and iliac arteries
D. Superficial femoral: mid to distal thigh
E. Popliteal artery
F. Tibial arteries: common in patients with diabetes

## PATHOPHYSIOLOGY OF PERIPHERAL VASCULAR DISEASE

**I. Peripheral Vascular Disease**
A. Arterial occlusive disease
    1. Obstruction or stenosis of vessel
        a. Decreased peripheral vessel blood flow
        b. Decreased vessel diameter
        c. Increased peripheral vascular resistance
        d. Decreased blood flow velocity
    2. Degenerative changes
        a. Reduced tissue oxygen and nutrient supply
            (1) Inadequate tissue integrity
            (2) Ischemic tissue
            (3) Destruction of muscle and elastic fibers
        b. Formation of calcium and/or cholesterol deposits
            (1) Thickening of arterioles
            (2) Loss of elasticity

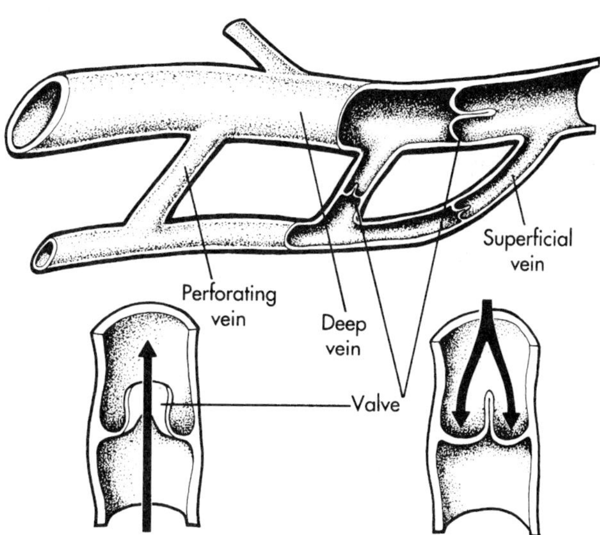


**FIGURE 19–3** Anatomy of the venous system of the leg. (From Price SA, Wilson LM: *Pathophysiology: Clinical Concepts of Disease Processes,* 5th Ed [p 542]. St. Louis, Mosby–Year Book, 1997.)

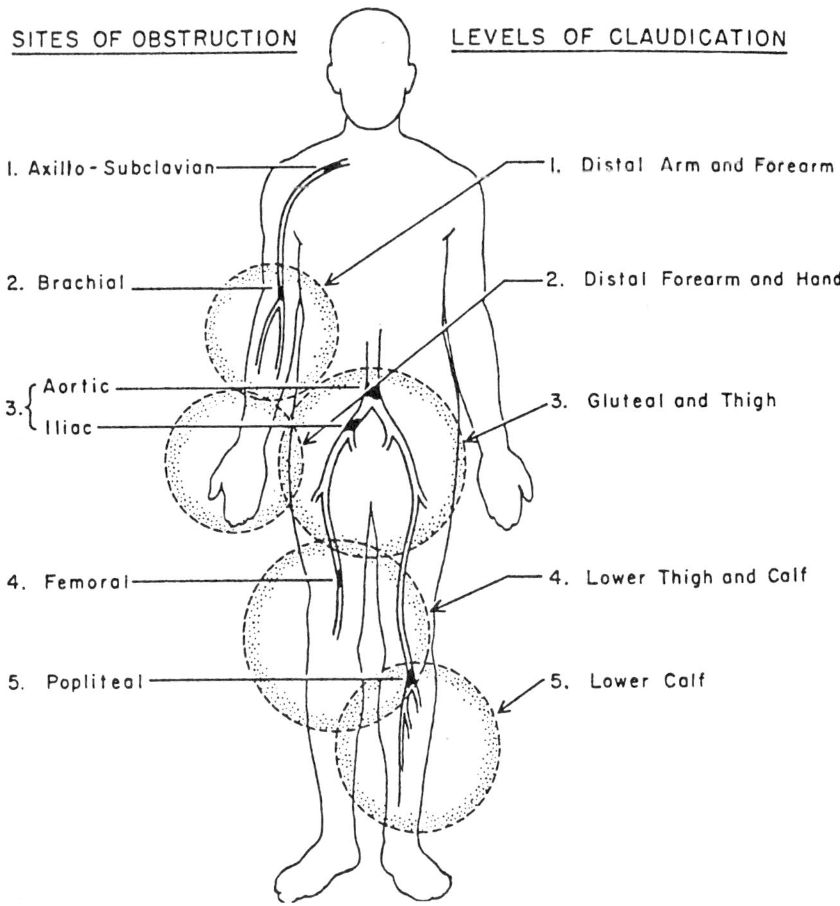


**FIGURE 19–4** Sites of arterial obstruction and corresponding levels of claudication. (From Fahey VA: *Vascular Nursing*, 2nd Ed [p 62]. Philadelphia, WB Saunders, 1994.)

B. Venous disease
   1. Deep vein thrombosis (DVT): disease of the deep veins of the lower extremity often accompanied by intraluminal clot
   2. Superficial thrombophlebitis: inflammation/clot in the superficial veins
   3. Virchow's triad: three factors that increase incidence of venous thrombosis
      a. Hypercoagulability due to alteration of platelet and clotting factors
      b. Venous stasis due to incompetent venous valves
      c. Intimal damage due to trauma, IV infusions, ischemia
   4. Pulmonary embolism: dislodged DVT with migration to pulmonary vasculature
   5. Varicose veins
      a. Structural weakness
      b. Vessel tortuosity
      c. Dilation
         (1) Incompetent venous valves
         (2) Reflux of blood results in venous pooling
   6. Venous hypertension: hereditary
      a. Incompetent valves results in reduced blood return to the heart
      b. Venous stasis and pooling of the blood results in venous hypertension

## II. Arterial Insufficiency: Arterial Occlusive Disease

A. Arteriosclerosis obliterans
   1. Atherosclerosis: most common form of arteriosclerosis obliterans
      a. Accumulation of lipids and connective tissue
      b. Intraluminal plaque formation
      c. Platelet aggregation
      d. Thrombus formation
      e. Loss of elasticity
   2. Möonckeberg's arteriosclerosis: arteriosclerosis of peripheral arteries characterized by calcium deposits within medial layer
   3. Arteriolosclerosis: sclerosis of arterioles

B. Aneurysm: abnormal dilation of vessel wall with high incidence of rupture and mortality when greater than 6 cm in diameter (Fig. 19–5)
   1. Fusiform: diffuse circumferential dilation of artery
   2. Saccular: area of pouching; affects localized part of arterial wall
   3. Dissecting: intimal layer torn; blood accumulates between layers
   4. False aneurysm: complete tear of all three layers of arterial wall caused by trauma, needle puncture, or suture failure at anastomosis site of prosthetic graft; palpable hematoma often present
   5. Pseudoaneurysm: dilated or tortuous segment of arterial wall without interruption of layers

## III. Vascular Diseases and Conditions

A. Acute
   1. Arterial embolism: sudden onset of symptoms of acute arterial insufficiency
      a. Originates in myocardium or arterial aneurysm
      b. May be secondary to external or iatrogenic trauma (catheter placement)
   2. Trauma: arterial wall tear or dissection

B. Chronic
   1. Diabetes mellitus: medial layer calcification; arteries become noncompressible

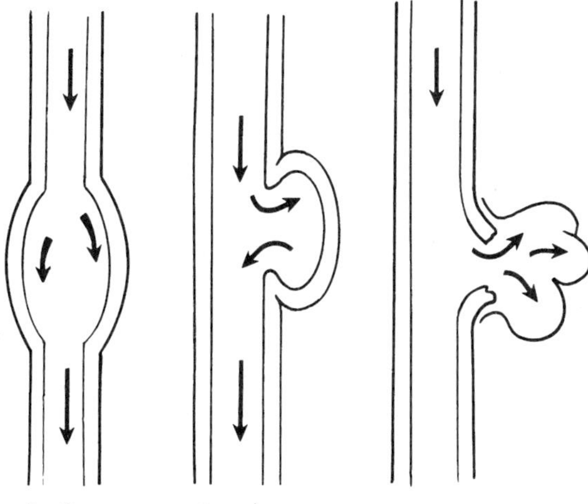


**FIGURE 19–5** Aneurysm types. (From Price SA, Wilson LM: *Pathophysiology: Clinical Concepts of Disease Processes,* 5th Ed [p 537]. St. Louis, Mosby–Year Book, 1997.)

2. Hypertension: increases permeability of intimal endothelium
3. Polycythemia: increased blood viscosity caused by increase in red blood cell count
4. Inflammatory processes: may cause occlusive lesions
   a. Arteritis: inflammation of arterial wall
      (1) Polyarteritis nodosa (PAN): systemic disease causing arterial inflammation and aneurysm rupture in adults
      (2) Kawasaki: similar to PAN, occurs in children
   b. Fibromuscular dysplasia (FMD): multiple areas of arterial stenosis and dilation
   c. Buerger's disease: thromboangiitis obliterans
      (1) Inflammation of arterial walls
      (2) Thrombus formation caused by intimal thickening
      (3) Affects plantar and digital vessels
      (4) Extremity cold, cyanotic, and painful
5. Raynaud's phenomenon: vasospastic disease
   a. Intense vasospasm of arteries and arterioles
   b. Precipitated by exposure to cold
   c. Ischemic changes: cyanosis, numbness, tingling
   d. Occurs in 40% of patients with systemic lupus erythematosus (SLE)

## IV. Clinical Signs and Symptoms

A. Arterial insufficiency: decreased blood flow may cause inadequate tissue oxygenation distal to lesion. A 70% to 90% occlusion of a large artery usually must occur before a decrease in blood flow or pressure causes symptoms at rest. A 60% obstruction may be sufficient to precipitate signs and symptoms during exercise.

1. Acute
   a. Peripheral pulses diminished, weak, or absent
   b. Cold and pale extremity (sudden onset)
      (1) Pallor when elevated
      (2) Rubor when dependent
   c. Sudden severe pain may occur during exercise or at rest
   d. Limited sensory and motor function
      (1) Possible paresthesia
      (2) Atrophied skeletal muscle: restricted limb movement
   e. Minimal edema: usually unilateral
   f. Bruit present with partial occlusion; no bruit with total occlusion
2. Chronic
   a. Diminished or weak distal pulses
   b. Pain at rest related to severe ischemia
   c. Tissue necrosis: gangrene
   d. Intermittent claudication
   e. Skin
      (1) Skin ulceration
      (2) Delayed healing of skin lesions
      (3) Skin texture: thin, shiny, dry
      (4) Cool skin: poikilothermic
   f. Color: pale extremity
      (1) Increased pallor when elevated
      (2) Rubor or cyanosis or both when dependent
   g. Possible paresthesia of limb
   h. Edema: none or mild
   i. Hair loss distal to occlusion
   j. Nails: thick, brittle
   k. Impotence: associated with aortoiliac disease

B. Venous insufficiency
  1. Acute
    a. Moderate pain localized to area of inflammation
    b. Pulses present or diminished (absent in presence of concomitant disease)
    c. Skin warm, cyanotic, mottled or pale
    d. Engorged veins when legs slightly dependent
    e. Moderate to severe peripheral edema
  2. Chronic
    a. Minimal to moderate pain
    b. Moderate to severe edema, unilateral or bilateral
    c. Sensation of heaviness at site of occlusion
    d. Muscle cramps, aching
    e. Ulceration of ankle area
    f. Superficial veins may be prominent
    g. Skin
      (1) Warm
      (2) Brawny (reddish brown) color
      (3) Pronounced lower leg pigmentation
      (4) Texture: thickening, scaling, and/or scarring

## INCIDENCE AND RISK FACTORS ASSOCIATED WITH PERIPHERAL VASCULAR DISEASE

**I. Incidence of Arterial Occlusive Disease**
  A. Highest incidence among elderly, male, diabetic smokers
  B. Gender
    1. More common in males
    2. Earlier onset in males
    3. Postmenopausal women susceptible
  C. Age
    1. Occurs beyond 30 years of age
    2. Symptoms worsen after 65 years of age

**II. Risk Factors of Atherosclerosis**
  A. Lifestyle habits
    1. Psychophysiologic stress triggers vasoconstriction
    2. Sedentary; lack of exercise
    3. Smoking
      a. Vasoconstrictive effect of nicotine
      b. Inhalation of carbon monoxide in cigarette smoke
        (1) Increases carboxyhemoglobin levels (carbon monoxide binds with hemoglobin)
        (2) Impaired oxygen transport
        (3) Hypoxic injury to intimal lining of artery
        (4) Increased platelet aggregation caused by enhanced platelet adhesiveness
    4. Diet
      a. Hyperlipidemia (hyperlipoproteinemia): accumulation of lipids in arterial wall
        (1) Elevated cholesterol: total serum levels
        (2) Elevated triglycerides
          (a) Low-density lipoproteins (LDL): high serum levels related to premature development of atherosclerotic process
          (b) High-density lipoproteins (HDL): high serum levels demonstrate protective effect against atherosclerosis
      b. Obesity

B. Positive family history
C. Disease processes
    1. Diabetes mellitus
    2. Hypertension

**III. Indications for Surgical Intervention**
A. Ischemic pain at rest
B. Significant limb ischemia
C. Limiting claudication

## DIAGNOSTIC ASSESSMENT

**I. Arteriography: Invasive Radiographic Procedure in Which Radiopaque Contrast Is Injected into Artery**
A. Purposes
    1. Depict location of stenosis, occlusion or view aneurysm
    2. Visualize collateral, proximal, and distal arterial circulation to determine surgical treatment options
B. Complications
    1. Intimal disruption
        a. Hematoma formation at puncture site
        b. Plaque dislodgment
        c. Arterial occlusion: thrombosis
        d. Distal embolization
        e. Arteriovenous fistula
        f. Arterial dissection
        g. Renal failure
    2. Transient ischemic attack (TIA) or cerebrovascular accident (CVA)
    3. Toxic reaction to contrast media: renal or cardiac
    4. Allergic reaction
        a. Skin rash
        b. Bronchospasm
        c. Altered consciousness
        d. Convulsions
        e. Anaphylaxis
        f. Cardiac arrest
C. Postarteriography assessment and intervention
    1. Assessment
        a. Vital signs
        b. Hematoma and/or bleeding at puncture site
        c. Signs and symptoms of acute arterial insufficiency
            (1) Skin: color, temperature
            (2) Pulses distal to puncture site
            (3) Pain
            (4) Urinary output
            (5) Neurologic status
            (6) Signs of heart failure or respiratory distress
    2. Intervention
        a. Observe for skin rash
        b. Maintain adequate hydration to flush dye
        c. Head of bed at 30 degrees or less
        d. Keep affected extremity straight for 4 to 6 hours after the procedure

**II. Computed Tomography (CT): A Tomograph Is an Image of a Cross-sectional Slice of a Body Part**

A. CT image is 3-D: a camera rotates around the selected body part taking 2-D images at multiple angles, which are converted to a composite 3-D image by a computer

B. Contrast material (usually iodine) is injected to heighten the contrast between the vessel wall and the blood

C. Used for diagnoses of aortic aneurysms and aortic dissection

D. Able to detect hematomas or thrombi better with CT than with arteriography

**III. Segmental Plethysmography: Measures Changes in Pulse Volume**

A. Pneumatic blood pressure cuffs are placed on the upper and lower thigh and ankle

B. The cuffs are inflated and the pressure changes during systole, which reflect blood volume, are monitored with a transducer. A pulse volume recording for each extremity site is recorded

C. Analysis of flow and pressure gradients reveal peripheral vascular disease sites

D. Flow abnormalities can be recorded during exercise and compared with resting flow patterns

**IV. Venous Tests**

A. Noninvasive laboratory studies

1. Venous Doppler ultrasonography examinations: used to determine blood flow patterns and velocity
   a. During inspiration intrathoracic pressure decreases and venous return to the heart increases
   b. During expiration venous flow to the lower extremities will increase
2. Air plethysmography (APG)
   a. Used to evaluate venous obstruction, reflux, and calf muscle pump function
   b. Able to differentiate deep and superficial venous insufficiency
3. Duplex imaging of valvular closing times indicate severity of venous reflux
4. Arm/foot pressure gradient measures outflow obstruction: normal difference between arm and foot is <4 mm Hg

B. Invasive testing

1. Ascending phlebography: used to assess venous patency
2. Descending phlebography: used to assess valvular function

## OPERATIVE PROCEDURES

**I. Endarterectomy**

A. Opening of occluded portion of artery

1. Removal of atheromatous material or plaque
2. Excision of artery's intimal lining

B. Performed on carotid, subclavian, iliac, or femoral artery

**II. Carotid-Subclavian Bypass**

A. Anastomosis of carotid and subclavian arteries to improve circulation

B. Common carotid used as donor for subclavian lesions

C. Subclavian used to restore circulation for carotid lesions

**III. Aortocarotid-Subclavian Bypass**

A. Insertion of bypass graft from ascending aorta to carotid or subclavian artery

B. For occlusive lesions of both common carotid or innominate and subclavian arteries

**IV. Carotid Artery Ligation**

A. Surgical occlusion of carotid artery

B. Temporary control of hemorrhaging during intracranial vessel surgery
C. Permanent control of intracranial or nasal hemorrhaging
D. Treatment of carotid-cavernous fistula

**V. Aorto-Innominate-Subclavian Bypass: Thoracic Aortic Graft to Innominate, Subclavian Arteries**

**VI. Aneurysectomy**
A. Excision of weakened dilated area of artery
B. Insertion of synthetic prosthesis to reestablish circulatory continuity
C. Usually occurring in abdominal aorta, thoracic aorta, or carotid, popliteal, or femoral artery

**VII. Thoracoabdominal Aortic Aneurysm Repair**
A. Clots are removed before anastomosis of Dacron graft
B. A spinal catheter is placed at L-1 to L-2 to allow for cerebrospinal fluid (CSF) drainage
C. Spinal cord ischemia is evaluated by monitoring CSF pressure

**VIII. Bypass Approaches for Aortoiliac Occlusions** (Fig. 19–6)
A. Aortoiliac bypass: insertion of vascular graft from distal aorta to iliac artery or arteries
B. Aortofemoral bypass (Fig. 19–6)
  1. Anastomosis of distal aorta to femoral arteries
  2. Lesion bypassed with vascular graft
C. Axillofemoral bypass (Fig. 19–7)
  1. Superficial flank placement
  2. Anastomosis of prosthetic graft from one axillary artery to one or both femoral arteries
  3. Restores blood flow beyond occlusive lesion
D. Femorofemoral bypass: femoral crossover graft (Fig. 19–8)
  1. Extraanatomic bypass procedure with subcutaneous placement across suprapubic area
  2. End-to-side anastomosis from patent femoral to stenotic femoral artery
  3. Diverts blood flow from one donor femoral artery to recipient stenotic artery

**IX. Aortorenal Bypass: Anastomosis of Abdominal Aorta to Renal Artery with Vascular Graft**

**X. Femoropopliteal Bypass**
A. Establishes adequate circulation to leg and foot through popliteal artery and branches
B. Graft used for superficial femoral artery occlusion

**XI. Femorotibial Bypass**
A. Autogenous saphenous vein graft from common femoral artery to proximal anterior tibial artery
B. Procedure indicated for superficial femoral and popliteal artery occlusion

**XII. Angioplasty: Percutaneous Insertion of Balloon-Tipped Catheter to Dilate Areas of Localized Vessel Stenosis**

**XIII. Vena Cava Ligation**
A. Partial or total surgical occlusion of vena cava to prevent emboli from entering pulmonary vasculature
B. Common ligation sites
  1. Superficial femoral
  2. Inferior vena cava below renal veins

**XIV. Vena Caval Umbrella Filter**
A. Insertion of intravascular device through jugular or femoral vein to occlude inferior vena cava
B. Prevents emboli from entering pulmonary vessels

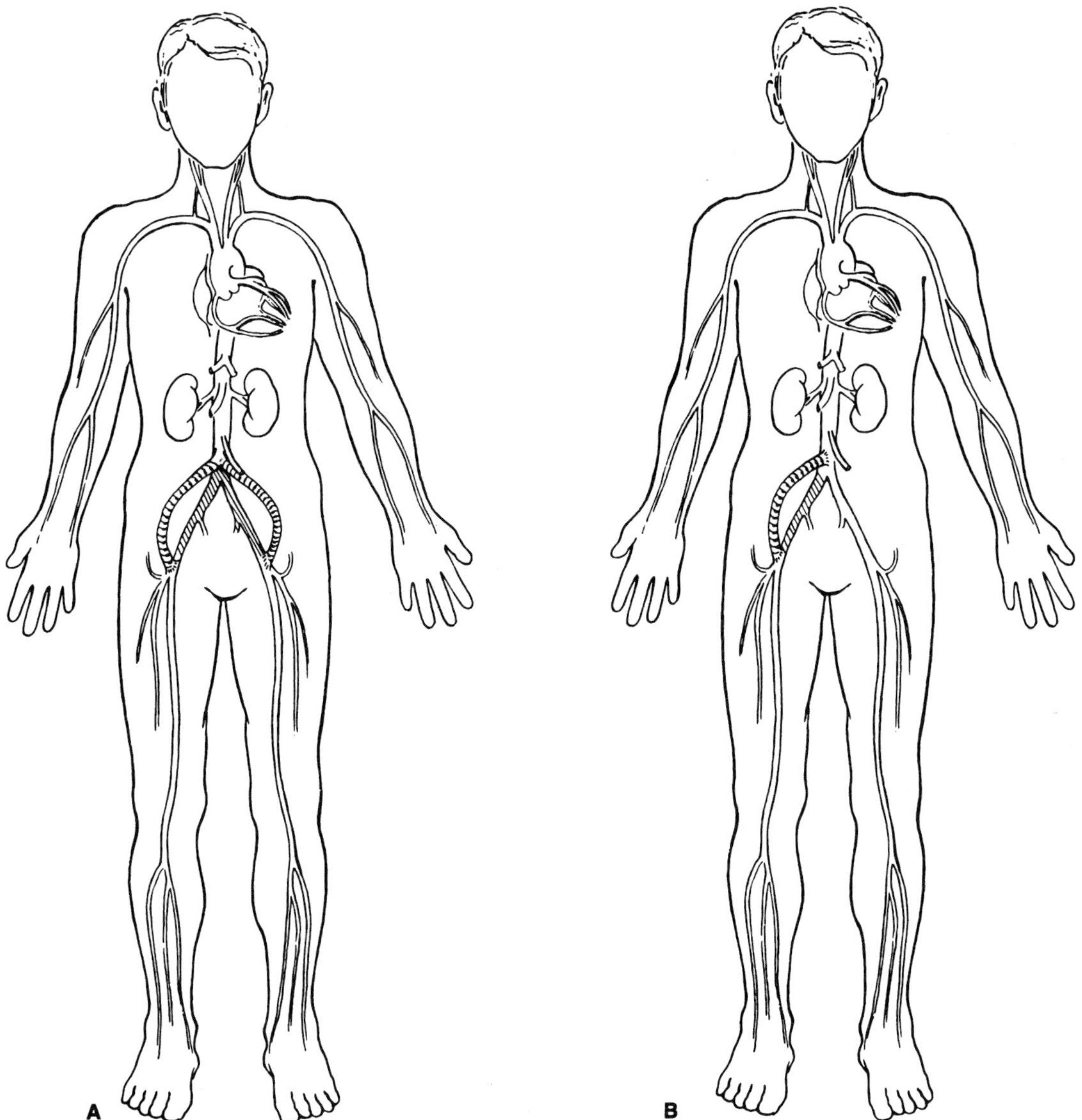


**FIGURE 19–6** Aortoiliac occlusion and revascularization. **A,** Aortobifemoral prosthetic bypass graft. **B,** Unilateral aortofemoral prosthetic bypass graft. (From Kinney MR, Packa DR, Dunbar SB: *AACN's Clinical Reference for Critical Care Nursing,* 3rd Ed [p 621]. New York, McGraw-Hill, 1993.)

**XV. Vein Ligation and Stripping: Surgical Ligation and Removal of Varicose Vein(s) of Leg(s)**

**XVI. Sympathectomy**

A. Interruption of some portion of sympathetic nervous system pathway

B. Causes vasodilation, improvement in circulation to extremity

C. Treatment for partial arterial obstruction with resultant distal trophic changes

## GENERAL SYSTEMS ASSESSMENT OF VASCULAR PATIENTS

**I. Cardiovascular: Myocardial Infarction Remains Leading Cause of Death After Peripheral Vascular Procedures Because of Coexisting Cardiovascular Disease**

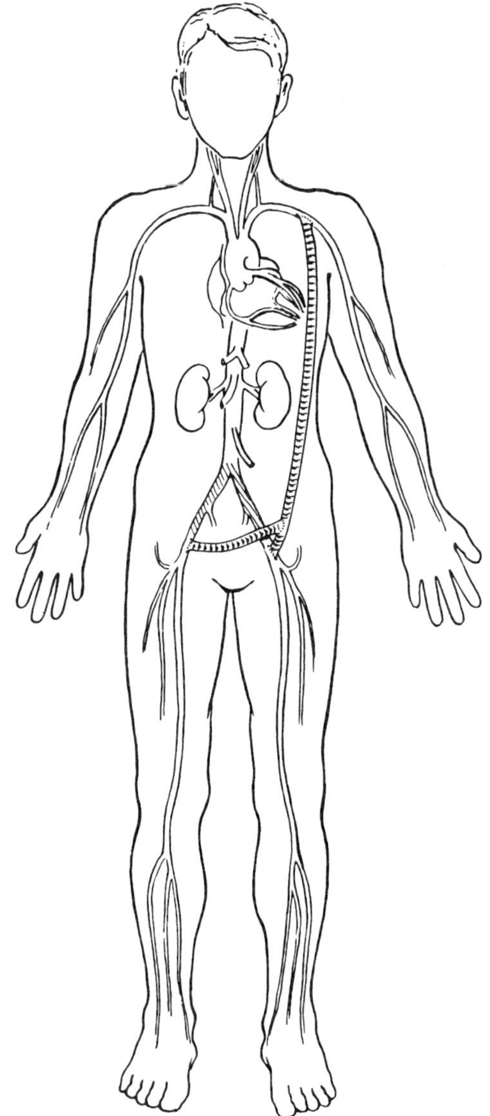

**FIGURE 19–7** Aortoiliac occlusion and revascularization. Left axillofemorofemoral prosthetic bypass graft. (From Kinney MR, Packa DR, Dunbar SB: *AACN's Clinical Reference for Critical Care Nursing*, 3rd Ed [p 622]. New York, McGraw-Hill, 1992.)

A. Evaluation of cardiac status
   1. Hemodynamic profile: cardiac output (CO), systemic vascular resistance (SVR)
   2. Electrocardiogram (ECG); dysrhythmias
      a. Increased myocardial oxygen demands
      b. Increased cardiac ischemia: angina
   3. Signs and symptoms of myocardial infarction
      a. Chest pain
      b. Dysrhythmias
      c. Diaphoresis
      d. Nausea and vomiting
      e. Dyspnea
      f. Hypotension
   4. Chest x-ray film to assess heart size and fluid status

B. Cardiac enzymes
   1. Creatine phosphokinase (CPK); lactic dehydrogenase (LDH); aspartate aminotransferase, serum (AST) also known as serum glutamic oxaloacetic transaminase (SGOT); alanine aminotransferase, serum (ALT), also known as serum glutamic pyruvic transaminase (SGPT)
   2. CPK isoenzyme
C. Serum electrolytes
   1. Hyperkalemia
      a. Oliguric renal failure
      b. Volume depletion
      c. Decreased effect of aldosterone: Addison's disease, chronic heparin administration
   2. Hypokalemia
      a. Diuretic or digitalis therapy

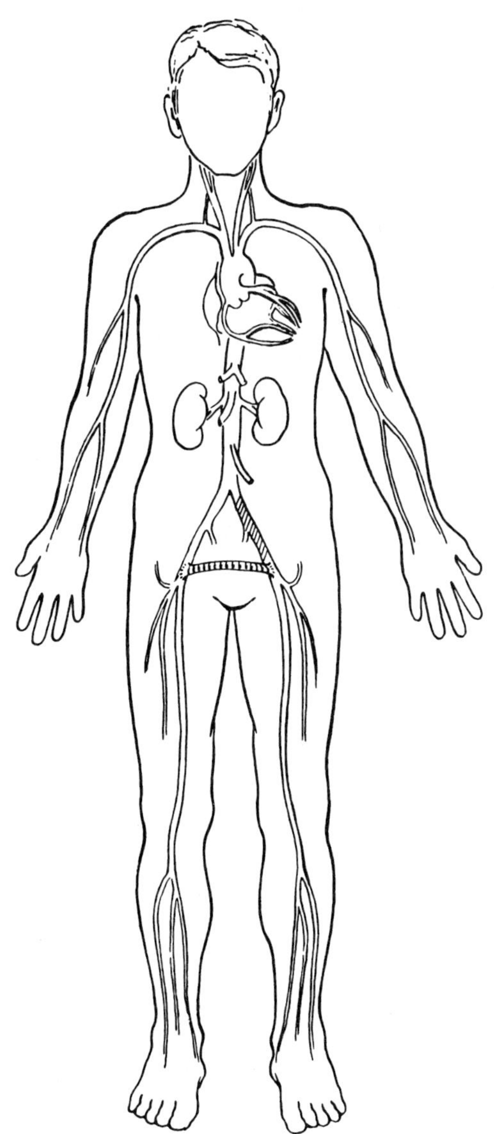

**FIGURE 19–8** Left iliac occlusion and revascularization. Right-to-left femorofemoral prosthetic bypass graft. (From Kinney MR, Packa DR, Dunbar SB: *AACN's Clinical Reference for Critical Care Nursing,* 3rd Ed [p 622]. New York, McGraw-Hill, 1992.)

b. Stress
c. Gastrointestinal disorders
(1) Long-term steroid therapy: arthritis, chronic obstructive pulmonary disease (COPD)
(2) Hypoaldosteronism
3. Hypernatremia
a. Mechanical ventilation without humidification
b. Fever
4. Hyponatremia
a. Diuretics
b. Gastrointestinal disorders
c. Hypotonic irrigating solutions
d. Hyperlipidemia
e. Hyperglycemia
5. Hypermagnesemia
a. Renal failure
b. Adrenal insufficiency
c. Shock
d. Hypothermia
6. Hypomagnesemia
a. Excessive loss of body fluids
b. Diuretics
c. Cardiac glycosides, aminoglycosides
d. Decreased intestinal absorption
e. Primary hyperaldosteronism
f. Hypercalcemia associated with hyperparathyroidism and hyperthyroidism
g. ECG reflects prolonged QT interval, decreased T-wave amplitude, shortened ST segment

**II. Accompanying Cardiovascular Disorders**

A. Hypertension
1. High incidence (40% to 60%) associated with PVD
2. Adds stress to anastomotic sites
3. Precipitates postoperative incisional bleeding

B. Hypotension
1. Decreases cerebral, coronary, and renal artery perfusion
2. Decreases stroke volume: decreased cardiac output

C. Valvular disease: associated with decreased cardiac output and left ventricular failure
1. Mitral valve stenosis: associated with pulmonary fibrosis and hypertension
2. Aortic insufficiency: associated with circulatory collapse with sudden hypotension

**III. Pulmonary Status**

A. Baseline parameters
1. Respirations
a. Rate, quality
b. Pattern, excursion
2. Auscultation of lungs
a. Wheezes
b. Rales
c. Rhonchi
d. Crackles
3. Arterial blood gases (ABGs), $Svo_2$ monitoring

4. Pulmonary function studies
   a. Forced vital capacity (FVC)
      (1) Measurement of volume of air expelled by fully inflated lung
      (2) Compromised FVC indicative of lung parenchymal restriction
   b. Forced expiratory volume (FEV)
      (1) Decreased FEV indicative of impaired elastic recoil (emphysema)
      (2) Increased FEV indicative of airway resistance (chronic bronchitis or asthma)
   c. Ventilation/perfusion ratio
5. Chest x-ray film
   a. Pulmonary infiltrate or lesion
   b. Heart size
   c. Congestive heart failure (CHF)
   d. Fibrosis or effusion

B. Pulmonary history
   1. Obstructive disorders (COPD, emphysema, asthma)
   2. Infections (bronchitis, tuberculosis)
   3. Presence of cough (lesions, smoking, bronchitis)
   4. Complaints of shortness of breath
   5. Orthopnea

## IV. Neurologic Status

A. Postoperative assessment: compare with preoperative baseline
   1. Level of consciousness
   2. Pupillary reactions
   3. Sensory and motor ability
   4. Evaluation of following cranial nerves
      a. Facial (VIII): controls facial muscles; affects ability to smile, show teeth, wrinkle forehead, raise eyebrows
      b. Hypoglossal (XII): most frequently traumatized; controls tongue; affects side-to-side motion of tongue
      c. Glossopharyngeal (IX): controls posterior third of tongue, uvula; affects gag reflex
      d. Vagus (X): controls pharynx, larynx, soft palate; affects gag reflex
      e. Spinal accessory (XI): controls trapezius and sternocleidomastoid muscles; affects strength and tone of shoulder muscles
      f. Phrenic nerve: controls diaphragm; affects diaphragmatic function in respiratory excursion

B. Neurologic history
   1. Vertigo
   2. Syncope
   3. TIA
   4. CVA
   5. Spinal cord ischemia with descending thoracic aorta repair

## V. Renal Status

A. Preoperative baseline studies
   1. Blood urea nitrogen (BUN)
   2. Creatinine
   3. Electrolytes
   4. Calcium
   5. Phosphorus
   6. Urinalysis

B. Specific renal function studies, if indicated
   1. Osmolar, free water, and sodium clearances

2. Creatinine or insulin clearance to evaluate glomerular filtration
3. Paraaminohippurate clearance to evaluate renal blood flow
4. Postangiographic renal function to evaluate possibility of renal failure caused by radioactive dye

C. Compromised renal system during vascular surgery caused by
1. Hemorrhage
2. Trauma
3. Renal vessel damage, tubular damage
4. Anoxia
5. Prolonged hypotension

**VI. Diabetes**

A. Relationship to PVD
1. High incidence of occurrence in patients with PVD
2. Higher incidence of postoperative complications
3. Altered fluid requirements

B. Management of diabetes in a surgical patient (insulin regimen dependent on institutional policy)
1. Preoperative dose: usually less than routine daily dose
2. Stress of surgery (with release of epinephrine and glucocorticoids) increases need for insulin
3. Diet-controlled diabetics may require insulin in immediate postoperative period

C. Laboratory assessment
1. Fasting glucose levels
2. Electrolyte series
3. Serum ketones/acetones
4. Renal function studies
5. ABGs

**VII. Hematologic Evaluation**

A. Laboratory studies
1. Prothrombin time, partial thromboplastin time
2. D-Dimer assay
3. Platelet count
4. Bleeding time, clotting time
5. Type and crossmatch
6. Complete blood count

B. Anticoagulant medications
1. Heparin/sodium warfarin (Coumadin)
2. Aspirin
3. Dipyridamole (Persantine)
4. Ticlopidine (Ticlid)

C. Previous postoperative bleeding/clotting problems
1. Disseminated intravascular coagulopathy (DIC)
2. Blood transfusion reactions
3. Thrombophlebitis
4. Pulmonary emboli
5. History of any postoperative bleeding

## INTRAOPERATIVE CONCERNS

**I. Carotid and Other Neck Vessel Procedures**

A. Anesthesia choices
1. Local anesthesia

a. Advantages
(1) Quick evaluation of level of consciousness and neurologic changes
(2) Minimizes risk of cerebral ischemia
b. Disadvantages
(1) Difficult to manage systemic complications (convulsions, dysrhythmias, hypotension, hypertension)
(2) Positional discomfort
2. General anesthesia
a. Advantages
(1) Facilitates control of hypertension, hypoxia, dysrhythmias, and blood loss
(2) Temperature control
b. Disadvantages
(1) Inability to assess immediate neurologic status
(2) May require postoperative ventilatory support
(3) Anesthetic side effects
B. Extubation as soon as possible allows for accurate neurologic evaluation
C. Maintenance of adequate cerebral blood flow: avoidance of hypotension
D. Intraoperative complications of carotid surgery
1. Hemorrhage
2. Acute CVA: higher incidence when stenosis of opposite carotid/vertebral artery prevents adequate cerebral perfusion
3. Facial/hypoglossal nerve damage (refer to neurologic assessment section)

**II. Intrathoracic Vascular Procedures**
A. Lung deflation during procedure
1. To protect lung from injury
2. For adequate exposure to operative site
B. Use of extracorporeal circulation, depending on location of lesion
C. Use of hypothermia and/or temporary shunts to minimize organ ischemia
D. Intraoperative complications
1. CVA
2. Pneumothorax, hemothorax
3. Myocardial injury
4. Severe hypotension
5. Renal failure
6. Spinal cord ischemia

**III. Abdominal Vessel Procedures**
A. Bowel preparation
1. Decrease incidence of ischemic bowel injury
2. Minimize postoperative ileus
B. Anesthesia choices
1. Spinal/epidural for elective lower abdominal procedures
a. Advantages
(1) Elimination of vasospasm
(2) Reduction of respiratory complications
b. Disadvantages
(1) Positional discomfort if procedure prolonged
(2) Anxiety increases tachycardia, dysrhythmias
(3) Prolonged decreased sensory and motor function
2. General anesthesia (as previously outlined)
C. Aortic crossclamping
1. Extreme hypertension can occur as aorta is clamped
2. Hypotension occurs after clamping released because of
a. Vasodilation of lower extremities

b. Third space fluid shifting
c. Metabolic acidosis: products of catabolism and ischemia released systemically

D. Renal status changes
1. Approximately 20% of postoperative abdominal vessel patients have acute renal failure develop
2. Transient oliguria if hypovolemia occurs
a. Fluid challenge
b. Mannitol: osmotic diuretic
c. Furosemide (Lasix): loop diuretic
3. Hematuria
a. Possible reaction to transfusion
b. Ureteral damage
c. Dislodged microemboli in renal arteries (renal failure)

E. Decreased core temperature related to
1. Massive fluid replacement
2. Length of procedure
3. Extensive viscera exposure
4. Cold irrigation fluid
5. Rapid heat loss in elderly patients
6. General anesthesia

F. Intraoperative complications
1. Hemorrhage: abdominal aorta, iliac vessels, inferior vena cava
2. Injury to ureters
3. Injury to duodenum, renal arteries/veins, kidney, or spleen
4. Hemiplegia
5. Ischemic bowel

G. Anticoagulation and reversal
1. Heparin administered during vessel clamping and anastomosis
2. Protamine sulfate administered to reverse effects of heparinization before completion of procedure

**IV. Sympathectomy: A Palliative Surgical Option for Patients with Peripheral Vascular Disease**

A. Peripheral blood vessels: under continuous control of sympathetic nervous system
1. With normal vasculature, sympathetic system regulates amount of vasoconstriction
a. To keep extremities warm, dry, and comfortable
b. To supply adequate amount of blood to periphery
2. With compromised peripheral circulation
a. Surgical division of sympathetic chain (variable response in patients with PVD)
(1) Permits permanent, maximal vasodilation
(2) Allows for maximal blood supply to affected extremity
(3) Not primary treatment for vascular obstructive disease
b. Benefits of sympathectomy
(1) Increases warmth and comfort of extremity
(2) Infection subsides, ulcers heal
(3) Small areas of gangrene or fibrosis improve
(4) Ischemic pain less severe

B. Surgical approaches
1. Lumbar sympathectomy: resection of ganglions L2, L3, L4
a. Indications for surgery
(1) Vasospastic disease
(2) Ischemic ulcers with pain at rest
(3) Certain forms of causalgia (severe sensation of burning skin)

b. Specific surgical risks
   (1) Hemorrhage caused by lumbar arterial or venous damage
   (2) Impotence related to genitofemoral nerve damage
   (3) Ureteral damage: inadvertent ligation or clipping during excision of lumbar sympathetic chain
c. Nursing considerations
   (1) Supine, lateral recumbent position
   (2) Increased sensitivity to position change, turning, elevating of head must be performed slowly
   (3) Flank dressing should remain dry
   (4) Presence of urine on dressing: ureteral damage
   (5) Presence of blood on dressing: lumbar vessel damage
   (6) Nasogastric decompression to prevent paralytic ileus
   (7) Pain: usually moderate, relieved by analgesics, severe flank pain indicative of ureteral ligation, hydronephrosis, requires surgical reexploration
   (8) Urine output: bladder distension and acute retention associated with operative discomfort
d. Neurovascular assessment: both lower extremities
   (1) Increase in warmth and vasodilation: desired result
   (2) Neuralgia may occur from damaged nerve

2. Cervical sympathectomy: resection of thoracic ganglia T2 to T6 and half of stellate ganglia C8 to T1
   a. Effectively denervates upper extremity of all extrinsic vasoconstrictor influences arising in sympathetic nervous system, permitting return of normal vasodilation
   b. Surgical approach: usually supraclavicular; may use thoracic, transaxillary, or transpleural approach
   c. Specific surgical risks
      (1) Hemothorax or pneumothorax
      (2) Phrenic nerve dysfunction: ipsilateral paralysis of diaphragm
      (3) Chylous leak caused by ligation of divided thoracic duct
   d. Nursing considerations: cervical sympathectomy
      (1) Elevation of head enhances respiratory exchange
      (2) Position on side opposite chest tube; permits optimal lung inflation
      (3) Chest tube drainage should be less than 200 ml in first 8 hours
      (4) Vital signs: changes may indicate intrathoracic or intercostal bleeding
   e. Cardiopulmonary assessment: includes care of mechanically ventilated patients and monitoring of cardiac parameters
   f. Neurovascular assessment
      (1) Palpable radial pulse: confirm with Doppler apparatus if necessary
      (2) Circulation to affected extremity: warm, dry, pink
      (3) Observe for Horner's syndrome: common after cervical sympathectomy
         (a) Ptosis of upper eyelid
         (b) Slight elevation of lower lid
         (c) Constriction of affected pupil
         (d) Increased salivation and drooping of mouth on affected side
   g. Pain management: per nursing diagnosis and intervention appropriate to unit policy
   h. Complications
      (1) Persistent pneumothorax: damage to underlying lung during thoracotomy
      (2) Intrathoracic bleeding: undetected intercostal vessel interruption
      (3) Radial nerve and artery damage
      (4) Pleural effusion

## POSTANESTHESIA CONCERNS

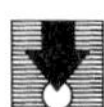

### NURSING DIAGNOSIS

Examples of related nursing diagnostic categories include:

- Ineffective airway clearance
- Pain
- Ineffective breathing pattern
- Altered peripheral tissue perfusion
- Decreased cardiac output
- Hypothermia
- Paralysis

**I. General PACU Care of Vascular Patient**

A. Postoperative report includes

1. Preoperative preparation
   a. Sedation: control of anxiety
   b. Anticholinergics for reduction of secretions
   c. Antibiotics
   d. Insulin: adjusted dose (according to regimen of institution)
   e. Heparin infusion rate
2. Preoperative medications: often continued until time of surgery
   a. Nitroglycerin
      (1) Increases coronary perfusion
      (2) Decreases peripheral resistance
   b. Antihypertensives
      (1) β-blocker
      (2) Calcium channel blocker
      (3) Ace inhibitors
   c. Antidysrhythmics
3. Background information
   a. Patient identification
   b. Baseline vital signs
   c. Procedure performed
   d. Anesthesia administered
   e. Drugs received
   f. Length of procedure
   g. Estimated blood loss
4. Intraoperative vital signs and monitoring data
5. Intraoperative problems encountered
6. Anticipated problems

B. Postoperative monitoring data: observe for compensatory mechanisms

1. ECG: rhythm, ST segment changes
2. Arterial line and/or noninvasive blood pressure
3. Central venous pressure (CVP)
4. Pulmonary artery pressures (Swan-Ganz catheter)
5. Core temperature
6. Ventilation and oxygen support
   a. Mechanical ventilation; parameters: $FIO_2$, mode-continuous mechanical ventilation (CMV), synchronous intermittent mechanical ventilation (SIMV), continuous positive airway pressure (CPAP), tidal volume (Tv), rate, positive end-expiratory pressure (PEEP), pressure support

b. Spontaneous ventilation: face mask
c. Oxygen saturation (pulse oximetry)
d. End-tidal $CO_2$
e. $Svo_2$

C. Vascular assessment
1. Skin
a. Temperature: warm, cool, or cold
b. Skin color: pink, ruddy, dusky, pale or mottled
2. Capillary refill
a. Normal color return after nail bed blanching
b. Color return should occur within 2 seconds
3. Peripheral pulses
a. Head and neck arteries
b. Carotid
c. Temporal
d. Upper extremity arterial pulses
(1) Radial
(2) Brachial
(3) Axillary
e. Lower extremity arterial pulses
(1) Femoral artery
(2) Popliteal artery
(3) Posterior tibial artery
(4) Dorsalis pedis artery
4. Quality of pulse
a. Reflection of cardiac output and peripheral vascular patency
b. Use of objective pulse quality scale for charting purposes

> 0 Absent pulse
> +1 Fleeting pulse
> +2 Weak, thready pulse
> +3 Normal quality
> +4 Increased volume, strong and bounding

5. Doppler ultrasound confirmation: device amplifies sound waves produced by pulsating blood flow in vessel and allows for detection of pulsatile flow in absence of palpable pulse
6. Marking of pulses: facilitates comparison of pulses and promotes continuity of care
7. Extraanatomic graft pulses: placed subcutaneously to improve recipient vessel circulation

D. Neurologic assessment (vital signs)
1. Level of consciousness: orientation to person, place, time
2. Motor and sensory function
a. Motion and sensation of all extremities
b. Bilateral and equal hand grasp
3. Pupillary function: equal reaction and accommodation to light
4. Abnormal findings
a. Tics
b. Tremors
c. Gazing
d. Seizures

E. Neurovascular assessment; evaluate the 6 Ps:
1. Pulses/pulselessness
2. Pain
3. Paresthesia
4. Paralysis

5. Pallor
6. Poikilothermia (coldness)

F. Fluid volume status
1. CVP, pulmonary artery pressures
2. Assessment of vital signs
3. Laboratory data
a. Hemoglobin, hematocrit
b. Serum $Na^+$, potassium
c. Coagulation studies
4. Replacement of blood and (third space) fluid loss
a. Colloid
b. Crystalloid
c. Plasma expanders

G. Operative site observation
1. Dressing site and condition
2. Drains and drainage
3. Presence of abnormalities
a. Hematoma formation
b. Discolorations
4. Changes in abdominal girth, diameter

H. Limb protection
1. Bed cradle
2. Heel and elbow padding
3. Lanolin for dry skin
4. Lamb's wool between toes
5. No pressure under knee
6. Avoidance of joint (graft) flexion at hip or knee

**II. PACU Care for Specific Vascular Procedures**

A. Carotid vessel procedures
1. Neurologic assessment
a. Presence of swallow and gag reflexes
b. Cranial nerve function: affected by intraoperative retraction and stretching of nerves
2. Respiratory concerns
a. Instruct patient to inhale deeply and minimize deep cough response to avoid elevation of venous pressure
b. Incentive spirometry encourages deep inhalation
c. Assess for possible respiratory obstruction
(1) Vocal cord edema/injury, surgical trauma
(2) Tracheal deviation: hematoma development at operative site, may present with stridor
3. Blood pressure concerns: maintain adequate blood pressure to maximize cerebral perfusion and minimize possible sequelae of hypertension or hypotension
a. Hypertension
(1) Sequelae
(a) Suture line disruption: tension at site of anastomosis may cause bleeding
(b) Hematoma formation: tracheal compression
(c) Cerebral hemorrhage, edema
(2) Nursing interventions
(a) Elevate head of bed to decrease venous pressure
(b) Comfort measures to minimize pain and maintain desired blood pressure parameters
(c) Ensure adequate ventilation

b. Hypotension
   (1) Sequelae resulting from hypersensitive carotid sinus
      (a) Sluggish blood flow through operative artery and graft
      (b) Difficult pulse assessment
      (c) Decreased cerebral or coronary artery perfusion
   (2) Nursing interventions
      (a) Increase fluids if indicated
      (b) Reduce high Fowler's to more moderate position
      (c) Titration of vasopressor
c. Pharmacologic intervention
   (1) Sodium nitroprusside (Nipride): vasodilator
      (a) Direct effect on arterial and venous smooth muscle
      (b) Used to treat severe acute hypertension: rapid onset
      (c) Reduces peripheral resistance and increases cardiac output
   (2) Nitroglycerin: vasodilator
      (a) Relaxes smooth muscle in small blood vessels
      (b) Causes venous and arterial dilation, increases coronary artery perfusion
      (c) Used for treatment of myocardial ischemia and hypertension
   (3) Trimethaphan (Arfonad): antihypertensive
      (a) Ganglionic blocking agent
      (b) Causes peripheral vasodilation; used to treat hypertension
   (4) Dopamine (Intropin): vasopressor
      (a) Directly stimulates $\beta$, and dopaminergic receptors
      (b) Low dose causes renal and mesenteric vasodilation and subsequently increases urine output
      (c) Midrange dose produces a positive inotropic effect on myocardium
      (d) High dose stimulates $\alpha$-adrenergic receptors and causes renal vasoconstriction, increased peripheral resistance, and increased blood pressure
   (5) Milrinone (Primacor)
      (a) Positive inotropic agent with vasodilator properties
      (b) Causes thrombocytopenia and may be contraindicated for some patients
   (6) Phenylephrine (Neo-Synephrine): vasopressor
      (a) Acts on $\alpha$-adrenergic receptors
      (b) Produces vasoconstriction and increased peripheral resistance
      (c) Increases systolic and diastolic blood pressure
      (d) Reflex bradycardia occurs because of increased vagal activity
   (7) Labetalol hydrochloride (Normodyne, Trandate): $\alpha$- and nonspecific $\beta$-receptor blocking agent
      (a) Used for treatment of hypertension
      (b) Administer supine to avoid orthostatic hypotensive effect
   (8) Esmolol (Brevibloc): $\beta$-blocking agent used to treat supraventricular tachyarrhythmias
      (a) Rapid onset of action, short half-life
      (b) Hypotension is most common side effect
   (9) Nifedipine (Procardia): calcium channel blocker used for treatment of chronic hypertension, acute hypertensive emergencies, and angina
      (a) Decreases systemic vascular resistance
      (b) Augments cardiac output

4. Bradycardia
   a. Causes
      (1) Altered baroreceptor responses
      (2) Vagal manipulation
      (3) Vagal pressure from hematoma formation
      (4) Myocardial infarction

- b. Interventions
  - (1) Pharmacologic
    - (a) Atropine (anticholinergic, parasympatholytic): inhibits action of acetylcholine; stimulates or depresses central nervous system depending on dose; used to treat bradycardia
    - (b) Glycopyrrolate (Robinul; anticholinergic): inhibits action of acetylcholine; used to treat bradycardia
  - (2) Surgical
    - (a) Excision of hematoma
    - (b) Reexploration of wound

5. Positioning: elevation of head
   - a. Decreases venous pressure
   - b. Facilitates respiratory excursion
6. Dressings/drains
   - a. Dressings: light, nonconstricting
   - b. Drains: Penrose, Jackson-Pratt, Hemovac

B. Intrathoracic vessel procedures

1. Respiratory support
   - a. Principles of care of intubated/mechanically ventilated patient
   - b. Head elevation permits respiratory excursion and allows proper chest tube function
   - c. Turn, cough, deep breathe every 2 hours and prn
2. Assess for complications
   - a. Atelectasis
   - b. Pneumothorax, hemothorax
   - c. Adult respiratory distress syndrome (ARDS)
   - d. CHF/pulmonary edema
3. Ensure proper chest tube functioning
   - a. Secure connections
   - b. Observe for air leaks
   - c. Measure drainage
   - d. Keep bottles below chest level
   - e. Auscultate lung sounds
   - f. Palpate for subcutaneous emphysema (crepitus)
4. Neurovascular assessment (as previously outlined)
   - a. Pulse assessment: upper and lower extremities
   - b. Motor and sensory function
     - (1) Spinal cord ischemia
       - (a) Paraplegia can occur with prolonged thoracic/aortic occlusion
       - (b) Decreased perfusion pressure to spinal cord
     - (2) Embolization to distal arteries, originating from aortic clot
5. Monitor for cardiac, pulmonary, renal function (as previously outlined)
6. Pain management (according to unit policy)
   - a. Prevent splinting and permit lung expansion
   - b. Allay apprehension and fear
   - c. Decrease tachycardia and hypertension
   - d. Enhance mechanical ventilation compliance

C. Abdominal vessel procedures

1. Continuous cardiopulmonary assessment (as previously outlined)
2. Observe for signs/symptoms of hypovolemic shock caused by hemorrhage
3. Gastrointestinal assessment
   - a. Nasogastric tube: decompresses stomach, prevents paralytic ileus
   - b. Complications
     - (1) Ileus

        (2) Occlusion of inferior mesenteric artery, causing colon ischemia
        (3) Hemorrhage: measure and monitor abdominal girth
4. Renal assessment (as previously outlined)
    a. Hematuria: aortic crossclamping, kidney and/or bladder trauma
    b. Oliguria: renal failure, tubular necrosis
5. Neurovascular status (as previously outlined)
    a. Pedal pulses may be absent for 6 to 12 hours postoperatively
        (1) Vascular spasm
        (2) Peripheral vasoconstriction
        (3) Vessel patency, verified by surgeon
        (4) Confirm absence with Doppler ultrasonography
    b. Absence of previously palpable pulse
        (1) Signifies occlusion of vessel or graft
        (2) Requires immediate surgical reexploration
6. Positioning
    a. Abdominal procedures: head elevation
        (1) Facilitates respiratory excursion
        (2) Decreases suture line stress
    b. Vena cava plication: supine to slight Trendelenburg
        (1) Prevents further reduction of venous return
        (2) Decreased venous return results in decreased cardiac output
7. Pain or vascular spasm
    a. Severe pain indicative of retroperitoneal bleeding
    b. Spasms
        (1) Usually follow aortic surgery
        (2) Aggravated by hypotension, hypothermia, pain, $CO_2$ retention
8. Hypothermia or shivering
    a. Sequelae
        (1) Increases oxygen requirement
        (2) ST segment depression can occur with increased myocardial oxygen requirement
        (3) Prolonged somnolence occurs with decreased cerebral perfusion
        (4) Increases vasoconstriction and vasospasm
            (a) Increases difficulty in palpating pulses
            (b) Aggravates hypertension
        (5) Increases patient anxiety and discomfort
    b. Corrective nursing interventions
        (1) Heated blankets, automatic hyperthermia blanket
        (2) Warming lights
        (3) Heated aerosol nebulizers with oxygen delivery
9. Complications
    a. Acute arterial occlusion
    b. Debris embolization: pulmonary, cerebral, peripheral
    c. Graft suture line hemorrhage
    d. Cardiopulmonary complications: dysrhythmias, myocardial infarction (MI), CHF
    e. Third space fluid accumulation
    f. Renal complications: failure, trauma

D. Extraanatomic vessel bypasses (femoral crossover, axillofemoral bypass)
1. Positioning: turn only to unoperated side
    a. Avoid external pressure on graft
    b. Avoid flexion of graft; careful pillow positioning
2. Pulse checks with femoral crossover
    a. Across symphysis pubis (femoral to femoral)
    b. Both lower extremities

3. Pulse checks with axillofemoral bypass: monitor donor arm and revascularized limb
   a. Avoid damage to donor artery; obtain blood pressure, draw blood from opposite arm
   b. Specific complications of axillofemoral bypass
      (1) Brachial plexus injury
      (2) Subclavian or axillary artery injury
      (3) Upper extremity embolization

E. Extremity vessel procedures (arterial bypass grafts, embolectomies; vein stripping and ligation)
1. Nursing concerns: arterial procedures
   a. Positioning: avoid severe joint flexion, crossing of legs, pillows under popliteal area
   b. Nonrestrictive dressings
   c. Neurovascular assessment
      (1) Comparison of both extremities
      (2) Doppler confirmation
      (3) If no pulses expected by surgeon, successful revascularization assessed by dry, pink, warm legs and feet
   d. Limb protection (as previously outlined)
   e. Laboratory data
      (1) Monitor glucose in diabetic patient: control of blood sugar can prevent infection
      (2) Monitor potassium: extracellular potassium increases with limb ischemia and infection
      (3) Monitor for metabolic acidosis: causes increased serum potassium
   f. Administer low-molecular weight dextran (500 ml over 10 to 24 hours)
      (1) Anticoagulation effect: interrupts action of fibrinogen and clotting factors
      (2) Reduces platelet accumulation and adhesiveness
      (3) Increases tissue perfusion
      (4) Reduces blood viscosity
      (5) Increases colloid osmotic pressure
   g. Control of pain to prevent spasms
2. Complications of extremity vessel procedures
   a. Graft occlusion
   b. Vein, nerve injury
   c. Pulmonary or cerebral emboli
3. Nursing concerns: vein procedures
   a. Positioning
      (1) Supine to slight head elevation with leg elevation
      (2) Avoidance of knee bending or leg crossing
   b. Dressing: multiple wounds covered by Ace bandages
   c. Neurovascular assessment: bilateral comparison as previously outlined
   d. Pain assessment: incisional discomfort vs. deep calf pain of thrombophlebitis
4. Complications of vein ligation, stripping procedures
   a. Hematoma and wound bleeding
   b. Femoral vein or femoral saphenous nerve damage
   c. Thrombophlebitis
   d. Edema

## BIBLIOGRAPHY

Allen A (ed): *Core Curriculum for Post Anesthesia Nursing Practice,* 2nd Ed. Philadelphia, WB Saunders, 1991.

Alspach, JG (ed): *Core Curriculum for Critical Care Nursing,* 4th Ed. Philadelphia, WB Saunders, 1991.

Bates B, Bickley LS, Hoekelman RA, Thompson JE: *A Guide to Physical Examination and History Taking,* 6th Ed. Philadelphia, JB Lippincott, 1995.

Bojar RM: *Manual of Perioperative Care in Cardiac and Thoracic Surgery,* 2nd Ed. Cambridge, Blackwell Science, 1994.

Boyer MJ: *Study Guide to Brunner and Suddarth's Textbook of Medical-Surgical Nursing,* 7th Ed. New York, JB Lippincott, 1992.

Bright LD, Georgi S: Peripheral vascular disease: Is it arterial or venous? *Am J Nurs,* Sept 1992.

Chulay M, Guzzetta C, Dosey B: *AACN Handbook of Critical Care Nursing.* Stamford, Conn, Appleton & Lange, 1997.

Civetta JM, Taylor RW, Kirby RR: *Critical Care,* 2nd Ed. Philadelphia, JB Lippincott, 1992.

Clochesy JM, Breu C, Cardin S, Whittaker AA, Rudy EB: *Critical Care Nursing,* 2nd Ed. Philadelphia, WB Saunders, 1996.

Dolan JT: *Dolan's Critical Care Nursing: Clinical Management Through the Nursing Process.* Philadelphia, FA Davis, 1991.

Eckman M, Priff N (eds): *Diseases,* 2nd Ed. Pennsylvania, Springhouse, 1997.

Emma LA: Chronic arterial occlusive disease. *J Cardiovasc Nurs* 7(1):14–24, 1992.

Estes MEZ: *Health Assessment and Physical Examination,* Albany, NY, Delmar Publishers, 1998.

Fahey VA: *Vascular Nursing,* 2nd Ed. Philadelphia, WB Saunders, 1994.

Fauci AS, Braunwald E, Isselbacher KJ, Wilson JD, et al (eds): *Harrison's Principles of Internal Medicine,* 14th Ed. New York, McGraw-Hill, 1998.

Guilmet D, Bachet J, Goudot G, et al: Aortic dissection: Anatomic types and surgical approaches. *J Cardiovasc Surg* 34(1):23–32, 1993.

Hoekstra JW (ed): *Handbook of Cardiovascular Emergencies,* 1st Ed. Boston, Little, Brown & Co, 1997.

Hollier LH, Procter CD, Naslund TC: Spinal cord ischemia. In Bernhard VM, Towne FB (eds): *Complications in Vascular Surgery.* St Louis, Quality Medical Publishing, 1991.

Hudak CM, Gallo BM, Benz JJ: *Critical Care Nursing: A Holistic Approach,* 5th Ed. Philadelphia, JB Lippincott, 1990.

Keller KB, Lemberg L: The importance of magnesium in cardiovascular disease. *Am J Crit Care* (2)4:348–350, 1993.

Kinney MR, Packa DR, Dunbar SB: *AACN's Clinical Reference for Critical-Care Nursing.* New York, McGraw-Hill, 1988.

Kuhn JK, McGovern M: Peripheral vascular assessment of the elderly client. *J Gerontol Nurs,* Dec, 1992.

Litwack K: *Post Anesthesia Care Nursing,* 2nd ed. St. Louis, Mosby–Year Book, 1995.

Luckman J: *Saunders Manual of Nursing Care.* Philadelphia, WB Saunders, 1997.

Meeker MH: *Alexander's Care of the Patient in Surgery,* 10th Ed. St. Louis, Mosby, 1995.

Owens MW, Daniel JL: IV magnesium sulfate in the treatment of ventricular tachycardia and acute myocardial infarction. *Crit Care Nurse* Dec 1993.

Pagana KD, Pagana TJ: *Diagnostic Testing & Nursing Implications: A Case Study Approach,* 4th Ed. St. Louis, Mosby, 1994.

Price SA, Wilson LM: *Pathophysiology: Clinical Concepts of Disease Processes,* 5th Ed. St. Louis, Mosby–Year Book, 1997.

Procter CD, Kazmier FJ, Hollier LH, Ramee SR: Selection of patients for peripheral revascularization surgery. *Med Clin North Am* 76(5):1159–1168, 1992.

Quaal SJ: Interactive hemodynamics of IABC. In Quaal SJ: *Comprehensive Intraaortic Balloon Counterpulsation,* 2nd Ed. St Louis, Mosby–Year Book, 1993.

Shettigar UR, Toole JG, Appunn DO: Combined use of esmolol and digoxin in the acute treatment of atrial fibrillation or flutter. *Am Heart J* 126(2):368–374, 1993.

Siedlecki B: Peripheral vascular disease. *Can Nurse* Dec 1992.

Stone DJ, Bogdonoff D, Leisure G, Spiekerman BF, Mathes DD: *Perioperative Care Anesthesia, Medicine and Surgery,* St. Louis, Mosby, 1998.

Stoney RJ, Effeney DJ: *Wylie's Atlas of Vascular Surgery: Thoracoabdominal Aorta and Its Branches.* Philadelphia, JB Lippincott, 1992.

Thomas CL (ed): *Taber's Cyclopedic Medical Dictionary,* 17th Ed. Philadelphia, FA Davis, 1993.

Veith FJ, Hobson RW, Williams RA, Wilson SE: *Vascular Surgery: Principles and Practice,* 2nd Ed. New York, McGraw-Hill, 1994.

Waugaman WR, Foster SD, Rigor BM (eds): *Principles and Practice of Nurse Anesthesia,* 2nd Ed. Norwalk, Conn, Appleton & Lange, 1992.

## REVIEW QUESTIONS

**1. Atherosclerosis develops as a response to which of the following:**
A. Vessel tortuosity
B. Incompetent valves
C. Thrombus formation
D. Thrombophlebitis

**2. The development of venous obstructive disease is related to:**
A. Decreased vessel diameter
B. Increased peripheral vascular resistance
C. Formation of calcium deposits
D. Incompetent valves

**3. Clinical manifestations of arterial insufficiency include which of the following:**
   A. Shiny, dry, warm skin
   B. Thick brittle nails; warm skin; hair loss
   C. Weak distal pulses; cool, pale skin; edema
   D. Hair loss; skin ulceration; cool skin

**4. The highest incidence of peripheral vascular disease is among:**
   A. Elderly, diabetic, postmenopausal females
   B. Elderly, diabetic, smoking males
   C. Middle-aged, diabetic, smoking males
   D. Middle-aged, diabetic, sedentary males

**5. A leading cause of death in patients undergoing peripheral vascular reconstructive surgery is:**
   A. Pulmonary embolism
   B. Myocardial infarction
   C. Congestive heart failure
   D. Occluded aortic graft

**6. The procedure of choice for a patient with left superficial femoral artery occlusion would be:**
   A. Femoropopliteal bypass
   B. Aortofemoral bypass
   C. Sympathectomy
   D. Aneurysectomy

**7. The sympathetic nervous system regulates the amount of vasoconstriction. A lumbar sympathectomy:**
   A. Would be the treatment of choice for a patient with aortoiliac disease
   B. Is a noninvasive, low-risk procedure with an excellent response rate
   C. Would be performed when permanent vasodilation of peripheral vessels is desired
   D. Is a primary treatment option for patients with vascular occlusive disease

**8. The foot of a patient with an acute arterial occlusion would:**
   A. Exhibit pallor when elevated, rubor when dependent
   B. Remain pulseless when elevated and become warm when dependent
   C. Be reddish brown in color and warm when elevated
   D. Become cyanotic when dependent but return to normal when elevated

**9. One hour after a carotid endarterectomy, Mrs. Green's blood pressure was stable at 130/70. She has been oriented to person, place, and time. She complains of neck pain and suddenly becomes confused and disoriented. Her arterial pressure is now 180/90. The appropriate nursing interventions would include:**
   A. Medicate for pain to control hypertension, continue to monitor, and notify physician
   B. Begin sodium nitroprusside (Nipride) infusion, and reevaluate blood pressure and neurologic vital signs in 10 minutes
   C. Notify physician, evaluate neurologic vital signs, check for incisional hematoma, and prepare (do not start) sodium nitroprusside
   D. Prepare (do not start) sodium nitroprusside infusion, medicate for pain, and continue to observe

**10. The disadvantages of using spinal or epidural anesthesia for abdominal vessel procedures include all of the following except:**
   A. Prolonged decreased sensory and motor function
   B. Positional discomfort if procedure prolonged
   C. Increased anxiety
   D. Elimination of vasospasm

**ANSWERS:** 1. C, 2. D, 3. D, 4. B, 5. B, 6. A, 7. C, 8. A, 9. C, 10. D

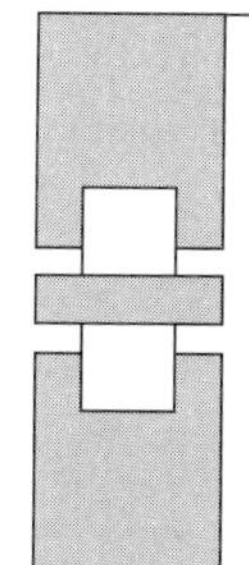

CHAPTER 20

# The Pulmonary Surgical Patient

Linda M. Bernard, MS, RN

## OBJECTIVES

**Study of the information represented by this outline will enable the learner to:**

1. Discuss the anatomy and physiology relevant to the care of the pulmonary surgical patient.
2. Identify systemic, orthopedic, neurologic, and primary pulmonary pathologic conditions that can cause pulmonary dysfunction.
3. Describe signs and symptoms of specific pulmonary pathologic conditions.
4. Describe components of preoperative assessment in the evaluation of a patient with a pulmonary disorder.
5. Explain surgical procedures used in the diagnosis and treatment of the pulmonary patient.
6. Identify special intraoperative considerations in the care of the pulmonary patient.
7. State the major complications seen postoperatively in the patient undergoing thoracic surgery.
8. Describe the key nursing assessments and interventions in the immediate postoperative phase of the patient undergoing thoracic surgery.

## ANATOMY AND PHYSIOLOGY

### I. Anatomy of Pulmonary System

A. Upper airway: nose and mouth to larynx—function of the upper airway is to warm, humidify, and filter inspired air
  1. Nose: bony and cartilaginous structure
  2. Pharynx: passageway for food and gas
    a. Nasopharynx: airway above soft palate
    b. Oropharynx: airway from soft palate to base of tongue
    c. Laryngopharynx: airway below base of tongue to larynx
  3. Larynx connects upper and lower airway; functions are gas conduction, protection against aspiration, and facilitation of cough and speech
    a. Thyroid cartilage: Adam's apple
    b. Glottis: opening of larynx
    c. Cricoid cartilage: narrowest part of airway in child
    d. Cricothyroid membrane: site for emergent cricothyroidotomy
    e. Epiglottis: cartilage that helps to prevent aspiration of foreign material during swallowing
    f. Vocal cords: vibration produces sound

B. Lower airway: tracheobronchial tree and parenchyma of lung (Fig. 20–1)—a series of connected tubes that provide a passageway for air to the alveoli
  1. Conducting airways: nose to terminal bronchioles; provide passageway for gas into and out of gas exchange airways; also called anatomic dead space
    a. Trachea
      (1) Carina: bifurcation point of trachea into right and left main-stem bronchi; important marker in endotracheal tube placement; anatomic landmark is the angle of Louis

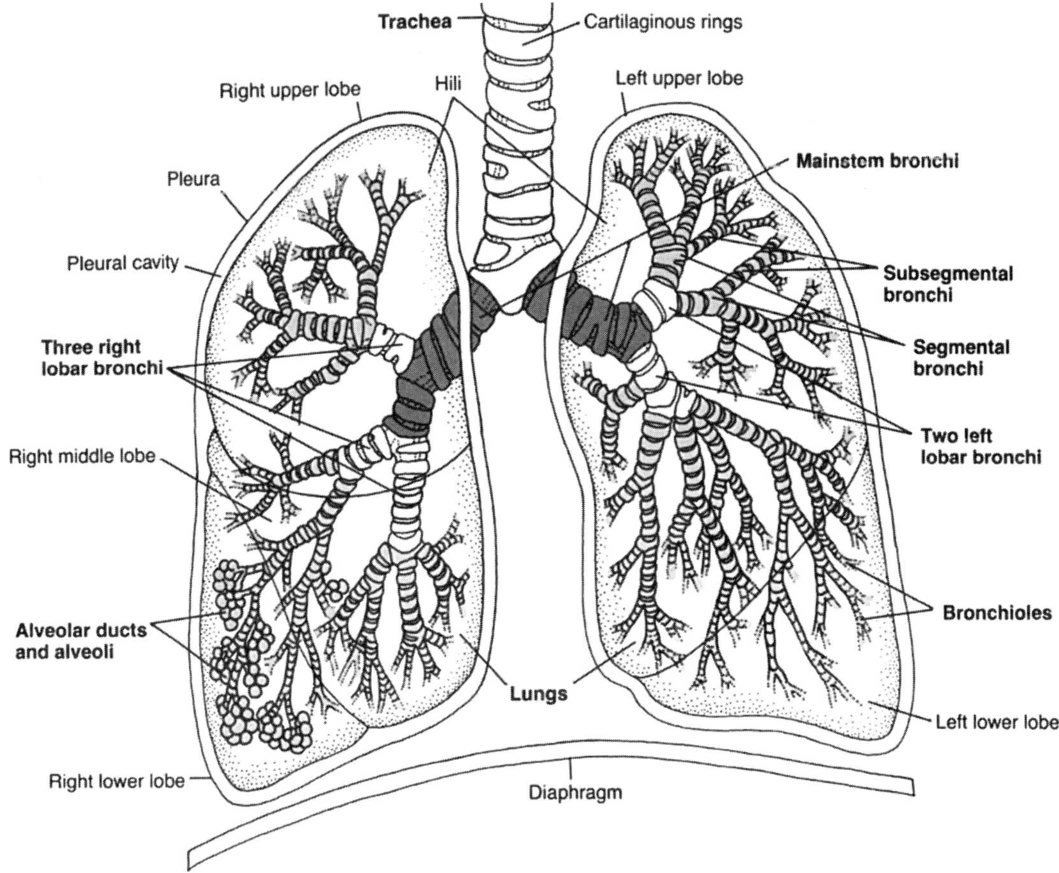


**FIGURE 20–1** Anatomy of lower respiratory tract. (From Ignatavicius DD, Bayne MV: *Medical-Surgical Nursing: A Nursing Process Approach* [p 1934]. Philadelphia, WB Saunders, 1991.)

b. Bronchi
   (1) Main stem: right and left
   (2) Lobar
   (3) Segmental
   (4) Subsegmental
c. Bronchioles
   (1) Terminal bronchioles: smooth muscle walls without cartilage

2. Gas exchange airways: area in which exchange of gases between pulmonary capillaries and alveoli occurs; volume is approximately 3 liters
   a. Respiratory bronchioles
   b. Alveolar ducts
   c. Alveoli (200 to 600 million in healthy lung)
      (1) Type 1 provide structure
      (2) Type 2 manufacture surfactant
      (3) Type 3 are alveolar macrophages

C. Thoracic cavity
   1. Bony structures
      a. Sternum, ribs, clavicle
      b. Vertebrae, scapulae
   2. Muscles of ventilation
      a. Inspiration
         (1) Major: diaphragm
         (2) Accessory: sternocleidomastoid, scalene, trapezius, and pectorals

b. Expiration (normally passive)
   (1) Active expiration: abdominal and intercostal muscles
3. Pleurae: two layers that normally slide easily over each other during ventilation
   a. Visceral: layer on lungs; no sensory innervation
   b. Parietal: layer on chest wall; sensory innervation
   c. Visceral and parietal pleurae meet at hilum to form pulmonary ligaments
   d. Pleural space: potential space; pressure within is normally subatmospheric
4. Mediastinum: anatomic space between lungs
   a. Structures within mediastinal space
      (1) Aortic arch and branches
      (2) Thymus
      (3) Innominate veins
      (4) Pulmonary artery and veins
      (5) Vena cava
      (6) Heart and pericardium
      (7) Lymphatic tissue and thoracic ducts
      (8) Trachea
      (9) Hilum of each lung
      (10) Azygos and hemizygous system
      (11) Esophagus
      (12) Vagus, cardiac, and phrenic nerves
      (13) Sympathetic nerve chains
5. Lungs
   a. Right: shorter and wider
      (1) Upper lobe
      (2) Middle lobe
      (3) Lower lobe
   b. Left
      (1) Upper lobe
      (2) Lower lobe

D. Pulmonary circulation
1. Purpose is to provide area for gas exchange
2. Pulmonary circulation acts as reservoir for left ventricle; only about 30% of pulmonary vessels are perfused at any given time
3. Low-pressure, low-resistance arterial system
   a. Arterioles perfuse each terminal bronchiole
   b. Alveolar-capillary membrane is area for gas exchange
   c. Bronchial circulation supplies lungs with oxygenated blood; responsible for anatomic shunt
4. Three-zone model of pulmonary blood flow
   a. Distribution of blood flow affected by posture; in upright position, blood flow decreases linearly from apex to base; in supine position, blood flow is greater to posterior (dependent) regions
   b. Zone I: ventilation exceeds perfusion
   c. Zone II: ventilation equals perfusion
   d. Zone III: perfusion exceeds ventilation

E. Neural control of ventilation
1. Respiratory center
   a. Medulla
      (1) Inspiratory area: responsible for basic ventilatory rhythm
      (2) Expiratory area: responsible for active expiration
   b. Pons
      (1) Pneumotaxic center: located in upper pons; stimulates expiratory center, which turns off inspiratory area to cause inspiration to end and expiration to begin

(2) Apneustic center: located in lower pons; prolongs inspiration by stimulation of inspiratory area

2. Chemical feedback mechanisms
   a. Central chemoreceptors
      (1) Located on ventrolateral surface of medulla
      (2) Influenced by pH of cerebrospinal fluid (CSF); increase in hydrogen ion concentration stimulates ventilation to increase in depth and rate
      (3) Responsible for normal control of ventilation
      (4) In chronic situations of hypercarbia, chemoreceptors become less sensitive to changes in $CO_2$ levels as reflected in hydrogen ion concentration
   b. Peripheral chemoreceptors
      (1) Located in aortic arch, bifurcation of internal and external carotid arteries
      (2) Have high metabolic rates so are sensitive to changes in oxygen supply
      (3) Hypoxemia causes stimulation of respiratory center of the medulla, resulting in increase in rate and depth of respiration, tachycardia, hypertension, and increase in minute ventilation, pulmonary resistance and cardiac output
3. Nerves
   a. Autonomic
      (1) Parasympathetic: main neural influence over airways in normal conditions; cause smooth muscle contraction
      (2) Sympathetic: cause smooth muscle dilation
   b. Phrenic: motor innervation for diaphragm
   c. Intercostals: motor innervation for intercostal muscles and muscles and skin of anterolateral thorax
4. Receptors
   a. Pulmonary stretch receptors: located in smooth muscle of airways; stimulation causes slowing of ventilatory rate
   b. Irritant receptors located between airway epithelial cells; sensitive to foreign gases and materials; stimulation initiates cough, bronchoconstriction, and increased respiratory rate
   c. Juxtacapillary (J) receptors: located in alveolar walls adjacent to capillaries; increase respiratory rate in response to fluid or inflammation
   d. Extrapulmonary receptors
      (1) Upper airway: respond to mechanical and chemical stimuli
      (2) Joint and muscle: increase ventilation during exercise
      (3) Chest wall: probably instrumental in sensation of dyspnea

## II. Components of Gas Exchange

A. Ventilation: movement of gas between atmosphere and alveoli
   1. Pressure changes during ventilation
   2. Volumes
      a. Tidal volume: amount of air in a resting breath; normal tidal volume range 400 to 700 ml
      b. Normal frequencies: 12 to 20 breaths per minute
      c. Minute ventilation: amount of air moving into and out of airway in 1 minute; normal minute ventilation is 4 to 8 L/min
      d. Alveolar ventilation: that part of ventilation that takes part in gas exchange; minute ventilation minus dead space ventilation
      e. Physiologic dead space: amount of air in a resting tidal breath that does take part in gas exchange; normal 2 ml/kg
   3. Distribution of ventilation: dependent regions of lungs ventilate better than uppermost regions except at low lung volumes, where ventilation then becomes greater at apices of lung

4. Work of breathing: energy required for ventilation can be divided into three components
   a. Compliance work: work required to overcome elastic forces of lung
   b. Tissue resistance work: work required to overcome tissues of lung and thoracic cage
   c. Airway resistance work: work required to overcome resistance to air movement in and out of lungs
5. Elastic recoil: tendency of lungs to collapse; tendency of chest wall to spring out
6. Critical closing volume: volume of alveolar distension at which force of recoil becomes greater than force of distension; below this volume, alveolus collapses
7. Compliance: a measurement of distensibility of chest and lung; how easily the elastic forces in the lung accept a volume of air; the volume change per unit of pressure change
   a. Conditions that increase compliance
      (1) Chronic obstructive pulmonary disease (COPD)
      (2) Aging process
   b. Conditions that decrease compliance (Reduced compliance requires that patient do more muscular work to achieve same minute ventilation.)
      (1) Adult respiratory distress syndrome (ARDS)
      (2) Bronchospasm
      (3) Pulmonary edema
      (4) Pulmonary fibrosis
      (5) Deformities of chest wall
      (6) Obesity, pregnancy, abdominal distension
      (7) Postoperative splinting, atelectasis, or pneumonia
8. Resistance: pressure difference required for a unit of air flow; airway resistance can be modulated by physical, neuronal, or chemical factors; dynamic measurement of pressure flow relationship affected by both length and radius of area; major sites of resistance are medium-sized airways
   a. Conditions that can increase resistance (Increased resistance requires that patient do more muscular work to achieve same minute volume.)
      (1) Edema of airways
      (2) Airway spasm
      (3) Obstruction: secretions, tumor, COPD
      (4) Endotracheal or tracheostomy tubes

B. Diffusion: movement of gas across alveolocapillary membrane
   1. Factors affecting diffusion
      a. Surface area of alveoli and capillaries available for diffusion
      b. Integrity of alveolocapillary wall; thickness of alveolocapillary membrane
      c. Hemoglobin level
      d. Difference of partial pressure of gas in alveolus vs. blood
      e. Solubility of gas
   2. Disease processes that decrease diffusion
      a. Interstitial disease
      b. COPD
      c. Pulmonary edema
      d. Decrease in lung tissue: pneumonectomy
   3. Oxygen transport: oxygen is transported either dissolved or bound to hemoglobin
      a. Dissolved: 3%
      b. Oxyhemoglobin: 97%
      c. Oxyhemoglobin dissociation curve graphically represents relationship of $Po_2$ to percentage of oxygen saturation of hemoglobin; upper flat curve indicates a relatively unchanged hemoglobin affinity at $Po_2$ levels greater than 70 mm Hg; steep slope of

curve (less than 60 mm Hg) indicates small decreases in $Po_2$ and results in massive unloading of oxygen from hemoglobin molecule
   (1) Factors favoring oxygen dissociation from hemoglobin (shift to right)
      (a) Acidosis
      (b) Hypercapnia
      (c) Hyperthermia
      (d) Increased levels of 2,3-DPG
   (2) Factors that decrease oxygen dissociation (shift to left)
      (a) Alkalosis
      (b) Hypocapnia
      (c) Hypothermia
      (d) Decreased levels of 2,3-DPG
  d. Oxygen content: $Cao_2 = Hb \times 1.34 \times Sao_2 + (Po_2 \times 0.003)$
  e. Oxygen transport: $Cao_2 \times 10 \times CO$
  f. Causes of hypoxemia
   (1) Hypoventilation
   (2) Diffusion abnormalities
   (3) Altered ventilation/perfusion ratios
   (4) Shunting
 4. Carbon dioxide transport
  a. Dissolved: 7% to 10%
  b. Carbaminohemoglobin: 30%
  c. Bicarbonate: 60% to 70%
C. Perfusion: movement of oxygenated blood to tissues
 1. Control of pulmonary circulation: hypoxic vasoconstriction
 2. Ventilation/perfusion ($\dot{V}/\dot{Q}$) ratios and abnormalities: normal $\dot{V}/\dot{Q}$ ratio is 0.85; changes in lung ventilation or pulmonary blood flow alter $\dot{V}/\dot{Q}$ relationships; this results in abnormalities of gas exchange
 3. Shunt: blood flow without alveolar ventilation

## ACID-BASE PHYSIOLOGY AND ARTERIAL BLOOD GASES

See Chapter 12.

## PATHOLOGIC DISORDERS OF CHEST

I. **Malignant Chest Disorders:** Most are symptomatic and advanced when diagnosed; symptoms include cough, change in voice, hemoptysis, chest pain and dyspnea; systemic symptoms are fatigue, fever, weight loss, and malaise; obstruction or compression of structures such as bronchi, blood vessels, and nerves are responsible for symptoms
 A. Lung cancer
  1. Non-small-cell lung cancer (NSCLC)
   a. Adenocarcinoma: characteristic development in peripheral site
   b. Squamous cell carcinoma: characteristic development in central location
   c. Large cell carcinoma: characteristic rapid growth
  2. Small cell lung cancer (SCLC)
   a. Oat cell carcinoma
   b. Characteristic central rapid growth
   c. Often metastatic to brain, liver, bone, bone marrow, and adrenal gland at diagnosis
  3. Carcinoid
   a. Characteristic central tracheobronchial tree location

4. Metastatic
    a. Malignant tumors from many body sites can metastasize to lung
    b. Breast, stomach, prostate, thyroid, and bone are common primary sites
    c. Metastatic lesions may occur in multiple sites

B. Pleural tumors
    1. Mesothelioma: primary pleural tumor related to asbestos exposure; most other pleural tumors are metastatic

C. Esophageal (see Chapter 28)
    1. Squamous cell
    2. Adenocarcinoma

D. Mediastinal
    1. Neurogenic
    2. Thymomas
    3. Lymphomas

**NURSING DIAGNOSIS**

Examples of related nursing diagnostic categories include:

- Ineffective breathing pattern
- Ineffective airway clearance
- Impaired gas exchange
- Pain

**II. Chronic Airflow Limitation:** Chronic diseases characterized by obstruction to airflow in lung parenchyma or airways; includes patients with chronic airflow obstruction (bronchitis and emphysema), destruction of alveolar tissue (emphysema), and potentially reversible airway disease (asthma); these diseases are seen commonly as secondary medical conditions in patient undergoing thoracic surgery.

A. Chronic bronchitis: Chronic inflammation results in hypertrophy and hyperplasia of mucus-secreting glands resulting in increased sputum production, narrowing of bronchioles and small bronchi by edema and mucous gland enlargement, and chronic cough
    1. Diagnosis
        a. Smoking history
        b. Chronic productive cough for most days of the year for at least 3 months for at least 2 years
    2. Signs and symptoms
        a. Dyspnea
        b. Cough
        c. Sputum production: mucopurulent or purulent
        d. Increased anteroposterior diameter of chest
        e. Cyanosis due to hypoxemia and polycythemia
        f. Increased inspiratory/expiratory (I/E) ratio
        g. Signs of right-sided heart failure
        h. Hypoxemia with hypercapnia
        i. Decreased excursion
        j. Increased fremitus due to secretions
        k. Crackles and wheezes
        l. Diminished breath sounds
    3. Treatment
        a. Improve airway clearance of secretions
            (1) Chest physiotherapy
            (2) Stir-up regimen

(3) Adequate hydration
(4) Mucolytic or expectorant medications
b. Oxygen therapy: assess arterial blood gases for hypoxemia and hypercapnia (elevated from patient's baseline)
c. Minimize airflow obstruction with bronchodilators, sympathomimetics, anticholinergics
d. Reduce inflammation
(1) Steroids
(2) Antibiotics if infection present
(3) Avoidance of smoking and other irritants
e. Emotional support

B. Emphysema: irreversible airway destruction distal to terminal nonrespiratory bronchioles; abnormal enlargement of distal air spaces increases compliance, impairs gas exchange; airways close prematurely, causing chronic air trapping; can coexist with chronic bronchitis
1. Diagnosis
a. Pulmonary function tests
(1) Increase in lung volumes
(2) Increase in airway resistance: decreased forced expiratory volume in 1 second ($FEV_1$)
b. Chest x-ray film
c. Arterial blood gases may show mild hypoxemia and hypercapnia
2. Signs and symptoms
a. Weight loss
b. Progressive exertional dyspnea
c. Cough productive of clear mucoid sputum
d. Tachypnea with prolonged I/E ratio
e. Increased anteroposterior diameter: barrel chest
f. Clubbing
g. Tachypnea
h. Decreased excursion
i. Decreased fremitus: diminished transmission of voice sounds to chest wall
j. Hyperresonance
k. Decreased breath sounds
l. Crackles and wheezes
3. Treatment
a. Improve airway clearance of secretions and mucus
(1) Chest physiotherapy
(2) Stir-up regimen
(3) Adequate hydration
b. Oxygen therapy: assess for hypoxemia and hypercapnia
c. Minimize bronchospasm with bronchodilators
d. Reduce inflammation
(1) Steroids
(2) Antibiotics if infection present
(3) Avoid smoking and inhaled irritants

C. Asthma: mild to severe, episodic, reversible airway bronchospasm; increased responsiveness of airways to variety of stimuli, both intrinsic and extrinsic; bronchospasm causes airway edema and production of thick, tenacious mucus; result is mucus plugging and hyperinflation of alveoli
1. Diagnosis: history of recurrent wheeze that responds to bronchodilators
2. Signs and symptoms
a. Dyspnea
b. Tachypnea, increased work of breathing
c. Prolonged I/E ratio

   d. Retractions if severe
   e. Diminished chest expansion
   f. Decreased breath sounds if severe
   g. Wheezing
3. Treatment
   a. Improvement may be spontaneous
   b. Bronchodilators
   c. Anti-inflammatory drugs
   d. Humidified oxygen

**NURSING DIAGNOSIS**

Examples of related nursing diagnostic categories include:
- Ineffective breathing pattern
- Ineffective airway clearance
- Impaired gas exchange

III. **Restrictive Disorders:** pulmonary disorders that impair respiratory function through decreased lung expansion and reduction in vital capacity
   A. Atelectasis: partial or total collapse of lung tissue; can be obstructive or compressive in nature; most common postoperative complication in thoracic surgical patient; consequences of atelectasis: increased work of breathing, impaired gas exchange, infection
      1. Etiology
         a. Mucus plugging
         b. Hypoventilation
         c. Bronchospasm
         d. Compression of lung tissue by blood, air, obesity
         e. Decreased compliance
         f. Postoperative splinting
         g. Postoperative decrease in functional residual capacity
      2. Who is at risk?
         a. Age >70 years
         b. Smoker
         c. Underlying pulmonary disease
         d. Debilitated preoperative condition
         e. Prolonged procedure with lung collapse
         f. Patient unable to cooperate with pulmonary stir-up regimen
         g. Patient with abnormal pulmonary function tests
      3. Diagnosis
         a. Chest x-ray film
         b. Physical examination
      4. Signs and symptoms (may vary depending on extent of atelectasis)
         a. Fever
         b. Dyspnea
         c. Tachypnea, increased work of breathing
         d. Hypoxemia may be present
         e. Change in level of consciousness; restlessness
         f. Decreased excursion, fremitus
         g. Dullness
         h. Diminished or absent breath sounds
         i. Crackles
      5. Treatment: see information on impaired airway clearance or impaired gas exchange

B. Chest trauma
   1. Flail chest: multiple rib fractures usually accompanied by sternal fracture; movement of injured chest is in response to pleural pressure changes that cause paradoxic breathing pattern
   2. Pulmonary contusion: blunt injury to lung parenchyma, airways, and alveoli, which may result in ventilation/perfusion mismatches

C. Pulmonary fibrosis: inflammatory response and diffuse scarring of alveolar walls caused by a number of disorders
   1. Sarcoidosis
   2. Collagen or vascular disorders
   3. Asbestos exposure

D. Pneumothorax: air in pleural space as result of traumatic or iatrogenic causes
   1. Etiology
      a. Trauma
      b. Surgical procedure or central venous line insertion
      c. Nerve block
      d. Positive-pressure ventilation
      e. Spontaneous bleb rupture
   2. Diagnosis: chest x-ray film
   3. Signs and symptoms depend on degree; symptomatic with >40% pneumothorax
      a. Dyspnea
      b. Tachypnea
      c. Chest pain
      d. Increased work of breathing
      e. Decreased fremitus
      f. Decreased excursion
      g. Tracheal deviation to contralateral side
      h. Decreased or absent breath sounds
   4. Treatment
      a. Maintain adequate oxygenation and ventilation
      b. Reexpand lung
         (1) Chest tube, water seal drainage
         (2) Heimlich valve: one-way valve attached to pleural tube that allows exit of fluid and air but inhibits entry of atmospheric air

E. Tension pneumothorax: life-threatening disorder in which air enters pleural space but cannot escape; as volume of air increases, lungs collapse and heart and mediastinal structures shift to contralateral side, impairing cardiac output
   1. Etiology: same as for pneumothorax
   2. Signs and symptoms
      a. Same as for pneumothorax but more pronounced
      b. Severe hypoxemia, progressive cyanosis
      c. Mediastinal shift, tracheal deviation to contralateral side
      d. Signs of shock
      e. Distant or absent breath sounds
   3. Treatment: goal is rapid decompression and release of air
      a. Chest tube
      b. Needle or intravenous catheter into second intercostal space

F. Pleural effusion: fluid in pleural space; may be exudative (high protein content) or transudative (low protein content)
   1. Etiology
      a. Infection
      b. Tumor
      c. Congestive heart failure

      d. Hepatic cirrhosis
      e. Pancreatic abscess
   2. Signs and symptoms
      a. Hypoxemia
      b. Tachypnea, dyspnea
      c. Dullness to percussion
      d. Decreased or absent fremitus
      e. Diminished breath sounds
   3. Treatment
      a. Thoracentesis
      b. Chest tube with water seal drainage

G. Hemothorax: blood in pleural space that compresses lung tissue
   1. Etiology
      a. Trauma
      b. Surgical procedure
      c. Neoplasm
      d. Pulmonary infarction
   2. Diagnosis: chest x-ray film
   3. Signs and symptoms: same as for effusion
   4. Treatment
      a. Depends on rate and volume of bleeding
      b. Thoracostomy and tube drainage
      c. Open thoracotomy and exploration

H. Empyema: pus in pleural space; may be acute or chronic
   1. Etiology
      a. Pneumonia
      b. Postpneumonectomy
   2. Diagnosis: chest x-ray film
   3. Signs and symptoms: signs of inflammation or infection
   4. Treatment
      a. Control of primary infection
      b. Thoracentesis
      c. Closed or open drainage
      d. Thoracostomy, decortication

I. Pulmonary edema (see Chapter 15)

IV. **Neuromuscular Disease:** may predispose surgical patient to ventilatory failure

A. Myasthenia gravis: disorder of neuromuscular transmission that results in weakness of voluntary muscles; thymectomy is a treatment

B. Guillain-Barré: disorder involving peripheral nerves; characteristic acute ascending weakness that can progress to paralysis

C. Muscular dystrophy: inherited myopathy

V. **Bronchiectasis:** irreversible dilation of airways caused by inflammation; inflammatory response may erode arteries, leading to hemoptysis

A. Etiology
   1. Infection
   2. Obstruction

B. Signs and symptoms
   1. Cough
   2. Sputum production
   3. Hemoptysis
   4. Signs of recurrent infection

C. Treatment
   1. Antibiotics
   2. Airway clearance
   3. Bronchodilators

**VI. Musculoskeletal Disease:** kyphoscoliosis: orthopedic disorder of thorax involving posterior and lateral curvature of spine; if severe enough, significant restriction of lung expansion may occur

**NURSING DIAGNOSIS**

Examples of related nursing diagnostic categories include:
- Ineffective breathing pattern
- Ineffective airway clearance
- Impaired gas exchange

## ASSESSMENT

**I. History**
A. Chief complaint
B. Current health status
C. Significant past medical history
   1. Respiratory disease
      a. Cancer
      b. Tuberculosis
      c. COPD, restrictive disease
      d. Pneumonia
      e. Abscess
   2. Acquired immune disease
   3. Cardiovascular disease
      a. Hypertension
      b. Recent myocardial infarction (MI)
   4. Diabetes
   5. Renal or hepatic dysfunction
   6. Smoking history
   7. Occupational or environmental exposure
D. Relevant symptoms of pulmonary pathologic conditions
   1. Cough or change in cough
   2. Sputum production
   3. Dyspnea
      a. Exertional
      b. Positional—orthopnea
      c. Paroxysmal nocturnal dyspnea
   4. Wheezing
   5. Hemoptysis
   6. Chest pain: may indicate chest wall, pleural, spinal, or mediastinal involvement
   7. Voice changes or hoarseness: may indicate recurrent laryngeal nerve damage or compression associated with tumor
   8. Dysphagia: may indicate esophageal involvement
   9. Constitutional signs
      a. Weakness or decreased exercise tolerance
      b. Weight loss; anorexia

c. Night sweats
d. Fever

10. Abnormal chest x-ray film
11. Superior vena cava syndrome: dyspnea; cough; dilation of veins on head, neck, and arms; and edema of face, arms, and upper body associated with compression of vena cava

## II. Physical Assessment

A. Inspection
1. General appearance
2. Level of consciousness
3. Temperature, turgor, moisture of skin
4. Color
    a. Peripheral cyanosis
    b. Central cyanosis
5. Nutritional status
6. Ability to speak
7. Chest configuration
    a. Congenital abnormalities
        (1) Chest wall, sternum: pectus excavatum or carinatum
        (2) Spine: lordosis, kyphosis, scoliosis
        (3) AP diameter
8. Rate, rhythm, depth of respirations
9. I/E ratio
10. Chest wall movement
    a. Excursion
    b. Symmetry
11. Clubbing
12. Use of accessory muscles

B. Palpation
1. Chest excursion
2. Tracheal position
3. Subcutaneous emphysema
4. Vocal fremitus

C. Percussion
1. Chest wall: normal tone is resonant
2. Diaphragmatic excursion

D. Auscultation
1. Bronchial
    a. Normally found at large airways
    b. Characteristic loud, high-pitched sound
    c. Expiratory phase equal to or longer than inspiratory phase
2. Vesicular
    a. Normally found in lung fields
    b. Soft, low-pitched sound
    c. Inspiratory phase longer than expiratory phase
3. Adventitious sounds—not heard in normal airway
    a. Discontinuous
        (1) Crackles: discrete, noncontinuous sounds
        (2) Heard primarily on inspiration
    b. Continuous
        (1) Wheezes: sibilant, high pitched
        (2) Rhonchi: sonorous, low pitched
        (3) Rub: grating sound

**III. Diagnostic Assessment**
- A. Laboratory
  1. Routine: complete blood count (CBC), chemistries, coagulation
  2. Arterial blood gases
  3. Sputum: culture, cytologic examination
  4. Pleural fluid: culture, cytologic examination
  5. Skin tests: diagnosis of fungal, bacterial infections
- B. Radiology
  1. Chest x-ray film
  2. Tomograms
  3. Bronchoscopy
  4. Lung scan
  5. Computed tomography (CT)
  6. Magnetic resonance imaging (MRI)
  7. Ventilation/perfusion scan: assessment of regional lung function
  8. Pulmonary angiography: diagnosis of vessel involvement by tumor
- C. Cardiac studies: electrocardiogram
- D. Pulmonary function tests: assess presence and severity of airway disease; measure lung volumes and estimate lung capacities; measure ventilatory mechanics; assist in predicting patient's ability to tolerate surgery
- E. Plethysmography: measures thoracic gas volumes
- F. Thoracentesis: percutaneous aspiration of pleural fluid; useful in diagnosis of cause of effusion or for symptomatic relief of effusion-associated dyspnea

## OPERATIVE PROCEDURES

**I. Diagnostic**
- A. Bronchoscopy: visualization of tracheobronchial tree; removal of secretions, fluid, foreign bodies; biopsy of tissue; lavage; application of medication or radiopaque medium
  1. Complications
     - a. Airway obstruction
       - (1) Laryngospasm
       - (2) Bronchospasm
       - (3) Glottic or subglottic edema
     - b. Hypoxemia
     - c. Pneumothorax
     - d. Bleeding
- B. Mediastinoscopy: visualization or biopsy of tumors or nodes at tracheobronchial junction, subcarina, or upper lobe bronchi
  1. Complications
     - a. Hemorrhage
     - b. Airway, esophageal injury
       - (1) Subcutaneous emphysema
       - (2) Chest pain
       - (3) Pneumothorax
     - c. Recurrent laryngeal nerve injury: hoarseness
- C. Laryngoscopy: visualization of vocal cords and airway; biopsy
  1. Complications: same as for bronchoscopy
- D. Thoracoscopy: visualization within pleural cavity to allow diagnosis of variety of pulmonary diseases and conditions; able to perform variety of procedures, including biopsy and resection of mediastinal nodes or masses, drainage of pleural effusion and pericardial effusion, sympathectomies, vagotomies, thymectomies
- E. Scalene node biopsy: positive biopsy indicates extramediastinal tumor involvement

F. Lung biopsy: may be percutaneous or open
   1. Complications
      a. Bleeding
      b. Pneumothorax

## II. Therapeutic

A. Repair of pectus excavatum: reconstructive repair of depression of sternum and lower costal cartilages
B. Chest wall reconstruction: closure and reconstruction of chest by use of adjacent tissue (i.e., musculocutaneous flap); reconstruction may be necessary after tumor excision, radiation necrosis
   1. Complication: flap ischemia—assessment of tissue perfusion every hour, including color, temperature, flap turgor
C. Thoracoplasty: removal of ribs or portions of ribs to reduce size of hemithorax or to collapse diseased lung; used to assist in obliteration of pleural space in chronic empyema
D. Decortication with pleurodesis: removal of restrictive fibrinous membrane or layer of tissue that interferes with ventilatory action; may be removed from lung, pleura, or diaphragm; may develop secondary to empyema, blood, or fluid in pleural space
E. Open window thoracostomy: surgical creation of an opening in the chest; involves resection of ribs to allow for drainage and irrigation of postpneumonectomy empyema. Opening may be closed surgically at completion of empyema treatment
F. Wedge resection: excision of pie-shaped section of lobe; used to remove small peripheral lesions
G. Segmentectomy: excision of individual bronchoalveolar segment of a lobe of lung; can be done if peripheral lesion is present without chest wall involvement
H. Lobectomy: removal of a lobe of lung
I. Pneumonectomy: removal of entire lung
   1. Right pneumonectomy removes 55% of vascular bed and breathing capacity so it is tolerated less well than left pneumonectomy
   2. Chest tube: may be clamped after surgery to allow serosanguineous effusion to fill hemithorax
      a. If bleeding suspected, chest film obtained to ascertain fluid level in chest
      b. Assess for tracheal deviation to ascertain excessive pressure in hemithorax
   3. Dysrhythmias: may be digitalized preoperatively
   4. Volume overload: extremely sensitive to volume administration
      a. Monitor for signs and symptoms of congestive failure
         (1) Crackles
         (2) Tachypnea
         (3) Dyspnea
         (4) Hypoxemia
         (5) Increased filling pressures
   5. Phrenic nerve may be severed on operative side to elevate hemidiaphragm
   6. Pericardium may be opened during procedure
      a. Ascertain whether pericardial closure was performed
      b. Check with physician regarding positioning restrictions
      c. Monitor for signs of cardiac herniation (acute cardiovascular compromise)
J. Sleeve resection: removal of tracheobronchial tree and associated lung segment or lobe and reattachment of remaining lung tissue; sleeve pneumonectomy may also be performed
K. Lung volume reduction surgery: removal of emphysematous lung tissue; procedure relieves pressure and increases expansion of functional lung tissue, increases thoracic expansion and improves respiratory mechanics and gas exchange; unilateral or bilateral and usually requires multiple chest tubes
L. Lung transplant: removal of recipient lung and replacement with donor lung

M. Thymectomy: removal of thymus; treatment for myasthenia gravis
    1. Preoperative pulmonary function testing may be done
    2. Will try to avoid or limit muscle relaxant during surgery
    3. Drugs that potentiate neuromuscular blockade are avoided
    4. Neurologist may help to assess ability to extubate and determine time to restart anticholinesterase drugs
    5. Complications
        a. Ineffective breathing pattern
        b. Ineffective airway clearance
        c. Myasthenic, cholinergic crisis
        d. Phrenic nerve injury
        e. Bleeding: innominate, internal mammary artery

## CARE OF PATIENT UNDERGOING PULMONARY SURGERY

**I. Preoperative Preparation:** goal is to decrease postanesthetic complications that may further compromise patient's status

A. Interventions
    1. Encourage patient to stop smoking before surgery (be aware many will not do so)
    2. Drug therapy
        a. Airway clearance
            (1) Mucolytics
            (2) Oral expectorants
        b. Infection resolution: antibiotics
        c. Bronchospasm control
            (1) Beta agonists
            (2) Anticholinergics
        d. Steroids
        e. Xanthine preparations
        f. Antidysrhythmics: digitalization for pneumonectomy
    3. Maneuvers to improve airway clearance and maximize ventilation
        a. Chest physiotherapy; postural drainage
        b. Incentive spirometry
        c. Pulmonary stir-up regimen
        d. Systemic hydration
    4. Identification of high-risk candidates
        a. Status of patient
        b. Stage of tumor or disease process
        c. Extent of procedure
    5. Manage anxiety; cautious use of preoperative sedation
    6. Minimize preoperative exposure to colds and flu

**II. Intraoperative Care**

A. Monitoring
    1. Noninvasive
        a. Blood pressure, electrocardiogram (ECG)
        b. Pulse oximetry
        c. End-tidal $CO_2$
    2. Invasive
        a. Arterial blood pressure catheter
        b. Central venous pressure
        c. Pulmonary artery catheter
        d. Esophageal temperature probe

   e. Cardiac output
   f. $Svo_2$
   g. Foley catheter

B. Positioning
   1. Facilitates exposure and surgical manipulation of lung tissue but may predispose to development of postoperative atelectasis because of side lying on nonoperative lung
   2. Attention to positioning necessary to prevent injury associated with pressure; in addition to prevent stretching or compression of nerve tissue
      a. Brachial plexus
      b. Peroneal nerve
      c. Ulnar nerve
      d. Radial nerve
         (1) Symptoms
            (a) Pain
            (b) Paresthesia
            (c) Impaired motor function

C. One-lung ventilation
   1. Provides unaffected lung protection from aspiration of blood and body fluids; also used during bilateral lung volume reduction surgery
   2. Provides greater access and motionless surgical field
   3. Methods
      a. Bronchial blockers
      b. Double-lumen endobronchial tube
   4. Special considerations
      a. Ventilate on 100%
      b. Replace with regular endotracheal tube at end of surgery
      c. Complications
         (1) Malposition
         (2) Hypoxemia

D. Jet ventilation: intermittent, high-frequency (60 to 200 bpm) ventilation delivered through small-bore injector cannula positioned within endotracheal tube; may also be used as alternate method of mechanical ventilation

E. Anesthesia
   1. General anesthesia
   2. Epidural or regional with inhalation; halogenated agents to bronchodilate and decrease airway irritability
   3. Intraoperative pain control measures to prevent postoperative splinting
      a. Intercostal nerve block
      b. Thoracic or epidural analgesia
      c. Narcotic into epidural space

F. Thoracic incisions
   1. Posterolateral
   2. Axillary
   3. Median sternotomy
   4. Anterior
   5. Thoracoabdominal
   6. Posterior
   7. Transverse anterior

G. Special intraoperative goals
   1. Bleeding stabilized before chest closure
   2. Chest cavity may be filled with saline while anesthesia hyperventilates to search for air leak from inadequate surgical closure
   3. Lung that has been collapsed is fully inflated with no atelectasis
   4. Chest closed with chest tube to water seal

5. Extubation desirable as soon as possible to avoid complications associated with positive-pressure ventilation

## III. Postoperative Care

A. Admission assessment
   1. Intraoperative vital sign trends
   2. History
   3. Anesthetic medications
   4. Special intraoperative events
   5. Airway patency and presence of artificial airways
   6. Oxygen therapy
   7. Vital signs, cardiac rhythm
   8. Oximetry, arterial blood gases
   9. Conditions of dressings, tubes
   10. Intravenous infusions and invasive monitoring
   11. Chest x-ray film to verify placement of chest tubes, resolution of pneumothorax; position of endotracheal tube if intubated

B. Physical assessment
   1. Inspection
      a. Airway patency and presence of artificial airways
      b. General condition
         (1) Level of consciousness
         (2) Confusion, restlessness, anxiety
            (a) Hypoxemia
            (b) Hypercapnia
      c. Respiratory rate
         (1) Tachypnea
            (a) Hypoxemia
            (b) Hypercapnia
            (c) Acidosis
            (d) Fever
         (2) Bradypnea
            (a) Hypercapnia
            (b) Residual anesthetic effect
      d. Rhythm
      e. I/E ratio: prolonged in respiratory distress
      f. Depth: hypoventilation common in early postoperative phase
      g. Chest wall movement
         (1) Decreased: hypoventilation
         (2) Asymmetric
            (a) Atelectasis
            (b) Consolidation
            (c) Effusion
            (d) Paralysis of diaphragm
            (e) Misplaced endotracheal tube
            (f) Splinting
            (g) Hemothorax, pneumothorax
      h. Cyanosis
         (1) Occurs when average concentration of unoxygenated hemoglobin exceeds 5 g/dl
         (2) Peripheral: associated with inadequate circulation
            (a) Vasoconstriction: hypothermia or stress response
            (b) Decreased blood flow: hypotension

(3) Central: associated with arterial desaturation in patients with adequate cardiac output
   (a) Decreased alveolar oxygen levels: hypoventilation, hypoxemia, ventilation/perfusion mismatch, atelectasis
   (b) Shunt: ARDS, congestive heart failure (CHF), pneumonia

i. Use of accessory muscles: indicative of reduced pulmonary reserve
   (1) Inspiratory muscles
      (a) Sternocleidomastoid
      (b) Scalene
      (c) Pectoralis major
      (d) Trapezius
   (2) Expiratory muscles
      (a) Intercostals
      (b) Abdominals

j. Retractions secondary to patient's effort to generate more negative pressure to improve ventilation

k. Nasal flaring

l. Sputum production

m. Abdominal paradox: retraction of abdomen during inspiration; indicates diaphragmatic fatigue and ventilatory failure

2. Palpation
   a. Chest expansion
   b. Trachea will deviate toward hemithorax with lowest intrathoracic pressure
   c. Trachea deviates away from pathologic conditions: space-occupying disorders
      (1) Tension pneumothorax
      (2) Hemothorax
      (3) Effusion
   d. Trachea deviates toward pathologic condition
      (1) Atelectasis
      (2) Phrenic nerve paralysis
      (3) Pneumonia (massive)
      (4) Pneumonectomy
   e. Subcutaneous emphysema: palpable crackling sensation that results from air that has escaped from lungs into subcutaneous tissue
      (1) Sources of air leak in postoperative patient
         (a) Pneumothorax
         (b) Tracheostomy site
         (c) Alveolar rupture from barotrauma
         (d) Tracheobronchial or esophageal injury
   f. Fremitus
      (1) Increased
         (a) Consolidation
         (b) Mucus in airways
      (2) Decreased
         (a) Atelectasis
         (b) Pneumothorax
         (c) Pneumonectomy
         (d) COPD
         (e) Effusion

3. Auscultation
   a. Absence of breath sounds, possibly from
      (1) Obstruction
         (a) Tongue

(b) Kink in endotracheal tube
(c) Spasm
(2) Secretions
(3) Pneumonectomy
(4) Effusion
(5) Pneumothorax
(6) Misplaced endotracheal tube
(7) Atelectasis

b. Diminished vesicular sounds from
(1) Obesity
(2) Hypoventilation
(3) COPD
(4) Misplaced endotracheal tube

c. Bronchial sounds in peripheral fields
(1) Increased tissue density: consolidation

d. Crackles
(1) Atelectasis
(2) Fluid

e. Wheezes
(1) High pitched: bronchospasm
(2) Low pitched (rhonchus): mucus in airways

f. Rhonchi
(1) Mucus in airways

g. Rub
(1) Grating or scraping sound of inflamed parietal visceral surfaces as they approximate at end inspiration
(2) Normal sound postthoracotomy

h. Voice sounds: amplified transmission of voice through thorax as a result of increased lung density of areas of atelectasis
(1) Bronchophony: increased transmission of spoken words "ninety nine"
(2) Egophony: spoken "ee" is auscultated "aa"
(3) Whispered pectoriloquy: auscultation of whispered voice is enhanced

C. Chest tube technology
1. Closed water seal drainage
a. Purpose
(1) Remove air and fluid from pleural space
(2) Reestablish pleural pressure

b. Components
(1) Chest tube; two tubes routinely placed
(a) Apex for air removal
(b) Base for fluid removal
(2) Water seal
(a) Extension of patient's pleura
(b) Allows for exit of fluid and water
(c) Acts as one-way valve and does not permit atmospheric pressure to equilibrate with the lung
(3) Collection chamber allows for collection and documentation of drainage
(4) Suction chamber
(a) Facilitates removal of air and water from pleural space
(b) Provides negative pressure to facilitate removal of air or drainage

c. Care of patients with chest tube
(1) Observe for intactness, i.e., all connections taped
(2) Position to facilitate drainage, i.e., no dependent loops
(3) Observe for "tidaling" or fluctuation of water seal column with respiration

(4) Monitor volume, color, and consistency of drainage
(5) Gently milk tubes as needed to maintain patency
(6) Maintain desired suction level; 20 cm is normal for adult patient
(7) Maintain suction so there is constant bubbling in suction chamber
(8) Assess for bubbling in water seal column, signaling air leak
(9) Assess for sudden cessation of drainage indicating clogged tube
(10) Assess for development or progression of subcutaneous emphysema indicating air leak

## POSTOPERATIVE NURSING CONCERNS

I. **Impaired Gas Exchange:** early extubation is goal to minimize barotrauma and development of bronchopleural fistula; most common causes of delayed extubation are concomitant pulmonary disease, cardiac dysfunction, multiorgan dysfunction, hemodynamic instability

A. Etiology
1. Residual anesthetic effects
2. Epidural effect: T3, T4 level of analgesia may impair intercostal function in borderline patient
3. Preoperative respiratory disease
4. Pain with splinting
5. Loss of lung parenchyma
6. Atelectasis
7. Decreased wall compliance resulting from surgery
8. ARDS
9. Misplaced endotracheal tube

B. Signs and symptoms
1. Shallow, rapid respirations
2. Dyspnea, increased work of breathing
3. Marginal pulse oximeter: oxygen saturation <90%
4. Hypoxemia: $Po_2$ <50 to 60 mm Hg
5. Hypercapnia with respiratory acidosis
6. Tachycardia
7. Change in mental status
8. Decreased breath sounds
9. Crackles
10. May progress to acute ventilatory failure

C. Nursing interventions
1. Incentive spirometry every hour
2. Assess level of consciousness, level of fatigue, work of breathing
3. Monitor rate, quality, depth of respiration
4. Auscultate breath sounds
5. Maintain ordered oxygen therapy (humidified)
6. Pulmonary stir-up regimen
7. Head of bed elevated 30 to 45 degrees
8. Reposition every 2 hours
9. Monitor pulse oximetry and arterial blood gases
10. Medicate for pain as ordered
11. If adequate ventilation and oxygenation cannot be achieved, prepare for reintubation
12. Reintubation criteria
    a. Hypercapnia with respiratory acidosis
    b. Hypoxemia: $Po_2$ <50 to 60 mm Hg
    c. Inability to speak short sentences
    d. Inability to maintain oxygen saturation >85%

e. Agitation
f. Symptomatic tachycardia or hypertension

**II. Ineffective Breathing Pattern** (vital capacity reduced 30% to 50% within first 24 hours after surgery)

A. Etiology
1. Splinting
2. Hypoventilation
3. Residual neuromuscular blockade, sedatives

B. Signs and symptoms
1. Shallow, rapid respirations
2. Hypoxemia (responsive to oxygen therapy)
3. Hypercapnia
4. Decreased breath sounds
5. May progress to acute ventilatory failure

C. Nursing interventions
1. Assess level of consciousness, level of fatigue, work of breathing
2. Monitor rate, quality, depth of respiration
3. Auscultate breath sounds
4. Maintain ordered oxygen therapy
5. Pulmonary stir-up regimen
6. Head of bed elevated 30 to 45 degrees
7. Reposition every 2 hours
8. Monitor pulse oximetry and arterial blood gases
9. Timely assessment and treatment of pain
10. If adequate ventilation and oxygenation cannot be achieved, prepare for reintubation

**III. Ineffective Airway Clearance**

A. Etiology
1. Pain
2. Residual sedatives, anesthesia
3. Inability of patient to follow directions

B. Signs and symptoms
1. Inability to expectorate secretions
2. Inability to perform adequate cough
3. Crackles and wheezes

C. Nursing interventions
1. Assess level of consciousness, level of fatigue, work of breathing
2. Monitor rate, quality, depth of respiration
3. Auscultate breath sounds
4. Maintain ordered oxygen therapy
5. Pulmonary stir-up regimen
6. Chest physiotherapy in patients with history of mucus production
7. Head of bed elevated 30 to 45 degrees
8. Reposition every 2 hours
9. Monitor pulse oximetry and arterial blood gases
10. Timely assessment and treatment of pain
11. Administer medication before pulmonary stir-up regimen
12. Suctioning as necessary
13. Prepare to assist with bedside bronchoscopy
14. If adequate ventilation and oxygenation cannot be achieved prepare for reintubation

## IV. Pain

A. See Chapter 32
B. Interventions
   1. Continuous intravenous narcotic
   2. Patient-controlled analgesia
   3. Epidural analgesia
   4. Intercostal nerve block

## V. Potential for Hemorrhage

A. Etiology
   1. Inadequate perioperative hemostasis
   2. Postoperative coagulopathy
   3. Pulmonary artery rupture
B. Signs and symptoms
   1. Chest tube drainage >200 ml/hr for 4 hours
   2. Hypotension
   3. Decreased filling pressures
   4. Tachycardia
   5. Restlessness
   6. Decreased cardiac output
C. Nursing interventions
   1. Establish drainage on admission
   2. Assess drainage at prescribed intervals
   3. Frequent vital sign assessment
   4. Inspect dressing for excessive drainage
   5. Notify physician of
      a. Chest tube drainage as above
      b. Sudden increase in drainage
      c. Abrupt decrease in drainage
      d. Falling hematocrit
   6. Prepare patient for surgical reexploration

## VI. Potential for Cardiac Dysrhythmias

A. Supraventricular most common
   1. Predisposing factors
      a. Advanced age
      b. Preexisting cardiac disease
      c. Extensive resection: pneumonectomy
      d. Intrapericardiac disease or dissection
   2. Etiology
      a. Mediastinal shifts
      b. Hypoxia, hypercapnia
      c. Vagal stimulation
      d. Atrial stretching, inflammation
      e. Alterations in pulmonary blood flow
      f. Increased sympathetic tone
      g. Acid-base disturbances
      h. Tachycardia
   3. Nursing interventions
      a. Assess hemodynamic stability
      b. Assess for precipitating factors
         (1) Acid-base disturbances
         (2) Alteration in oxygenation and ventilation

(3) Electrolyte imbalance
(4) Adverse effect of bronchodilators

4. Treatment
   a. Electrocardiographic diagnosis
   b. Pharmacologic therapy for stable rhythms
   c. Cardioversion, pacing for unstable rhythms

**VII. Potential for Acute Myocardial Infarction (MI)**

A. Predisposing factors
   1. Age
   2. MI within preceding 3 months
   3. History of coronary artery disease

**VIII. Potential for Cardiac Herniation**

A. Etiology
   1. Displacement of heart through pericardial defect
   2. Twisting of great vessels obstructs inflow and outflow tracts of heart
   3. May be precipitated by
      a. Change in position
      b. Coughing
      c. Positive-pressure ventilation

B. Signs and symptoms
   1. Cardiovascular collapse
   2. Jugular venous distension, upper body cyanosis
   3. Tachycardia, myocardial ischemia
   4. Displaced point of maximum intensity
   5. Cyanosis

C. Nursing interventions
   1. Check for positioning restrictions, especially with pneumonectomy patient or any time that pericardium has been opened
   2. Alert physician of precipitating factors of cardiovascular collapse
   3. Prepare patient for emergent surgical reduction

D. Treatment
   1. Reposition patient if turning causes symptoms
   2. Surgical reduction

## BIBLIOGRAPHY

Beattie EJ, Bloom N, Harvey J: *Thoracic Surgical Oncology*. New York, Churchill Livingstone, 1992.

Bird G, Macaluso S: Lung volume reduction surgery for emphysema. *Crit Care Clin North Am* 8:323–331, 1996.

Brandt H, Loddenkemper R, Mai J: *Atlas of Diagnostic Thoracoscopy*. New York, Theime, 1985.

Cooper JD, Trulock EP, Triantafillou A, et al: Bilateral pneumonectomy (volume reduction) for chronic obstructive pulmonary disease. *J Thorac Cardiovasc Surg* 109:106–119, 1995.

Caretti D: Care of the patient with Clagett open window thoracostomy. *Medsurg Nurs* 6:18–23, 1997.

Carroll P: Nursing the thoracotomy patient. *RN* 55: 34–43, 1992.

Des Jardin T, Burton C: *Clinical Manifestations and Assessment of Respiratory Disease,* 3rd Ed. St Louis, Mosby, 1995.

Farzan S, Farzan D: *A Concise Handbook of Respiratory Disease*. Stamford, Conn. Apple & Lange, 1997.

Finkelmeier B: Difficult problems in postoperative management. *Crit Care Q* 9:59–70, 1986.

Fishman A: *Pulmonary Diseases and Disorders,* 2nd Ed. New York, McGraw-Hill, 1988.

Foster J: Intensive care of the patient after reconstructive surgery. *Focus Crit Care* 19:122–127, 1992.

Graling P, Hetrick V, Kiernan P: Bilateral lung volume reduction surgery. *AORN J* 63:389–412, 1996.

Kryger M (ed): *Introduction to Respiratory Medicine,* 2nd Ed. New York, Churchill Livingstone, 1990.

Langstrom W: Surgical resection of lung cancer. *Nurs Clin North Am* 27:665–679, 1992.

Majid A, Hanzah H: Pain control after thoracotomy. *Chest* 101:981–984, 1992.

Matthay M, Weiner-Kronish J: Respiratory management after cardiac surgery. *Chest* 95:424–434, 1992.

McCance K, Huether S: *Pathophysiology: The Biological Basis for Disease in Adults and Children,* 2nd Ed. St Louis, Mosby–Year Book, 1997.

McGregor R, Schakenbach L: Lung volume reduction surgery: A new breath of life for emphysema patients. *Medsurg Nurs* 5:245–252, 1996.

Mentzer SJ, DeCamp MM, Harpole DH, Sugarbaker DJ: Thoracoscopy and video-assisted thoracic surgery in the treatment of lung cancer. *Chest* 107 (6 Suppl):298S–301S, 1995.

Meyer S et al: Postoperative care of the lung transplant patient. *Crit Care Nurs Clin North Am* 8:239–252, 1996.

O'Byrne C: Postoperative care and complications in the thoracotomy patient. *Crit Care Q* 8:53–58, 1985.

Shapiro B, Kacmark R, Cane R, et al: *Clinical Application of Respiratory Care,* 4th Ed. St Louis, Mosby–Year Book, 1991.

Shields T (ed): *General Thoracic Surgery,* 3rd Ed. Philadelphia, Lea & Febiger, 1989.

Simpson T, Wahl G, De Traglia M, et al: The effects of epidural versus opioid analgesia on postoperative pain and pulmonary function in adults who have undergone thoracic and abdominal surgery: A critique of research. *Heart Lung* 21:125–140, 1992.

Tampinco-Golos I: Endoscopic thoracotomy. *AORN J* 55:1167–1180, 1992.

Tager A, Ginns L: Complications of lung transplantation. *Crit Care Clin North Am* 8:273–292, 1996.

Waldenhausen J, Orringer M: *Complications in Cardiothoracic Surgery.* St Louis, Mosby–Year Book, 1991.

West J: *Pulmonary Pathophysiology,* 4th Ed. Baltimore, Williams & Wilkins, 1994.

Wilkens R, Sheldon R, Krider S: *Clinical Assessment of Respiratory Care.* St Louis, Mosby–Year Book, 1990.

Witkowski A: *Pulmonary Assessment: A Clinical Guide.* Philadelphia, JB Lippincott, 1985.

Wolfe W: *Complications of Thoracic Surgery: Recognition and Management.* St Louis, Mosby–Year Book, 1992.

## REVIEW QUESTIONS

**1. In evaluating the pulmonary patient, what parameters are assessed?**

A. Chest x-ray film
B. Previous history of pulmonary disease
C. CBC, chemistries, arterial blood gases
D. All of the above

**2. Type 2 alveolar cells are important in the production of:**

A. Oxyhemoglobin
B. Surfactant
C. Mucus
D. Lactic acid

**3. The central chemoreceptors respond to:**

A. Changes in CSF pH
B. Changes in dissolved oxygen
C. Changes in work of breathing
D. Changes in compliance

**4. All of the following are common presenting signs in the patient with lung cancer except:**

A. Cough
B. Dyspnea
C. Hemoptysis
D. Night sweats

**5. Which procedure removes fibrinous deposits of restrictive membranes of the pleural lining?**

A. Wedge resection
B. Decortication
C. Sleeve resection
D. Thoracoplasty

**6. Which are clinical manifestations of chronic obstructive disease?**
A. Increased anteroposterior diameter, prolonged expiration, wheezes
B. Moist cough, tachypnea, hypotension
C. Absent breath sounds, dullness to percussion
D. Dyspnea, tracheal deviation

**7. Causes of impaired gas exchange in the pulmonary patient include all the following except:**
A. Residual anesthetic effect
B. Inadequate pain relief causing hypoventilation
C. Atelectasis
D. Vagal stimulation

**8. Which of the following put the pulmonary patient at risk for postoperative dysrhythmias?**
A. Mediastinal shifts
B. Vagal stimulation
C. Atrial stretching or inflammation
D. All of the above

**9. Thymectomy is the surgical intervention of choice for the patient with:**
A. Graves' disease
B. Bronchiectasis
C. Guillain-Barré syndrome
D. Myasthenia gravis

**10. Pneumonectomy patients are at high risk for the development of:**
A. Pleural friction rubs
B. Complete heart block
C. Fluid overload
D. Asthma

**ANSWERS:** 1. D, 2. B, 3. A, 4. D, 5. B, 6. A, 7. D, 8. D, 9. D, 10. C

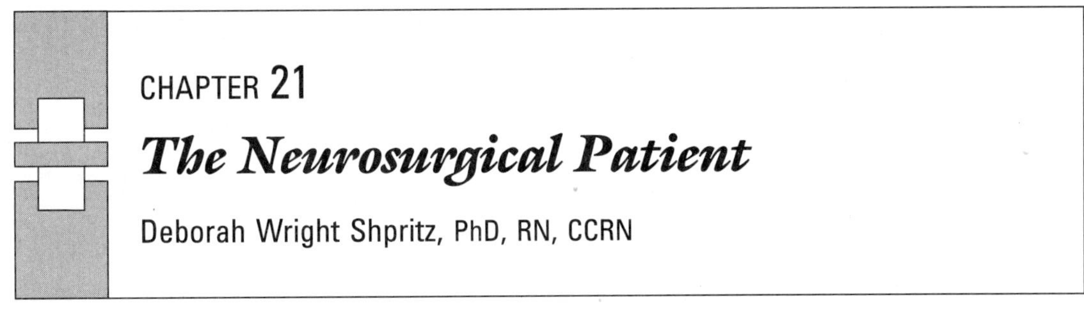

CHAPTER 21

# The Neurosurgical Patient

Deborah Wright Shpritz, PhD, RN, CCRN

## OBJECTIVES

**Study of the information represented by this outline will enable the learner to:**

1. Describe salient aspects of the anatomy and physiology of the nervous system as it relates to the patient undergoing neurologic surgery.
2. Explain the pathophysiology of increased intracranial pressure (ICP).
3. Discuss the medical and nursing management of the patient with increased ICP.
4. Describe the pathophysiology, diagnosis, and treatment of the most common conditions requiring neurologic surgery.
5. Discuss neurodiagnostic testing procedures.
6. Compare the most common neurologic procedures.
7. Identify potential complications of patients undergoing neurologic surgery.
8. Perform a nursing neurologic assessment.
9. Formulate a care plan for the postanesthesia neurosurgical patient.
10. Demonstrate competency in the care of the postanesthesia neurosurgical patient.

Nursing care of the neurosurgical patient in the postanesthesia care unit (PACU) requires attention to all body systems and their interaction with the central nervous system (CNS). In particular, the PACU nurse must understand the pathophysiology, signs, and symptoms of increased ICP and the appropriate medical and surgical interventions. Neurologic assessment and regular patient monitoring for potential complications are essential components of PACU care of the neurosurgical patient whether the surgery involves the head or the spinal cord.

## ANATOMY AND PHYSIOLOGY OF THE BRAIN

I. Cellular Structure
  A. Neuron: basic structural unit
    1. Excitable nerve cell: receives and conducts impulses
    2. Functions
      a. Afferent, or sensory, neurons conduct impulses from receptors to CNS
      b. Efferent, or motor, neurons conduct impulses from CNS to effector organs
    3. Structure
      a. Cell body contains nucleus, cytoplasm, cell membrane
      b. Nerve cell processes
        (1) Dendrites: short processes with multiple projections that conduct impulses to cell body
        (2) Axon: longest process of cell body; conducts impulses away from cell body
      c. Synapses: communication points between two neurons

- d. Neurotransmitters: protein substances that facilitate or inhibit impulse transmission across synapses
  - (1) Adrenergic
    - (a) Dopamine
    - (b) Norepinephrine
    - (c) Epinephrine
  - (2) Cholinergic: acetylcholine
  - (3) Serotonin
  - (4) Gamma-aminobutyric acid (GABA)
  - (5) α- and β-endorphins
  - (6) Histamine
  - (7) Substance P

B. Gray matter: cortex of brain; contains cell bodies and dendrites of CNS

C. White matter: contains myelinated axons and neuroglia

D. Neuroglia: support cells of CNS

1. Nonexcitable
2. More numerous than neurons
   - a. Astrocytes
     - (1) Small cell bodies with numerous projections
     - (2) Projections end on blood vessels, ependyma, and pia mater
   - b. Oligodendrocytes
     - (1) Smaller and more delicate than astrocytes
     - (2) Responsible for formation of myelin
   - c. Microglia: smallest neurologic cell
   - d. Ependyma
     - (1) Lines cavities of brain and spinal cord
     - (2) Single layer of cuboid cells with villi
     - (3) Facilitates movement of cerebrospinal fluid (CSF)

## II. Extracerebral Structures

A. Scalp: protects integrity of skull

B. Skull

1. Protects brain from external forces
2. Composition
   - a. Frontal bone (1)
   - b. Parietal bones (2)
   - c. Temporal bones (2)
   - d. Occipital bone (1)
   - e. Ethmoid bone (1)
   - f. Sphenoid bone (1)
3. Compartments
   - a. Anterior fossa: contains frontal lobes, olfactory nerves
   - b. Middle fossa: contains temporal, parietal, occipital lobes
   - c. Posterior fossa: contains cerebellum, brainstem (composed of midbrain, pons, medulla)

C. Meninges (Fig. 21–1)

1. Function
   - a. Protection for brain and spinal cord
   - b. Support underlying structures
2. Layers from outermost layer inward
   - a. Dura mater ("tough mother")
     - (1) Dense, fibrous, inelastic

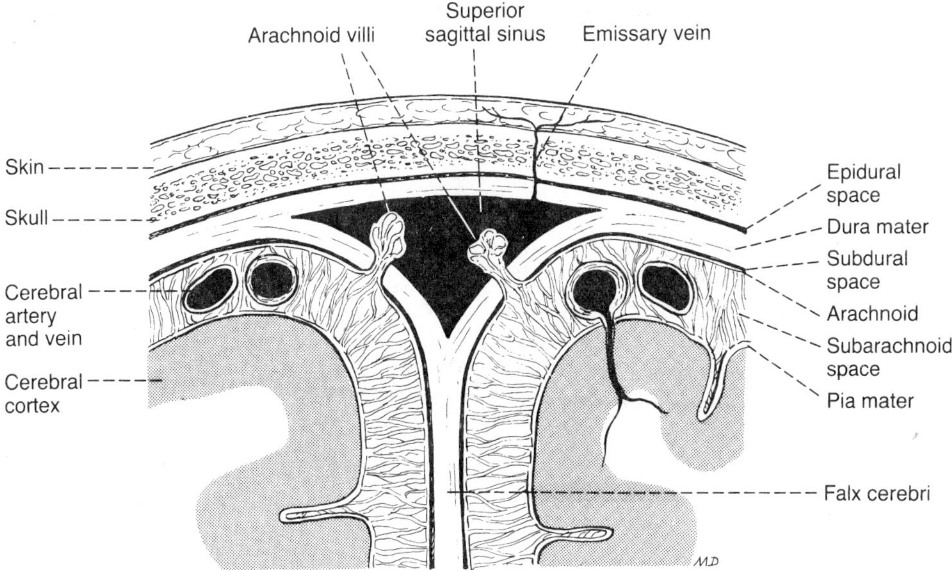


**FIGURE 21–1** Meninges (coronal section through superior sagittal sinus). (From Black JMN, Matassarin-Jacobs E: *Luckmann and Sorensen's Medical Surgical Nursing*, 4th Ed [p 624]. Philadelphia, WB Saunders, 1993.)

(2) Double layered
- (a) Outer layer (periosteal): periosteum of skull
- (b) Inner layer (meningeal): creates intracranial compartments

(3) Dural folds: divide cranial vault into compartments
- (a) Falx cerebri: separates right and left cerebral hemispheres
- (b) Tentorium cerebelli: separates basal surfaces of occipital and temporal lobes from cerebellum
- (c) Falx cerebelli: separates right and left cerebellar hemispheres

b. Arachnoid membrane
- (1) Thin, delicate, elastic, fibrous
- (2) Closely adheres to dura mater
- (3) Separated from dura mater by subdural space
- (4) Contains blood vessels of varying sizes
- (5) Connects to pia mater by trabeculae
- (6) Arachnoid granulations enable CSF to move from subarachnoid space to venous system

c. Pia mater
- (1) Innermost layer
- (2) Meshlike, vascular membrane
- (3) Follows sulci and fissures
- (4) Inseparable from brain's surface

3. Spaces

a. Epidural
- (1) Potential space
- (2) Must be created by force (e.g., trauma, surgical dissection)

b. Subdural
- (1) Potential space
- (2) Below dura, above arachnoid

c. Subarachnoid: contains CSF, arteries, and veins
d. Cisterns: pockets of arachnoid filled with CSF

## III. Cerebral Vasculature

A. Arterial system: two paired systems of blood vessels (anterior and posterior) that combine to form circle of Willis (Figs. 21–2 and 21–3)
  1. Anterior arterial circulation
    a. Common carotid: branches into external and internal carotid arteries
    b. Internal carotid artery (ICA): enters cranial cavity at petrous portion of temporal bone; supplies most of hemispheres (except occipital lobe, basal ganglia) and upper two thirds of diencephalon
    c. External carotid artery (ECA): supplies skin and muscles of face, scalp
    d. Anterior cerebral artery (ACA): supplies medial surfaces of frontal and parietal lobes
    e. Anterior communicating artery: connects anterior cerebral arteries
    f. Middle cerebral artery (MCA)
      (1) Largest branch of ICA
      (2) Supplies two-thirds of cerebral hemispheres
    g. Posterior communicating artery (PCA): connects anterior with posterior circulation
  2. Posterior arterial circulation
    a. Vertebral arteries
      (1) Paired arteries arising from subclavian artery
      (2) Enter cranial vault through foramen magnum
      (3) Branches supply spinal cord, underside of cerebellum, medulla, and choroid plexus of fourth ventricle
      (4) Two arteries merge to form basilar artery
    b. Basilar artery
      (1) Branches into posterior cerebral arteries and smaller vessels supplying posterior fossa
    c. Posterior cerebral artery (PCA): supplies brainstem, occipital lobe, inferior and medial surfaces of temporal lobe

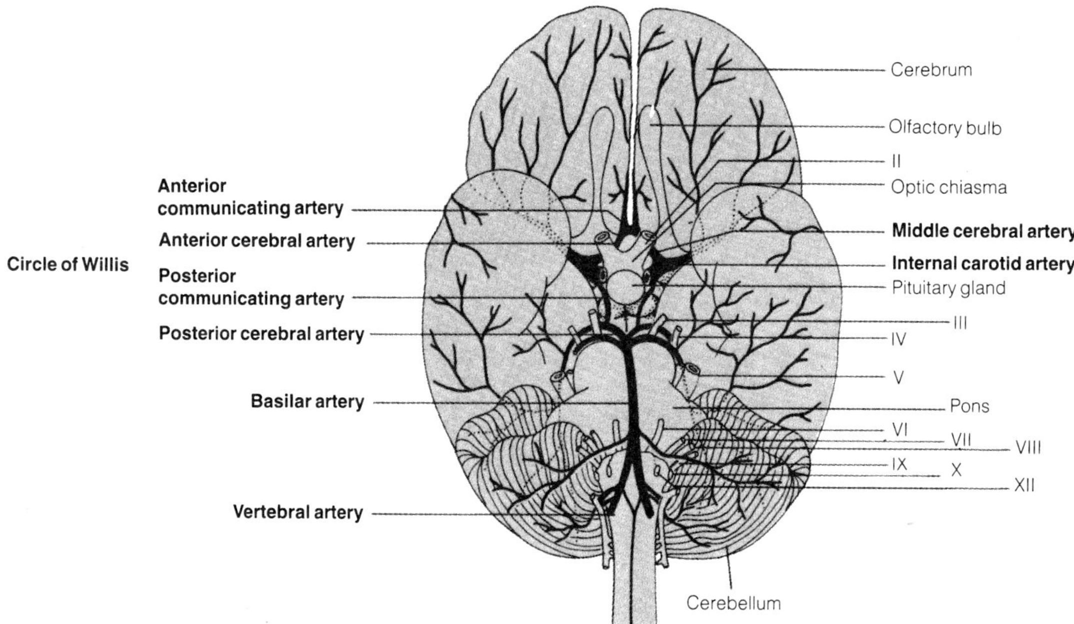


**FIGURE 21–2** Arterial circulation to brain. Circle of Willis is prominent area of interconnections from carotid and vertebral arteries. (From Gaudin AJ, Jones KC: *Human Anatomy and Physiology* [p 592]. San Diego, Harcourt Brace Jovanovich, 1989.)

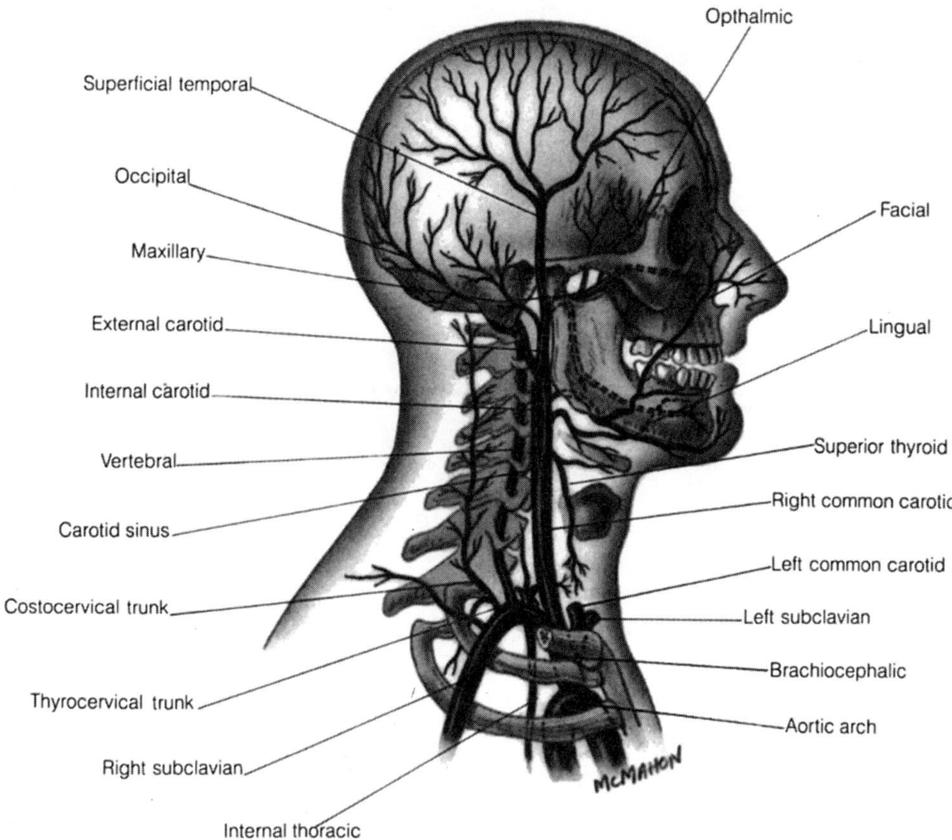


**FIGURE 21–3** Major arteries of head and neck. (From Gaudin AJ, Jones KC: *Human Anatomy and Physiology* [p 592]. San Diego, Harcourt Brace Jovanovich, 1989.)

B. Venous drainage: valveless, thin-walled system of superficial and deep veins and venous sinuses (Fig. 21–4)
  1. Superficial veins: drain external surfaces of brain into superior sagittal, cavernous, sphenoparietal, and petrosal sinuses
    a. Superior cerebral veins
    b. Middle cerebral veins
    c. Inferior cerebral veins
  2. Deep veins: drain internal areas of brain
    a. Basal veins: connect superficial and deep cerebral veins
    b. Vein of Rosenthal
    c. Great cerebral vein (great vein of Galen)
  3. Venous sinuses: located between two layers of dura mater
    a. Posterior (superior) group
      (1) Superior sagittal
      (2) Inferior sagittal
      (3) Straight
      (4) Transverse
      (5) Sigmoid
      (6) Occipital
    b. Anterior (interior) group
      (1) Cavernous
      (2) Superior petrosal (2)
      (3) Inferior petrosal (2)
      (4) Basilar plexus

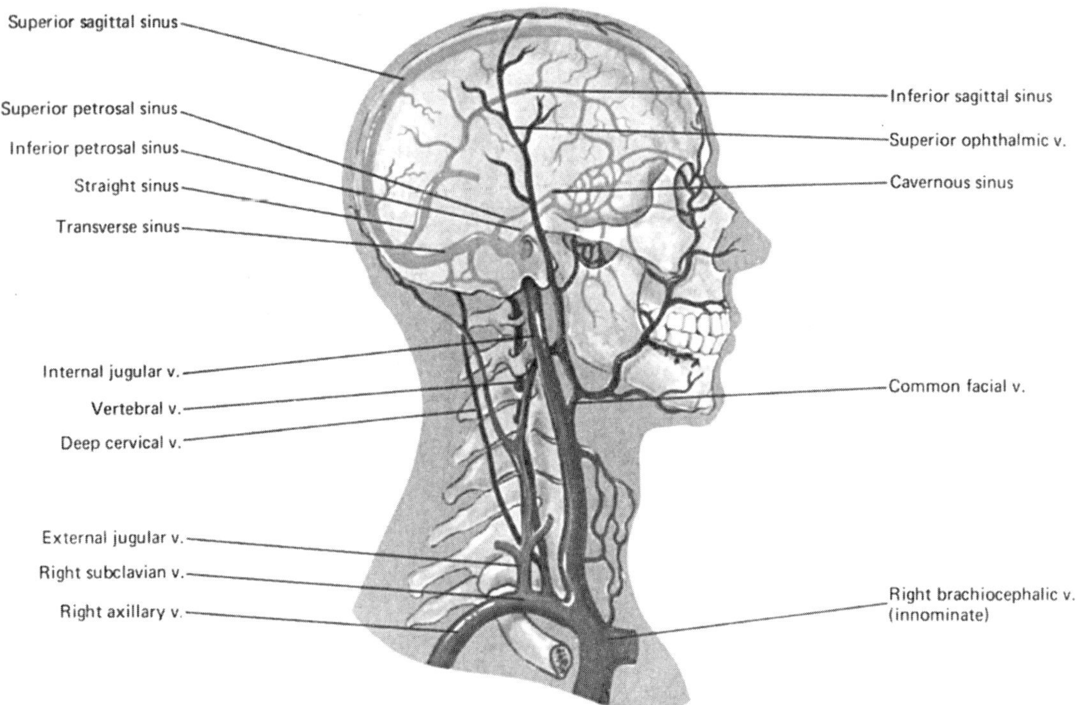


**FIGURE 21–4** Venous drainage of brain. (From Solomon EP, Phillips GA: *Understanding Human Anatomy and Physiology* [p 232]. Philadelphia, WB Saunders, 1987.)

IV. **Ventricular (CSF) System** (Fig. 21–5)
   A. Formation of CSF
      1. Approximately 500 ml/d produced (0.37 ml/min)
      2. 150 ml in system at one time
      3. Formed in choroid plexus
      4. Choroid plexus located in temporal horns of lateral ventricles, posterior portion of third ventricle, and roof of fourth ventricle
   B. Function
      1. Supports and cushions CNS
      2. Provides for excretion pathways for cerebral metabolic wastes
      3. Maintains stable chemical environment
      4. Facilitates intercerebral transport
   C. CSF properties
      1. Appearance
         a. Clear
         b. Colorless
         c. Odorless
      2. Protein: 15 to 45 mg/ml
      3. Glucose
         a. 50 to 75 mg/dl
         b. Two thirds of serum glucose
      4. White blood cells: 0 to 5/mm$^3$
      5. Red blood cells: none
      6. pH: 7.35 to 7.40
      7. Specific gravity: 1.005 to 1.009
      8. Pressure: 0 to 15 mm Hg or 50 to 150 mm $H_2O$
   D. Blood-brain barrier (BBB)

1. Composed of network of endothelial cells (cells of capillaries) and projections from astrocytes close to neurons
   a. Located throughout brain except in hypothalamus, pineal gland area, and floor of fourth ventricle in upper medulla
   b. More permeable in newborn than adult
2. Tight junctions between endothelial cells and astrocytes

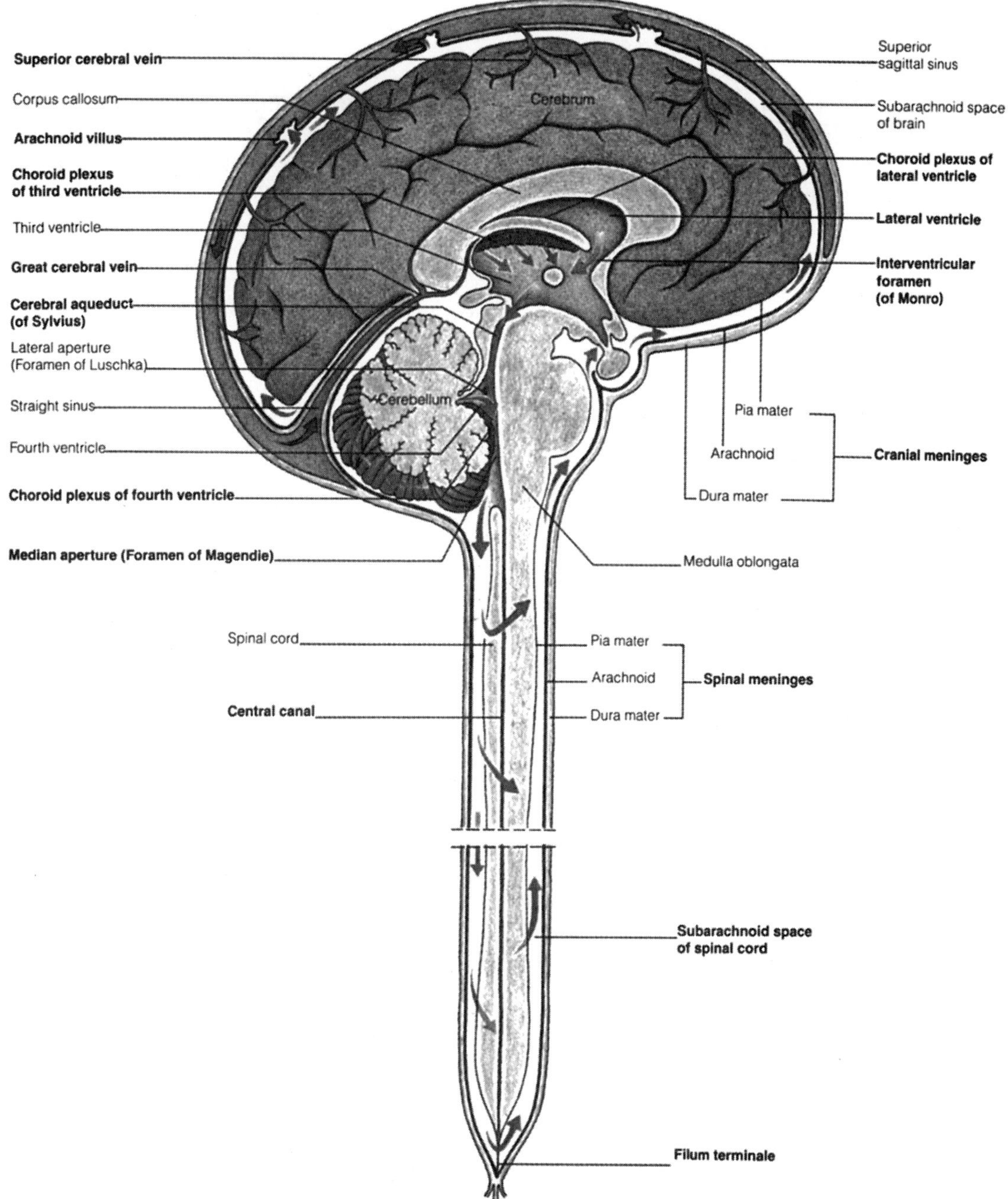


**FIGURE 21–5** Cerebrospinal fluid circulates around and within brain and spinal cord in intermeningeal spaces. It is secreted by choroid plexuses and reabsorbed in dural sinuses. Arrows indicate direction of flow. (From Gaudin AJ, Jones KC: *Human Anatomy and Physiology* [p 592]. San Diego, Harcourt Brace Jovanovich, 1989.)

3. Functions
   a. Preserve homeostasis of CNS
   b. Selectively permeable to facilitate entry of needed metabolites and remove toxic or unnecessary metabolites
   c. Permeable to water, oxygen, carbon dioxide, other gases, glucose, and lipid soluble substances
4. Breakdown of BBB by inflammation, tumors, and toxins allows large molecules to pass directly into CNS

E. Cerebral hemispheres (Fig. 21–6)
1. Cerebral cortex: outermost layer, composed of gray matter
   a. Gyri: raised projections
   b. Sulci: grooves between gyri
   c. Left cortex: deals with symbols and symbolic material, including language, mathematics, abstractions, reasoning; analytic aspect
   d. Right cortex: deals with visual-spatial tasks, processing of whole sensory experiences such as dancing, art appreciation; creative aspect
2. Lobes
   a. Frontal lobes (2)
      (1) Motor cortex: controls voluntary and fine motor movement
      (2) Sensory cortex: sensory association areas integrate and interpret sensory input
      (3) Memory
      (4) Personality and emotional behavior
      (5) Complex intellectual functioning
   b. Parietal lobes (2): posterior to central sulcus of Rolando
      (1) Sensory discrimination
      (2) Tactile receptive and association areas
      (3) Body image
   c. Temporal lobes (2): located under fissure of Sylvius
      (1) Hearing
      (2) Olfaction
      (3) Sensory speech (Wernicke's area)
      (4) Short-term memory
   d. Occipital lobe (1): integrates visual reception
3. Corpus callosum
   a. Bundle of nerve fibers
   b. Connects cerebral hemispheres
   c. Allows transfer of information from one hemisphere to the other
4. Basal ganglia
   a. Group of subcortical gray matter
   b. Buried deep in hemispheres near thalamus and lateral ventricle
   c. Links cerebral cortex to certain thalamic nuclei
   d. Modulates voluntary body movements, especially hands and legs
   e. Extrapyramidal system component
5. Internal capsule
   a. White matter pathways
   b. Carries ascending and descending motor and sensory fibers

F. Limbic system
1. Looks like a ring of tissue surrounding ventricles
2. "Visceral" or "emotional" brain
3. Interconnections with other brain structures
4. Damage affects emotional responses, sexual behavior, motivation, biologic rhythms

G. Diencephalon: located within cerebrum and continuous with midbrain
1. Epithalamus
   a. Narrow band forming roof of diencephalon

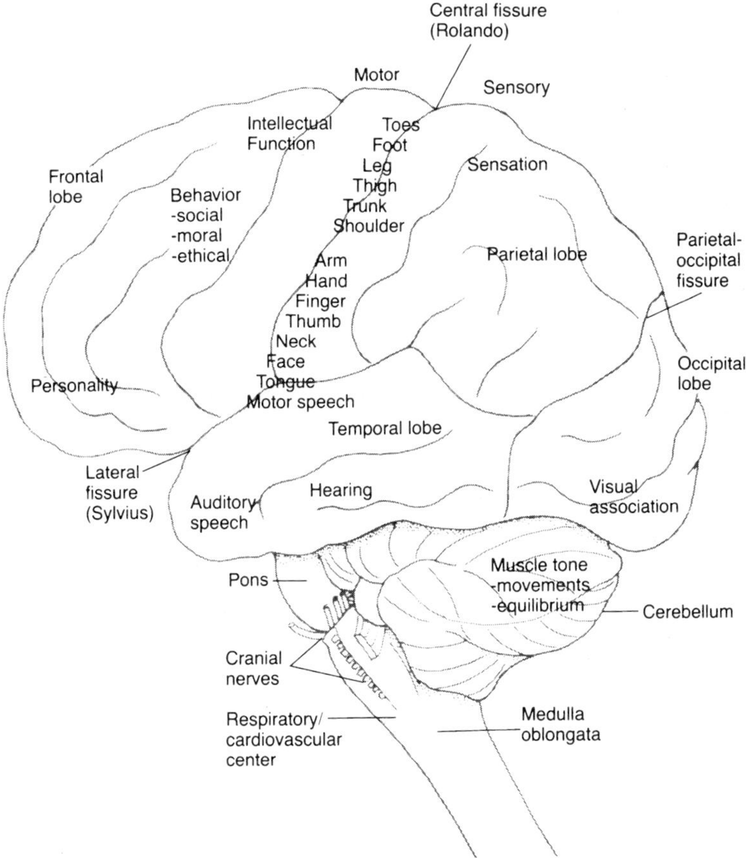


**FIGURE 21–6** Cerebral hemispheres.

   b. Associated with limbic system, optic reflexes, reproductive activity, inhibition of gonadal development
2. Thalamus
   a. Located on both sides of third ventricle
   b. Acts as relay point for most sensory and motor tracts
   c. Perception of primary sensations of pain, touch, pressure, temperature
   d. Contributes to emotions, behavioral expression
   e. Coordinates and regulates functional activity of cerebral cortex
3. Hypothalamus
   a. Anterior to brainstem
   b. Connected to pituitary gland by hypophyseal stalk (infundibulum)
   c. Forms base of diencephalon
   d. Maintains internal body homeostasis
      (1) Regulates body temperature, endocrine activities, body water
      (2) Appestat: controls and regulates appetite
      (3) Has role in maintaining awake state
      (4) Secretes neurohormones (hypothalamic releasing and inhibiting factors), oxytocin, vasopressin (antidiuretic hormone)
   e. Influences behavior patterns
      (1) Helps control primitive responses such as fear, instinct, self-preservation
      (2) Physical expression of emotions
      (3) Enhances CNS activity
   f. Cardiovascular regulation
   g. Uterine contractility and milk ejection

H. Brainstem (Fig. 21–7)
 1. Contains reticular activating system (RAS)
 2. Relays messages between cerebral structures and spinal cord
 3. Gives rise to cranial nerves III through XII
 4. Composition
  a. Midbrain (mesencephalon)
   (1) Connects to cerebrum through diencephalon
   (2) Control of various visual, auditory, postural reflexes
  b. Pons
   (1) Connects to cerebellum
   (2) Contains apneustic, pneumotaxic respiratory centers
  c. Medulla oblongata
   (1) Bottom structure of brainstem
   (2) Connects to cervical spinal cord
   (3) Contains critical centers for cardiac, respiratory, vasomotor, rhythmicity functions
   (4) Center for protective reflexes: coughing, sneezing, swallowing, gagging, vomiting
   (5) Decussation (contralateral crossing) of motor tracts descending from cerebrum occurs in pyramids

I. Cerebellum (see Fig. 21–7)
 1. Located at base of brain below occipital lobes
 2. Right and left hemispheres connected at midline
 3. Connected to brainstem by three sets of cerebellar peduncles
  a. Superior
  b. Middle
  c. Inferior
 4. Receives input from brainstem and spinal cord nuclei
 5. Functions
  a. Maintain muscle tone
  b. Coordinate muscle movement with sensory input
  c. Control equilibrium

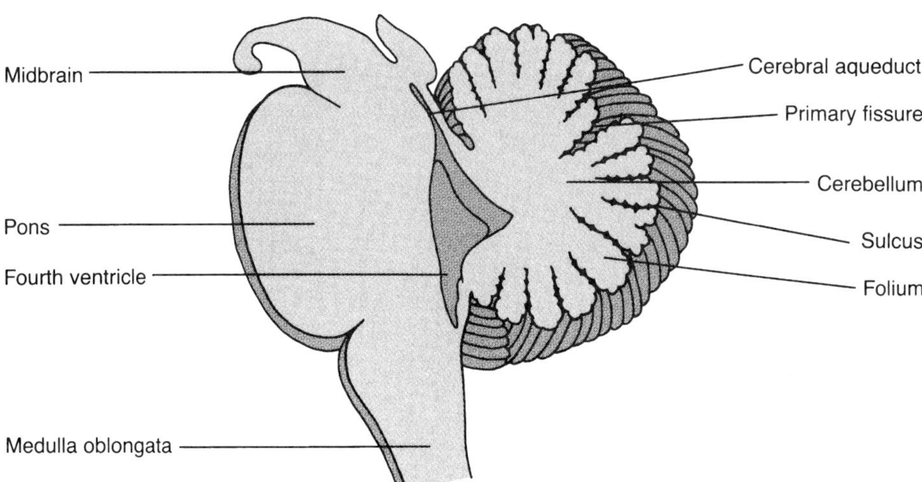


**FIGURE 21–7** Sagittal view of brainstem, fourth ventricle, and cerebellum. (From Black JM, Matassarin-Jacobs E: *Luckmann and Sorensen's Medical Surgical Nursing,* 4th Ed [p 624]. Philadelphia, WB Saunders, 1993.)

J. Cranial nerves (Table 21–1)
   1. Help in remembering names of cranial nerves (CN)

| *Mnemonic* | *CN Number and Name* |
|---|---|
| O (n) | I Olfactory |
| O (ld) | II Optic |
| O (lympus′) | III Oculomotor |
| T (owering) | IV Trochlear |
| T (ops) | V Trigeminal |
| A | VI Abducens |
| F (inn) | VII Facial |
| A (nd) | VIII Auditory |
| G (erman) | IX Glossopharyngeal |
| V (iewed) | X Vagus |
| S (ome) | XI Spinal accessory |
| H (ops) | XII Hypoglossal |

   2. Help in remembering whether nerves are sensory, motor, or both (S, M, B)

| *Mnemonic* | *CN Number and Name* |
|---|---|
| S (ome) | I Olfactory |
| S (ay) | II Optic |
| M (arry) | III Oculomotor |
| M (oney) | IV Trochlear |
| B (ut) | V Trigeminal |
| M (y) | VI Abducens |
| B (rother) | VII Facial |
| S (ays) | VIII Auditory |
| B (ad) | IX Glossopharyngeal |
| B (usiness) | X Vagus |
| M (arry) | XI Spinal accessory |
| M (en) | XII Hypoglossal |

K. Autonomic nervous system
   1. Part of peripheral nervous system
   2. Implications for patient undergoing intracranial surgery should be considered (Table 21–2)
   3. Overall purpose: regulation of involuntary functions of internal organs
   4. Sympathetic nervous system
      a. Originates in thoracic area of spine and upper lumbar segments of spinal cord
      b. Impulses travel from CNS to ganglia (relay stations outside spinal column) along postganglionic (adrenergic) fibers to effector organs where catecholamines are released (norepinephrine)
      c. Regulates body's energy expenditures
      d. Prepares body for stress (fight or flight)
   5. Parasympathetic nervous system
      a. Cell bodies located in extreme ends of spinal cord (brainstem, sacrum)
      b. Transmits impulses from CNS along preganglionic fibers to ganglia located in or near effector organs
         (1) Nerves are cholinergic
         (2) Acetylcholine released
      c. Helps in conservation of body's energy
      d. Affects localized, discrete areas rather than whole body

**TABLE 21–1 Rapid Neurologic Evaluation of Cranial Nerve Function**

| NERVE | ORIGIN | FUNCTION | METHOD OF TESTING |
|---|---|---|---|
| I Olfactory | Olfactory bulb | Sensory—sense of smell | Identify odors, one nostril at a time |
| II Optic | Lateral geniculate body | Sensory—vision and circuit for light reflex | Acuity—Snellen chart or newspaper; test each eye separately<br>Visual fields—confrontation method, each eye separately; move finger from eight cardinal points and indicate when it is seen |
| III Oculomotor | Midbrain | Motor—pupillary constriction, elevation of upper eyelid, extraocular movements conjointly with III, IV, and VI | Light flashed in affected eye<br>Light flashed in unaffected eye |
| IV Trochlear | Midbrain | Motor—extraocular movements of eye downward and inward (oblique muscles) | Follow fingers, using eight cardinal points |
| V Trigeminal | Pons | Sensory—ophthalmic: cornea of eye and above; maxillary: cheek and upper lips; mandibular: lower lip and chin | Touch cotton to both sides along divisions, corneal reflex |
| | | Motor—masseter and temporal muscles: biting down and chewing; lateral movement of jaw | "Bite down, chew" |
| VI Abducens | Pons | Motor—extraocular movements of eyes laterally | Follow fingers using eight cardinal points; test III, IV, VI together |
| VII Facial | Pons | Motor—facial muscles around eyes, mouth, and forehead | "Wrinkle your forehead" |
| | | Sensory—taste receptors on anterior two thirds of tongue | Identify flavors—does food taste the same? |

Adapted from Davis J, Mason CB: *Neurologic Critical Care,* (p 32). New York, Van Nostrand Reinhold, 1979.

| SITES OF INVOLVEMENT | ABNORMAL FINDINGS | FREQUENCY |
|---|---|---|
| Fracture of cribriform plate or in ethmoid area | Anosmia | Uncommon |
| Direct trauma to orbit or globe or fracture involving optic foramen | Loss of both direct and consensual pupillary constriction when light flashed in affected eye; unaffected eye has normal direct and consensual response | Common |
| Pressure on geniculate body; laceration or intracerebral clot in temporal, parietal, occipital lobes | Absence of blink when hand brought suddenly from side; indicates visual field defect (always homonymous) | Common |
| Pressure of herniating uncus on nerve just before it enters cavernous sinus or fracture involving cavernous sinus | Dilated pupil, ptosis; eye turns down and out<br>Direct pupil reflex absent; consensual reflex present<br>Direct pupil reflex present; consensual reflex absent | Very frequent |
| Course of nerve around brainstem | Eye fails to move down and out | Infrequent |
| Direct injury to terminal branches, particularly second division in roof of maxillary sinus | Loss of sensation of pain and touch<br>Paresthesias | Uncommon (exception: trigeminal neuralgia) |
| | Palpated masseter and temporalis fail to contract | |
| As with III, IV | Eyes fail to move laterally | Infrequent |
| Supranuclear: intracerebral clot | Forehead wrinkles because of bilateral innervation of frontalis; otherwise, paralysis of facial muscles as below | Frequent |
| Peripheral: laceration or contusion in parotid area | Paralysis of facial muscles; eye remains open; angle of mouth droops; forehead fails to wrinkle | Frequent |
| Peripheral: fracture of temporal bone | As above plus associated involvement of acoustic nerve (see below), dry cornea, and loss of taste on anterior two thirds of tongue | Frequent |

*Table continued on following page*

**TABLE 21–1 Rapid Neurologic Evaluation of Cranial Nerve Function** *(Continued)*

| NERVE | ORIGIN | FUNCTION | METHOD OF TESTING |
|---|---|---|---|
| VIII Acoustic | Pons | Sensory—cochlear division: hearing; vestibular division: maintenance of equilibrium and posturing of head | In children and unresponsive patients, clap hands close to ears<br>Weber's test: bone conduction with tuning fork; Rinne's test: air conduction using mastoid process<br>Caloric test |
| IX Glossopharnygeal | Medulla | Motor—constrictors of pharynx used in swallowing<br>Sensory—taste receptors on posterior one third of tongue | Touch walls of pharynx with tongue blade<br>Identify tastes |
| X Vagus | Medulla | Sensory—pharynx and larynx<br>Motor—pharnyx and larynx, movement of soft palate and uvula; conjointly with IX—ability to speak clearly | Touch with tongue blade to emit gag reflex<br>Watch movement of uvula when patient says "ahhh" |
| XI Spinal accessory | Medulla | Motor—sternocleidomastoid, trapezius, and rhomboid muscles | Shrug shoulders against resistance, turn head against resistance, flex chin |
| XII Hypoglossal | Medulla | Motor—tongue | "Stick out tongue, wiggle tongue" |

## NEUROLOGIC ASSESSMENT

I. **Baseline Status:** necessary to determine improvement or deterioration in patient's condition
   A. Level of consciousness (LOC)
      1. Reflects functional integrity of brain
      2. Most sensitive indicator of neurologic function
      3. Alertness mediated by RAS and cortex of cerebral hemisphere
      4. Involves awareness of environment and appropriate response to stimuli
   B. Assessment technique
      1. Arouse patient to maximum level of wakefulness
      2. Begin by calling patient by familiar name
      3. If no response, shake patient vigorously
      4. If no response, apply noxious stimuli, being careful not to injure patient
         a. Nail bed pressure
         b. Supraorbital pressure
         c. Pinching trapezius muscle
         d. Sternal pressure
      5. Assess orientation to environment
         a. Ask alert, verbal patient to tell you where he or she is
         b. Use yes or no questions to assess intubated patients
         c. For patients who may be confused, give choices similar to yes or no questions for intubated patients (i.e., "Is this place a hospital? Is this place your home?")
         d. Ask the date, year

| SITES OF INVOLVEMENT | ABNORMAL FINDINGS | FREQUENCY |
|---|---|---|
| Fracture of petrous portion of temporal bone; CN VII often involved | Startle reflex<br>Sound not heard by involved ear | Common |
| Herniation | Caloric test negative | |
| Brainstem or deep laceration of neck | Loss of taste to posterior one third of tongue<br>Loss of sensation on affected side of soft palate | Rare |
| Brainstem or deep laceration of neck<br>Compression by herniation | Sagging of soft palate; deviation of uvula to normal side<br>Hoarseness from paralysis of vocal cords<br>Loss of gag reflex | Rare |
| Laceration of neck | Inability to shrug shoulders or turn head | Rare |
| Neck laceration, usually associated with major vessel damage | Tongue protrudes toward affected side; dysarthria | Rare |

e. Avoid using "squeeze my hand" to assess strength or ability to follow commands
   (1) Patients with diffuse cerebral injury, particularly frontal lobe problems, retain strong hand grasp reflex similar to infant's
   (2) Give patient a single step command (e.g., "Show me two fingers")
   (3) If you do ask patient to squeeze your hand, also ask patient to let go of your hand

f. Assess for behavioral changes such as restlessness, irritability, combativeness

C. Pupillary reactivity
   1. Oculomotor nerve (CN III) and brainstem control pupil size and reaction
   2. Sluggish pupils indicate pressure on CN III, which runs parallel to brainstem
   3. Assessment technique
      a. Observe size, shape, equality, and reaction to light
      b. Assess and compare pupils bilaterally
      c. Record pupil size as small, medium, or large unless reference is available to measure exact size
   4. Be aware of effect of anesthetic agents and preoperative medications on pupil size and reactivity
      a. Constricting agents (miotic)
         (1) Opiates and narcotics
         (2) Cholinergic agents
            (a) Optical miotics (pilocarpine)
            (b) Neostigmine bromide (Prostigmin)
            (c) Barbiturates
            (d) Edrophonium chloride (Tensilon)
            (e) Pyridostigmine bromide (Mestinon)

**TABLE 21–2 Effects of Autonomic Nervous System**

| EFFECTOR ORGAN | SYMPATHETIC (ADRENERGIC EFFECT) | PARASYMPATHETIC (CHOLINERGIC EFFECT) |
|---|---|---|
| Pupil | Dilates | Constricts |
| Salivary glands | Decreases secretion | Increases secretion |
| Bronchi | Dilates | Constricts |
| Respiratory rate | Increases | Decreases |
| Heart | | |
| Pulse | Increases | Decreases |
| Contraction | Strengthens | Weakens |
| Blood pressure | Increased | Decreased |
| Stomach | Decreases contractions | Increases contractions |
| Adrenal glands | Stimulates secretion of epinephrine, norepinephrine | Decreases secretions |
| Digestive tract | Decreases motility | Increases motility |
| | Contracts sphincters | Relaxes sphincters |
| | Inhibits secretions | Stimulates secretions |
| Bladder | Relaxes | Contracts |
| | | Relaxes sphincter |
| Sweat glands | Increases activity | Decreases activity |
| Hair | Piloerection | Relaxes |
| Blood vessels | | |
| Coronary | Dilates | No significant effect |
| Skeletal muscle | Dilates | Constricts |
| Skin | Constricts | No significant effect |

b. Dilating agents (mydriatic)
   (1) Anticholinergic agents
      (a) Atropine sulfate
      (b) Naloxone hydrochloride
      (c) Scopolamine hydrobromide
c. Topical mydriatics
d. Adrenergic agents
   (1) Catecholamines
      (a) Dobutamine (Dobutrex)
      (b) Dopamine (Intropin)
      (c) Epinephrine (Adrenalin)
      (d) Isoproterenol (Isuprel)
      (e) Norepinephrine (Levophed)
   (2) Noncatecholamine agents
      (a) Ephedrine
      (b) Metaraminol (Aramine)
      (c) Phenylephrine (Neo-Synephrine)

5. Pupil size can be altered by direct eye trauma or congenital malformations
6. Any change in pupil size or reactivity should be reported to physician at once

D. Motor function
1. Voluntary motor movement controlled by fibers originating in frontal lobes of cerebral cortex
2. Fibers descend through brainstem; most cross and continue to spinal cord
3. Assessment technique for alert patient
   a. Test strength of all muscle groups against resistance and gravity
   b. Upper extremities: palmar (pronator) drift method
      (1) Ask patient to close eyes and extend arms in front with palms up
      (2) Paretic arm will slowly drift downward and palm will turn upward
   c. Muscle strength assessed by testing active, passive, and active resistive movements

d. Lower extremities: grading of muscle strength
   (1) 0: no evidence of contractility
   (2) 1: trace of contractility, no movement
   (3) 2: full range of motion with gravity eliminated
   (4) 3: full range of motion against gravity
   (5) 4: full range of motion against gravity with some resistance
   (6) 5: full range of motion against gravity with full resistance (normal power)

4. Assessment technique for nonalert patient: apply noxious stimuli and observe response
   a. Purposeful movement such as pushing away stimulus indicates intact neuraxis
   b. Localization of gross location of stimulus indicates cortical dysfunction
   c. Nonpurposeful responses indicate dysfunction deeper in cerebral hemispheres and midbrain area
      (1) Incomplete removal of stimulus
      (2) Slight movement without moving away from stimulus
      (3) Withdrawal of only the part stimulated
      (4) Lower extremities flex at knees
   d. Decorticate posturing (flexion response)
      (1) Occurs with disruption of corticospinal pathways
      (2) Loss of cerebral cortex influence over movement (Fig. 21–8)
   e. Decerebrate posturing (extension response)
      (1) Indicates damage in deeper cerebral hemispheres and upper brainstem
      (2) Indicative of more severe brain dysfunction with poor prognosis

E. Reflexes that reflect integrity of neuroaxis
   1. Oculocephalic reflex (Doll's eyes)
      a. Can only be elicited in patients with depressed LOC
      b. Alert patients override reflex
      c. Tests integrity of brainstem between CN III and CN VIII
      d. Technique
         (1) Hold patient's eyes open
         (2) Briskly turn patient's head side to side
         (3) Pause to assess eyes on each side
      e. Interpretation
         (1) Normal (Doll's eye reflex present)
            (a) Conjugate eye deviation to direction opposite direction head is turned; eyes move in orbits
            (b) In comatose patient indicates brainstem is intact between CN III and CN VIII
         (2) Abnormal (Doll's eye reflex absent)
            (a) Dysconjugate eye movements
            (b) Eyes move with head; eyes do not move in orbits
            (c) Eyes appear fixed like painted eyes of a china doll
            (d) Indicative of severe lesion in brainstem
            (e) Contraindicated in actual or suspected cervical injuries
   2. Oculovestibular reflex (cold calorics)
      a. Provides information about integrity of brainstem and connections to cerebral cortex
      b. Contraindicated in patients with ruptured tympanic membrane
      c. Technique
         (1) Assess integrity of tympanic membrane
         (2) Cold water (50 ml) slowly injected into external auditory canal
         (3) Observe eye movement (two phases)
            (a) Normal: eyes initially deviate to side of stimulus followed by rapid component of nystagmus deviating toward opposite side

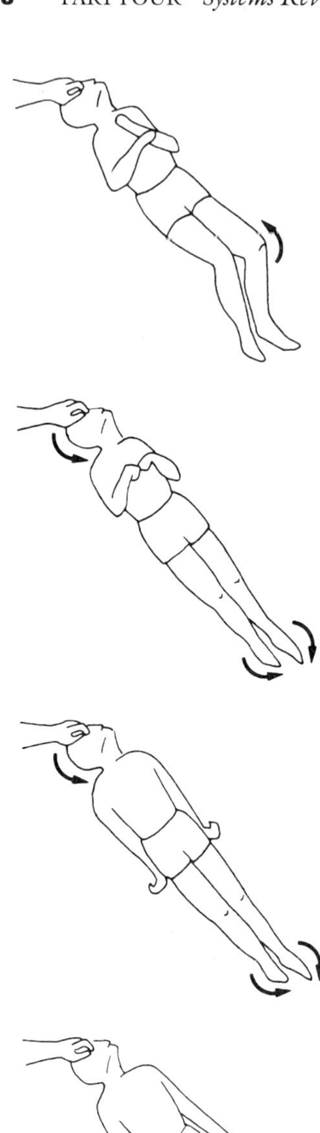

Bilateral Withdrawal
(Flexion)

Arms flexed
Legs flexed
Knees come up

Bilateral Decortication
(Abnormal Flexion)

Arms flexed
Wrists flexed
Legs extended

Bilateral Decerebration
(Extension)

Arms extended
Wrists externally rotated
Legs extended
Feet internally rotated

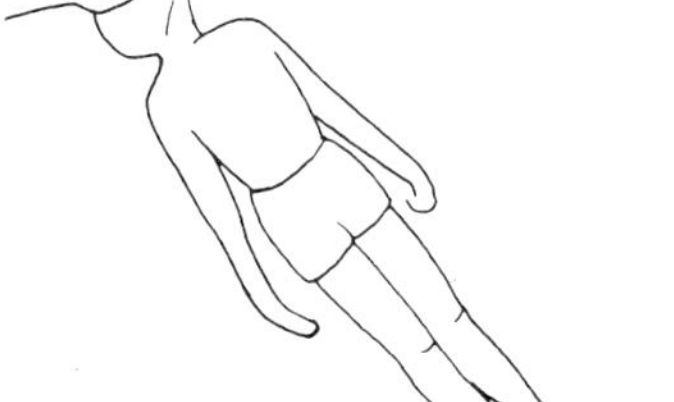

Bilateral Flaccidity

No response in any extremity to noxious stimuli
*Note:* Spinal cord injury must be ruled out as cause of flaccidity before patient is considered brain dead.

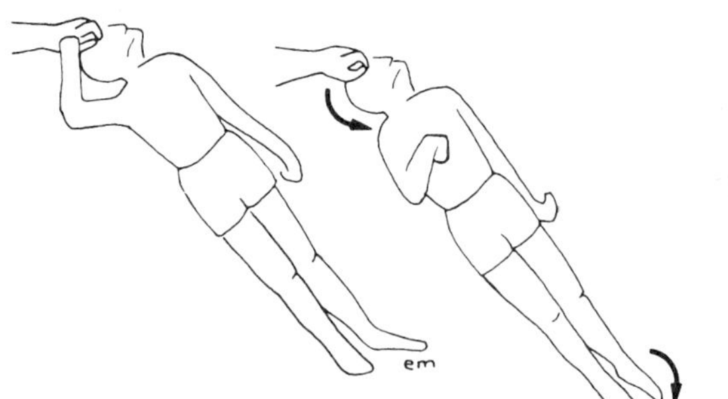

Lateralization*

Left Figure: Purposeful right side
Decorticate left side

Right Figure: Decorticate right side
Decerebrate left side

*These figures show how responses can vary from limb to limb and stress the importance of checking all extremities for motor response.

**FIGURE 21–8** Motor signs in response to noxious stimuli. (From Marshall SB, Marshall LF, Vos HR, Chesnut RM: *Neuroscience Critical Care.* Philadelphia, WB Saunders, 1990.)

(b) Abnormal: any deviation from pattern described indicates pathologic condition in brainstem or higher structures; prognosis very poor

F. Vital signs
1. Changes usually seen late in clinical course; should not be relied on to signal impending neurologic clinical problems
2. Observe for Cushing's triad (reflex), a sign of increased ICP
   a. Increased systolic blood pressure
   b. Decreased diastolic blood pressure
   c. Decreased pulse rate (bradycardia)
3. Observe for widening pulse pressure: systolic blood pressure increases while diastolic pressure decreases
4. Observe for changes in respiratory rate and rhythm
5. Assessment of cranial nerve function may be needed depending on underlying neurologic problem (see Table 21–1)

G. Documentation
1. Variety of assessment tools available, but most include parameters of Glasgow Coma Scale (Fig. 21–9)
2. Frequency of neurologic assessment may be dictated by unit protocol and patient condition
   a. Report abnormal findings to physician
   b. Be alert to subtle changes in any of the above parameters
3. Give specific descriptions of stimulus used and resulting response of patient

| | | |
|---|---|---|
| EYES OPEN | Spontaneously | 4 |
| | To Speech | 3 |
| | To Pain | 2 |
| | None | 1 |
| BEST VERBAL RESPONSE | Oriented | 5 |
| | Confused | 4 |
| | Inappropriate Words | 3 |
| | Incomprehensible Sounds | 2 |
| | None | 1 |
| BEST MOTOR RESPONSE | Obeys Commands | 5 |
| | Localizes Pain | 4 |
| | Flexion to Pain | 3 |
| | Extension to Pain | 2 |
| | None | 1 |

**FIGURE 21–9** Glasgow coma scale.

## DYNAMICS OF INCREASED ICP

I. **Monro-Kellie Hypothesis:** skull is closed container with fixed volume of blood, CSF, and brain tissue contained within nondistensible skull
   A. Contents of skull
      1. Blood: 10%
      2. CSF: 10%
      3. Brain tissue: 80%
   B. Volume-pressure relationship (elastance)
      1. Small increases in volume more readily compensated for in uninjured or noncompromised brain
      2. Increases in volume over extended period of time more readily compensated for than comparable volume over shorter period of time
      3. Little room in skull for slack
      4. In traumatized or injured brain even small increases in volume can produce drastic elevations in ICP
   C. Compensatory mechanisms: increase in one intracranial volume must be compensated for by a decrease in one of the remaining volumes
      1. Displacement and reduction of CSF volume
      2. Reduction in blood volume
      3. Displacement of brain tissue
   D. Normal intracranial pressure
      1. 0 to 15 mm Hg—with invasive monitoring
      2. 50 to 150 mm $H_2O$—with external manometer
   E. Causes of increased ICP
      1. Abnormal production, circulation, or absorption of CSF
         a. Hydrocephalus
            (1) Communicating
            (2) Noncommunicating
         b. Congenital abnormalities: hydrocephalus, Arnold-Chiari malformation
         c. Obstructive masses: tumors, abscesses
      2. Increase in intracranial blood volume
         a. Hemorrhage
         b. Hyperthermia: increases metabolic demands and thus blood volume
         c. Venous drainage impairment
         d. Hypercapnia—increases in $Paco_2$ or $H^+$ levels
         e. Vascular abnormalities
            (1) Aneurysms
            (2) Arteriovenous malformations (AVMs)
         f. Vasodilating drugs
            (1) Anesthetic gases
               (a) Halothane
               (b) Enflurane
               (c) Isoflurane
               (d) Nitrous oxide
            (2) Some antihypertensives
            (3) Some histamines
      3. Increase in brain tissue volume
         a. Tumors
         b. Infectious processes
         c. Edema
      4. Other
         a. Respiratory procedures: suctioning, PEEP, intubation, increased airway pressure

b. Body positions: Trendelenburg, prone, extreme hip flexion, neck flexion
c. Coughing
d. Isometric muscle exercises
e. Valsalva maneuver
f. Noxious stimuli
g. Emotional upset
h. Seizure activity
i. Rapid eye movement (REM) sleep or arousal from sleep
j. Clustering care activities

F. Autoregulation: ability of cerebral circulation to maintain relatively constant cerebral blood flow and pressure needed to provide oxygen and nutrients to brain tissue
1. Cerebral perfusion pressure (CPP)
a. Determines cerebral blood flow
b. CPP = Mean arterial blood pressure (MABP) – ICP
c. $\text{MABP} = \dfrac{(\text{Diastolic BP} \times 2) + \text{Systolic BP}}{3}$
d. Interpretation of CPP values
(1) 80 to 100 mm Hg: normal
(2) 60 mm Hg: provides minimally adequate blood supply
(3) <50 mm Hg: autoregulation begins to fail
(4) <40 mm Hg: cerebral blood flow decreases by 25%
(5) <30 mm Hg: incompatible with life; neuronal hypoxia and cell death
2. Invasive ICP monitoring needed to calculate CPP
3. CPP calculation should be part of neurologic assessment

G. Clinical presentation of signs of increased ICP
1. Depends on location, cause, and degree of compensation
2. Damage to brain tissue
a. Tissue ischemia due to decreased cerebral blood flow
b. Brain structures compressed by increasing pressure
3. Symptoms
a. Deterioration in LOC
b. Pupillary dysfunction
c. Changes in motor status
d. Changes in vital signs: Cushings triad (reflex)
e. Seizures
f. Headaches
g. Vomiting
h. Papilledema
i. CN palsies
j. Sensory changes
k. Impaired brainstem reflexes

H. Herniation syndromes: increasing pressure causes displacement of brain tissue
1. Transcalvarial herniation
a. Occurs at surgical incision site or through site of gunshot or stab wound or fracture site
2. Cingulate herniation
a. One of cerebral hemispheres displaced laterally across midline with blood vessels and tissue compressed
3. Central transtentorial herniation
a. Downward displacement of cerebral hemispheres through tentorial notch located at level of tentorium cerebelli, which separates cerebellum from cerebral hemispheres

4. Uncal (lateral) herniation
   a. Displacement of medial tip of temporal lobe (uncus) through tentorium, compressing midbrain
   b. Most common herniation syndrome
5. Infratentorial herniation
   a. Compression of brainstem, cerebellum
   b. Medullary collapse

## II. Medical Interventions

A. Direct: remove cause
B. Indirect
   1. Maintain patent airway
   2. Maintain normal fluid and electrolyte balance
      a. Adequate fluid management with saline to avoid dehydration and hypotension
      b. Serum osmolarity kept between 290 and 320 mOsm/kg
      c. Monitor serum glucose, electrolytes
   3. Avoid administration of narcotics; use acetaminophen (Tylenol) or codeine for pain
   4. Give diuretics
      a. Osmotic diuretics: mannitol
         (1) Draws water from extracellular space of edematous brain into plasma
         (2) Does not cross blood-brain barrier
         (3) Can cause fluid and electrolyte imbalances
      b. Furosemide (Lasix)
         (1) Thought to decrease CSF production
         (2) Decreases systemic fluid volume
         (3) Manage rebound effect of mannitol
   5. Administer corticosteroids
      a. Controversial with head trauma or cerebral infarction with edema but useful with brain tumors
      b. Dosage tapered before discontinued
   6. Initiate therapeutic hyperventilation
      a. Maintain $P_{CO_2}$ between 27 and 33 mm Hg
      b. Should be done with mechanical ventilation
      c. Short-term use recommended (<72 hours); not for prophylaxis
      d. Manual hyperventilation with AMBU recommended only emergently for patients with "pressure signs" until ventilator available
   7. Reduce cerebral stimulation and metabolic demand
      a. Control pain
      b. Maintain normothermia: if using hypothermia blankets, prevent shivering, which will increase metabolic demands and ICP
      c. Control seizures with phenytoin sodium
      d. Control hyperactivity with sedation
      e. Barbiturate coma
         (1) Used with uncontrolled refractory increased ICP
         (2) Pentobarbital or thiopental used
         (3) Reduces brain's metabolic requirements and produces arteriolar constriction
         (4) Sophisticated monitoring capabilities required
      f. Neuromuscular blockade for severe agitation
C. Ventriculostomy to drain CSF
D. Operative decompression: surgical removal of tip of temporal lobe, portion of frontal lobe, or portion of cranial bone

## III. Nursing Interventions

A. Goals
   1. Protect patient at risk from sudden increases in ICP

2. Prevent permanent brain damage
   a. Maintenance of patent airway
   b. Ongoing neurologic assessment

B. Positioning
   1. Elevate head of bed 30 to 45 degrees
   2. Maintain head in neutral position with sandbags or Philadelphia collar
   3. Avoid prone position
   4. Patients with infratentorial craniotomies may be positioned flat or slightly elevated

C. Prevent Valsalva's maneuver by having patient exhale

D. Prevent isometric muscle contraction by assisting patient in turning

E. Avoid clustering of nursing activities: space nursing care to give patient frequent rest periods, which decreases stimulation

## IV. ICP Monitoring

A. Purpose
   1. Monitor trends in ICP
   2. Measure CPP
   3. Test intracranial compliance

B. ICP monitoring techniques (Fig. 21–10)

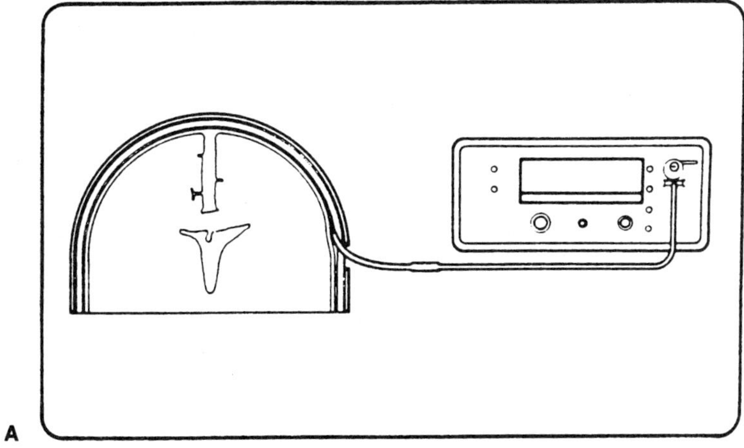


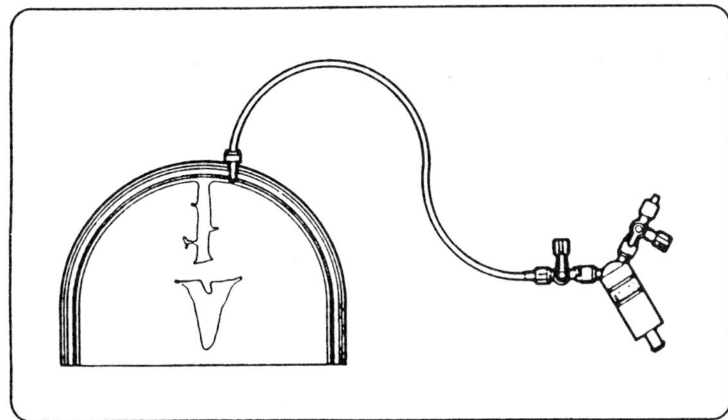


**FIGURE 21–10** **A,** Epidural monitoring system. **B,** Subdural monitoring system.

*Illustration continued on following page*

1. Intraventricular catheter: inserted through anterior horn of lateral ventricle on non-dominant side
   a. Advantages
      (1) Most accurate measurement of ICP
      (2) Allows for sampling of CSF
      (3) Allows for calculation of CPP and determination of intracranial compliance
      (4) Intrathecal administration of medications
      (5) Use as ventriculostomy to decrease increased ICP
   b. Disadvantages
      (1) Increased risk of infection and hemorrhage
      (2) Catheter placement difficult with small ventricles
      (3) Catheter obstruction by cerebral tissue
2. Subarachnoid bolt (Richmond or Becker bolt): inserted into subarachnoid space through cranial burr hole
   a. Advantages
      (1) Less risk of infection
      (2) Placement is easier and can be used in patients with small ventricles
   b. Disadvantages
      (1) Inability to sample CSF

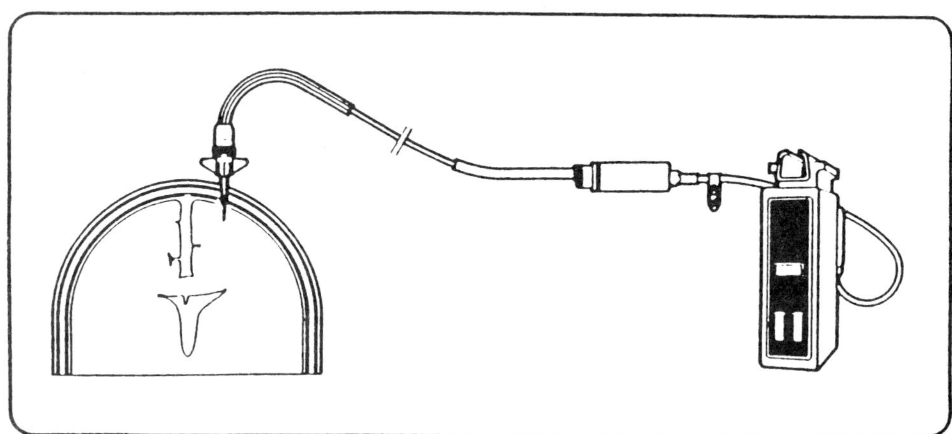


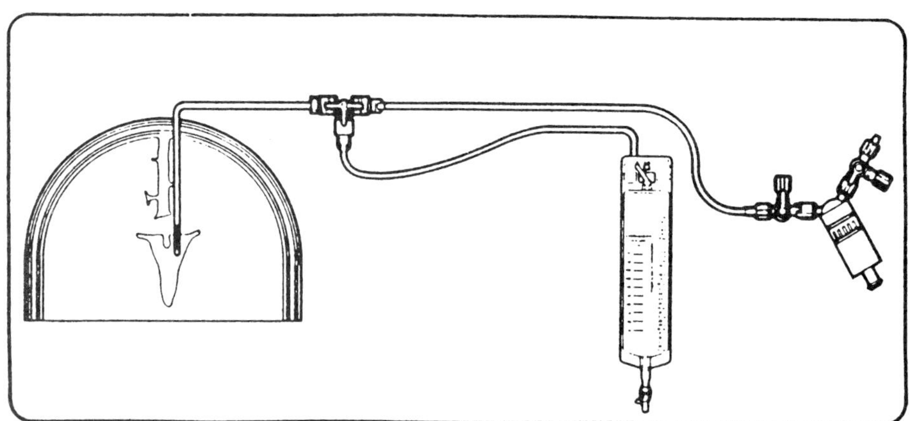


**FIGURE 21–10** *Continued* **C,** Intraparenchymal monitoring system. **D,** Intraventricular monitoring system. (From Marshall SB, Marshall LF, Vos HR, Chesnut RM: *Neuroscience Critical Care* [pp 369–370]. Philadelphia, WB Saunders, 1990. Courtesy of Camino Laboratories, San Diego, California.)

(2) Inability to test compliance
(3) Does not allow for intrathecal administration of medications
(4) Questionable reflection of actual ICP
(5) Brain tissue can herniate into monitoring device if ICP is very high

3. Epidural or subdural sensors or catheters: inserted into epidural or subdural space
   a. Advantages
      (1) Easily inserted
      (2) Decreased risk of infection
      (3) Brain or subarachnoid space not penetrated
      (4) Recalibration may not be necessary, depending on type of device used
   b. Disadvantages
      (1) Questionable reflection of actual ICP because of pressure from adjacent dura
      (2) Inability to sample CSF
      (3) Requires specialized monitoring
4. Fiberoptic transducer-tipped catheter
   a. Advantages
      (1) Easily inserted and requires small hole
      (2) Versatile: can be inserted into ventricles, subarachnoid space, brain parenchyma, subdural space
      (3) Zero balancing required only at time of insertion
      (4) Unit contains its own monitor so patient can be transported while getting accurate ICP readings
      (5) Baseline drift minimal over time
      (6) Decreased risk of infection
   b. Disadvantages
      (1) Does not allow for CSF sampling or drainage
      (2) Fiberoptic cable very delicate and can break easily
      (3) Periodic replacement of probe may be necessary
      (4) Expensive

C. ICP waveforms
   1. Mechanism is transmission of pressure to transducer that converts pressure waves into waveform visible on oscilloscope

D. Nursing interventions
   1. Strict aseptic technique
   2. Observe for leaks and breaks in system
   3. Close observation of waveforms
   4. Troubleshooting of dampened waveforms
   5. Recalibration of system according to unit protocol
   6. Never irrigate system
   7. Calculation of intracranial compliance is physician responsibility
   8. Removal of system is physician responsibility

## DISORDERS POTENTIALLY REQUIRING SURGICAL INTERVENTION

**I. Brain Tumors**

A. Pathologic condition: damage to brain tissue through expansion, infiltration, or destruction

B. Classification: no universally accepted system
   1. Benign vs. malignant
      a. Malignancy depends on
         (1) Rate of growth
         (2) Infiltration
         (3) Location

   b. Benign tumors may be "malignant" by location (i.e., malignant effects as result of surgical inaccessibility)
   c. Benign tumors can degenerate into malignant tumors
2. Primary vs. secondary
   a. Primary
      (1) Arise from CNS tissue or supporting cells of CNS (glial cells)
      (2) Account for 90% of diagnosed tumors
      (3) Rarely metastasize outside CNS
      (4) Examples: glioma, astrocytoma, oligodendroglioma, glioblastoma, glioblastoma multiforme
   b. Secondary
      (1) Metastasis of tumors from another part of body
      (2) Most common primary site is lungs in both males and females
      (3) Multiple lesions common
      (4) Prostate, skin, and ovarian malignancies rarely metastasize to brain
3. Location
   a. Tentorium used as anatomic landmark
      (1) Thick band of dura mater separating cerebral hemispheres from cerebellum
      (2) Forms small, circular opening around upper part of brainstem (tentorial notch)
   b. Supratentorial (above tentorium)
      (1) 70% of adult tumors
      (2) Deficits variable: paralysis, seizures, language deficits, memory loss, visual field cuts, personality changes
   c. Infratentorial (below tentorium)
      (1) Posterior fossa: contains brainstem and cerebellum
      (2) 70% of pediatric tumors
      (3) Deficits can include ataxia, cranial nerve deficits, autonomic nervous system dysfunction, vomiting, drooling, hearing loss, visual disturbances
   d. Intracerebral (arising within brain tissue)
      (1) May be supratentorial or infratentorial
      (2) Gliomas, metastatic lesions, astrocytomas
      (3) Usually malignant
   e. Extracerebral (arising from meninges)
      (1) May be supratentorial or infratentorial
      (2) Meningiomas
      (3) Usually benign
      (4) Slow growing, encapsulated
      (5) Can recur after surgical excision
4. Histologic classification
   a. Tumors can arise from supporting cells of brain (gliomas) or extracerebral structures (meningiomas) or metastasize from malignancies in other body systems
   b. Described by specific cell contained in tumor (glioma, astrocytoma)
   c. Gliomas graded according to degrees of malignancy or differentiation of cell of origin
      (1) Grade I
         (a) Well differentiated
         (b) Closely resembles normal cells
         (c) Long-term survival
      (2) Grade II
         (a) Moderately differentiated
         (b) 4- to 5-year survival
      (3) Grade III
         (a) Poorly differentiated
         (b) 1-year survival

(4) Grade IV
(a) Very poorly differentiated
(b) Has lost characteristics of cell of origin
(c) Poor prognosis

C. Clinical findings: dependent on location of tumor and degree of increased ICP
1. Headache
a. Characteristically worse in morning
b. Intensified by activity
2. Seizures: adults with first-time seizure are considered to have brain tumor until proven otherwise
3. Papilledema
4. Vomiting
5. Sensory and motor dysfunctions
6. Speech impairments
7. Changes in personality or mental function

D. Diagnostic tools
1. History and physical assessment
2. Skull films
3. Computed tomography (CT) scan
4. Magnetic resonance imaging (MRI)
5. Angiography

E. Treatment modalities
1. Radiation therapy: often initially to shrink tumor
2. Chemotherapy
3. Craniotomy
4. Radiosurgery: gamma knife

## II. Brain Abscess

A. Pathologic condition: pocket(s) of exudate formed from infections of adjacent tissue or hematogenous spread

B. Clinical findings
1. Headache
2. Focal signs
3. Signs of increased ICP

C. Diagnostic tools
1. History and physical assessment
2. Skull films
3. CT scan
4. MRI
5. Culture of abscess exudate through stereotactic approach
6. Routine laboratory studies

D. Treatment modalities
1. Aspiration or excision of abscess
2. Intravenous antibiotic therapy
3. Treatment of increased ICP

## III. Trigeminal Neuralgia

A. Pathologic condition
1. Cause unknown
2. Most common in middle and later life

B. Clinical findings
1. Explosive, severe pain in distribution of CN V
2. Pain may spontaneously remit and recur
3. Pain may cause patient to avoid activities that intensify it, such as eating, hygiene

C. Treatment modalities
   1. Pharmacologic
      a. Carbamazepine (Tegretol)
      b. Phenytoin (Dilantin)
   2. Alcohol block of one or more branches
   3. Surgical retrogasserian rhizotomy
   4. Sensory root decompression (Taarnhoj procedure)
   5. Microsurgical decompression of trigeminal root (Jannetta procedure)
   6. Radiofrequency percutaneous electrocoagulation
   7. Vascular decompression of CN V through posterior fossa craniotomy

**IV. Craniocerebral Trauma**

A. Mechanism of injury
   1. Deceleration: head hits stationary object
   2. Acceleration: head struck by moving object
   3. Acceleration-deceleration (coup-contracoup): head hits object, brain rebounds inside cranium against opposite cranial bones
   4. Shear-strain: twisting, sliding motions of brainstem

B. Types of injuries
   1. Primary (impact) injury: damage produced by blow
      a. Concussion: transient loss of consciousness lasting several minutes
      b. Contusion: actual bruising of brain tissue resulting in structural damage
      c. Laceration: actual tearing of brain tissue
      d. Fractures
         (1) Linear
         (2) Comminuted
         (3) Depressed
         (4) Basilar
   2. Intracranial secondary injury: damage that follows impact injury
      a. Hematomas
         (1) Epidural: bleeding, usually from middle meningeal artery; accumulates between skull and dura
         (2) Subdural: venous bleeding beneath dura mater; may be acute, subacute, or chronic
      b. ICP
      c. Brain swelling
      d. Cerebral edema
   3. Extracranial secondary injury
      a. Hypoxia
      b. Systemic hypotension

C. Clinical findings
   1. Epidural hematoma
      a. Momentary loss of consciousness
      b. "Lucid interval"
      c. Rapid deterioration
      d. Signs of increased ICP
   2. Subdural hematoma
      a. Drowsiness
      b. Agitation
      c. Slow cerebration and confusion
      d. Signs of increased ICP
   3. Intracerebral hematoma
      a. Immediate neurologic deficits

b. Signs of increased ICP
c. Loss of consciousness usually occurs from onset of injury
4. Skull fractures
a. Basilar fracture most common
(1) Involves bones of floor of cranial vault
(2) Otorrhea, rhinorrhea
(3) Battle's sign: ecchymosis over mastoid process
(4) Raccoon's eyes: periorbital ecchymosis
(5) Otorrhagia
(6) Test ear or nasal drainage for glucose and observe for concentric circles (halo or ring sign) on dressing or linens
5. Open head injuries
a. Gunshot and stab wounds
b. Potential for infection is high

D. Diagnostic tools
1. History and physical assessment
2. Skull films
3. CT scan
4. MRI (not for initial diagnosis; may be used for follow-up)
5. Routine laboratory studies
a. Alcohol and drug screen
b. Arterial blood gases (ABGs)
6. Cervical spine films to rule out accompanying cervical fracture
7. Radiographs to rule out other injuries

E. Treatment modalities
1. Surgical evacuation of hematomas usually needed depending on size and presence of signs of increased ICP
2. Debridement
a. Removal of bone fragments, foreign objects, infarcted tissue
b. Permits inspection of skull fractures and penetrating wound

**V. Intracranial Hemorrhage**

A. Pathologic condition
1. Arterial aneurysm rupture: dilation of weakened arterial wall causing blood-filled sac
2. AVM rupture
a. Congenital communication of arteries and veins without intervening capillaries
b. Forms tangled, interwoven mass
c. Occurs more often in younger patients
d. Vessels rupture more easily than normal vessels
3. Hypertensive hemorrhage

B. Clinical findings
1. Subarachnoid hemorrhage
a. Sudden, violent headache: "worst headache of my life"
b. Altered LOC
c. Signs of increased ICP
d. Nausea and vomiting
e. Meningeal irritation
(1) Kernig's sign: resistance and pain when patient's leg is flexed at hip and knee
(2) Brudzinski's sign: flexion of hips and knees in response to passive flexion of neck
f. Focal signs depending on location of bleeding
g. Bloody CSF
h. Hunt and Hess classification of aneurysms (Table 21–3)

**TABLE 21–3 Hunt and Hess Classification of Aneurysms**

| | |
|---|---|
| Grade 0 | Unruptured aneurysm |
| Grade I | Asymptomatic or minimal headache, slight nuchal rigidity |
| Grade I-A | Fixed neurologic deficit but no acute meningeal signs |
| Grade II | Moderate to severe headache; nuchal ridigity present; CN III palsy but no other neurologic deficits |
| Grade III | Drowsy, confused, mild focal deficits |
| Grade IV | Stupor, moderate to severe hemiparesis; early decerebrate rigidity; vegetative disturbances |
| Grade V | Deep coma; decerebrate rigidity; moribund |

2. Intracerebral hemorrhage
   a. Abrupt changes in LOC
   b. Signs of increased ICP
   c. Headache
   d. Nausea and vomiting
   e. Focal signs dependent on site of bleeding

C. Diagnostic tools
   1. History and physical assessment
   2. Lumbar puncture and CSF analysis
   3. Arteriogram, magnetic resonance angiography (MRA)
   4. CT scan
   5. Routine laboratory studies

D. Treatment modalities
   1. Medical
      a. Minimize increases in ICP
      b. Promote cerebrovascular perfusion
      c. Prevent complications
   2. Surgical
      a. Craniotomy for evacuation of hematomas, clipping of aneurysm
      b. Carotid endarterectomy
      c. Extracranial-intracranial bypass
      d. Embolization of AVM, aneurysm
      e. Gamma knife radiosurgery
      f. Interventional neuroradiology
         (1) Insertion of balloons and coils
         (2) Angioplasty and stenting

**VI. Hydrocephalus**

A. Pathologic condition
   1. Noncommunicating hydrocephalus
      a. Obstruction of CSF flow within ventricular system resulting in lack of communication within subarachnoid space
      b. Etiology
         (1) Congenital malformation of ventricular system
         (2) Adhesions caused by inflammatory processes (e.g., meningitis)
         (3) Obstructive, space-occupying lesions
   2. Communicating hydrocephalus
      a. Obstruction of CSF flow in subarachnoid space or basilar cisterns
      b. Too few or nonfunctioning arachnoid villi cannot reabsorb CSF sufficiently
      c. Etiology
         (1) Congenital malformations
         (2) Adhesions caused by inflammatory disorders

(3) Overproduction of CSF
(4) Occlusion of arachnoid villi by particulate matter (blood, pus)

B. Clinical findings: dependent on patient's age and type of hydrocephalus
   1. Infants
      a. Enlarged head
      b. Thin, fragile, shiny-looking scalp
      c. Weak, underdeveloped neck muscles
      d. Poor sucking reflex
      e. "Sunset" eyes
      f. Signs of increased ICP
   2. Older children and adults
      a. Impaired mental function
      b. Gait disturbances
      c. Signs of increased ICP
      d. Papilledema
      e. Incontinence
      f. Nausea and vomiting
C. Diagnostic tools
   1. History and physical assessment
   2. Skull series
   3. CT scan
   4. MRI
   5. Isotope cisternogram (flow study)
   6. Lumbar puncture
   7. Transillumination of infant's skull
D. Treatment modalities
   1. Removal of obstruction
   2. Ventriculostomy with external ventricular drainage for temporary relief
   3. Insertion of shunt (Fig. 21–11)

## DIAGNOSTIC TOOLS

**I. Neuroimaging Techniques**

A. Skull series
   1. Indications
      a. Fractures
      b. Skull erosions
      c. Deviated pineal gland
   2. No contraindications
B. Cerebral angiography (conventional and MRA)
   1. Purpose
      a. To detect abnormalities of cerebral circulation
      b. To locate lesions distorting cerebral vessels
   2. Indications
      a. Cerebral vascular abnormalities
      b. Aneurysms
      c. AVMs
      d. Visualization of cerebral arteries and veins
   3. Contraindications
      a. Allergy to contrast dye
C. Radionuclide scan
   1. Uses gamma scintillation counter and injection of radioisotope
   2. Radioisotope uptake increased in pathologic tissue

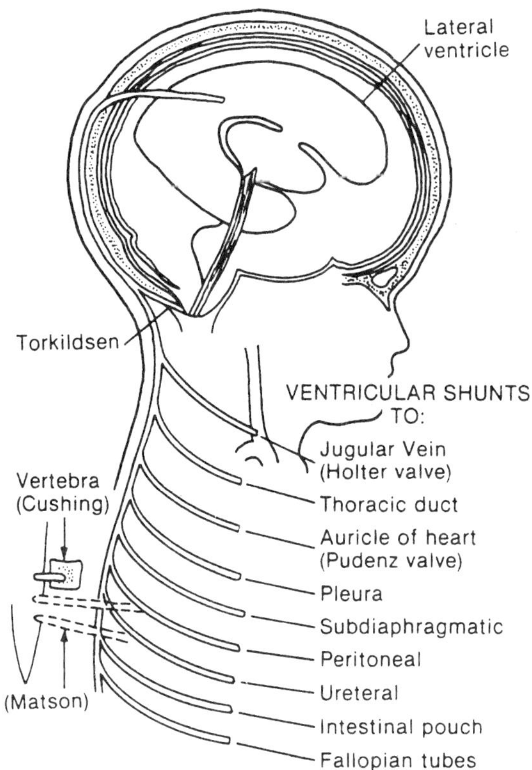


**FIGURE 21–11** Surgical hydrocephalic shunting procedures that have been used in the past to reduce CSF volume by facilitating CSF removal from craniospinal space. (From Ransohoff J, et al: Hydrocephalus: A review of etiology and treatment. *J Pediatr* 56:399–411, 1960.)

3. Indications
   a. Brain tumors or masses
   b. Cerebral infarction
   c. Headaches
   d. Seizure disorders
   e. Other major neurologic disorders
4. Contraindications
   a. Uncooperative patient
   b. Pregnancy

D. CT scan
1. Noninvasive test, but contrast media may be injected to facilitate visualization of vasculature
2. Provides clear, cross-sectional brain images
3. Uses computer reconstruction
4. Contrast media, gadolinium, may be used for enhancement
5. Contraindications
   a. Uncooperative patient
   b. Allergy to contrast dye or shellfish

E. MRI/MRA
1. Tomography technique using magnetic properties of protons in body tissues
2. High-resolution images are very clear
3. Indications: any neurologic condition
4. Contraindications
   a. Pregnancy

b. Uncooperative patient
c. Any metallic implants (e.g., pacemakers, orthopedic devices, clips)
5. Sedation may be required because of claustrophobic nature of scanner

F. Positron emission tomography (PET) scan
1. Uses principles of CT scan and radionuclide scanning
2. Evaluation of biochemical brain substances
3. Maps metabolic brain activity
4. Expensive
5. Indications—limited diagnostic purposes
a. Psychiatric disorders
b. Epilepsy
c. Alzheimer's disease
d. Cerebrovascular disease
e. Cerebral injuries

G. Evoked potentials
1. Measure changes in brain's electrical activity in response to variety of sensory stimulation (visual, auditory, somatosensory)
2. Indications
a. Neuromuscular disorders
b. Cerebrovascular disease
c. Head and spinal cord injury
d. Tumors
e. Peripheral nerve disease

H. Other diagnostic tools
1. Lumbar puncture
2. Electrocardiogram (ECG)
3. Electroencephalogram (EEG): assists in diagnosis of seizure activity, brain death
4. Echoencephalogram: detects shifts of midline structures
5. Radiographs of other body systems as indicated
6. Cerebral blood flow studies
7. Electromyogram (EMG)
8. Laboratory testing
a. Blood
b. Urine
c. Cultures (as needed)
d. CSF studies

## OPERATIVE PROCEDURES

### I. Burr Holes (Trephination)

A. Procedure: removal of isolated or multiple small circular portions of cranium for purposes of clot removal or in preparation for craniotomy where a series of burr holes are made and connected

B. Purpose
1. Removal of subdural fluid or blood
2. Drainage of CSF
3. Aspiration of abscess
4. Instillation of medications
5. Instillation of air for ventriculography

### II. Craniotomy

A. Procedure
1. Series of burr holes made into skull

2. Burr holes connected with saw
3. Bone flap removed
4. Opening kept as small as possible without restricting surgical approach
5. Bone flap may or may not be replaced

B. Purpose
1. Excision of pathologic lesions with preservation of vital structures
2. Repair of CSF leaks
3. Repair of aneurysm, AVMs
4. Revascularization procedures (superficial temporal artery to middle cerebral artery anastomosis)
5. Decompression of cranial contents to decrease ICP and relieve symptoms
6. Histologic identifications of lesions
7. Improvement of neurologic status and quality of survival

**III. Cranioplasty**

A. Procedure
1. Repair of skull defects
2. Materials used
   a. Autogenous bone grafts
   b. Cartilage
   c. Metal (tantalum, stainless steel mesh)
   d. Celluloid or synthetic resins (methyl methacrylate)
   e. Synthetic dura

B. Purpose
1. Protection of cranial contents
2. Improvement of cosmetic appearance
3. Usually done only in supratentorial area because neck muscles protect infratentorial areas

**IV. Craniectomy: Removal of Portion of Cranial Bone for Operative Decompression to Decrease ICP**

**V. Transsphenoidal Hypophysectomy**

A. Procedure
1. Removal of pituitary gland through subnasal midline rhinoseptal approach
2. Often requires collaboration of neurosurgery and ENT

B. Purpose
1. Removal of pituitary tumors
2. Preservation of pituitary gland, infundibular stalk, and normal vital structures
3. Palliation for breast cancer
4. Identification of tumor tissue
5. Decompression

**VI. Shunts**

A. Procedure
1. Placement of reservoir under scalp
2. Connection of reservoir to tubing emptying into distal site

B. Purpose
1. Improvement or preservation of neurologic status by providing alternative CSF pathway
2. Emergency reduction of increased ICP in presence of rapid neurologic deterioration
3. Instillation of antibiotics, analgesics, chemotherapeutic agents
4. Sampling of CSF

C. Types (see Fig. 21–11)
1. Ventriculoperitoneal
2. Ventriculoatrial

3. Lumbar-peritoneal
4. External lumbar drain
5. Multiple shunt sites (ureter, pleura, etc.)

D. Components of shunting system
1. Primary catheter: into lateral ventricle through burr hole
2. Reservoir: rests on mastoid bone to collect CSF
3. One-way valve: at reservoir to prevent CSF reflux
4. Terminal catheter: tunneled under skin to termination point and secured in position

## VII. Stereotactic Procedures

A. Procedure
1. Precise localization of lesion through use of three-dimensional coordinates, stereotactic frame, and instrumentation
2. Involves intraoperative use of CT scans, radiographs

B. Purpose
1. Precise localization of deep brain lesions for biopsy
2. Destruction of intracranial sensory pathways
3. Especially useful with intractable, chronic pain

## VIII. Application of Silverstone Clamp or Carotid Ligation or Both

A. Procedure
1. Incision into anterolateral area of neck
2. Application of clamp or ligature on carotid artery

B. Purpose
1. Reduction of flow and intravascular pressure on aneurysm, AVM, or fistula
2. Promote spontaneous clotting of lesion
3. Partial elimination of lesion from cerebral circulation
4. Evaluation of collateral circulation

## IX. Carotid Endarterectomy

A. Procedure
1. Incision made in neck area
2. Heparinization and clamping of artery above and below obstruction
3. Small incision made into artery
4. Obstruction removed
5. End-to-end anastomosis, suturing of artery, or patching of artery with autologous vein or Gortex graft

B. Purpose
1. Removal of stenotic vessel area
2. Removal of plaques in vessels
3. Primarily involves carotid bifurcation and junction of carotid and vertebral vessels with aorta or subclavian and innominate arteries
4. Bypass of occlusion by use of grafts
5. Primary purpose is to restore flow to cerebral circulation

## X. Microradiosurgery

A. Procedure
1. Gamma knife
   a. Precise destruction of deep and inaccessible lesions during single session using 201 sharply focused sources of cobalt 60 radiation; surrounding healthy tissue not harmed
   b. Minute measurement and precise patient positioning
   c. Indications
      (1) Excessive risk for conventional surgical procedure
      (2) Surgical inaccessibility of lesion

- (3) Prior surgical failure
- (4) Patient refusal to undergo conventional craniotomy

d. Uses
- (1) AVMs
- (2) Tumors
- (3) Other intracranial lesions for which conventional surgery is inappropriate

e. Time between treatment and results long
f. Time required for treatment limits centers to one or two patients per day
g. Procedure can be done with local anesthesia, but patient needs to be cooperative

2. Lasers
   a. Types
      - (1) Carbon dioxide
      - (2) Argon
      - (3) Nd:YAG
   b. Allows for precise dissection without traumatizing surrounding tissues
   c. Formerly inaccessible anatomic areas can be reached

B. Limited general application at this time
C. Patient selection important aspect

**XI. Seizure Surgery**

A. Procedure
1. Phase 1: noninvasive scalp monitoring
2. Phase 2: placement of depth electrodes
3. Phase 3: placement of grids and resection of seizure focus

B. Purpose
1. Localization of seizure focus
2. Removal of epileptogenic focus without causing neurologic deficits

C. Selection criteria
1. Refractory to medical management
2. Unilateral focus
3. Significant alteration in quality of life

## INTRAOPERATIVE ANESTHESIA CONCERNS

**I. Effects of Anesthetics and Other Drugs**

A. ICP
1. Factors contributing to increased ICP
   a. Halogenated agents (enflurane) dilate cerebral vasculature
   b. Ketamine hydrochloride and tubocurarine chloride initially increase ICP
   c. "Bucking" during intubation or extubation
2. Factors contributing to decreased ICP
   a. Hyperventilation used alone or in combination with nitrous oxide and/or barbiturates
   b. Intravenous (IV) anesthetic agents and other drugs (thiopental sodium, barbiturates, droperidol, fentanyl citrate, osmotic diuretics)
   c. Hypothermia
   d. Nondepolarizing neuromuscular blocking agents

B. Blood pressure
1. Marked reduction observed with halothane or enflurane use, in posterior fossa approaches and preoperative increased ICP, with droperidol (Innovar) use
2. Sitting position predisposes patient to hypotension
3. Reflex hypertension may occur after nitroprusside infusion
4. Controlled hypotension may be used in aneurysm surgery
5. Invasive monitoring (arterial lines, pulmonary artery catheter) necessary

C. Pulse rate
   1. May increase or decrease with stimulation of autonomic nervous system
   2. Decreased with increased ICP, droperidol use, depolarizing neuromuscular blocking agents
   3. Increased with autoregulatory failure, nondepolarizing neuromuscular blocking agents, ketamine use

D. Electrolyte balance
   1. Dehydration as result of
      a. Fluid restriction
      b. Diabetes insipidus
      c. Diuresis as result of osmotic diuretic administration
   2. Hypokalemia after diuretic administration
   3. Varying degrees of electrolyte imbalances resulting from endocrine dysfunction
   4. Hyponatremia as result of syndrome of inappropriate antidiuretic hormone secretion (SIADH) or cerebral salt wasting

**II. Hypothermia**

A. May be caused by low ambient room temperature (60° to 65° F), resulting in body heat loss, especially if large body surfaces are exposed

B. Anesthetic agents
   1. Peripheral vasodilation
   2. Synergistic actions with hypothermia
   3. Paralyze hypothalamic thermoregulatory mechanisms

C. Shivering
   1. Can cause increase in oxygen consumption as much as 500%
   2. Can occur as anesthetic agents wear off, resulting in hyperexcitability
   3. Increases basal metabolic rate, which increases ICP
   4. Use of muscle relaxants as prophylaxis

**III. Sitting Position Considerations**

A. Potential complications
   1. Palsies
      a. Types
         (1) Brachial plexus
         (2) Peroneal nerve
      b. Prevention
         (1) Meticulous padding of bony prominences
         (2) Careful positioning with good body alignment (within constraints of procedure)
   2. Hypotension precipitates cerebral hypoxia
   3. Air embolism
      a. Results from opening of negative-pressure venous channels, causing atmospheric air to enter
      b. Air in diploic veins can be demonstrated on skull films
      c. Increased risk with use of nitrous oxide
      d. Air embolus can travel to right side of heart and pulmonary circulation
      e. Can cause obstructed ventricular outflow and ventricular dysrhythmias

B. Prophylaxis
   1. Close observation
      a. Right atrial or pulmonary catheter
      b. Esophageal stethoscope
      c. Doppler ultrasonographic sensor
      d. End-expired $CO_2$
   2. Auscultation of right side of heart with Doppler ultrasonography to detect air turbulence
   3. Application of antiembolic stockings: Ace elastic wraps or sequential compression air boots to lower extremities

4. Maintenance of adequate blood volume
5. Positive end-expiratory pressure (PEEP)
6. Intermittent compression of internal jugular vein
7. Frequent flushing of surgical wound with saline or lining with Cottonoids

## IV. Neuroanesthesia

A. No ideal anesthetic agent for use with neurologic surgery patients
B. Choice of anesthetic agent must take into consideration effect on
   1. Cerebral metabolism (cerebral metabolic oxygen requirement)
   2. Cerebral blood flow
   3. ICP
   4. Vasomotor tone
      a. Vasoconstriction
      b. Vasodilation
C. Additional considerations
   1. Nonflammability
   2. Ease of administration
   3. Effect on hemostasis and blood pressure
   4. Adequate brain relaxation
   5. Nonirritability so as to reduce coughing and retching
   6. Minimal side effects and adverse reactions
D. Combination of drugs used should counter side effects
E. Mannitol solution started to reduce brain volume
F. CSF may be removed to decrease ICP
G. Other medications used intraoperatively
   1. Phenytoin (Dilantin) for seizure prophylaxis
   2. Dexamethasone to control cerebral edema
   3. Antibiotics to decrease risk of infection
   4. Cardiac drugs for hypotension, hypertension, or dysrhythmias
H. Controlled hypothermia may be used to decrease brain's metabolic rate, cellular metabolism, and oxygen demand
I. Controlled hypotension may be used to decrease vascularity (e.g. aneurysm, AVM)

## V. Potential Intraoperative Sequelae

A. Increase in neurologic deficits
B. Increased ICP
C. Altered endocrine function (diabetes insipidus, SIADH)
D. Formation of hematoma at surgical site
E. Leakage of CSF
F. Compromised circulatory status
   1. Hypotension or hypertension
   2. Bradycardia
G. Intraoperative blood loss
H. Cardiac compromise: dysrhythmias

## POSTANESTHESIA CARE

### NURSING DIAGNOSIS

Examples of related nursing diagnostic categories include:
- Hyperthermia
- Hypothermia
- Altered cerebral tissue perfusion
- Fluid volume excess
- Fear
- Anxiety
- Alteration in comfort
- Potential alteration in elimination
- Potential impaired skin integrity
- Potential for infection
- Potential alteration in gas exchange
- Potential for ineffective airway clearance
- Potential for sensory-perceptual alterations

I. **Report of Operative Procedure**
   A. Surgical procedure
   B. Pathologic findings
   C. Complete or subtotal resection (if tumor)
   D. Was bone flap replaced or left out
   E. Was any brain tissue sacrificed that may produce other than expected neurologic deficits
   F. Intraoperative problems or complications
   G. Expected deficits
   H. Medications administered during operative procedure

II. **Goals**
   A. Prompt recognition of potential complications
   B. Implementation of preventive measures

III. **Assessment** (see p. 374 for more complete assessment)
   A. Ongoing, frequent, and careful observations
   B. Temperature
      1. Hyperthermia: patient may have temperature up to 101° F as result of pressure on hypothalamus
      2. Hypothermia: may be aggravated by certain anesthetic agents and low ambient temperature in operating room
   C. Hemodynamic monitoring
      1. Pulmonary artery catheter
      2. Arterial line
      3. CVP
   D. Neurologic assessment
      1. Invasive ICP monitoring
      2. Cranial nerve assessment if infratentorial surgery was performed

IV. **Postoperative Complications**
   A. Structural
      1. Cerebral edema
      2. Intracranial bleeding
      3. Hydrocephalus
      4. Cerebral infarction

5. Tension pneumocephalus
6. CSF leakage

B. Metabolic
1. Hypoxia
2. Water and electrolyte disturbances
3. Hypoglycemia
4. Selected endocrine disorders
    a. Diabetes insipidus
        (1) Most common with supratentorial surgery
        (2) Lack of ADH
        (3) Increased urine output (polyuria): 4 to 10 L/d; >200 ml/hr
        (4) Serum hypernatremia
        (5) Decreased urine specific gravity (<1.001 to 1.005)
        (6) Decreased urine osmolality (<300 mOsm/L, usually 50 to 100 mOsm/L)
        (7) Increased serum osmolality (>290 mOsm/kg)
    b. SIADH
        (1) Increased ADH secretion
        (2) Decreased serum osmolality (<280 mOsm/kg)
        (3) Increase in total body water
        (4) Increased weight gain
        (5) Dilutional hyponatremia
        (6) Increased urine osmolality (>900 mOsm/L)
        (7) Oliguria (<400 to 600 ml/24 hr)
        (8) Urine appears concentrated
        (9) Elevated specific gravity

C. Other
1. Hyperthermia
2. Seizures
3. Infection

**V. Signs of Neurologic Deterioration**

A. Decrease in LOC
B. Increased restlessness
C. Appearance of new neurologic deficit
D. Increased severity of existing neurologic deficits
E. Decorticate or decerebrate posturing
F. Elevated baseline ICP
G. Seizures
H. CSF leaks
I. Changes in routine vital signs
1. Temperature >101° F
2. Increase in systolic blood pressure >30 mm Hg
3. Decrease in pulse rate of >20 bpm
4. Respiratory rate <12/min or appearance of irregular pattern
5. Development of cardiac dysrhythmias

**VI. Nursing Interventions After Cranial Surgery**

A. Maintain patent airway
1. Encourage deep breathing, use of incentive spirometer
2. Avoid coughing (increases ICP)
3. Administer oxygen
4. Provide ventilatory assistance if needed to establish greater control over $P_{CO_2}$ levels and ICP
5. Pulse oximetry

6. Perform serial ABGs to monitor $Po_2$ and $Pco_2$
7. Provide oral and nasal airways as needed
8. Position to prevent aspiration and obstruction
9. Suction as necessary

B. Positioning
  1. Supratentorial craniotomy
    a. Elevate head of bed 30 to 45 degrees
      (1) Facilitates venous drainage
      (2) Reduces cerebral edema
      (3) Promotes CSF circulation
    b. Maintain neutral head position and avoid neck flexion
    c. Turn side to side; may be positioned supine
    d. If large cranial cavity exists, position on nonoperative side to prevent shifting and displacement of intracranial contents by gravity
    e. Provide small pillow under nape of neck
    f. Position and support paralyzed limbs
  2. Infratentorial craniotomy
    a. May be kept flat or slightly elevated depending on physician preference
    b. Body in neutral alignment
    c. May be turned side to side
    d. Do not position supine
      (1) Avoid pressure on surgical incision
      (2) Prevent shifting and displacement of intracranial contents by gravity
  3. Transphenoidal surgery
    a. Elevate head of bed 30 to 45 degrees
    b. Body in neutral alignment
  4. Shunt insertion
    a. Flat on nonoperative side
    b. Body in neutral alignment

C. Maintain skin and mucous membrane integrity
  1. Mouth care frequently, especially with infratentorial surgery, because patients are given nothing by mouth for 24 hours
  2. Turn carefully, padding bony prominences
  3. Instill artificial tears to prevent corneal damage, especially if corneal reflex is absent
  4. Apply cool compresses to eyes for periorbital edema

D. Prevent infection
  1. Aseptic technique when dealing with invasive monitoring devices
  2. Observe for CSF drainage
    a. Halo or ring sign: blood-tinged center surrounded by lighter colored concentric rings on linen or dressings
    b. Check drainage with dextrose stick
      (1) CSF contains glucose, mucus does not
      (2) CSF glucose level is two thirds serum glucose
  3. Use sterile technique with dressing changes, especially with CSF leaks
  4. Initial dressing changes are usually done by physician

E. Prevent fluid and electrolyte imbalances
  1. Monitor fluid balance carefully to minimize cerebral edema—maintain euvolemia with saline
  2. Serum osmolality 290 to 320 mOsm/kg
  3. Maintain urinary output at ≥30 ml/hr
  4. Observe for excessive urinary output
  5. Monitor urine specific gravity, skin turgor
  6. Administer antiemetics to avoid vomiting, which can increase ICP

F. Maintain normothermia
   1. Treat hyperthermia
      a. Oxygen
      b. Remove excessive bed covers
      c. Administer antipyretics
      d. Sponge baths using tepid water
      e. Hypothermia blanket may be more effective in neurogenic hyperthermia
         (1) Set thermostat 1° F less than patient temperature to avoid shivering, which raises ICP
         (2) Reset thermostat as patient's temperature decreases
         (3) Shivering raises ICP but may be treated with chlorpromazine hydrochloride (Thorazine)
   2. Treat hypothermia
      a. Avoid sudden elevation of limbs to prevent infusion of cold blood into heart
      b. Could precipitate dysrhythmias
      c. Initiate rewarming therapy

G. Support patient having seizure
   1. Protection during seizure activity
      a. Head
      b. Intravenous (IV) and monitoring lines
      c. Paralyzed limbs
   2. Avoid restraining patient (contributes to agitation)
   3. Maintain patent airway
   4. Administer oxygen and anticonvulsants as ordered

H. Minimize headache
   1. Elevate head of bed
   2. Reduce environmental stimulation
   3. Administer analgesics (codeine or acetaminophen) to prevent the following
      a. Respiratory depression
      b. Depression of LOC
      c. Masking of pupillary signs

I. Minimize effect of periorbital edema
   1. Apply small ice bags or compresses during early phase
   2. Apply petroleum jelly to protect skin before application of ice bags if edema is severe
   3. Alternate warm and cold compresses as ordered

J. Minimize increases in ICP

K. Psychologic and emotional support
   1. Speak quietly, even if it appears patient is unconscious
   2. Provide explanations and reassurance
   3. Assist mobilization of coping mechanisms
   4. Communicate with family
      a. Provide frequent updates on patient condition
      b. Answer questions as honestly as possible
      c. Provide reassurance and support
      d. Assist mobilization of coping mechanisms

## ANATOMY AND PHYSIOLOGY OF THE SPINAL CORD

**I. Vertebral Column** (Fig. 21–12)

A. Purpose
   1. Support and protection of spinal cord
   2. Flexibility for movement

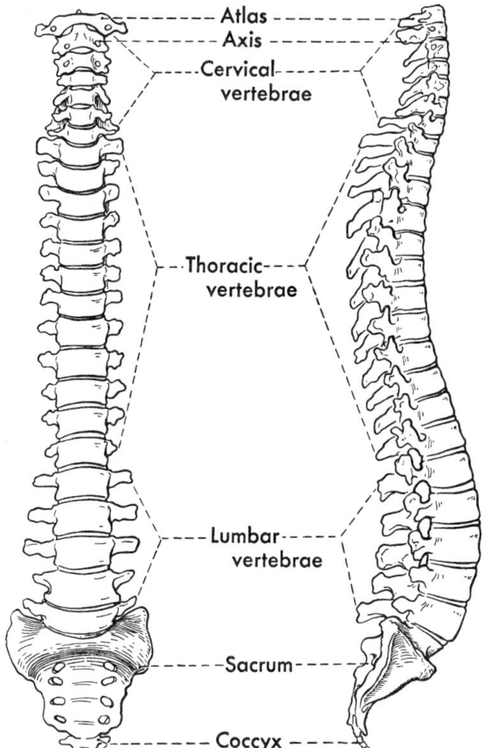


**FIGURE 21–12** Anterior and lateral views of vertebral column. (Reprinted with permission from Hollinshead WB, Jenkins DB: *Functional Anatomy of the Limbs and Back,* 5th Ed. Philadelphia, WB Saunders, 1981.)

B. Unique aspects
   1. Atlas (C1): sits on odontoid process
   2. Axis (C2)
   3. Odontoid process (dens): projects up from axis
C. Divisions
   1. Cervical (7)
   2. Thoracic (12)
   3. Lumbar (5)
   4. Sacral (5)
   5. Coccygeal (4, fused as 1)
D. Parts of vertebrae (Fig. 21–13)
   1. Body: separated by disks
   2. Arch
      a. Pedicles (2): short, thick pieces of bone; spinal nerves exit between pedicles of adjacent vertebrae
      b. Laminae (2): broad plates on either side of spinous process
      c. Spinous process (1): projects from rear of arch
      d. Articulating processes (4): facet joints; connect each vertebral arch to arches of vertebrae above and below
      e. Transverse processes (2): points of attachment for muscles and ligaments
   3. Foramen
      a. Opening where vertebral arch meets vertebral body
      b. Allows for passage of spinal cord

- E. Spinal ligaments
  - 1. Anterior longitudinal ligament
    - a. Attaches to anterior surface of vertebral body and intervertebral disks
    - b. Broad, strong
    - c. Extends from occipital bone and anterior tubercle of atlas to sacrum
  - 2. Posterior longitudinal ligament
    - a. Attaches to posterior surface of vertebral bodies within spinal cord
    - b. Thick, strong
    - c. Extends from occipital bone to coccyx
  - 3. Ligamenta flava
    - a. Elastic fibers connecting lamina of adjacent vertebrae
    - b. Extend from axis to first segment of sacrum
    - c. Help hold body erect
    - d. Thin, broad, and long in cervical area
    - e. Thicker in thoracic area
    - f. Thickest in lumbar region
- F. Intervertebral disks (Fig. 21–13)
  - 1. Sit between vertebral bodies
  - 2. Fibrocartilaginous
  - 3. Vary in size, thickness, and shape at different spinal levels
  - 4. Serve as cushions between bony surfaces of vertebral bodies
  - 5. Parts
    - a. Nucleus pulposus
      - (1) Central, spongy core
      - (2) Loses resiliency with age
    - b. Anulus fibrosus
      - (1) Fibrous capsule that surrounds nucleus pulposus
      - (2) Degenerative changes can occur in middle and later life

## II. Spinal Cord

- A. Characteristics (Fig. 21–14)
  - 1. 1 cm in diameter; average length of 42 to 45 cm
  - 2. Originates at foramen magnum and ends at L2
  - 3. Elongated mass of nerve tissue that is continuous with medulla oblongata
  - 4. 31 segments, each with a pair of spinal nerves
  - 5. Surrounded by meninges for protection
  - 6. Central canal contains CSF
- B. Purposes
  - 1. Conducts sensory and motor impulses to and from brain
  - 2. Controls many reflexes
- C. Arterial blood supply
  - 1. From vertebral arteries
  - 2. Anterior spinal artery (1): runs full length of cord, midventrally
  - 3. Posterior spinal arteries (2): run full length of spinal cord along each row of dorsal roots
- D. Venous drainage
  - 1. Intradural vein: follows arterial pattern
  - 2. Extradural intravertebral veins: form plexus from cranium to pelvis with communication to veins of neck, thorax, abdomen
- E. Transverse section (Fig. 21–15)
  - 1. White matter
    - a. Myelinated fibers
    - b. Comprise bulk of spinal cord

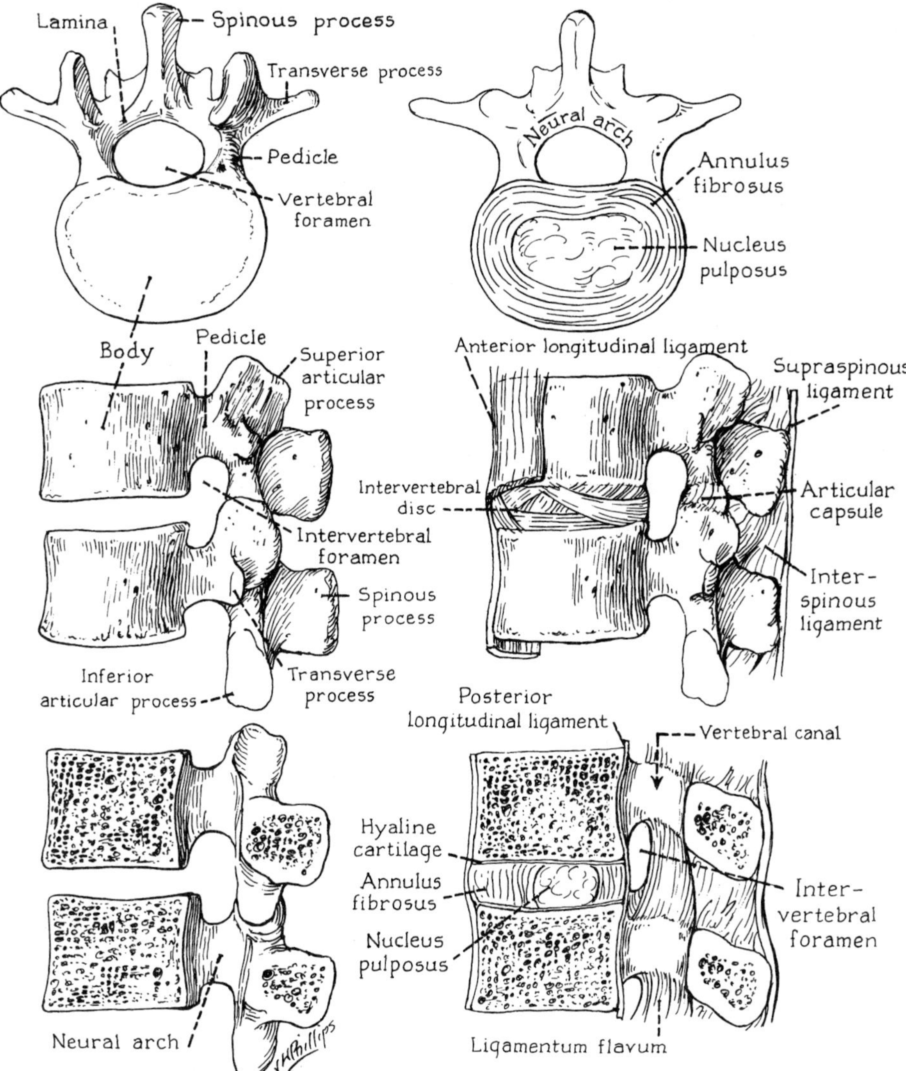


**FIGURE 21–13** Anatomy of vertebra and intervertebral joints with associated ligaments. (Reprinted with permission from Rosse C, Clawson DK: *The Musculoskeletal System in Health and Disease.* New York, Harper & Row, 1980.)

c. Encases gray matter
d. Each half divided into columns (funiculi) containing ascending (sensory) and descending (motor) tracts

2. Gray matter
   a. Unmyelinated fibers
   b. H-shaped appearance of inner core
   c. H divided into columns (horns) containing ascending (sensory) and descending (motor) tracts
      (1) Anterior (ventral) horns: motor, efferent
      (2) Posterior (dorsal) horns: sensory, afferent, axons from peripheral sensory neurons
      (3) Lateral horns
         (a) Thoracic and upper lumbar segments only
         (b) Sympathetic nervous system cell bodies

F. Ascending tracts
   1. Spinothalamic
      a. Carry sensations of pain, temperature, light touch, pressure
      b. Originate in posterior gray column on opposite side and terminate in thalamus
   2. Spinocerebellar
      a. Carry impulses of proprioception (knowledge of position and body parts) or kinesthesia from lower body
      b. Originate in posterior gray horns and terminate in cerebellum
   3. Fasciculus gracilis and fasciculus cuneatus
      a. Carry impulses of proprioception from muscles, joints; light touch from skin, discrete localization, two-point discrimination, vibratory sense, stereognosis
      b. Originate in posterior white columns and terminate in medulla where they cross and continue to thalamus

G. Descending tracts
   1. Lateral corticospinal (pyramidal)
      a. Voluntary motor movement, especially contraction of small muscle groups such as hands, fingers, feet, toes
      b. Originate in motor areas of cerebral cortex on opposite side and terminate in anterior gray columns

H. Upper motor neurons
   1. Located entirely in CNS

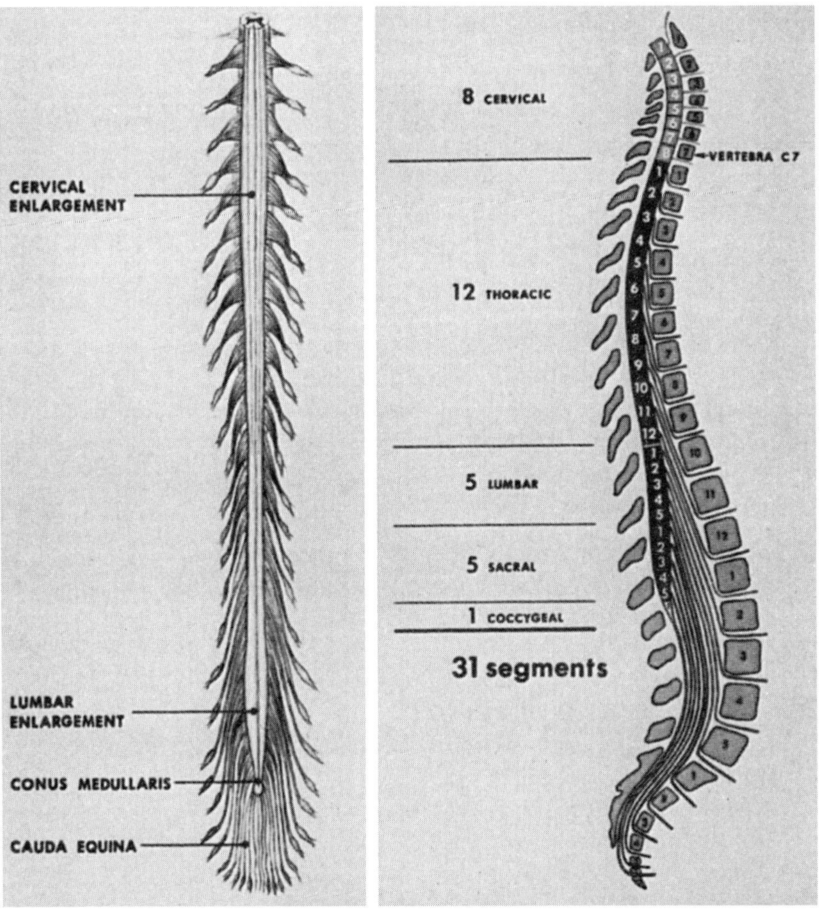


**FIGURE 21–14** Gross anatomy of spinal cord and relationship between spinal cord segments, spinal nerves, and vertebral column. (Reprinted with permission from Dunkerley GB: *A Basic Atlas of the Human Nervous System.* Philadelphia, FA Davis, 1975.)

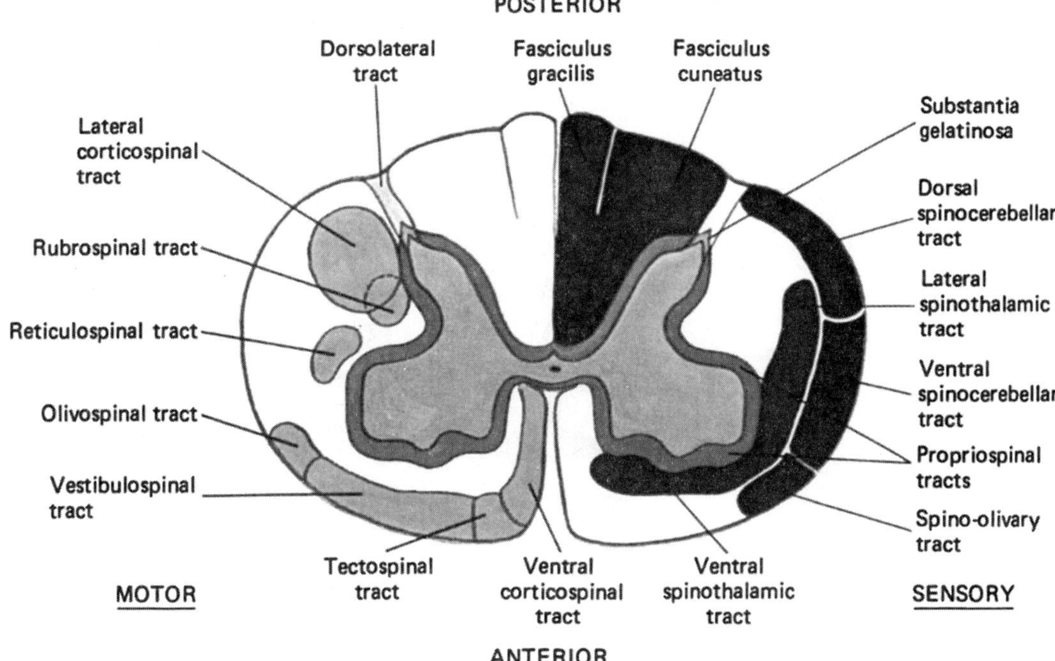


**FIGURE 21–15** Cross-sectional view of major long nerve fiber pathways of spinal cord. (From Guyton A: *Basic Neuroscience*, 2nd Ed. Philadelphia, WB Saunders, 1991.)

2. Neurons and their fibers
3. Extend from cerebral centers to cells in spinal cord
4. Facilitating and inhibitory descending pathways that modify lower motor neurons
5. Paralysis
   a. Increased muscle tone and spasticity
   b. Little to no atrophy of muscles involved
   c. Hyperactive deep tendon reflexes
   d. Babinski's sign

I. Lower motor neurons
   1. Located in anterior horn cells and spinal and peripheral nerves
   2. Receive impulses from different levels of CNS and channels to muscles
   3. Paralysis
      a. Total loss of voluntary muscle control with complete transection
      b. Decreased muscle tone and flaccidity
      c. Diminished or absent reflexes
      d. Absence of pathologic reflexes
      e. Local twitching of muscle groups
      f. Progressive atrophy of atonic muscles

J. Spinal roots (Fig. 21–16)
   1. Dorsal (posterior) roots: afferent (sensory) impulses from skin segments (dermatomal areas) to dorsal root ganglia
   2. Ventral (anterior) roots: convey efferent (motor) impulses from spinal cord to body
   3. Dorsal and ventral roots meet and join to form spinal nerve

K. Spinal nerves
   1. 31 pairs exit from spinal cord
      a. Cervical (8): exit above corresponding vertebrae
      b. Thoracic (12): exit below corresponding vertebrae
      c. Lumbar (5): exit below corresponding vertebrae

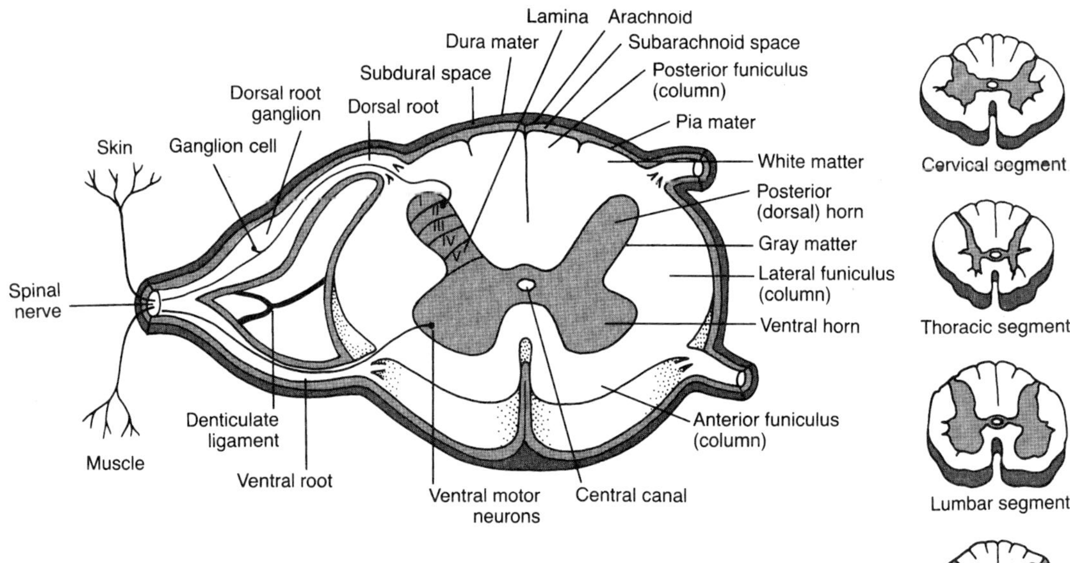


**FIGURE 21–16** Spinal cord and surrounding meninges. (From Black JM, Matassarin-Jacobs E: *Luckmann and Sorensen's Medical Surgical Nursing*, 4th Ed [p 622]. Philadelphia, WB Saunders, 1993.)

- d. Sacrum (5): exit below corresponding vertebrae
- e. Coccyx (1): exits below corresponding vertebrae

2. Formed by union of anterior and posterior roots attached to spinal cord
3. Spinal segment made up of corresponding spinal cord segment plus spinal nerves

L. Plexus
1. Network of interlacing nerves formed by primary branch of nerves or by terminal funiculi
2. Cervical
   - a. Innervates muscles of neck and shoulders
   - b. Gives rise to phrenic nerve, which supplies diaphragm
3. Brachial: radial and ulnar nerves merge
4. Lumbar: gives rise to femoral nerve
5. Sacral: gives rise to sciatic nerve

## ASSESSMENT OF SPINAL CORD FUNCTION

**I. Motor Function**

A. Muscle size: inspect for atrophy, hypertrophy
B. Muscle strength: as described in neurologic assessment
C. Muscle tone
D. Coordination
1. Rapid alternating movements
2. Heel to shin
3. Finger to nose

**II. Sensory Function**

A. Superficial sensation
1. Light touch (cotton wisp)
2. Pain (pinprick)

B. Deep sensation
   1. Proprioception: move big toe and fingers in various positions and have patient identify position with eyes closed
C. Technique
   1. Have patient close eyes
   2. Begin at feet and work upward systematically
   3. Compare findings on both sides
   4. Ask patient to tell you when sensation is felt
   5. Note dermatome level

**III. Reflexes**
   A. Superficial
      1. Abdominal
      2. Cremasteric
      3. Bulbocavernosus
      4. Perianal reflex (anal wink)
      5. Plantar
   B. Deep tendon reflexes (DTR)
      1. Biceps
      2. Triceps
      3. Brachioradial
      4. Patellar
   C. Pathologic
      1. Corticospinal tract involvement
         a. Babinski reflex positive

**IV. For Patients with Spinal Cord Injuries:** many units have specific spinal cord assessment forms that differentiate muscle groups, motor and sensory levels (Fig. 21–17)

## DISORDERS REQUIRING SPINAL SURGERY

**I. Herniated Intervertebral Disc**
   A. Major cause of severe and chronic back pain
      1. Disruption of anulus with leakage of nucleus pulposus
      2. May extrude into epidural space and compress nerve roots
   B. Often referred to as HNP (herniated nucleus pulposus)
   C. Cervical and lumbar areas most susceptible to injury and stress (especially lumbar disc disease)
   D. Patients often admitted with diagnosis of radiculopathy, disease of spinal nerve root
   E. Occurs more in men
   F. Occurs most often in 30- to 50-year-old age group
   G. Etiology
      1. 50%: trauma
      2. Degenerative processes such as osteoarthritis, aging
      3. Congenital anomalies (scoliosis) can predispose to disc injury
   H. Signs and symptoms
      1. Lumbar (90% to 95% at L4–S1 level)
         a. Pain aggravated by stooping, straining, or standing or by jarring movements such as sneezing or coughing
         b. Postural deformity
            (1) Lumbar lordosis absent
            (2) Restriction in lateral flexion
            (3) Limited lumbar spine movement

UNIVERSITY OF MARYLAND
MIEMSS—UMMS
**SPINAL CORD INJURY FLOW SHEET**

Muscle Strength

5 Normal
4 Active movement through range of motion against resistance
3 Active movement through range of motion against gravity
2 Active movement through range of motion with gravity eliminated
1 Palpable or visible contraction
0 Total paralysis
U Unable to test strength of extremity

Rectal Tone, Proprioception, Diaphragm
P–Present A–Absent U–Untestable

| Medication | Sensation |
|---|---|
| S—Sedation | N—Normal |
| PL—Paralytic | ABN—Abnormal |
| T—Tranquilizer | A—Absent |
| P—Pain | U—Untestable |

| | |
|---|---|
| Level of bony/ ligamentous injury | |
| Anatomical Classification | |

MOTOR LEVEL *Circled entry means to refer to nurses note*

| | | | | | | | | | | | | | |
|---|---|---|---|---|---|---|---|---|---|---|---|---|---|
| Date | | | | | | | | | | | | | |
| Time | | | | | | | | | | | | | |
| Medications | | | | | | | | | | | | | |
| Diaphragm (R/L) | $C_4$ | | | | | | | | | | | | |
| Deltoid (raise arms) (R/L) | $C_5$ | | | | | | | | | | | | |
| Biceps (elbow flexion) (R/L) | $C_{5,6}$ | | | | | | | | | | | | |
| Wrist extensors (R/L) | $C_6$ | | | | | | | | | | | | |
| Triceps (elbow extension) (R/L) | $C_7$ | | | | | | | | | | | | |
| Flexer digitorum profundus (finger flexion) (R/L) | $C_8$ | | | | | | | | | | | | |
| Hand intrinsics (finger abduction) (R/L) | $T_1$ | | | | | | | | | | | | |
| Iliopsoas (hip flexion) (R/L) | $L_2$ | | | | | | | | | | | | |
| Quadriceps (knee extension) (R/L) | $L_3$ | | | | | | | | | | | | |
| Tibialis anterior (dorsiflex foot) (R/L) | $L_4$ | | | | | | | | | | | | |
| Extensor hallucis longus (great toe extension) (R/L) | $L_5$ | | | | | | | | | | | | |
| Gastrocnemius (ankle plantar flexion) (R/L) | $S_1$ | | | | | | | | | | | | |
| Function | Level | | | | | | | | | | | | |
| Proprioception (finger) (R/L) | | | | | | | | | | | | | |
| Proprioception (toe) (R/L) | | | | | | | | | | | | | |
| Rectal Tone (P/A) | | | | | | | | | | | | | |
| Initials | | | | | | | | | | | | | |
| Initials/signature | | | | | | | | | | | | | |

Medical Records No.

**FIGURE 21–17** Spinal cord injury assessment tool. (From Cardona VD, Hurn PD, Mason PJB, Scanlon AM, Veise-Berry SW: *Trauma Nursing,* 2nd Ed. Philadelphia, WB Saunders, 1994.)

c. Motor deficits
   (1) Hypotonia
   (2) Paresis
   (3) Footdrop
   (4) Atrophy of affected muscles

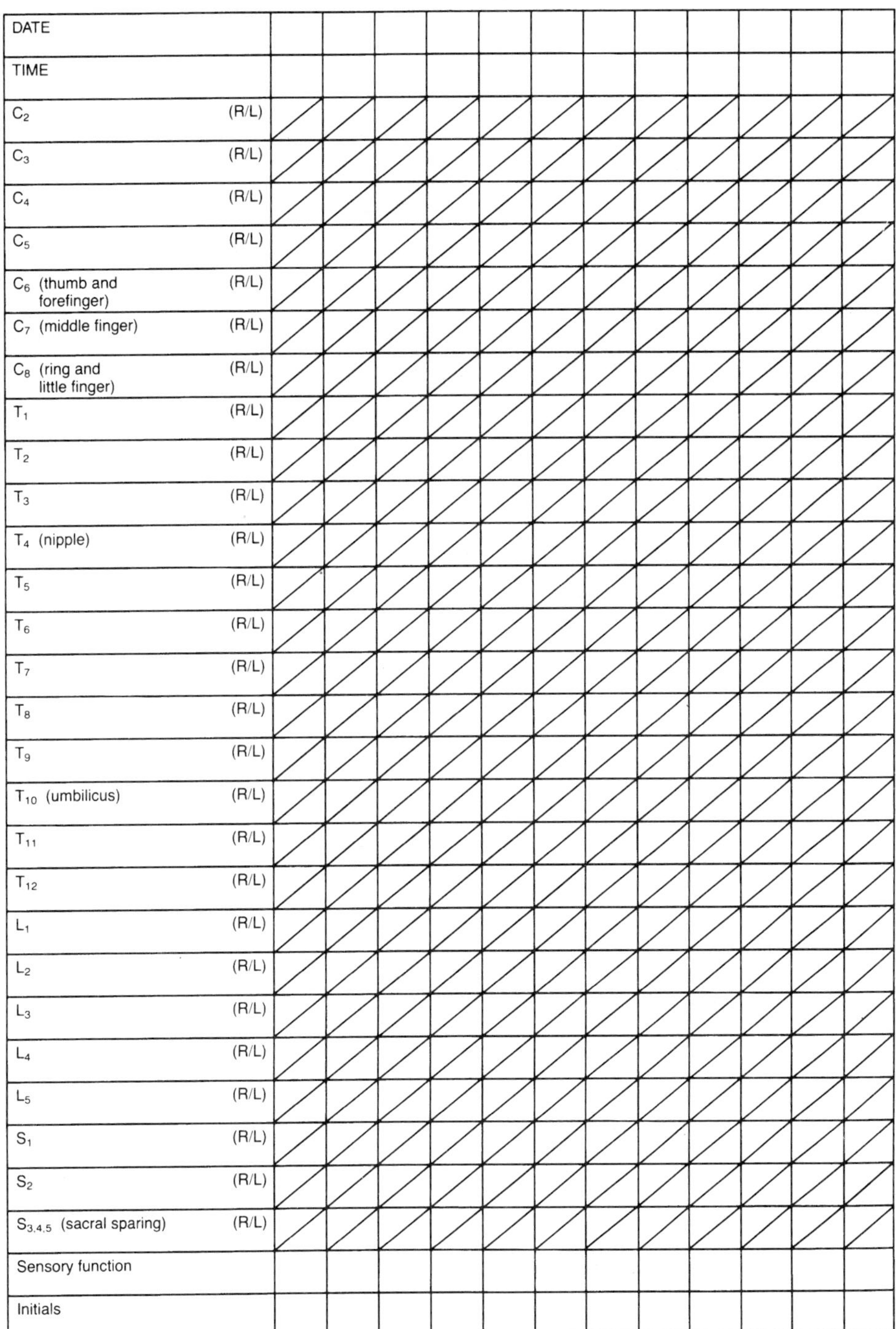

SENSATION

| DATE | | | | | | | | | | | | | |
|---|---|---|---|---|---|---|---|---|---|---|---|---|---|
| TIME | | | | | | | | | | | | | |
| $C_2$ | (R/L) | | | | | | | | | | | | |
| $C_3$ | (R/L) | | | | | | | | | | | | |
| $C_4$ | (R/L) | | | | | | | | | | | | |
| $C_5$ | (R/L) | | | | | | | | | | | | |
| $C_6$ (thumb and forefinger) | (R/L) | | | | | | | | | | | | |
| $C_7$ (middle finger) | (R/L) | | | | | | | | | | | | |
| $C_8$ (ring and little finger) | (R/L) | | | | | | | | | | | | |
| $T_1$ | (R/L) | | | | | | | | | | | | |
| $T_2$ | (R/L) | | | | | | | | | | | | |
| $T_3$ | (R/L) | | | | | | | | | | | | |
| $T_4$ (nipple) | (R/L) | | | | | | | | | | | | |
| $T_5$ | (R/L) | | | | | | | | | | | | |
| $T_6$ | (R/L) | | | | | | | | | | | | |
| $T_7$ | (R/L) | | | | | | | | | | | | |
| $T_8$ | (R/L) | | | | | | | | | | | | |
| $T_9$ | (R/L) | | | | | | | | | | | | |
| $T_{10}$ (umbilicus) | (R/L) | | | | | | | | | | | | |
| $T_{11}$ | (R/L) | | | | | | | | | | | | |
| $T_{12}$ | (R/L) | | | | | | | | | | | | |
| $L_1$ | (R/L) | | | | | | | | | | | | |
| $L_2$ | (R/L) | | | | | | | | | | | | |
| $L_3$ | (R/L) | | | | | | | | | | | | |
| $L_4$ | (R/L) | | | | | | | | | | | | |
| $L_5$ | (R/L) | | | | | | | | | | | | |
| $S_1$ | (R/L) | | | | | | | | | | | | |
| $S_2$ | (R/L) | | | | | | | | | | | | |
| $S_{3,4,5}$ (sacral sparing) | (R/L) | | | | | | | | | | | | |
| Sensory function | | | | | | | | | | | | | |
| Initials | | | | | | | | | | | | | |

**FIGURE 21–17** *Continued*

d. Sensory deficits
  (1) Paresthesias
  (2) Numbness
e. Problems with micturition
f. Sexual dysfunction
g. Alteration in reflexes

2. Cervical (most commonly C6–7 and C5–6)
   a. Pain
   b. Paresthesias
   c. Reflex loss
   d. Motor weakness in hand, forearm
   e. Restricted neck movement
   f. Atrophy of affected muscles
   g. Tenderness when pressure exerted over cervical area of spine

I. Diagnostic tools
   1. History and physical assessment
   2. Spinal films
   3. Contrast myelography
   4. MRI
   5. CT scan

## II. Spinal Cord Injury

A. Mechanisms of injury
   1. Hyperflexion
   2. Hyperextension
   3. Deformation
   4. Axial loading
   5. Excessive rotation

B. Classification of injury
   1. Concussion
   2. Contusion
   3. Laceration
   4. Transection
   5. Hemorrhage

C. Spinal cord injury syndromes
   1. Quadriplegia
      a. Lesion involves one or more cervical segments
      b. Loss of motor and sensory function below level of lesion, usually upper and lower extremities
      c. Bowel, bladder, and sexual dysfunction
   2. Paraplegia
      a. Lesion involves one or more of thoracic, lumbar, or sacral regions
      b. Loss of motor and sensory function below level of lesion, usually lower extremities
      c. Bowel, bladder, and sexual dysfunction
   3. Complete lesion: implies total loss of motor and sensory function below level of lesion
   4. Incomplete lesion
      a. Preservation of motor or sensory function or both below level of lesion
      b. Classified according to area of damage
         (1) Central cord syndrome
            (a) More pronounced motor deficits in upper extremities than lower extremities
            (b) Sensory loss varies
            (c) Bowel, bladder dysfunction variable or function may be totally preserved
            (d) Injury to central area of spinal cord, usually cervical area
         (2) Anterior cord syndrome
            (a) Loss of pain, temperature, and motor function below level of lesion
            (b) Light touch, position, vibration intact
            (c) Injury to anterior spinal artery through HNP, trauma, hyperflexion
            (d) Injury in anterior part of spinal cord including spinothalamic tracts, corticospinal tracts, anterior gray horn cells

(3) Brown-Séquard syndrome
(a) Ipsilateral paralysis or paresis
(b) Ipsilateral loss of touch, pressure, and vibration
(c) Contralateral loss of pain and temperature
(d) Transverse hemisection of cord, usually as a result of knife or missile injury
(4) Posterior cord syndrome
(a) Rare syndrome
(b) Position and vibration senses of posterior columns are affected
(5) Root syndrome
(a) Tingling, pain, motor weakness of selected muscles; absent or decreased reflexes
(b) Sacral roots: bowel and bladder dysfunction
(c) Cervical roots: tingling and weakness in arm; pain radiating down arm and into shoulder
(d) Compression resulting from HNP or vertebral subluxation with compression of nerve roots
(6) Horner's syndrome
(a) Seen with partial transection at T1 level or above
(b) Associated with miosis, ptosis, loss of sweating on ipsilateral side
(c) Lesions of preganglionic sympathetic trunk or cervical postganglionic sympathetic neurons

D. Treatment
1. Medical: dependent on patient's symptoms and severity of injury
2. Surgery
a. May be delayed
(1) Allow for decrease in cord edema
(2) Allow for immobilization and realignment of vertebral column
(3) Allow for reduction of fracture dislocation
b. May occur within 12 to 72 hours if any of following are present
(1) Compression of spinal cord
(2) Progressive neurologic deficits
(3) Bony fragments with compound fractures because they could penetrate cord
(4) Penetrating wounds
(5) Bone fragments in spinal cord
c. Purpose
(1) Decompress spinal cord or spinal nerves to prevent the following
(a) Pain
(b) Loss of neurologic function
(c) Ischemia or necrosis of neural tissue
(2) Stabilization
d. Procedures
(1) Decompression laminectomies with fusion
(2) Posterior laminectomy using acrylic wire mesh and fusion
(3) Insertion of Harrington rods or instrumentation for stabilization

E. Complications: affect all body systems
1. Neurologic
a. Spinal shock
b. Autonomic dysreflexia
c. Spinal instability
d. Pain
e. Syringomyelia
f. Spasticity

2. Respiratory
   a. Hypoxia
   b. Aspiration
   c. Pulmonary embolus
   d. Pneumonia
   e. Atelectasis
3. Cardiovascular
   a. Bradydysrhythmias
   b. Orthostatic hypotension
   c. Superior mesenteric artery syndrome
   d. Deep vein thrombosis
4. Orthopedic, musculoskeletal, integumentary
   a. Heterotopic ossification
   b. Contractures
   c. Osteoporosis
   d. Pressure ulcers
5. Gastrointestinal
   a. Bleeding
   b. Fecal impaction or incontinence
   c. Paralytic ileus
6. Genitourinary
   a. Urinary tract infections
   b. Urinary calculi
   c. Urinary retention or incontinence
   d. Sexual dysfunction

F. Spinal shock
1. Condition occurring immediately after injury; may last hours to months depending on severity of injury
2. Commonly lasts 1 to 6 weeks after injury
3. Characteristics
   a. Loss of motor, sensory, autonomic, and reflex activity below level of lesion
   b. Flaccid paralysis
   c. Bradycardia
   d. Paralytic ileus
   e. Hypotension
4. Resolution of spinal shock
   a. Gradual process
   b. Varies with patient and level of injury
   c. Characteristics
      (1) Return of perianal reflex (anal wink)
      (2) Return of motor, sensory, reflex, and autonomic activity depending on completeness of lesion
      (3) Isolated cord segment may develop its own reflex activity

G. Autonomic dysreflexia
1. Usually occurs after resolution of spinal shock and return of reflex activity
2. Occurs most often with lesions at T6 or above
3. Results from uninhibited sympathetic discharge
4. Causes
   a. Bladder distension
   b. Fecal impaction
   c. Noxious stimuli (vary with individual patient)
5. Symptoms
   a. Pounding headache

b. Hypertension (can be dangerously high)
   (1) Changes in mental status
   (2) Seizures
   (3) Intracerebral hemorrhage
c. Profuse sweating above level of lesion
d. Nasal congestion
e. Flushed skin above level of lesion
f. Pallor below level of lesion
g. Piloerection (goose pimples) below level of lesion
h. Anxiety
i. Visual disturbances

6. Treatment
   a. Assess patient
   b. Remove stimulus
   c. Elevate head of bed
   d. Notify physician immediately
   e. Fast-acting antihypertensive medications may be ordered

## III. Spinal Cord Tumors

A. Less common than brain tumors
B. Usually occur in young and middle-aged adults, with men and women equally affected
C. Sites
   1. Cervical: 30%
   2. Thoracic: 50%
   3. Lumbosacral: 20%
D. Classification
   1. Intramedullary
      a. Within spinal cord tissue
      b. May compress cord and nerve roots and destroy cord tissue
      c. Usually malignant
      d. Types
         (1) Astrocytoma
         (2) Ependymoma
         (3) Oligodendroglioma
         (4) Hemangioblastoma
      e. Characteristics
         (1) Slow growing
         (2) May extend over more than one spinal segment
         (3) Loss of pain and temperature
         (4) Caudal area tumors may precipitate sexual, bladder, and bowel dysfunction
      f. Compression is usually on central portion of spinal cord rather than on nerve roots
   2. Extramedullary
      a. Can occur inside or outside dura but do not occur within spinal cord parenchyma
      b. Types
         (1) Extradural: occur outside dural sac
            (a) Symptoms occur rapidly
            (b) Mostly malignant
            (c) Pain a common symptom and may occur before signs of spinal cord compression
            (d) Metastatic tumors (from lungs, breast, prostate, kidneys, gastrointestinal tract)
            (e) Multiple myeloma
            (f) Lymphoma

(2) Intradural: occur inside dural sac
(a) Most common spinal cord tumor
(b) Most frequently seen in thoracic area
(c) Gradual onset of symptoms of cord compression
(d) Pain may not always be present
(e) Meningioma
(f) Neurofibroma
(g) Congenital: dermoid, epidermoid

E. Symptoms
1. Etiology
a. Destruction of spinal cord parenchyma
b. Compression of spinal cord or spinal nerves
c. Compression or occlusion of spinal blood vessels
d. Obstruction of CSF flow
2. Dependent on the following
a. Level of lesion
b. Tumor type

F. Diagnostic tools
1. History and physical assessment
2. Spinal films
a. Assess destruction of bony structures
b. Assess presence of vertebral column lesions
3. Contrast myelography
a. Identifies obstruction of spinal CSF pathway (subarachnoid space)
b. Identifies location, size, boundaries of lesion
c. Considered hallmark of diagnostic armamentarium
d. May be scheduled immediately before surgery so patient may proceed directly from myelogram to operating room
4. CT scan: identifies location, size, boundaries of lesion
5. MRI
a. Identifies location, size, boundaries of lesion
b. Identifies destruction of bony structures
6. CSF analysis
a. Routine analysis as discussed with cranial space-occupying lesions
b. CSF collected from below level of lesion may show increases in protein, absence of large amounts of cells, rapid coagulation
7. Spinal angiogram: assists in differentiating vascular lesions
8. Electromyogram: used for differential diagnosis
9. Other laboratory test or x-ray films as indicated by patient's symptoms and condition

## OPERATIVE PROCEDURES

**I. Laminectomy**
A. Most frequent surgical procedure
B. Procedure
1. Removal of laminae, part of posterior arch of vertebrae, and attached ligamentum flavum
2. Hemilaminectomy: excision of part of laminae
C. Purpose
1. Decompression of spinal cord or spinal nerves
2. Allow for discectomy

D. Spinal fusion may be performed at same time for stability of spinal column
E. Approaches
   1. Posterior (traditional): with cervical surgery, incision is made through back
   2. Anterior: with cervical surgery, incision is made anteriorly through throat and neck area

## II. Discectomy

A. Procedure
   1. Lumbar
      a. Posterior approach used
      b. Entire disc removed
   2. Cervical
      a. Posterior approach: only extruded disc fragments removed
      b. Anterior approach: total disc removed
B. Purpose: removal of nucleus pulposus done with or without laminectomy

## III. Microdiscectomy

A. Procedure or purpose: microscopic surgical technique
   1. Allows for easier identification of anatomic structures
   2. Improves precision in removing small fragments
   3. Decreases tissue trauma and pain: smaller incision
B. Patient able to ambulate sooner
C. Advantages
   1. Decreases risk of CSF leak through dural laceration
   2. Improved hemostasis: decreases vascular trauma and hematoma formation
   3. Decreases spasms by decreasing traction on spinal nerve roots
   4. Less risk of stripping muscle from fascia

## IV. Percutaneous Discectomy

A. Procedure/purpose: endoscopic lumbar surgical technique
   1. Posterolateral approach
   2. High power suction shaver and cutter system
   3. Local anesthesia
B. Alternative to microdiscectomy
C. Indicated in disc-related root compression with deficits but anulus fibrosis intact

## V. Spinal Fusion—With or Without Instrumentation

A. Procedure: insertion of bone chips, usually from iliac crest, between vertebrae; variety of surgical hardware (rods, screws, bolts) may also be used
B. Purpose
   1. Immobilization of vertebral column
   2. Stabilization of weakened vertebral column
C. Types
   1. Lumbar
      a. Motion increases above level of fusion
      b. Patient often unaware of permanent area of stiffness
   2. Cervical
      a. Increased limitation of movement
      b. Anterior approach: used when cervical area of spine is unstable
      c. Often performed with anterior laminectomy and discectomy

## VI. Foraminotomy

A. Procedure: surgical enlargement of intervertebral foramen to accommodate spinal nerves

B. Purpose
    1. Decrease pressure on spinal nerve
    2. Release entrapped spinal nerve
C. Most often done in cervical area where foramen is smaller in diameter

**VII. Chemonucleolysis**

A. Procedure
    1. Injection of chymopapain, enzyme found in papaya plant, into nucleus pulposus
    2. Fluoroscopy and local anesthesia used
B. Purpose
    1. Decreases size of disc by hydrolysis
    2. Decreases pain
C. Fallen out of favor
    1. Increased incidence of pain recurrence
    2. Adverse reactions to chymopapain

**VIII. Rhizotomy**

A. Procedure: destruction of sensory nerve roots at entrance to spinal cord
B. Purpose: interruption of transmission of pain
C. Types
    1. Closed: percutaneous insertion of catheter to destroy nerve root through coagulation, injection of neurolytic chemicals, or cryodestruction
    2. Open
        a. Requires laminectomy
        b. Nerve roots isolated and destroyed

**IX. Chordotomy**

A. Procedure: pain pathways transected at midline portion of spinal cord before impulse ascends through spinothalamic tract
B. Purpose: interruption of transmission of pain

## POSTANESTHESIA CARE

### NURSING DIAGNOSIS

Examples of related nursing diagnostic categories include:

- Altered spinal cord tissue perfusion
- Alteration in comfort
- Impaired physical mobility
- Fear/anxiety
- Potential for infection
- Potential ineffective breathing patterns
- Potential alteration in gas exchange
- Potential alteration in urinary elimination
- Potential alteration in bowel elimination
- Knowledge deficit

**I. Report of Operative Procedure**

A. Surgical procedure
    1. Fusion
        a. Donor site if autologous bone used
        b. Cadaveric bone
    2. Insertion of hardware for stabilization

B. Pathologic findings
C. Complete or subtotal resection (if tumor)
D. Intraoperative problems
E. Existing deficits
F. Expected deficits
G. Medication administered during procedure

**II. Goals**

A. Prompt recognition of potential complications
B. Implementation of preventive measures
C. Maintenance of functional integrity of spinal cord

**III. Assessment**

A. Ongoing, frequent, and careful observation
B. Specific spinal cord assessment form may assist in consistent documentation of improvement or deterioration (see Fig. 21–17)
C. Assess for signs of meningeal irritation
   1. Headache
   2. Photophobia
   3. Nuchal rigidity
   4. Kernig's sign: resistance and pain when patient's leg is flexed at hip and knee
   5. Brudzinski's sign: flexion of hips and knees in response to passive flexion of neck
D. Hemodynamic monitoring: especially useful for patient with spinal cord injury who may be in spinal shock
   1. Swan-Ganz catheter
   2. Arterial lines
   3. CVP line
E. Respiratory status
   1. Especially important with cervical lesions
   2. Assess rate, use of accessory muscles, nasal flaring
   3. Breath sounds
   4. Ability to handle secretions
   5. For patients with anterior cervical approach (may have damage to laryngeal nerves, vocal cords, hematoma formation)
      a. Hoarseness
      b. Tracheal deviation (edema)
   6. Pulse oximetry
   7. ABGs
F. Neurovascular checks
G. Urinary elimination
   1. Voiding pattern
   2. Intake and output
   3. Palpate abdomen for distension
H. Auscultate bowel sounds, presence of distension

**IV. Postoperative Complications**

A. Increase in existing deficits
B. Motor loss: paralysis of upper or lower extremities
C. Sensory loss
D. Urinary retention
E. Paralytic ileus
F. Leakage of CSF through dural tear or fistula
G. Hematoma at operative site (will increase neurologic deficits)
H. Arachnoiditis
I. Infection

J. Respiratory distress
K. Spinal cord–injured patients may experience any of the complications indicated in discussion of spinal cord injury

## V. Signs of Deterioration in Status

A. Increase in existing deficits
B. Appearance of new deficits
C. Spinal shock
D. Autonomic dysreflexia

## VI. Nursing Interventions After Spinal Injury

A. Maintain patent airway
   1. Coughing and deep breathing
   2. Use of incentive spirometry
   3. Supplemental oxygen
   4. Assistance with mechanical ventilation may be needed with cervical lesions
B. Frequent assessment of neurologic status: note deviations from patient's baseline
C. Positioning
   1. Factors
      a. Type of surgery
      b. Type of lesion
      c. Site of lesion
      d. Presence of complications
   2. Reduce pressure on operative site
   3. Reposition every 2 hours once specified by surgeon
   4. Log rolling
      a. Maintain alignment
      b. Decrease pain
      c. Decrease muscle spasms
      d. Use of turning sheet decreases stress on care giver and helps ensure alignment
   5. Avoid twisting
   6. Proper body alignment
   7. Stryker frame
      a. May be used for variety of spinal surgeries depending on patient condition and severity of injury
      b. May be used in conjunction with halo apparatus or Gardner-Wells tongs
         (1) Maintain traction
         (2) Observe pin sites
         (3) Assess stability of halo apparatus and security bolts
      c. Physician must be present first time patient is turned down
      d. Psychosocial and emotional support needed because patients frequently are afraid and anxious on frame
   8. Cervical collar or Philadelphia collar
D. Maintain skin and mucous membrane integrity
   1. Monitor incision site
      a. Hematoma development
      b. Edema at surgical site
      c. CSF leakage
         (1) Test for glucose
         (2) Look for halo or ring sign
   2. Pad bony prominences
   3. Frequent repositioning for paralyzed patients

E. Pain control
   1. Assess pain
      a. Level, location, duration
      b. Use of pain scale
   2. Patient-controlled analgesia (PCA) often used with spinal surgery
   3. Frequent repositioning
   4. Maintenance of stabilizing devices
   5. Administration of pain medications if patient-controlled analgesia not used
   6. Alternative methods of pain relief
      a. Relaxation
      b. Imagery

F. Antiembolic stockings or sequential compression devices

G. Psychosocial and emotional support
   1. Reassure patient frequently
   2. Inform patient when assessing, performing procedures
   3. Keep family informed of patient's condition
   4. Answer patient's and family's questions as honestly as possible

## BIBLIOGRAPHY


American Association of Neurological Surgeons. *Guidelines for the Management of Severe Head Injuries.* Chicago, American Association of Neuroscience Nurses, 1995.

American Association of Neuroscience Nurses. *Clinical Guidelines Series: Intracranial Pressure Monitoring.* Chicago, The Association, 1997.

Arsenault L: Selected postoperative complications of cranial surgery. *J Neurosurg Nurs* 17(3):155–163, 1985.

Barker E: *Neuroscience Nursing.* St. Louis: Mosby, 1994.

Cammermeyer M, Appledorn C: *AANN's Core Curriculum for Neuroscience Nursing,* 3rd Ed. Chicago, American Association of Neuroscience Nurses, 1996.

Cardona VD, Hurn PD, Mason PJB, Veise-Berry SW: *Trauma Nursing: From Resuscitation Through Rehabilitation.* Philadelphia, WB Saunders, 1993.

Chipps E, Clanin N, Campbell V: *Neurologic Disorders.* St Louis, Mosby–Year Book, 1992.

German K. Intracranial pressure monitoring in the 1990's. *Crit Care Nurs Q* 17(1):21–32, 1994.

Guyton AC: *Basic Neuroscience,* 2nd Ed. Philadelphia, WB Saunders, 1991.

Hickey J: *The Clinical Practice of Neurological and Neurosurgical Nursing.* Philadelphia, JB Lippincott, 1997.

Ignatavicius D, Workman L, Mishler MA: *Medical-Surgical Nursing: A Nursing Process Approach.* Philadelphia, WB Saunders, 1995.

Laws ER, Thaper K. Brain tumors: *CA* 43(5):263–271, 1993.

Marshall SB, Marshall LF, Vos HR, Chesnut RM: *Neuroscience Critical Care: Pathophysiology and Patient Management.* Philadelphia, WB Saunders, 1990.

Osborn I: The neurosurgical patient in the postanesthesia unit. *Anesthesiol Clin North Am* 8(2):355–364, 1990.

Schultz DL: The role of the neuroscience nurse in lumbar fusion. *J Neurosci Nurs* 27(2):90–95, 1995.

Shpritz D: Brain tumor basics. *Crit Care Nurse* 6(5): 94–96, 1986.

Shpritz D: Craniocerebral trauma. *Crit Care Nurse* 3(2):48–61, 1983.

Shpritz D: *Delmar's Rapid Nursing Interventions: Neurologic.* Albany, NY, Delmar Publishers, 1996.

Shpritz D: Emergency neurologic assessment. *Crit Care Nurse* 5(5):66–68, 1985.

Spetzler RF: Gamma knife radiosurgery. *BNI Q* 13(1): 4–48, 1997.


## REVIEW QUESTIONS

**1. Which of the following factors interact to maintain normal intracranial pressure (ICP)?**

A. Brain tissue, plasma, cerebrospinal fluid (CSF)
B. Lymphatic fluid, CSF, blood
C. Brain tissue, lymphatic tissue, blood
D. Brain tissue, CSF, blood

2. **What is the normal value for intracranial pressure?**
   A. 5 to 10 mm Hg
   B. 10 to 20 mm Hg
   C. 0 to 15 mm Hg
   D. 15 to 25 mm Hg

3. **Which of the following nursing interventions is of the highest priority for a patient with increased intracranial pressure?**
   A. Administration of corticosteroids
   B. Maintenance of a patent airway
   C. Elevation of the head of the bed 30 to 45 degrees
   D. Maintenance of an ICP monitoring system

4. **Which of the following is the most sensitive indicator of neurologic deterioration?**
   A. Decorticate or decerebrate posturing
   B. Decreased level of consciousness
   C. Increase in systolic blood pressure greater than 30 mm Hg over baseline
   D. Seizures

5. **In caring for a patient who has just had a supratentorial craniotomy, which of the following positions is most appropriate?**
   A. Allow the patient to assume a position of comfort
   B. Elevate the head of the bed 30 to 45 degrees
   C. Maintain the head of the bed flat
   D. Position the patient flat with the head turned to the side

6. **Which of the following assessment parameters and anatomic correlates are correct?**
   A. Decorticate posturing (flexion) is associated with lower motor neuron damage
   B. Decreased level of consciousness is associated with pressure on the reticular activating system (RAS)
   C. Pupil dilation is associated with pressure on the optic nerve and the sympathetic nerve fibers
   D. Widened pulse pressure is associated with constriction of the cerebral arteries supplying the brainstem

7. **Mr. Jones is admitted to the PACU after a craniotomy for evacuation of a subdural hematoma. He is being hyperventilated on a ventilator through an endotracheal tube that is part of the protocol used to lower intracranial pressure. What is the underlying physiologic rationale for this therapeutic intervention?**
   A. Low levels of oxygen ($Po_2$) constrict cerebral blood vessels
   B. Low levels of carbon dioxide ($Pco_2$) constrict cerebral blood vessels
   C. Low levels of oxygen ($Po_2$) dilate cerebral blood vessels
   D. Low levels of carbon dioxide ($Pco_2$) dilate cerebral blood vessels

8. **As part of Mr. Jones' care you must calculate his cerebral perfusion pressure (CPP) with the intraventricular catheter inserted in the operating room. His admitting CPP is 83 mm Hg. Which of the following nursing actions is the most appropriate?**
   A. Notify the physician because this value indicates neuronal death has occurred
   B. Do nothing, because this value is normal
   C. Increase his CPP by increasing his IV fluids
   D. Increase his CPP by elevating the head of the bed

9. **Mr. Jones has a temperature of 101.4° F. You notify the physician who tells you to do nothing. What is the possible cause of the elevated temperature in Mr. Jones?**
   A. Mr. Jones has meningitis but was given antibiotics in the OR
   B. Mr. Jones is probably dehydrated
   C. Pressure on the hypothalamus during surgery produces temporary elevations in temperature
   D. Part of the neurosurgical anesthesia protocol produces hyperthermia

**10. A Janetta procedure is done to:**
A. Evacuate a subdural hematoma
B. Decompress CN V
C. Relieve pressure on the spinal cord
D. Relieve sciatic pain

**11. In a patient with hydrocephalus, which of the following procedures will most likely be performed as a curative measure?**
A. Lumbar puncture
B. Lumbar drain
C. Ventriculoperitoneal shunt
D. Arteriovenous shunt

**12. A patient who has had a transsphenoidal hypophysectomy has had the removal of:**
A. Adrenal glands
B. Uterus
C. Pituitary gland
D. Thyroid gland

**13. Patients who have cranial surgical procedures in the sitting position are at risk for which of the following complications?**
A. Decubitus ulcers
B. Air emboli
C. Extensive blood loss
D. Hypertension

**14. Of the following statements, which is correct concerning upper or lower motor neuron lesions?**
A. Lower motor neuron lesions result in hyperreflexia
B. Lower motor neuron lesions originate in the brain
C. Upper motor neuron lesions result in significant muscle atrophy
D. Upper motor neuron lesions result in spasticity

**15. Incomplete spinal cord lesions as a result of trauma imply:**
A. There is total loss of motor and sensory function below the level of the lesion
B. There is some preservation of motor and/or sensory function below the level of the lesion
C. Surgical repair will restore all motor and sensory function
D. There is loss of sensory function only

**16. Spinal shock is characterized by:**
A. Areflexia below the level of the lesion
B. Bradycardia and hypertension
C. Unconsciousness and hypotension
D. Spastic paralysis

**17. During an acute episode of autonomic dysreflexia, sodium nitroprusside is administered. The rationale for administering this medication is to:**
A. Decrease renal perfusion
B. Decrease vascular resistance
C. Increase cardiac output
D. Increase venous return

**18. Mr. Ford is admitted to the PACU after removal of a thoracic intramedullary spinal cord tumor. You know that this type of tumor is usually:**
A. Benign
B. Malignant
C. Totally resectable
D. One that will recur quickly

**19. What is the most frequent surgical procedure performed on the spine?**

A. Discectomy
B. Foraminotomy
C. Laminectomy
D. Spinal fusion

**20. A spinal fusion may involve the use of which of the following to stabilize the spine?**

A. Abdominal fascia
B. Bone chips from iliac crest
C. Harrington rods
D. Transposition of muscle from the thigh

**21. The most important nursing intervention in caring for a patient with spinal surgery is:**

A. Pain control
B. Inspection of incision site every 2 hours
C. Log rolling
D. Prevention of constipation

**ANSWERS:** 1. D, 2. C, 3. B, 4. B, 5. B, 6. B, 7. B, 8. B, 9. C, 10. B, 11. C, 12. C, 13. B, 14. D, 15. B, 16. A, 17. B, 18. B, 19. C, 20. B, 21. C

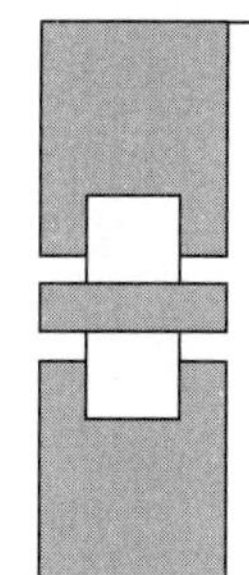

CHAPTER 22

# The Urologic Surgical Patient

William M. Kiefner, RN

Gratia M. Nagle, BA, CRNFA, CURN

### OBJECTIVES

**Study of the information represented by this outline will enable the learner to:**

1. Identify the structure and function of the genitourinary system.
2. Understand the pathophysiologic implications of each urologic disorder reviewed.
3. Synthesize principles of physical assessment with the principles of the nursing process.
4. Identify the specific postanesthesia care unit (PACU) considerations in patient care after each urologic procedure discussed in the chapter.
5. Incorporate biologic, psychologic, social, and cultural assessment of the patient.

The genitourinary system includes the adrenal glands, kidneys, ureters, bladder, urethra, genital organs (Fig. 22–1), and the most important structure, the nephron, within the kidney (Fig. 22–2). The nephron is responsible for urine formation and general homeostasis (Fig. 22–3). The entire system and its related anatomy are capable of succumbing to a host of disorders. It is essential to possess adequate knowledge of how these units function in interrelationships under normal circumstances. This chapter addresses many of the genitourinary disorders commonly encountered in the PACU. The treatment of acute renal failure is beyond the scope of this chapter's objectives. The reader is urged to consult the Bibliography for more information.

## ANATOMY AND PHYSIOLOGY OF THE GENITOURINARY SYSTEM

**I. Adrenal Gland**

- A. Enclosed by Gerota's (perirenal) fascia
- B. Caps each kidney superiorly
  1. Right is triangular, between liver and vena cava
  2. Left is rounded and crescent shaped, close to aorta, and partially covered by pancreas
- C. Composed of cortex and medulla
- D. Secretions influenced by pituitary gland
  1. Cortex secretes steroids, hormones
  2. Medulla secretes adrenaline (epinephrine)
- E. Arterial blood supplied by the inferior phrenic artery, renal artery, and aorta
- F. Venous blood supply
  1. Right has short vein that empties into vena cava
  2. Left terminates in left renal vein
- G. Lymphatics
  1. Accompany suprarenal vein
  2. Drain into lumbar lymph nodes
- H. Adrenal disease often directly affects renal function (refer to information on pathophysiology for descriptions)

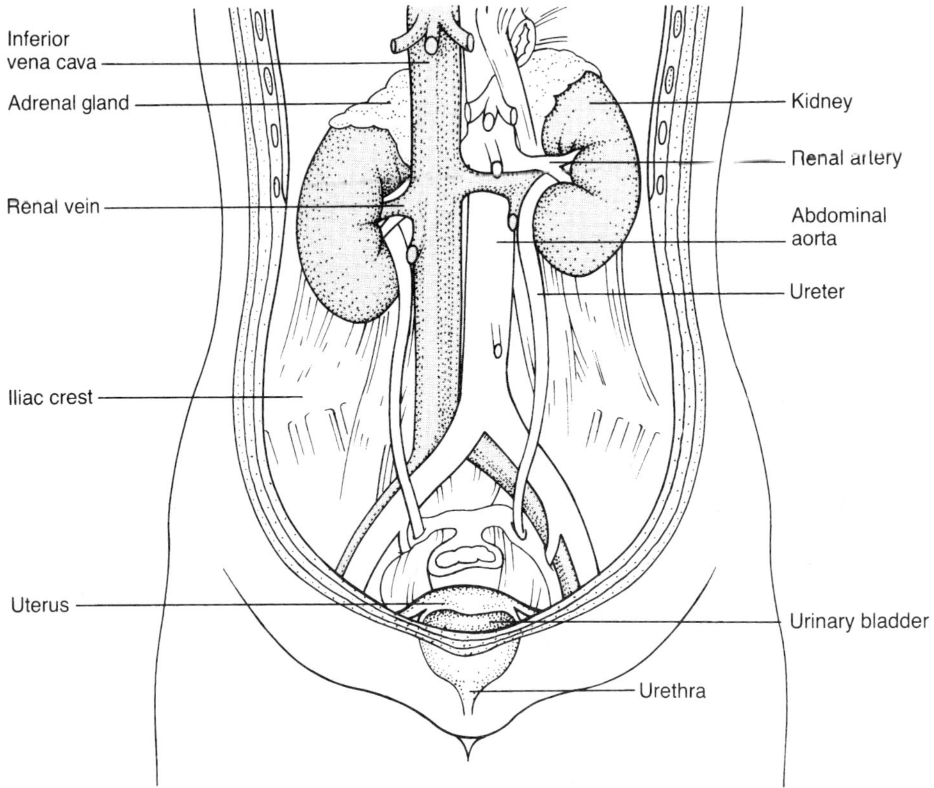


**FIGURE 22–1** Anatomy of urinary system. (From Ignatavicius DD, Bayne MV: *Medical-Surgical Nursing.* Philadelphia, WB Saunders, 1991, p 1800.)

1. Alport's syndrome
2. Cushing's disease
3. Pheochromocytoma
4. Adenoma
5. Carcinoma

**II. Kidney**

A. Comprised of cortex, medulla, calices, nephron, and pelvis
   1. Two or three major calices join renal pelvis
   2. Renal pelvis may be intrarenal and extrarenal
      a. Left lies at level of first or second lumbar vertebra
      b. Tapers to form ureter
      c. Right is lower than left

B. Retroperitoneal, parallel to vertebrae and psoas muscle

C. Autonomic innervation with intraperitoneal organs accounts for gastrointestinal symptoms that accompany genitourinary disease, including nausea, vomiting, and pain

D. Arterial blood supply
   1. End arteries (absence of collateral connections)
   2. Renal artery enters hilum between pelvis and renal vein
      a. Divides into anterior and posterior branches
      b. Anterior supplies upper and lower poles and anterior surface
      c. Posterior supplies posterior surface
      d. Divides again into interlobar arteries to glomeruli

E. Venous blood supply
   1. Renal veins paired with renal arteries
   2. Left renal vein is three times longer than right

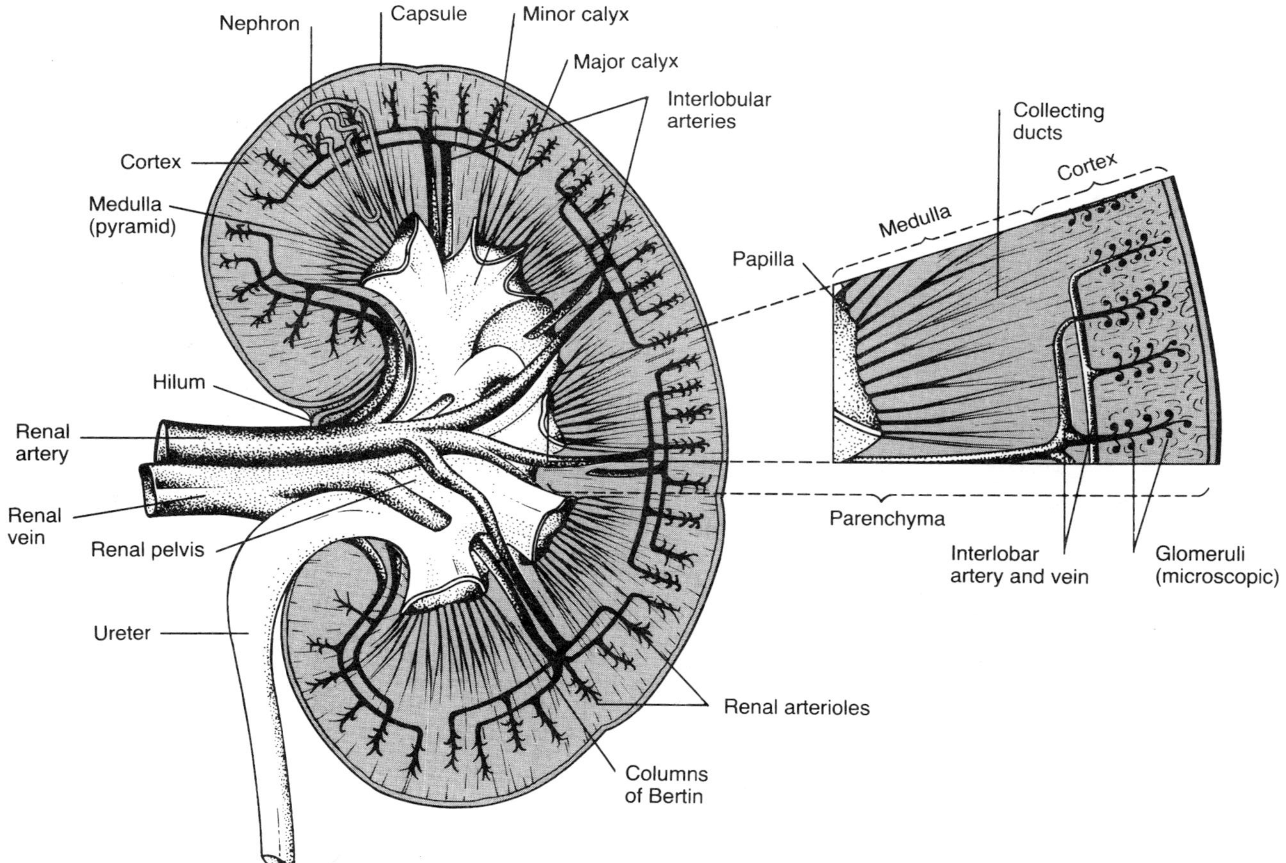


**FIGURE 22–2** Major structures of kidney. (From Ignatavicius DD, Bayne MV: *Medical-Surgical Nursing*. Philadelphia, WB Saunders, 1991, p 1801.)

**WHAT HAPPENS IN THE NEPHRON (THE KIDNEY'S FUNCTIONAL UNIT)?**

Blood enters the afferent arteriole on its way to the glomerulus for filtration. In the glomerulus, hydrostatic pressure and other forces promote the filtration of water, electrolytes, and other substances out of the capillaries and into the space within Bowman's capsule. The blood components remaining in the capillaries are returned to the systemic circulation through the efferent arteriole and the peritubular capillary network. Meanwhile, the filtered substances—known as filtrate—pass through the proximal convoluted tubule, the loop of Henle, and the distal convoluted tubule and are altered by tubular reabsorption and tubular secretion. The final filtrate that remains after passage through the tubules is excreted through the collecting duct as urine.

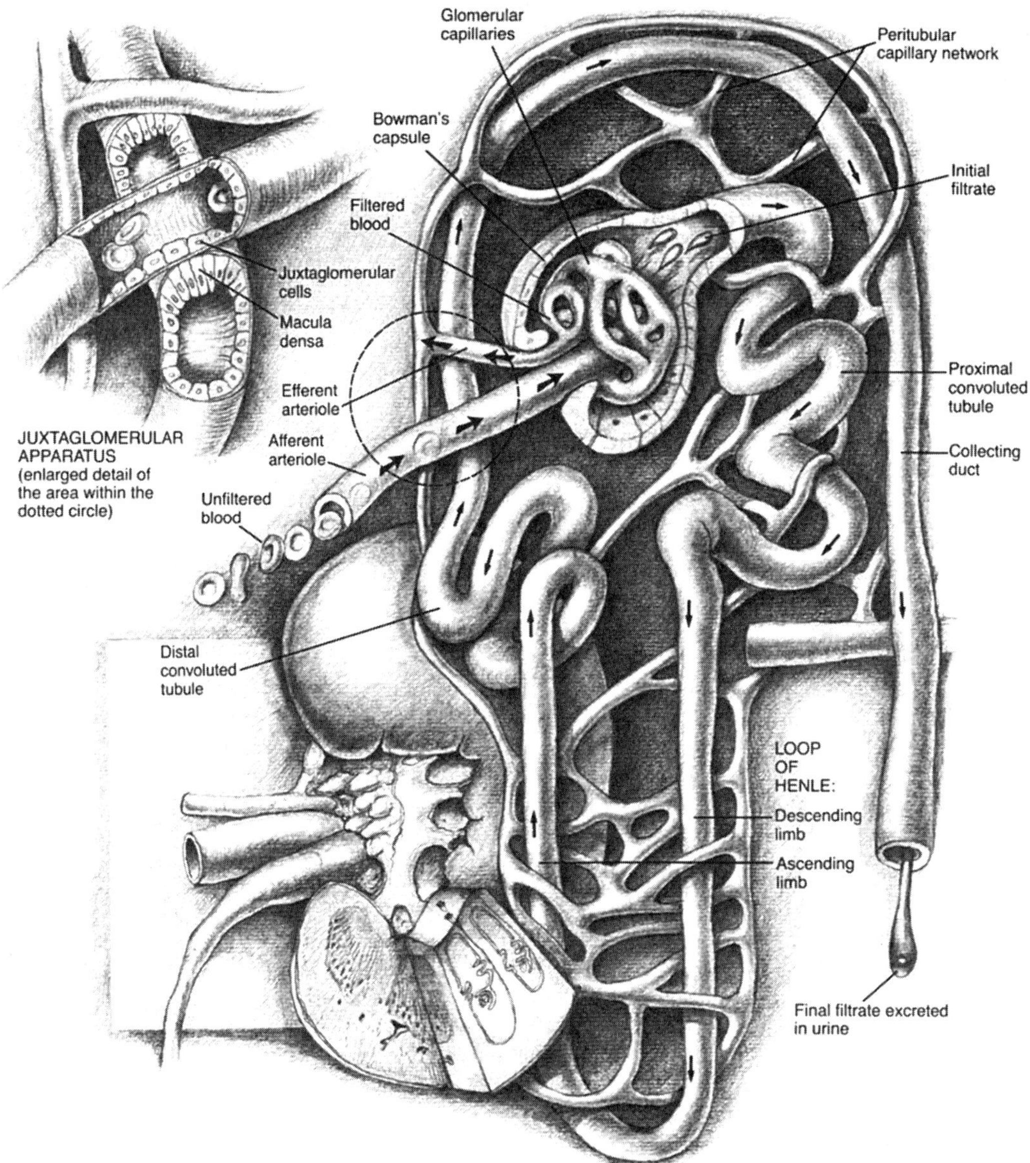


The specialized cells of the juxtaglomerular apparatus—juxtaglomerular cells in the afferent and efferent arterioles and macula densa in the distal convoluted tubule—regulate the flow of blood into and out of the nephron by dilating or constricting as they sense changes in blood volume and pressure. Dilation of the afferent arteriole together with constriction of the efferent arteriole increases glomerular capillary blood volume and hydrostatic pressure to promote filtration and increase urinary output. Constriction of the afferent arteriole with dilation of the efferent arteriole promotes the opposite effect: decreased filtration and decreased urinary output.

**FIGURE 22–3** Nephron function. (From Ignatavicius DD, Bayne MV: *Medical-Surgical Nursing*. Philadelphia, WB Saunders, 1991, p 1803.)

F. Accessory renal vessels
   1. Common, although renal artery and vein are usually sole blood supply
   2. May compress ureter to cause hydronephrosis
G. Lymphatics drain into lumbar lymph nodes
H. Nephron
   1. Functional unit of kidney
   2. Approximately 1 million tiny nephrons in each kidney
   3. Each nephron is composed of secretory or excretory tubules lined with thin epithelial cells
      a. Secretory tubule
         (1) Within cortex
         (2) Consists of renal corpuscle and secretory portion of renal tubule
      b. Renal corpuscle
         (1) Vascular glomerulus projects into Bowman's capsule
            (a) Selectively permeable membrane
            (b) Permeable to water and solutes (crystalloids)
            (c) Impermeable to large molecules and plasma proteins
         (2) Continuous with epithelium of proximal convoluted tubule
      c. Secretory renal tubule
         (1) Proximal convoluted tubule is extension of Bowman's capsule
         (2) Loop of Henle
            (a) Reabsorbs 25% of glomular filtrate
            (b) Ascending limb impermeable to water
               (i) Actively reabsorbs electrolytes (especially chloride, sodium)
               (ii) Generates medullary hypertonicity by formation of hypotonic tubular fluid
            (c) Descending limb permeable to water and salts
               (i) Diffusion of NaCl from ascending limb across interstitial space
               (ii) NaCl recycles through loop of Henle multiple times
            (d) Essential for water conservation with dehydration and hemorrhage
         (3) Distal convoluted tubule
            (a) Tiny collecting ducts that form larger duct
            (b) Empty into renal pelvis at base of kidney
            (c) Urine flows from renal pelvis into ureters to bladder
      d. Excretory tubule
         (1) Lies in medulla
         (2) Collecting tubule, continuous with ascending limb of proximal convoluted tubule
         (3) Empties into minor calyx

## III. Ureter

A. Follows smooth S curve
B. Lies on psoas muscle, passes medial to sacroiliac joints and lateral near ischial spines
C. Penetrates base of bladder medially at oblique angle
   1. Posteroinferior to bladder dome
   2. 5 cm apart
D. Areas of narrowing
   1. At ureteropelvic junction
   2. As it crosses over external iliac vessels
   3. As it passes through bladder wall
E. Averages 26 to 30 cm long in adult

## IV. Bladder

A. Hollow, muscular, pelvic organ

B. Reservoir for urine
   1. Adult capacity: 350 to 700 ml
   2. Urge to urinate common at 400 ml
C. Lies behind symphysis pubis in adult, slightly higher in child
   1. When full, rises above symphysis pubis, especially in children
   2. Easily palpated, especially when full
   3. If overdistended may cause visible lower abdominal bulge
   4. Postponing urination strains bladder capacity
D. Ureteral orifices are on proximal trigone at extremities of interureteric ridge
   1. 2.5 cm apart
   2. Trigone located between ridge and bladder neck
E. Bladder neck (internal sphincter) formed of interlaced muscle fibers of detrusor
   1. Muscle fibers converge
   2. Pass distally to form smooth musculature of urethra
F. Dome and posterior surface covered by peritoneum
G. Arterial blood supply comprised of superior, middle, inferior vesical arteries
   1. From trunk of internal iliac (hypogastric) artery
   2. From obturator and inferior gluteal arteries
   3. In females, also has branches from uterine and vaginal arteries
H. Venous blood supply rich and empties into internal iliac (hypogastric) veins
I. Lymphatics drain into vesical, external and internal iliac, and common iliac lymph nodes

**V. Adult Male Anatomy**

A. Prostate gland
   1. Glandular, fibromuscular organ lying below and behind bladder
      a. Produces seminal fluid
      b. Transports spermatozoa to ejaculate
      c. Posterosuperior surface adjacent to vas deferens and seminal vesicles
   2. Doughnut configuration around bladder outlet
   3. Contains 2.5 cm posterior urethra and prostatic urethra
   4. Supported by puboprostatic ligaments and urogenital diaphragm
   5. Ejaculatory ducts pierce prostate posteriorly and empty through verumontanum
      a. On floor of prostatic urethra
      b. Proximal to striated external urinary sphincter
   6. Consists of five lobes or zones
      a. Anterior, posterior, median, right lateral, and left lateral lobes
      b. Peripheral, central, transitional, anterior, and preprostatic sphincteric zones
   7. Periurethral glands at median and lateral lobes are usual site of prostatic adenoma
   8. Posterior lobe prone to malignancy
   9. Blood supply
      a. Arterial blood supply from inferior vesical, internal pudendal, and middle rectal arteries
      b. Venous blood supply drains into periprostatic plexus
         (1) Connects to deep dorsal vein of penis
         (2) Connects to internal iliac (hypogastric) veins
   10. Nerve supply derived from sympathetic and parasympathetic nerve systems
   11. Lymphatics drain into internal iliac, sacral, vesical, and external iliac lymph nodes
B. Seminal vesicles
   1. Lie under base of bladder and above prostate gland
   2. Each joins corresponding vas deferens to form ejaculatory duct
   3. Nerve supply is mainly from sympathetic system
   4. Lymphatics supply prostate gland
C. Spermatic cord
   1. Extends from internal inguinal ring through inguinal canal to testis bilaterally

2. Contents of each cord
   a. Vas deferens
   b. Internal and external spermatic arteries
   c. Artery of vas (deferential artery)
   d. Venous pampiniform plexus (forms spermatic vein superiorly)
   e. Lymph vessels that empty into external iliac lymph nodes
   f. Nerves
3. Enclosed in layers of thin fascia
4. Serves to suspend testis
5. Some cremaster nerve fibers penetrate cords in inguinal canal

D. Epididymis
1. Coiled duct that is continuous with vas deferens at its lower pole
2. Consists of head (upper pole), central body, and tail (lower pole)
3. Connected to posterior surface of testis at upper pole
4. Appendix often found on upper pole
5. Efferent ductules in head carry spermatozoa from testis to vas deferens
6. Sperm mature during transportation to vas

E. Testis
1. Essential for male reproductive system
   a. Produces spermatozoa
   b. Secretes testosterone
   c. Housed in scrotal sac to provide lower temperature for sperm viability
2. Covered by thick fascial layer of tunica albuginea
   a. Posteriorly forms mediastinum testis
   b. Fibrous septa separate testis into approximately 250 lobules
3. Covered with and separated from scrotal wall by tunica vaginalis
4. Appendix testis, similar to epididymis testis, located at upper pole
5. Seminiferous tubules contain interstitial Leydig's cells essential for testosterone production
6. Shares common embryologic origin with kidney and closely associated blood supply
   a. Internal spermatic artery originates in aorta just below renal artery
   b. Internal spermatic artery joins deferential artery
   c. Right spermatic vein enters vena cava just below right renal vein
   d. Left spermatic vein empties into left renal vein
7. Lymphatics drain into paraaortic lymph nodes, which are connected to mediastinal nodes

F. Scrotum
1. Relaxation and contraction of muscular layer regulate internal temperature
   a. Temperature generally 1° to 2° F lower than body temperature
   b. Temperature regulation necessary for fertility
2. Septum of connective tissue divides internal sac into two pouches
3. Provides support to testes
4. Arterial blood supply from femoral, internal pudendal, and inferior epigastric arteries
5. Veins are paired with arteries
6. Lymphatics drain into subinguinal and superficial inguinal lymph nodes

G. Urethra
1. 15 to 30 cm long
2. Mucosal tissue

H. Penis
1. Composition
   a. Glans or tip
      (1) Before circumcision, prepuce forms hood over glans (foreskin)
      (2) Prepuce may be smoothed back to expose glans

(3) Contains nerve endings
(4) Glans formed by distal, expanded end of bulbospongiosus muscle

b. Shaft or body
(1) Suspensory ligament from pubic symphysis
(2) Ligament inserts into fascia of corpus cavernosa

c. Two corpus cavernosa and corpus spongiosum underlie glans and shaft
(1) Corpus cavernosa run along either side of corpus spongiosum
(2) Urethra surrounded by corpus spongiosum
(3) All contain vascular cavities
(4) Corpus spongiosum fills with blood during sexual arousal and produces erection

2. Arterial blood supply from internal pudendal arteries
   a. Deep artery of penis supplies corpus cavernosa
   b. Dorsal artery of penis
   c. Bulbourethral artery supplies corpus spongiosum, glans, and urethra
3. Venous blood supply
   a. Superficial dorsal vein
   b. Deep dorsal vein
   c. Drains into internal pudendal vein
4. Lymphatic system
   a. Lymphatics from penile skin drain into subinguinal and superficial inguinal nodes
   b. Lymphatics from glans drain into external and subinguinal iliac nodes

I. Organs of reproduction
1. Prostate gland
2. Seminal vesicles
3. Testes
4. Penis

## VI. Adult Female Anatomy

A. Urethra

1. 4 cm long in adult female and slightly curved
   a. Lies anterior to vagina beneath symphysis pubis
   b. Short length is common cause of frequent cystitis
2. Comprised of submucosa of connective and elastic tissue
   a. Filled with spongy venous spaces
   b. Contains many periurethral glands
      (1) Glands of Skene
         (a) Open on floor of urethra inside meatus
         (b) Stimulate mucus secretion during sexual arousal
         (c) Inflammation may contribute to urethritis or cystitis
      (2) Bartholin's gland
         (a) Salivary ducts opening on inner aspects of labia minora within vagina
         (b) Inflammation may contribute to chronic urethritis or cystitis
3. Arterial blood supply
   a. Inferior vesical artery
   b. Vaginal artery
   c. Internal pudendal artery
4. Venous blood supply empties into internal pudendal veins
5. Lymphatic system
   a. Lymphatics from external urethra drain into subinguinal and inguinal lymph nodes
   b. Lymphatics from deep urethra drain into internal iliac lymph nodes

B. Organs of reproduction
   1. Uterus
   2. Fallopian tubes
   3. Ovaries
   4. Vagina

## RENAL PHYSIOLOGY

Fluid and electrolyte balance within the kidney is maintained through a complex, and not fully understood, interaction of hormonal systems, electrolyte balance, renal blood flow, glomular filtration, red blood cell formation, and calcium formation. Renal shutdown may quickly ensue with hypovolemia, because the nephrons become unable to adequately manufacture urine as a result of the decreased blood supply to the kidney. When this occurs measures must be taken to reverse the situation.

**I. Endocrine Function (Hormonal Interactions)**
- A. RAAS (renin-angiotensin-aldosterone system) cascade is major renal hormonal regulator for:
  1. Systemic blood pressure
  2. Regional blood flow
  3. Sodium and potassium balance
- B. Renin
  1. Enzyme-catalyzing agent
  2. Manufactured in specialized lining of afferent renal arterioles
     a. Volume receptors
     b. Response to reduced arterial blood pressure or renal perfusion as a result of
        (1) Hemorrhage
        (2) Sodium depletion
        (3) Heart failure
     c. Responsible for formation of angiotensin
- C. Angiotensin
  1. Powerful vasoconstrictor
  2. Raises blood pressure
  3. Stimulates aldosterone release
  4. Feedback mechanisms have limited compensatory ability to affect alterations in volume
  5. Medical management directed toward external efforts
     a. Replacement of blood, fluids, electrolytes
     b. Drug therapies
- D. Aldosterone
  1. Release from adrenal cortex stimulated by:
     a. Decreased sodium levels
     b. Increased potassium levels
  2. Prompts kidney to
     a. Absorb more sodium
     b. Excrete more potassium
  3. Net effect of release
     a. Conserve sodium and water
     b. Raise blood volume
  4. Potential adverse effects
     a. Systemic vasoconstriction
     b. Decreased organ perfusion
- E. Prostaglandins
  1. Produced, metabolized, and acted on in renal medulla

2. Maintain renal function by effect on afferent and efferent arterioles of glomerular capillary
3. Modulate renin release
4. Affect urine concentration through synergistic activity with AVP (an antidiuretic hormone)
5. Nonsteroidal anti-inflammatory agents must be cautiously used
   a. Cause salt and water retention
   b. Acute renal failure can occur in states of dehydration

F. Erythropoietin
1. Secreted by kidney in response to decrease in tissue oxygen tension
2. Stimulates production of new red blood cells
3. Exerts effect directly on bone marrow
4. Insufficient levels often found in patient with impaired renal function

G. ADH (antidiuretic hormone)
1. Exerts effect on distal tubules of nephrons
2. Acts as messenger in tubules, informing of body's need for water
3. Secreted by posterior pituitary gland when significant loss of body water occurs
4. Results in increased reabsorption of water and decrease in urine output

H. Vitamin D
1. Activated in kidney
2. Deficiency plays major role in chronic renal failure
   a. Losses in urine with nephrotic syndrome
   b. Defective enzyme activity in kidney caused by
      (1) Renal disease
      (2) Diminished parenchymal function
3. Decreased levels with hypocalcemia
4. Stimulates intestinal absorption of calcium and phosphate
5. Increases reabsorption of calcium and phosphorus by kidney

## II. Fluid-Electrolyte Balance (Electrolyte Interactions)

A. Sodium
1. Kidney regulates total body sodium by varying urinary excretion in relation to intake
2. Secretion adjusted in response to alterations in blood volume
3. Reabsorption accounts for most of energy consumed by kidney

B. Potassium
1. Filtration and excretion are independent of one another
   a. Once filtered, is almost totally reabsorbed in proximal tubules and loop of Henle
   b. Excreted is derived from tubular secretions in distal nephron
2. Secretion enhanced by tubular fluid flow rate and increases in sodium reabsorption

C. Calcium
1. Renal excretions and net intestinal absorption must be equal for proper calcium balance
2. Calcium phosphates crystallize in alkaline urine (hereditary distal tubular acidosis)
3. Ionized in plasma
4. Two thirds reabsorbed in proximal tubules by bulk flow with sodium and fluids
5. Direct relation to sodium balance

D. Phosphates
1. 90% reabsorbed in proximal tubule through sodium-dependent process
2. Balance reabsorbed in distal tubule
3. Plasma level constant when renal function is normal
   a. Excess concentrations of saline decrease proximal reabsorption
   b. Phosphate depletion raises reabsorption
   c. Excretion depressed with hyperparathyroidism and vitamin D deficiencies
4. At saturation point, excess load is excreted in urine

E. Glucose in glomerular filtrate completely reabsorbed at normal blood concentrations

### III. Glomerular Filtration

A. Nephrons operate in highly sophisticated pressure system

B. Pressure gradients affect filtration

1. Blood reaches glomerulus through renal artery at forward pressure of about 90 mm Hg
2. Fluid in Bowman's capsule creates hydrostatic pressure at about 15 mm Hg, resisting filtration
3. Presence of protein in plasma and not in capsule creates opposing force
   a. Uneven distribution of protein causes water concentration of plasma to be lower than capsule's
   b. Difference in water concentration induces osmotic flow of fluid from capsule into capillary
      (1) Water
      (2) Crystalloids
4. Osmotic gradient creates difference in hydrostatic pressure of about 30 mm Hg
5. When opposing forces are subtracted from original renal artery pressure, forward pressure is decreased to 45 mm Hg
6. Net filtration pressure
   a. Protein-free filtrate forced through glomerulus into Bowman's capsule
   b. Filtrate passes down into tubules
   c. Urine production initiated

### IV. Urine Production

A. Originates in glomerulus (filtering agent)

1. Selectively permeable membrane leaves filtrate virtually protein free
2. Composed basically of water and solutes (crystalloids)

B. Filtrate passes through proximal convoluted tubule

1. Water and crystalloids reabsorbed according to body's need
2. Loop of Henle concentrates urine
3. Distal convoluted tubule can reabsorb or excrete water and solutes
   a. Reabsorbs only what body requires
   b. Excretes remainder

### V. Key Points

A. Kidneys depend on minimum blood flow and on pressure regulated by renal arteries

B. Net filtration pressure can be affected by change in renal artery pressure

C. Pressure has direct effect on urine production

D. Sustained changes in pressure cause compromise in system function

E. Kidneys maintain electrolyte balance

F. End products of metabolism excreted in urine

## PATHOPHYSIOLOGY

### I. Upper Genitourinary System

A. Adrenal gland

1. Alport's syndrome
   a. Hereditary nephritis accompanied by deafness
   b. Managed with diet and medication
   c. Generally progresses to require dialysis and subsequent renal transplantation
2. Cushing's disease
   a. Caused by overproduction of cortisol (hydrocortisone) as a result of
      (1) Bilateral adrenocortical hyperplasia from overproduction of ACTH in pituitary gland (85%)

(2) Adrenal adenoma (10%)
(3) Adenocarcinoma of adrenal gland (5%)

b. Signs and symptoms
   (1) Marked muscle weakness, especially in quadriceps
   (2) Obesity with abnormal fat distribution that leaves extremities unaffected
      (a) Moon face
      (b) Cervical vertebral hump ("buffalo hump")
      (c) Clavicular fat pads
      (d) Pendulous abdomen
   (3) Striae of thighs and abdomen, often resulting in skin ulcerations
   (4) Hypertension
   (5) Calcium loss
      (a) Osteoporosis with compression fractures of lumbar spine and ribs
      (b) Renal calculi
   (6) Sleep disturbances with irritability and sometimes psychosis
   (7) Diabetic glucose tolerance curve
   (8) Slow wound healing
c. Surgical intervention usually alleviates symptoms with exception of osteoporosis
   (1) Total bilateral adrenalectomy
   (2) Transsphenoidal hypophysectomy

3. Pheochromocytoma
   a. Surgically curable hypertensive syndrome
      (1) Systolic and diastolic hypertension
      (2) Hypertension may be sustained, or, more commonly, paroxysmal
      (3) Other frequent symptoms
         (a) Headache (severity directly related to degree of hypertension)
         (b) Unprovoked diaphoresis with flushing or blanching
         (c) Tachycardia with palpitations from epinephrine excess
         (d) Postural hypotension
            (i) From diminished plasma volume and ganglionic blockage
            (ii) May result in profound weakness
         (e) Weight loss
            (i) Anorexia resulting from elevated blood glucose and fatty acid levels
            (ii) Decreased gastrointestinal motility: nausea, vomiting, constipation
   b. Tumor may be bilateral or extraadrenal
   c. Often occurs in combination with other glandular diseases
   d. Laboratory analysis
      (1) Elevated hematocrit (HCT), white blood cells (WBCs), serum protein
      (2) Few lymphocytes
      (3) Elevated fasting glucose level with diabetic glucose tolerance curve
      (4) Urine hormonal analysis reveals elevated epinephrine and sometimes norepinephrine
   e. Administration of 1 mg intravenous (IV) glucagon will raise blood pressure and catecholamine in 2 minutes

B. Kidney
   1. Agenesis
      a. Absence of one kidney
      b. Presence of atrophic kidney (not fully developed)
   2. Hypoplasia
      a. Presence of small kidney with small renal artery
      b. Contributes to renal hypertension
   3. Polycystic kidneys (hereditary)
      a. Occurs in renal cortex from defective collecting system
      b. Bilateral cystic disease leading to progressive functional impairment as cysts enlarge

c. Symptoms
   (1) Bilateral flank pain, often with colic
   (2) Hematuria
   (3) Hypertension
   (4) Nodular, palpable kidneys, often tender
d. Usually results in need for dialysis and possible transplantation

4. Congenital ureteropelvic junction obstruction
5. Glomerulonephritis
   a. Inflammatory process that attacks glomerulus
   b. Possible immune reaction
   c. Contributing causes
      (1) Infectious organisms
         (a) Streptococci
         (b) Staphylococci
      (2) Systemic diseases
         (a) Lupus erythematosus
         (b) Polyarteritis nodosa
            (i) Result of trauma, anticoagulants, or tumor
            (ii) Cause of spontaneous subcapsular hematoma
         (c) Diabetic glomerulosclerosis
         (d) Amyloidosis
         (e) Alport's syndrome
6. Nephrotic syndrome (combination of symptoms)
   a. Massive edema
   b. Proteinuria
   c. Hypoalbuminemia
   d. Hyperlipidemia
   e. Lipiduria
7. Renal artery stenosis
   a. Plaque formation
   b. Embolism
   c. Thrombosis
   d. Contributes to renal hypertension
8. Simple (solitary) renal cyst
9. Pyelonephritis
10. Perinephric abscess
11. High-output renal failure (oliguria)
   a. Urine output volume insufficient relative to body's excretory need
      (1) Occurs with urine volumes less than 400 ml/d if kidney can concentrate to normal specific gravity (1.010 to 1.025)
      (2) Occurs with urine volumes of 1000 to 1500 ml/d when concentrating ability impaired causing low specific gravity
   b. Metabolites retained
   c. High loss of body water
   d. Etiology
      (1) Inadequate plasma volume with vasodilation and substantially decreased protein levels
      (2) Normal kidney function compromised by poor perfusion
         (a) Decreased plasma volume results in decreased perfusion
         (b) Poor perfusion accompanies decrease in cardiac contractility
      (3) Prerenal azotemia (rising serum urea blood levels)
12. Acute renal failure
   a. Substantial decrease in glomerular filtration rate results in decrease in clearance of metabolites excreted by kidneys: urea, potassium, phosphate, creatinine

b. Body retains metabolites in bloodstream
   (1) Abnormally high creatinine level in bloodstream (best indicator of renal failure)
   (2) Retention produces state known as azotemia (excess of urea in blood)
   (3) Azotemia can be tolerated until treatment interventions are instituted
   (4) Uremia characterized by progressively higher levels of circulating metabolites
   (5) Uremia (intoxication) seen in advanced nephritis and anuria, incompatible with life
c. Causes
   (1) Prerenal
      (a) Dehydration (volume depletion)
         (i) Hemorrhage
         (ii) Gastrointestinal losses (vomiting, diarrhea)
         (iii) Renal losses (excessive diuretic therapy)
         (iv) Burns
         (v) Heat prostration
      (b) Volume shifts
         (i) "Third space" losses
         (ii) Vasodilating drugs
         (iii) Gram-negative sepsis
      (c) Volume expansion
         (i) Congestive heart failure
         (ii) Nephrotic syndrome
         (iii) Cirrhosis with ascites
      (d) Vascular anomalies
         (i) Dissecting arterial aneurysms
         (ii) Malignant hyperthermia
         (iii) Atheroembolism
   (2) Intrarenal (parenchymal) conditions
      (a) Glomerulonephritis
      (b) Ischemic reaction to vascular compromise
      (c) Acute tubular necrosis
      (d) Acute cortical necrosis
      (e) Antibiotic nephrotoxicity
   (3) Postrenal conditions
      (a) Calculus in patients with solitary kidney
      (b) Bilateral ureteral obstruction: stricture
      (c) Bladder outlet obstruction: benign prostatic hypertrophy
      (d) Postrenal trauma

13. Chronic renal failure
   a. Irreversible destruction of renal tissue
   b. Reduced metabolite clearance requiring peritoneal dialysis or hemodialysis
   c. Chief parameters indicative of renal failure
      (1) Elevated blood urea nitrogen (BUN)
      (2) Elevated serum creatinine
      (3) Decreased creatinine clearance
   d. Lengthy disease course
      (1) Azotemia
      (2) End-stage renal disease
   e. Etiology
      (1) Primary causes
         (a) Glomerulonephritis

(b) Pyelonephritis
(c) Congenital hypoplasia
(d) Polycystic kidney disease
(2) Secondary causes
(a) Diabetes
(b) Hypertension
(c) Systemic lupus erythematosus
(d) Alport's syndrome
(e) Amyloidosis
(i) Idiopathic, often malignant condition
(ii) Increased protein levels
(iii) May also involve bladder and prostate
f. Treatment modalities
(1) Maintenance hemodialysis
(2) Peritoneal dialysis
(3) Renal transplantation

C. Ureter
1. Congenital abnormalities
a. Incomplete ureter
b. Duplication of ureter
(1) Y formation
(2) Double ureter on one or both sides
c. Ureterocele
d. Ureteral stricture
e. Ureterovesical reflux
f. Ureteral stenosis
2. Acquired condition
a. Stenosis
(1) Surgical trauma
(2) External trauma
b. Metastatic lymph node enlargement
c. Endometriosis
d. Tumors
e. Calculi

## II. Lower Genitourinary System

A. Bladder
1. Exstrophy
a. Congenital fusion of bladder wall
b. Bladder eversion
2. Interstitial cystitis
a. Fibrotic condition of bladder wall
b. Loss of normal bladder capacity develops
3. Stress incontinence
a. Leakage of urine with sneezing, coughing, laughing, straining
b. Common in older females and after multiple pregnancies
4. Bladder diverticulum
5. Bladder tumors

B. Prostate gland
1. Benign prostatic hypertrophy (BPH)
a. Gland enlarges
b. Evident bladder outlet obstruction necessitates surgical intervention

2. Carcinoma
   a. Nonsurgical treatments
      (1) Androgen therapy
      (2) Radiation
   b. Surgical modalities
      (1) Orchiectomy
         (a) Testosterone production eliminated
         (b) Alternative to hormonal therapies
      (2) Prostatectomy

C. Penis and male urethra
   1. Phimosis
      a. Foreskin unretractable over glans
      b. Tendency for infection and fibrosis
      c. Circumcision indicated
   2. Balanoposthitis
      a. Inflamed glans and mucous membrane
      b. Purulent discharge
      c. Circumcision indicated
   3. Urethral stricture (stenosis)
      a. Congenital or acquired condition
      b. Surgical interventions
         (1) Urethral dilatation
         (2) Meatotomy
         (3) Urethroplasty
   4. Hypospadias
      a. Congenital anomaly
      b. Opening of meatus proximal to its normal glandular position at tip of penis
      c. Requires surgical reconstruction of urethra
   5. Epispadias
      a. Congenital anomaly (often associated with bladder exstrophy)
      b. Absence of dorsal urethral wall
      c. Requires surgical correction
   6. Carcinoma of penis and/or urethra
   7. Trauma (i.e., fractured urethra)

D. Testis, spermatic cord, and scrotum
   1. Cryptorchidism (undescended testis)
      a. Evident at birth
      b. Absence of one or both testis in scrotum
      c. Requires surgical intervention by the age of 1 to 2 years
         (1) Sterility ensues when left untreated much beyond this time
         (2) Maturation will not occur
         (3) Tendency for cancerous development increases over time if left untreated
   2. Testicular tumors
      a. Usually malignant
      b. Common in 18- to 35-year age group
      c. Enlargement of testis occurs, usually painless
      d. Requires metastatic workup, orchiectomy, and chemotherapy
   3. Spermatocele
      a. Intrascrotal cystic mass
      b. Attached to superior head of epididymis
      c. Caused by obstruction of sperm-carrying tubular system
      d. Most commonly occurs after vasectomy
   4. Varicocele
      a. Most often seen on left side

- b. Veins of spermatic cord become engorged because of venous backflow
- c. Often painful
- d. Uncorrected can affect fertility

5. Hydrocele
   - a. Collection of fluid within scrotal sac
   - b. May compromise testicular blood supply
6. Torsion of testis or spermatic cord
   - a. Strangulation of testicular blood supply
   - b. Usually of traumatic origin
   - c. Patient presents with extreme pain
   - d. Requires immediate surgery

E. Female urethra
1. Urethrovaginal fistula (vesicovaginal fistula)
   - a. Abnormal passageway between urethra and vagina
   - b. Develops after trauma
     - (1) Pelvic fracture
     - (2) Surgery
     - (3) Radiotherapy
   - c. Vaginal urethroplasty performed to correct condition
2. Urethral diverticulum
   - a. Urethral pouch develops
   - b. Associated with trauma
     - (1) Cystitis
     - (2) Urethritis
     - (3) Obstetric
   - c. Requires excision and plastic repair
3. Urethral carcinoma
4. Urethral caruncle

## III. Voiding Dysfunctions

A. Frequency
1. Perception of urge to urinate at more frequent intervals
2. Causes
   - a. Residual urine
   - b. Inflamed bladder mucosa or submucosa
   - c. Bladder capacity inadequate
   - d. Bladder instability
   - e. Interstitial cystitis
   - f. Bladder infection

B. Urgency
1. Strong sensation of having to void immediately
2. Causes
   - a. Cystitis
   - b. Bladder instability

C. Nocturia
1. Need to urinate often during normal sleep time
2. Often symptom of renal or prostate disease
3. Causes
   - a. Fluid retention (shift of circulating fluids to kidneys during rest)
   - b. Excess fluid intake before bedtime
   - c. BPH
   - d. Renal calculi
   - e. Cystitis

D. Dysuria
   1. Painful urination
   2. Causes
      a. Prostatitis
      b. Cystitis
      c. Urethritis
      d. Pyelonephritis
E. Enuresis
   1. Involuntary urination, often during sleep
   2. Normal in first 2 to 3 years of life
   3. Causes
      a. Delayed neuromuscular maturation
      b. Organic disease: infection, urethral stenosis, neurogenic bladder, pituitary malfunction
      c. Emotional or behavioral problems
F. Incontinence (includes stress, urge, mixed, and paradoxic or overflow types)
   1. Inability to control urination
   2. Causes
      a. Exstrophy of bladder
      b. Epispadias
      c. Vesicovaginal fistula
      d. Trauma: childbirth, prostatectomy
      e. Bladder instability: detrusor, sphincter
G. Hematuria
   1. Presence of gross or microscopic blood in urine
   2. Causes
      a. Tumors or cysts
      b. Calculi
      c. Infection
      d. Sickle cell disease
      e. Glomerulonephritis
H. Obstruction and stasis
   1. Backflow of urine may occur leading to hydronephrosis
   2. Normal urinary flow blocked or arrested
      a. Prostatic obstruction
      b. Urethral obstruction
      c. Vesicoureteral reflux
      d. Pyelonephritis
      e. Calculi
   3. Contributing causes
      a. Hypercalciuria
         (1) Increased calcium intake
         (2) Increased vitamin D intake
      b. Hyperphosphatemia
      c. Hyperparathyroidism
      d. Gout
      e. Cushing's disease
         (1) Increased cortisol production
         (2) Protein loss in urine
I. Infection
   1. Specific (organisms capable of causing clinical disease)
      a. Tuberculosis
      b. Gonorrhea
      c. Actinomycosis

2. Nonspecific (similar manifestations among several conditions)
   a. Gram-negative rods
   b. Gram-positive cocci
3. Venereal diseases
   a. Gonorrhea
   b. Syphilis
   c. Lymphogranuloma venereum
   d. Granuloma inguinale
   e. Herpes genitalis
   f. Condylomata acuminata

## THE NURSING PROCESS

PACU nursing is a planned process, achieved through a series of integrated steps. The focus in the PACU is on total patient care through a team effort. The nursing process is therefore of key importance. By utilizing the nursing process, PACU nurses focus on the patient, incorporating their skills and knowledge to optimize patient outcomes. Because of the relatively short duration of patient contact, the nurse must adapt this process to the setting.

The nursing process consists of four phases: assessment, planning, intervention, and evaluation. On the basis of the data collected during the assessment phase, a nursing diagnosis is formulated and all pertinent patient information is recorded.

**I. Assessment**

A. Inspect (consistent with observation)
   1. Observe for visible signs of pathologic conditions
      a. Abdomen (kidneys, bladder, lungs)
         (1) Costovertebral fullness
         (2) Distension
         (3) Oxygen perfusion
      b. Penis
         (1) Edema
         (2) Discharge
         (3) Inflammation, rash
         (4) Ulcerations, lesions
      c. Scrotum
         (1) Edema, crepitus
         (2) Discoloration
         (3) Alteration in testicular shape, size, or position
      d. Operative wounds
         (1) Bleeding
         (2) Drainage
         (3) Assess frequently
   2. Interview patient for presence of postoperative sequelae
      a. Collaborate with other perioperative care givers to promote optimum follow-through
      b. Compare findings with preoperative psychosocial assessment
         (1) All patients
            (a) Use comprehensive assessment tools
            (b) Establish presence of preexisting physical impairments and disease processes
            (c) Note allergies and need for ancillary drug therapies
         (2) Pediatric patient
            (a) Age crucial to proper assessment and intervention
            (b) Establish cognitive level of child; note phobias, peculiarities, emotional maturity

        (c) Allow treasured toy or other "security blanket" to be nearby
        (d) Evaluate merit of parental comfort
   c. Expand on preoperative and intraoperative teaching
      (1) Initiate deep breathing, coughing, mobilization
      (2) Explain presence of any invasive devices resulting from operative experience
         (a) Urinary catheters: urge to void, application of traction
         (b) Wound drains
         (c) IV and arterial lines
      (3) Offer medications to control discomfort or agitation frequently
      (4) Alleviate fears of embarrassment because of altered body image
         (a) Promote calming environment
         (b) Provide privacy
         (c) Provide warmth
      (5) Communicate as care is being given to patient
         (a) Wound and drain inspections
         (b) Frequent vital signs
         (c) $O_2$ therapy

B. Auscultate (first step after inspection of urologic patient)
   1. Abdomen
      a. Palpation alters normal peristalsis
      b. Evaluation of bowel sounds important after abdominal and flank surgeries
   2. Lungs
      a. Evaluate presence and character of breath sounds
      b. Absence of sounds may infer blockage of airway or abnormal screening in pleural cavity
   3. Heart
      a. Detection of murmurs or bruits associated with aneurysms and renal artery stenosis
      b. Note rate and character of apical beats

C. Palpate (not part of routine nursing assessment)
   1. Kidneys
      a. Realistic only in thin adult
      b. Normal kidney is firm and smooth
         (1) Tenderness should be expected after renal surgery
         (2) Tenderness or pain may also indicate renal abnormality
      c. Palpate deeply anteriorly as supine patient inhales deeply
         (1) Use left hand for left kidney
         (2) Use right hand for right kidney
      d. Place palm of hand over costovertebral angle posteriorly and deliver light blow
         (1) Necessary for patient to be sitting
         (2) Angle formed by lower thoracic vertebrae and eleventh and twelfth ribs
         (3) Lower poles of kidneys below rib cage bilaterally
            (a) Should be perceived by patient as dull thud
            (b) Sharp tenderness or pain may require further evaluation
   2. Abdomen
      a. Patient should be in supine position
      b. Note any resistance to light palpation over lower abdomen and suprapubic region
         (1) May indicate bladder distension
         (2) May indicate bladder infection
         (3) Pelvic mass may elicit similar reaction
   3. Penis
      a. Palpate shaft with patient in supine position
      b. Note tenderness or nodules
   4. Testes
      a. Determine presence of testis in each hemiscrotum
      b. Testis is oval with C-shaped tube dorsally

c. Should be sensitive to pressure
 (1) Tenderness to light palpation may indicate further evaluation
 (2) Distinct nodules should not be present
5. Prostate gland
 a. Rectal examination with patient in lateral recumbent position
 b. Establish symmetry, smooth consistency, size, contour, and mobility
  (1) Normal size 4 cm
  (2) BPH: symmetric enlargement and boggy consistency common
  (3) Adenocarcinoma: asymmetric enlargement, discrete nodule or lobular induration often
  (4) Inflammation and prostatitis: symmetric enlargement and moderate to extreme tenderness
  (5) Neurologic impairment: inability to tighten anal sphincter common
 c. Urethral secretions may be obtained and analyzed for bacterial infection

D. Percuss
1. Kidneys
 a. Rarely achievable
 b. May be possible on child
2. Bladder
 a. Tympany normal over bladder because of proximity of bowel
 b. Dullness occurs with distension
3. Lungs
 a. Anterior aspects and apices should be resonant
 b. Posterior aspect resonant to ninth rib
 c. Bases reveal gradual transition from resonance to dullness over borders
 d. Bases should move downward 5 to 6 cm on inspiration

E. Review pertinent preoperative diagnostic data
1. Laboratory studies
 a. Urinalysis
  (1) Most fundamental and valuable of all screening methods
  (2) Value dependent on
   (a) Proper specimen collection
   (b) Prompt delivery of specimens
  (3) Components
   (a) pH (4.6 to 8)
   (b) Appearance (color, clarity)
    (i) Normal clarity is clear
    (ii) Normal color is straw to amber
   (c) Odor (aromatic)
   (d) Specific gravity (1.010 to 1.025)
    (i) Infant (1.001 to 1.020)
    (ii) Elderly (values decrease with age)
   (e) Protein (albumin, 0 to 8 mg/dl)
   (f) Glucose (sugar, 0)
   (g) Ketones (0)
   (h) Blood (red blood cells [RBCs], 0 to 2; casts, 0)
   (i) Leukocytes (WBCs, 0)
   (j) Microscopic evaluation
    (i) Casts, crystals, bacteria
    (ii) RBCs, WBCs
 b. Creatinine clearance
  (1) Urine collected for 24 hours
  (2) First AM voiding discarded and first voiding of following morning collected
  (3) Requires refrigeration

c. Urine culture and sensitivities
d. BUN, 10 to 20 mg/dl
   (1) Infant or child, 5 to 18 mg/dl
   (2) Above 100 mg may infer renal function impairment
e. Urine osmolality
   (1) Monitors electrolyte and water balance
   (2) Evaluate dehydration
f. Serum creatinine (0.5 to 1.2 mg/dl)
   (1) Range for females slightly lower
   (2) Above 1.5 mg/dl indicates impairment of renal function
g. Complete blood count (CBC) and differential
h. Serum electrolytes
i. Cholesterol (150 to 200 mg/dl)
j. Coagulation studies (prothrombin time [PT], partial thromboplastin time [PTT], platelets, bleeding time)

2. Diagnostic procedures
   a. Ultrasonography
      (1) Able to focus on particular organ
      (2) Picture of organ displayed on screen
         (a) Measure shape and size
         (b) High-frequency sound waves
      (3) Affected areas alter image by response to sound waves
   b. Intravenous pyelogram (IVP)
      (1) Visualizes entire urinary system through IV administration of contrast dye
      (2) Isolates abnormalities
      (3) Mortality has decreased with use of nonionic dyes
      (4) Dye may prove nephrotoxic when certain abnormalities are present
   c. Renal scan (renal isotope studies)
      (1) Evaluates renal flow and function
      (2) Displays space-occupying lesions
   d. Computed tomography (CT scan)
      (1) Retroperitoneal lymph nodes can be evaluated
      (2) Intraabdominal and prostate abnormalities revealed
   e. Cystogram
      (1) Radiopaque dye instilled into bladder through cystoscopy or catheterization
      (2) Usually performed when reflux is suspected
   f. Retrograde pyelogram
      (1) Done with cystoscopy using radiopaque dye
      (2) Ureters catheterized
   g. Angiograms
      (1) Renal arteries catheterized under fluoroscopy
      (2) Demonstrates integrity of renal circulation and great vessels
      (3) Renal artery stenosis and pheochromocytoma may be identified
   h. Chest x-ray film
   i. Electrocardiogram (ECG)

F. Establish nursing diagnosis based on data retrieval
G. Develop care plan according to findings
H. Implement care using criteria of nursing process
I. Evaluate patient outcomes

**NURSING DIAGNOSIS**

Examples of related nursing diagnostic categories include:

- Fluid volume imbalance
- Altered tissue perfusion
- Alteration in urinary elimination
- Potential for infection
- Electrolyte imbalance
- Disturbance of self-esteem
- Pain
- Impaired pulmonary exchange
- Anxiety
- Potential for positional injury

## OPERATIVE PROCEDURES

Intraoperatively, as well as preoperatively and postoperatively, the overall well-being of the patient is the primary concern. When any surgery is performed, all body functions are in some way affected and must be closely monitored. This section focuses on operative procedures most often encountered and explicit concerns, exclusive to each procedure, that have the greatest impact on the patient's welfare. Many of the alterations in patient status are interrelated.

It is beyond the scope of this chapter to give detailed accounts of the surgical procedures discussed. The reader is urged to consult the Bibliography for more information.

**I. Renal Surgery**

A. Adrenalectomy

1. Purpose or procedure
   a. Correct hypersecretion of adrenal hormones
   b. Remove neoplasms
   c. Secondary treatment of hormonal-dependent carcinomas
      (1) Breast
      (2) Prostate
2. Intraoperative concerns
   a. Damage to liver, pancreas, or spleen
   b. Maintenance of appropriate cortisone levels
   c. Fluid volume imbalance
   d. Inadequate pulmonary perfusion
   e. Hypotension with pheochromocytoma
3. Postanesthesia priorities
   a. Cortisone administration indicated if bilateral
   b. Counteract preoperative antihypertensive agents
   c. IV fluids to maintain blood volume
   d. Alertness to signs of hemorrhage and shock
   e. Maintain adequate pulmonary perfusion
   f. Closely monitor cardiovascular status
   g. Hourly urine and electrolyte values
   h. Increased susceptibility to infection requires strict dressing and drain techniques
   i. Judicious use of narcotics (heightened effect with decreased adrenal function)
4. Psychosocial concerns
   a. Change in lifestyle
   b. Threat of cancer

5. Complications
   a. Hypovolemic and hyponatremic shock
   b. Hemorrhage
   c. Dehydration
   d. Infection

B. Renal transplantation
1. Purpose or procedure
   a. Reverse end-stage renal disease
   b. Transplantation from cadaver or living donor
   c. Includes anastomosis of renal artery of donor organ to hypogastric or common iliac artery of recipient
   d. Kidney placed in pelvic fossa
   e. Continuity of urinary tract established by implanting donor ureter into recipient bladder
2. Intraoperative concerns
   a. Preoperative elimination of potential sources of infection
      (1) Dialysis cannulas
      (2) Bladder infection
      (3) Dental abscesses
      (4) Upper respiratory infection
      (5) Skin conditions
   b. Minimize shock that adversely affects new kidney's function
   c. Control hypertension
   d. Avoid agents metabolized by kidney
   e. Monitor and control electrolyte balance
3. Postanesthesia priorities
   a. Preparation and assembly of patient care supplies
      (1) Blood collection tubes
         (a) CBC
         (b) Clotting factors
         (c) Electrolytes
         (d) BUN
         (e) Creatinine
         (f) Liver enzymes
         (g) Glucose
         (h) Arterial blood gases (ABGs)
      (2) Urine collection containers
      (3) Sterile specimen tubes
      (4) Hemodynamic monitoring equipment
      (5) Intravenous solutions
         (a) D5, ½NS
         (b) D5, ¼NS
         (c) Ringer's lactate
         (d) Plasmanate
         (e) $D_5W$
      (6) Medications
         (a) Furosemide (Lasix)
         (b) Sodium bicarbonate
         (c) Methylprednisolone (hydrocortisone)
         (d) Antihypertensive agents
         (e) Immunosuppressive drugs as per hospital protocol (i.e., cyclosporin A)
      (7) Sterile irrigating solutions and syringes
      (8) Protective isolation measures as per hospital protocol (patient immunosuppressed)

b. Data retrieval
   (1) Establish presence of hepatitis or serum-positive antigens
   (2) Note times of last steroids and antibiotics
c. Monitor all vital signs frequently
   (1) Patients generally hypertensive
   (2) Temperature may fluctuate
d. Monitor central venous pressure lines frequently
   (1) Assess blood volume
   (2) Ensure adequate kidney perfusion
e. Replace crystalloids and colloids
   (1) Urinary output may be massive (especially with living donor kidney)
   (2) Measure urinary output scrupulously and at specified intervals
   (3) Insensible body fluid loss
f. Maintain patency of catheters
g. Initiate pulmonary toilet to combat upper respiratory complications
h. Collect ordered laboratory specimens
   (1) Blood
   (2) Urine
i. Administer medications as indicated
   (1) Steroids
   (2) Antibiotics
   (3) Immunosuppressants
   (4) Antihypertensive agents

4. Psychosocial and interfamily concerns
   a. Patient has undergone extreme physical, mental, and psychologic strain
      (1) Hemodialysis
      (2) Transplant seen as last chance for health
      (3) Fear of rejection
      (4) May display excessive concern about renal function
   b. Nurse will need to maintain inner calm and tolerance
5. Complications
   a. Early onset
      (1) Anuria or oliguria from hypovolemia
         (a) Acute tubular necrosis
         (b) Thrombosis (especially renal artery)
         (c) Operative difficulties
      (2) Hyperacute rejection (immediate nephrectomy mandated)
   b. Delayed onset
      (1) Acute or chronic rejection
      (2) Ureteral obstruction
      (3) Infection
         (a) Constant threat to success of transplant
         (b) Nonpathogenic bacteria and viruses may become opportunistic organisms
      (4) Steroid reaction
         (a) Gastric bleeding or perforation
         (b) Emotional disturbances or altered body image
         (c) Aseptic bone necrosis
            (i) Position and turn patient gently
            (ii) Minimal use of tape on tissue-fine skin
         (d) Nephrotoxicity to cyclosporin A

C. Nephrectomy (radical nephrectomy, nephroureterectomy)
   1. Purpose or procedure
      a. Reasons for removal of kidney
         (1) Malignancy

(2) Extensive renal calculi
(3) Trauma
(4) Renal vascular disease
(5) Infection
(6) Polycystic disease
(a) Medical management and eventual transplant are preferred method
(b) Carcinoma may develop from long-term dialysis, requiring organ removal
b. May include excision of ureter or adrenal gland or both
c. Surgical approaches
(1) Flank or lumbar incision
(2) Transabdominal
(3) Thoracoabdominal
2. Intraoperative concerns
a. Flank and lumbar approaches
(1) Position causes compression of dependent side
(a) Altered pulmonary perfusion
(b) Pressure points on bony prominences
(c) Brachial plexus injuries
(d) Compromise of arterial and venous circulation
(e) Pneumothorax
(2) Potential injury to peritoneum
b. Transabdominal (not commonly used)
(1) Potential injury to liver, pancreas, or spleen
(2) Proximity to aorta and vena cava
(3) Fluid volume and electrolyte depletion
(a) Increased incidence of third space losses with this approach
(b) Altered tissue perfusion
c. Thoracoabdominal approach
(1) Same concerns as flank approach
(2) Dependent lung deflated intraoperatively, requiring postoperative chest tube
3. Postanesthesia priorities
a. Accurate intake and output records
b. Skin integrity
c. Adequate pulmonary perfusion
d. Fluid volume and electrolyte replacement
e. Maintain comfort level
(1) Position on affected side to limit stress on suture line
(2) Pain medication
4. Psychosocial concerns
a. Threat of disease to remaining kidney
b. Anxiety over potential metastases
5. Complications
a. Hemorrhage
b. Atelectasis
D. Extracorporeal shock wave lithotripsy (ESWL)
1. Purpose or procedure
a. Noninvasive treatment modality for obstructive renal stone disease
(1) Involves water bath or water-filled cushions
(2) External shock waves directed at renal and ureteral calculi
(3) Calculi selectively disintegrated
b. Remnants pass in urine through forced diuresis
c. Ureteral stent placed to maintain patency of ureter (not always required)
2. Intraoperative concerns
a. Hemorrhage

   b. Ureteroscopy or percutaneous nephroscopy may be necessary
   c. Maintenance of pulmonary exchange
      (1) General or spinal anesthesia common
      (2) Position may hamper accessibility to patient
3. Postanesthesia priorities
   a. Maintain adequate fluid replacement
   b. Management of postoperative pain
   c. Strain all urine for stone debris (patient to go home with strainer)
4. Psychosocial concerns
   a. Altered body image if nephrostomy tube present
   b. Bruising over areas of shock entry
   c. Anxiety over potential alteration in facial appearance
      (1) Facial edema common following position in sling
      (2) Facial bruising common following position in sling
   d. Anxiety over potential postoperative hematuria
   e. Anxiety about safety of procedure
5. Complications
   a. Hemorrhage
   b. Subcapsular hematoma
   c. Steinstrasse (street of stones, often resulting in obstruction)
   d. Renal colic
   e. Sepsis
   f. Hypertension

E. Ureterolithotomy or nephrolithotomy
1. Purpose or procedure
   a. Surgical removal of large and adherent renal and ureteral calculi
   b. Flank or prone approach
   c. Ureteral stent placed to maintain patency of ureter
2. Intraoperative concerns
   a. Compression of dependent side (see information on nephrectomy)
   b. Hemorrhage
   c. Renal ischemia and parenchymal damage
   d. Hypertension
3. Postanesthesia priorities
   a. Meticulous maintenance of ureteral stents and catheters
   b. Pain management
   c. Adequate pulmonary ventilation
   d. Fluid volume replacement
   e. Intake and output
4. Psychosocial concerns
   a. Fear of developing more stones necessitating further surgery
   b. Often extreme pain postoperatively
5. Complications
   a. Hemorrhage
   b. Occlusion of ureteral and urethral catheters
   c. Paralytic ileus

F. Ureteral reimplantation or dismembered pyeloplasty
1. Purpose or procedure
   a. Repair of ureteral junction obstructions or reflux
   b. Ureter repositioned at newly created hiatus in bladder or renal pelvis
      (1) Abdominal approach for reimplantation
      (2) Flank approach for pyeloplasty
2. Intraoperative concerns
   a. Minimize trauma to involved ureter

- b. Avoid injury to renal vessels
- c. Maintenance of pulmonary and circulatory perfusion in flank position
- d. Strong fixation of ureter
- e. Integrity of ureteral blood supply

3. Postanesthesia priorities
   - a. Management of catheters, drains, and ureteral stents
     - (1) Collection bags labeled
     - (2) All drainage devices properly secured
   - b. Monitor urinary output
     - (1) Separate record for each catheter
     - (2) Assess for blood and sediment
     - (3) All drainage may not equal 30 ml/hr
     - (4) Report any significant drops in output volume
   - c. Administer antibiotics as ordered
4. Psychosocial concerns
   - a. Patients are frequently children
   - b. Concern over long-term prognosis of repair
   - c. Potential for infection high in early stages of recovery
5. Complications
   - a. Infection
   - b. Hemorrhage
   - c. Hydronephrosis
   - d. Hypertension
   - e. Ureteral leak or stricture

G. Ureteroscopy/EHL (electrohydraulic lithotripsy) or laser disintegration of calculi

1. Purpose/procedure
   - a. Diagnose and evaluate patency of ureter
   - b. Removal of obstructing calculi
   - c. Involves rigid or flexible instrumentation
   - d. High volumes of saline irrigation used
2. Intraoperative concerns
   - a. Extravasation of irrigating fluids
   - b. Peripheral vascular circulation
   - c. Ureteral spasm and perforation
   - d. Radiation exposure
3. Postanesthesia priorities
   - a. Monitor electrolyte balance
   - b. Maintenance of stents and catheters
   - c. Pain management
4. Psychosocial concerns
   - a. Recurrence of calculi
   - b. Threat of long-term treatment for retained stone fragments
5. Complications
   - a. Avulsion or perforation of ureter
   - b. Ileus
   - c. Urinoma
   - d. Ureteral stricture
   - e. Alteration in vascular supply to ureter

## II. Genitourinary Surgery

A. Cystoscopy

1. Purpose or procedure
   - a. Evaluation of bladder, urethra, trigone, prostate, and ureteral orifices
   - b. Involves flexible or rigid instrumentation

c. Biopsies may be accomplished
d. Method to instill bladder medications
e. Possible to crush bladder or prostate calculi (litholapaxy)
f. Commonly an outpatient procedure

2. Intraoperative concerns
a. Anesthetic may be local, general, or spinal
b. Bladder perforation, urethral trauma

3. Postanesthesia priorities
a. Catheter patency and output
b. Observe for hemorrhage
c. Monitor for dysuria
d. Unaltered urinary elimination after procedure or catheter removal

4. Psychosocial concerns
a. Fear of cancer
b. Concern about process of urination

5. Complications
a. Incontinence
b. Hemorrhage
c. Bladder perforation
d. Infection

B. Transurethral resection of bladder tumor or bladder neck

1. Purpose or procedure
a. Resection of lesions and contractures
b. Cystoscopy approach

2. Intraoperative concerns
a. Electrocautery safety
b. Peripheral vascular integrity
c. Bladder perforation may lead to extravasation of irrigating fluids (very low incidence)
d. Blood volume and electrolyte balance
e. If laser is used, implementation of appropriate precautions
f. Hypothermia (irrigation warming units)

3. Postanesthesia priorities
a. Catheter patency
b. Continuous irrigation may be indicated
c. Monitor urinary output and character
d. Infection
e. Hypothermia

4. Psychosocial concerns
a. Fear of cancer
b. Fear of recurrence

5. Complications
a. Urinary retention
b. Hemorrhage
c. Electrolyte imbalance

C. Cystectomy (partial/radical)

1. Purpose or procedure
a. Removal of malignancy
b. Radical required when widespread
(1) Involves urinary diversion techniques
(2) Entire bladder removed with lymphadenectomy
(3) Lengthy surgery

2. Intraoperative concerns
a. Abdominal approach
b. Pulmonary and renal function

c. Fluid and electrolyte balance
d. Control of body temperature
3. Postanesthesia priorities
a. Fluid and electrolyte replacement
b. Pulmonary perfusion
c. Catheter maintenance
d. Nasogastric tube or gastrostomy tube may be present
e. Maintenance of wound drains and ureteral stents
4. Psychosocial concerns
a. Altered body image
b. Change in lifestyle
c. Fear of metastases
5. Complications
a. Shock
b. Hemorrhage

D. Urinary diversion
1. Purpose or procedure
a. Divert ureters before or following radical cystectomy, for neuropathic bladder, or noncompliant interstitial cystitis
(1) Diverted to abdominal stoma generally
(2) Newer techniques create neobladder with internal ureteral diversion
(3) Ureteral stents placed to maintain ureteral patency
b. Segment of ileum generally used
c. Various types of diversion
(1) Ileal conduit
(2) Bladder replacement with section of colon, sigmoid, or ileum
(3) Continent diversion (Kock pouch, Indiana pouch)
2. Intraoperative concerns
a. Fluid and electrolyte balance
b. Gastric control
c. Pulmonary and renal function
d. Patient's body temperature
e. Peripheral vascular integrity
3. Postanesthesia priorities
a. Nasogastric or gastrostomy tube
b. Stomal care
c. Maintenance of ureteral stents and catheters
d. Measure intake and output hourly
e. Pulmonary perfusion and peripheral circulation
f. Fluid and electrolyte balance (metabolic acidosis or alkalosis)
g. Pain management
h. Central venous pressure and arterial lines
4. Psychosocial concerns
a. Depression caused by poor body image
b. Prognosis may be poor
5. Complications
a. Distension
b. Mucous plugs
c. Hemorrhage
d. Intestinal leaks, ulcers
e. Infection
f. Stomal necrosis, obstruction, herniation, or fistula
g. Vitamins $B_{12}$, A, and D and iron deficiencies

E. Bladder augmentation
  1. Purpose or procedure
    a. Increase bladder capacity
    b. Neuropathic bladder
    c. Segment of small or large bowel or stomach anastomosed to bladder at dome
  2. Intraoperative concerns
    a. Fecal spills
    b. Fluid and electrolyte balance
    c. Gastric control
  3. Postanesthesia priorities
    a. Nasogastric or gastrostomy tube
    b. Hourly urinary output measurements
    c. Pulmonary perfusion
    d. Peripheral vascular circulation
    e. Fluid and electrolyte imbalance
    f. Urinary catheters and irrigations
  4. Psychosocial concerns
    a. Need for intermittent catheterization
    b. Copious mucous discharge
  5. Complications
    a. Metabolic disorders
    b. Hyperchloremic acidosis
    c. Vitamin $B_{12}$ deficiency
    d. Bladder rupture
    e. Urinary retention

F. Bladder neck suspensions
  1. Purpose or procedure
    a. To correct urinary stress incontinence
    b. Various endoscopic techniques entail lithotomy position
      (1) Raz sling
      (2) Stamey or Pereyra endoscopic suspension procedure
      (3) Pubovaginal sling
      (4) Laparoscopic-modified Burch procedure
    c. Traditional abdominal approach: supine frog-legged or modified lithotomy position
      (1) Marshall-Marchetti-Krantz
      (2) Endoscopy not performed
  2. Intraoperative concerns
    a. Pressure on bony prominences
    b. Peripheral vascular circulation
    c. Bladder perforation
  3. Postanesthesia priorities
    a. Maintenance of urinary catheters
    b. Urinary output
  4. Psychosocial concerns
    a. Fear that procedure will be ineffective
    b. Body image
  5. Complications
    a. Urinary retention
    b. Wound infection
    c. Urinary tract infection
    d. Continued incontinence

G. Artificial urinary sphincter implantation
  1. Purpose or procedure
    a. To correct persistent incontinence and urinary leakage

b. Most often performed on post prostatectomy patient
c. Mechanical device placed around bladder neck or bulbous uretha
(1) Inflation pump in scrotal sac or labia majora
(2) Reservoir placed behind rectus abdominis muscle
2. Intraoperative concerns
a. Maintain body temperature
b. Strict adherence to aseptic technique
c. Prevent urethral damage
3. Postanesthesia priorities
a. Catheter care and maintenance
b. Wound and skin care (skin often raw from persistent leakage of urine)
c. Fluid and electrolyte balance
d. Administration of antibiotics as required
4. Psychosocial concerns
a. Embarrassment
b. Low self-esteem
5. Complications
a. Infection
b. Recurrence of persistent stress incontinence
c. Urinary retention
d. Cuff erosion

H. Pelvic lymph node dissection (lymphadenectomy)
1. Purpose or procedure
a. Histologic staging of prostatic and bladder carcinomas
b. Adjunct surgery for testicular carcinomas
c. Abdominal approach through laparotomy or laparoscopy
d. Nodes along external iliac, obturator, and hypogastric veins removed
e. May include removal of nodes along aorta and vena cava (retroperitoneal lymph node dissection)
2. Intraoperative concerns
a. Bowel perforation or herniation with laparoscope
b. Damage to arteries, veins, nerves
c. Pulmonary perfusion, especially with laparoscopy
d. Increased intraabdominal pressure with laparoscopy (pneumoperitoneum)
e. Hemorrhage
f. Adequate tissue retrieval
3. Postanesthesia priorities
a. Adequate pulmonary perfusion
b. Intraabdominal hemorrhage
4. Psychosocial concerns
a. Fear of cancer and metastases
b. Altered body image related to possible future surgery
c. Anticipation of impotence and sterility
5. Complications
a. Lymphocele
b. Lymph obstruction
c. Ileus
d. Wound infection
e. Pneumonia
f. Retrograde ejaculation
g. Infertility and impotence
h. Scrotal hematoma or pneumoscrotum

I. Prostatectomies
  1. Purpose or procedure
    a. Transurethral resection of prostate (TURP)
      (1) For BPH
      (2) Done endoscopically with resectoscope
      (3) Laser may be incorporated into procedure for ablation of bleeders
    b. Suprapubic
      (1) For BPH when prostate too large to remove endoscopically
      (2) Low abdominal incision to expose and enter bladder
      (3) Enucleation of lateral and medial lobes
    c. Radical (retropubic)
      (1) For carcinoma of prostate (simple retropubic may be done for BPH)
      (2) Abdominal approach to expose and open bladder at urethral juncture with prostate
      (3) Entire gland and seminal vesicles removed, penile vessels ligated
      (4) Nerve-sparing approach has become more common
      (5) Significant blood loss generally involved
    d. Perineal (simple and radical)
      (1) For carcinoma and BPH
      (2) Patient in lithotomy position
      (3) Incision made behind scrotum between ischial fossae
      (4) Blood loss more easily controlled
  2. Intraoperative concerns
    a. TURP
      (1) Fluid and electrolyte balance
        (a) Extravasation or extraperitoneal or intraperitoneal absorption of irrigants (Sorbitol, Glycine)
          (i) Transurethral resection syndrome
          (ii) Newer irrigants have decreased risk
          (iii) Abdominal pain, restlessness, pallor, and diaphoresis often first indicators
        (b) Blood loss
      (2) Cardiac and pulmonary status
        (a) Hypertension or hypotension
        (b) Bradycardia or tachycardia
        (c) Dyspnea
      (3) Pressure on bony prominences because of lithotomy position
      (4) Peripheral vascular circulation
      (5) Perforation of bladder neck, prostatic capsule, or bladder wall
    b. Suprapubic
      (1) Suture line integrity
      (2) Bleeding because of vascular nature of gland
    c. Retropubic (radical and simple)
      (1) Bleeding
      (2) Fluid volume depletion
      (3) Hypothermia
      (4) Cardiac status
      (5) Integrity of urethral anastomosis
      (6) Damage to nerves
    d. Perineal (radical and simple)
      (1) Pressure on bony prominences
      (2) Peripheral vascular perfusion

(3) Integrity of urethral anastomosis
(4) Pulmonary and cardiac status altered by extreme position
(5) Bleeding

3. Postanesthesia priorities (consistent for all; radical and TURP patient at increased risk)
   a. Catheter maintenance and irrigation
      (1) Traction on catheter to promote hemostasis of prostatic fossa
      (2) Observe for occlusion from clots
      (3) Sudden, excessive bleeding could indicate balloon has slipped into prostatic fossa
   b. Urinary output
      (1) Alertness to signs of hemorrhage (pink to frank blood)
      (2) Record hourly output volumes
      (3) Observe for massive diuresis with TURP patient
   c. Fluid or electrolyte replacement
      (1) Evaluate serum osmolality and other pertinent laboratory data
         (a) Hemoglobin and hematocrit
         (b) Potassium
         (c) Sodium
      (2) Decreased sodium values may indicate dilutional hyponatremia (transurethral resection syndrome/water intoxication, TURP patient at increased risk)
         (a) Other hyponatremic signs
            (i) Shortness of breath, hypoxemia
            (ii) Mental disorientation (confusion)
            (iii) Nausea and vomiting
            (iv) Muscle twitch, apprehension
         (b) Treatment
            (i) Furosemide to mobilize edema and diurese excess fluid combined with saline drip
            (ii) Infuse hypertonic saline (3% to 5%) in 100 ml/hr increments for 2 to 4 hours if serum osmolality is low
            (iii) Untreated, transurethral resection syndrome has led to seizures and vascular collapse
   d. Monitor cardiac and pulmonary status
      (1) Sedate to combat restlessness
      (2) Evaluate for hypoxemia
   e. May have nasogastric tube
   f. May have epidural catheter for postoperative pain control
4. Psychosocial concerns
   a. Impotence
   b. Infertility
   c. Fear of metastases
5. Complications
   a. Urinary retention
   b. Incontinence
   c. Fistula formation
   d. Urethral calculi formation
   e. Congestive heart failure or pulmonary edema
   f. Dilutional hyponatremia
   g. Delayed wound healing or infection
   h. Hemorrhage
   i. Transurethral resection syndrome (often manifested in PACU)
   j. Erectile dysfunction
   k. Bladder neck contracture

l. Epididymitis
m. Osteitis pubis

J. Penile implant or penile vein ligation
1. Purpose or procedure
a. Correct erectile dysfunction through implant or venous diversion
b. Techniques for arterial revascularization also being accomplished
2. Intraoperative concerns
a. Infection
b. Hemorrhage
3. Postanesthesia priorities
a. Frequent dressing assessment for hemorrhage
b. Maintenance of urinary catheter
c. Compression dressings with venous ligations
4. Psychosocial concerns
a. Impotence anxiety
b. Loss of self-esteem
5. Complications
a. Wound infection
b. Erosion of implant
c. Mechanical failure of implant
d. Hemorrhage
e. Persistent pain

K. Circumcision
1. Purpose or procedure
a. Correction of constricting foreskin
b. Surgical excision of redundant foreskin
2. Intraoperative concerns
a. Bleeding
b. Suture line integrity
3. Postanesthesia priorities
a. Frequent dressing assessment
(1) Edema
(2) Hemorrhage
b. Ice applications as needed
c. Pain management
4. Psychosocial concerns
a. Embarrassment
b. Loss
5. Complications
a. Excessive scarring
b. Hemorrhage

L. Hypospadias repair or urethroplasty
1. Purpose or procedure
a. Urethral or meatal reconstruction and repositioning
b. Often a staged procedure
c. High percentage are children
2. Intraoperative concerns
a. Urethral damage
b. Infection
c. Peripheral circulation or body temperature
3. Postanesthesia priorities
a. Catheter care and maintenance
b. Monitor urinary output
c. Fluid/electrolyte balance

d. Body temperature
e. Frequent dressing assessment or changes
4. Psychosocial concerns
a. Anxiety (most are children)
b. Parental separation in PACU
5. Complications
a. Infection
b. Urethral stricture
c. Excessive scarring
d. Urinary retention

M. Orchiectomy (radical, simple)
1. Purpose or procedure
a. Removal of diseased testis
b. Scrotal or inguinal approach
c. Adjunct therapy for prostatic carcinoma
d. Radical may include retroperitoneal lymphadenectomy
2. Intraoperative concerns
a. Cardiac dysrhythmias from traction on spermatic cord
b. Hypothermia
c. Hemorrhage
d. Third space losses
3. Postanesthesia priorities
a. Compression dressings
b. Ice packs
c. Catheter and drain care
d. Fluid/electrolyte balance
e. ECG changes
4. Psychosocial concerns
a. Altered body image (loss of manhood)
b. Concern over fertility
c. Concern over sexual ability
5. Complications
a. Hemorrhage
b. Shock
c. Infection

N. Orchidopexy
1. Purpose or procedure
a. Placement of undescended testis in normal anatomic position within scrotum
b. Inguinal approach usually including hernia repair
2. Intraoperative concerns
a. Body temperature (most are small children)
b. Burns
(1) Warming blankets
(2) Prep solutions
(3) Electrocautery
c. Bleeding
3. Postanesthesia priorities
a. Maintenance of traction on testis
(1) May have rubber band attached to leg with tape
(2) May be attached with suture to dental roll on distal aspect of scrotum
b. Titrate small doses of pain remedies as ordered
c. Examine frequently for edema and hemorrhage
d. Ice packs to scrotum

4. Psychosocial concerns
    a. Anxiety separation from parents
    b. Fear of surroundings
    c. Promote calm environment to limit activity of child
5. Complications
    a. Compromise of testicular blood supply
    b. Torsion of spermatic cord
    c. Hemorrhage
    d. Dislodgment of traction device

O. Varicocelectomy or spermatocelectomy
1. Purpose or procedure
    a. Collection of large dilated veins ligated
    b. Commonly in left scrotum
    c. Varicosities affect fertility
    d. Necessary for pain relief
    e. Scrotal or low inguinal incision
    f. May be performed laparoscopically
2. Intraoperative concerns
    a. Damage to companion arteries
    b. Bleeding
3. Postanesthesia priorities
    a. Edema (ice)
    b. Pain (medication)
    c. Hemorrhage (compressive dressings)
4. Psychosocial concerns
    a. Infertility
    b. Concern about long-term pain relief
5. Complications
    a. Scrotal hematoma
    b. Hemorrhage
    c. Continued persistent pain

P. Hydrocelectomy
1. Purpose or procedure
    a. Excision of tunica vaginalis
    b. Expression of excessive accumulation of normal fluid between testis and tunica
    c. Generally scrotal incision
2. Intraoperative concerns
    a. Infection (cultures often done)
    b. Testicular damage
    c. Drain insertion
3. Postanesthesia priorities
    a. Pressure dressings
    b. Assess character and amount of drainage
    c. Scrotal support
    d. Ice to area
        (1) Edema
        (2) Pain
        (3) Hemorrhage
4. Psychosocial concerns
    a. Embarrassment (often young boys and men)
    b. Concern about sexual function
5. Complications
    a. Hematoma
    b. Compromise of testicular blood supply

Q. Detorsion of spermatic cord/testis
  1. Purpose or procedure
    a. Spermatic cord brought into proper position and sutured to scrotal wall
    b. Highest incidence in teenage boys
    c. Bilateral often done to avoid same occurrence in unaffected testis
  2. Intraoperative concerns
    a. Compromise of blood supply to testis
    b. Testicular hypertrophy
  3. Postanesthesia priorities
    a. Observe for sudden severe pain
    b. Maintain compressive dressings
  4. Psychosocial concerns
    a. Anxiety about testicular integrity
    b. Embarrassment
  5. Complications
    a. Hemorrhage (orchiectomy could result if strangulation ensues)
    b. Persistent pain
    c. Sterility

R. Vasectomy
  1. Purpose or procedure
    a. Elective sterilization
    b. Scrotal approach with patient under any type of anesthesia
  2. Intraoperative concerns
    a. Adequate ligation of bilateral vas deferens
    b. Too high a ligation results in extreme chronic pain
  3. Postanesthesia priorities (see information on hydrocelectomy)
  4. Psychosocial concerns
    a. Ambivalence over decision
    b. Fear of impotence
    c. Questionable association with prostate cancer
    d. Concern about continued presence of viable sperm
  5. Complications
    a. Varicocele
    b. Chronic pain
    c. Migration of vas causing reconnection and resumption of fertility

S. Vasovasostomy or epididymovasostomy
  1. Purpose or procedure
    a. To reverse previous vasectomy
    b. To correct stenosis of vas deferens or epididymis
    c. Involves microscopic techniques
  2. Intraoperative concerns
    a. Presence of live sperm cells
    b. Stress on anastomosis because of inadequate length
  3. Postanesthesia priorities
    a. Compression dressings
    b. Assess for bleeding
    c. Ice to control edema
  4. Psychosocial concerns
    a. Desire for fertility
    b. Fear that procedure will not help
  5. Complications
    a. Infection
    b. Fibrosis at anastomosis site

## III. Laparoscopy

A. Recent surgical modality used as alternate operative approach

B. Purpose or procedures
1. Large incisions are avoided
2. Postoperative course tends to be shorter
3. Procedures currently being performed
   a. Nephrectomy, nephroureterectomy
   b. Pelvic lymph node dissection
   c. Bladder neck suspension
   d. Spermatocelectomy, varicocelectomy
   e. Orchidopexy, orchiectomy

C. Intraoperative concerns
1. Improper trocar placement
   a. Subcutaneous emphysema
   b. Preperitoneal insufflation
   c. Vascular injury
   d. Organ perforation
2. Incorrect positioning can lead to peripheral nerve damage
   a. Well-padded bony prominences
   b. Pronated hands
   c. Shoulder braces placed over bony aspects, not soft tissue
   d. Extreme hip or sacral positions done cautiously
3. Cardiac dysrhythmias (bradycardia, premature ventricular contractions, sinus tachycardia)
4. Blood pressure fluctuations (hypotension, hypertension)
5. Central venous pressure irregularities
6. Venous gas embolus caused by needle insertion into blood vessel
7. Hypoxemia from restricted movement of diaphragm or pulmonary blood pooling
8. Aspiration from increased abdominal pressure
9. Pneumothorax if $CO_2$ enters pleural space
10. Pneumoscrotum—most common postoperative complaint

D. Postanesthesia priorities
1. $O_2$ to assist pulmonary exchange
2. Pain management to lessen effects of abdominal distension and muscular soreness from position (patient may experience referred shoulder pain from $CO_2$ mobilization)
3. Frequent vital signs with attention to blood pressure and respiration
4. Monitor urinary output
5. ECG monitor to assess cardiac status

E. Psychosocial concerns
1. Fear of cancer
2. Anxiety over potential internal injury resulting from surgery

F. Complications
1. Fever or peritonitis from bowel perforation
2. Hemorrhage from vessel injury intraoperatively
3. Incisional hernias
4. Ascites, hyponatremia or azotemia from unrecognized bladder perforation
5. Abdominal adhesions caused by excessive manipulation
6. Pneumoscrotum, pneumothorax, lymphocele, or lymph obstruction

## BIBLIOGRAPHY

Bagley DH et al: *Ureteroscopy.* Washington, DC, American Urological Association Office of Education, 1992 (abstract).

Barrett DM et al: *Artificial Urinary Sphincters.* Washington, DC, American Urological Association Office of Education, 1992 (abstract).

Brundage DJ: *Renal Disorders.* St Louis, Mosby–Year Book, 1992.

Chisholm GD, Fair WR: *Scientific Foundations of Urology,* 3rd Ed. Chicago, Year Book Medical Publishers, Inc./Heinemann Medical Books, 1990.

Clayman RV et al: *Laparoscopy.* Washington, DC, American Urological Association Office of Education, 1992 (abstract).

Drain CB: *The Post Anesthesia Care Unit: A Critical Care Approach to Post Anesthesia Nursing,* 3rd Ed. Philadelphia, WB Saunders, 1994.

Gillenwater JY et al: *Adult and Pediatric Urology.* St Louis, Mosby–Year Book, 1991.

Gillenwater JY et al: *Current Practice and Controversies in ESWL.* Washington, DC, American Urological Association Office of Education, 1992 (abstract).

Gray M: *Genitourinary Disorders.* St Louis, Mosby–Year Book, 1992.

Horne MM, Swearingen PL: *Fluid, Electrolytes, and Acid-Base Balance.* St Louis, Mosby–Year Book, 1993.

Lytton B et al: *Intraureteral Disintegration of Urinary Calculi.* Washington, DC, American Urological Association Office of Education, 1992 (abstract).

Marshall FF: *Urologic Complications.* Chicago, Year Book Medical Publishers, 1986.

Meeker MH, Rothrock JC: *Alexander's Care of the Patient in Surgery,* 9th Ed. St Louis, Mosby–Year Book, 1991.

Mulcahy JJ et al: *Complications of Prosthetic Penile Surgery.* Washington, DC, American Urological Association Office of Education, 1992 (abstract).

Nagle GM et al: *Genitourinary Surgery.* St Louis, Mosby–Year Book, 1997.

Pagana KD, Pagana TJ: *Mosby's Diagnostic and Laboratory Test Reference.* St Louis, Mosby–Year Book, 1992.

Tanagho EA, McAninch JW: *Smith's General Urology,* 13th Ed. East Norwalk, Conn, Appleton & Lange, 1992.

## REVIEW QUESTIONS

**1. A characteristic of angiotensin is:**

A. Powerful vasodilation
B. Prevention of aldosterone release
C. Powerful vasoconstriction
D. Lowering of blood pressure

**2. Patients with chronic renal insufficiency are anemic because:**

A. Erythropoietin is not produced in sufficient amounts
B. Renin is not produced in sufficient quantity
C. The glomerulus is unable to properly filter the plasma
D. Aldosterone is secreted in excessive amounts

**3. Azotemia results from an abnormally high level of what metabolite?**

A. Phosphate
B. Urea
C. Potassium
D. Sodium

**4. Aldosterone raises blood volume by:**

A. Causing glomeruli to reabsorb crystalloids
B. Conserving sodium and water
C. Increasing clearance of metabolites
D. Increasing excretion of proteins

**5. Volume shifts may lead to acute renal failure. Which of the following may cause volume shifts?**

A. Vasodilation
B. Malignant hyperthermia
C. Glomerulonephritis
D. Acute tubular necrosis

**6. A condition that contributes to the formation of urinary calculi is:**
A. Acute cystitis
B. Vomiting and diarrhea
C. Interstitial nephritis
D. Hyperparathyroidism

**7. A contributing cause of renal vascular hypertension is:**
A. Proteinuria
B. Embolism
C. Hyperlipidemia
D. Renal artery stenosis

**8. Postoperative nursing care of the urologic patient should always include which of the following?**
A. Maintenance of adequate fluid replacement
B. Monitoring of catheter patency
C. Monitoring of urinary output
D. All of the above

**9. Applying traction to a catheter:**
A. Decreases the need for periodic irrigation
B. Prevents catheter occlusion
C. Creates hemostasis of prostatic fossa
D. Assists monitoring of urinary output

**10. What parameters must be closely monitored in the postoperative cystectomy patient?**
A. Fluid
B. Electrolyte balance
C. Central venous pressure
D. All of the above

**11. The most significant symptom of crisis in the patient with pheochromocytoma is:**
A. Headaches
B. Profuse diaphoresis
C. Severe malignant hypertension
D. Tachycardia

**12. The best indicator of renal fracture is:**
A. Extravasation on IVP
B. Elevated creatinine
C. Extravasation on CT scan
D. Debilitating flank pain

**13. The minimum acceptable urinary output per hour in the adult and child is:**
A. Adult, 50 ml/hr; child, 30 ml/hr
B. Adult, 1 ml/kg/hr; child, 1.5 ml/kg/hr
C. Adult, 1.5 ml/kg/hr; child, 2 ml/kg/hr
D. Adult, 50 ml/hr; child, 40 ml/hr

**14. After laparoscopy, the most commonly observed postoperative complaint is:**
A. Pneumoscrotum
B. Pneumothorax
C. Abdominal distension
D. Cardiac dysrhythmias

**15. What nursing precaution is key in the care of the dialysis patient?**

A. Sterile technique
B. Universal precautions
C. Intake and output monitoring
D. All of the above

**16. Potential sources of infection in the dialysis patient include:**

A. Dialysis catheters
B. Skin lesions
C. Dental abscesses
D. All of the above

**17. TUR syndrome is caused by:**

A. Hyponatremia
B. Hemorrhage
C. Retained prostate chips
D. Hypothermia

**18. When treating post TUR syndrome it is most important to monitor:**

A. ABGs and $O_2$ saturation
B. Serum osmolality and electrolytes
C. Hemoglobin and hematocrit
D. White blood count and urine catecholamines

**ANSWERS:** 1. C, 2. A, 3. B, 4. B, 5. A, 6. D, 7. D, 8. D, 9. C, 10. B, 11. C, 12. C, 13. B, 14. A, 15. D, 16. D, 17. A, 18. B

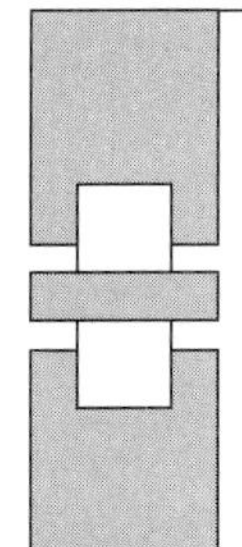

CHAPTER 23

# The Gastrointestinal Surgical Patient

Denise O'Brien, BSN, RN, CPAN, CAPA

## OBJECTIVES

**Study of the information represented by this outline will enable the learner to:**

1. Describe the fluid and electrolyte problems most frequently encountered in the patient with a gastrointestinal disorder.
2. Incorporate the care of the other body systems into the postoperative management of the gastrointestinal surgery patient.
3. Describe two specific system complications of the gastrointestinal surgery patient.
4. State the rationale for placement of tubes and drains in the gastrointestinal surgery patient.
5. State the rationale for observations necessary in postanesthesia care of the patient undergoing gastrointestinal surgery.

The gastrointestinal system is one of the longest systems in the human body, offering many opportunities for pathology. Many operative procedures are performed on this system. The most frequently encountered procedures in the adult population will be discussed. A few references will be made to those pediatric gastrointestinal procedures performed primarily for congenital defects.

## ANATOMY AND PHYSIOLOGY

Before using this review text, the reader will have independently reviewed the anatomy and physiology for this system (Fig. 23–1) and be able to do the following:

1. Correctly name and locate the major anatomic components of the gastrointestinal tract and the accessory organs of digestion
2. Identify the major functions of each of the divisions of the gastrointestinal system and the accessory organs of digestion

## PATHOPHYSIOLOGY

A list of causes of gastrointestinal pathophysiologic conditions follows. The causes are varied, and therefore this list is not inclusive. Examples of disease processes or operative procedures are included parenthetically for clarification.

**I. Neoplasms/growths**

A. Malignancies, either primary or metastatic

B. Polyps: protrusions from mucous membrane

C. Calculi or stones (e.g., cholelithiasis), primarily resulting from supersaturation of bile with cholesterol

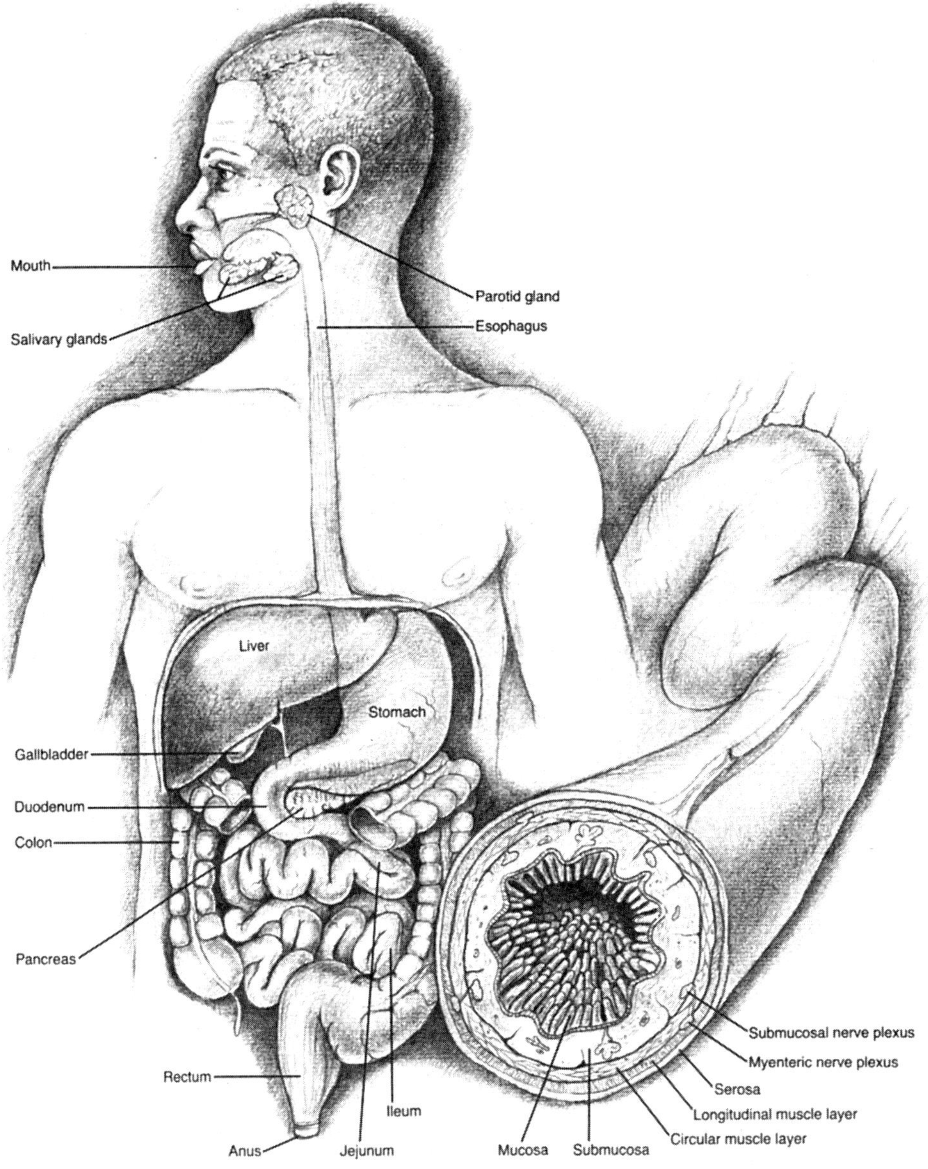


**FIGURE 23–1** The gastrointestinal system. (From Ignatavicius DD, Bayne MV: *Medical-Surgical Nursing,* [p 1221]. Philadelphia, WB Saunders, 1991.)

## II. Strictures or Obstructions

A. Stricture: abnormal narrowing of gastrointestinal passage

B. Obstruction: blockage of gastrointestinal passage

C. Adhesions: union of two normally separate surfaces or a fibrous band that connects them, occasionally producing obstruction or malfunction of an organ

1. Abdominal surgery sometimes results in adhesions of scar tissue

2. Approximately 5% of cases associated with adhesions occur in persons who have had no previous abdominal surgery
   a. Congenital origins
   b. Result of prior inflammatory processes that have resolved without surgical intervention (e.g., pelvic inflammatory disease, diverticulitis, and appendicitis)

## III. Ulceration

A. Ulcer disease
B. Ulcerative colitis (also an inflammatory process)
C. Stress ulceration, resulting from the following:
   1. Surgical stress
   2. Burns
   3. Cranial trauma
   4. Sepsis associated with multisystem failure
   5. Alcohol
   6. Medications (e.g., aspirin, steroids, nonsteroidal antiinflammatory agents [NSAIDs])

## IV. Herniations

A. Incisional
B. Inguinal or femoral
C. Hiatal
D. Umbilical

## V. Perforations

A. Caused by ulceration
B. Resulting from trauma

## VI. Inflammations

A. Regional enteritis (Crohn's disease)
B. Cholecystitis
C. Pancreatitis
D. Appendicitis
E. Diverticulitis
F. Esophagitis
G. Gastritis

## VII. Altered Innervation

A. Acquired megacolon
B. Achalasia
C. Hiatal hernia

## VIII. Congenital Defects

A. Hirschsprung's disease
B. Tracheoesophageal fistula
C. Imperforate anus
D. Pyloric stenosis
E. Arteriovenous malformation

## IX. Ischemia: Arterial or Venous Infarction

A. Complication after abdominal aortic aneurysmectomy
B. After repair of coarctation of aorta
C. After coronary artery bypass

**X. Gastroesophageal Reflux Disease (GERD)**
   A. Symptomatic clinical condition or change in tissue structure
   B. Results from the reflux of stomach or duodenal contents into the esophagus
   C. Symptoms may include heartburn, gastric regurgitation, dysphagia, pulmonary manifestations (asthma, coughing, wheezing, laryngeal inflammation)

## ASSESSMENT PARAMETERS

**I. Diagnostic Tests or Procedures: Tests Ordered Depend on Gastrointestinal Area Thought to be Involved**
   A. Laboratory tests
      1. Basic hematology and electrolyte studies
      2. Serum enzyme levels
      3. Serum markers (e.g., carcinoembryonic antigen)
         a. CA 19-9 for pancreatic cancer
         b. Alpha-fetoprotein (AFP) for hepatocellular cancer
      4. Coagulation studies if liver involvement suspected
      5. Bilirubin studies, liver function tests, alkaline phosphatase
      6. Gastric analysis studies
         a. 24-hour pH monitoring with probe for reflux
      7. Microbiologic studies
      8. Urinalysis
   B. Endoscopic procedures
      1. Motility studies (e.g., esophageal motility studies and manometry)
      2. Esophagoscopy
      3. Gastroscopy
      4. Esophagogastroduodenoscopy (EGD)
      5. Endoscopic retrograde cholangiopancreatography (ERCP), with or without stents
      6. Colonoscopy
      7. Sigmoidoscopy
   C. Radiologic examinations
      1. Barium swallow
      2. Upper gastrointestinal series
      3. Gallbladder series (oral cholecystogram)
      4. Cholangiogram (intravenous and operative)
      5. Percutaneous transhepatic cholangiography
         a. Tubes and stents placed
      6. Barium enema
      7. Flat plate of abdomen
      8. Visceral angiography
         a. $CO_2$ angiography
      9. Chest x-ray film
   D. Scans
      1. Endoscopic ultrasonography
         a. Endoscopic ultrasonography of pancreas and biliary system
      2. Transanal ultrasonography
      3. Computed tomography (CT)
      4. Radionuclide
         a. Gastrointestinal, liver, spleen
         b. Labeled red blood cells (RBCs) to check site of bleeding
         c. Tracer enzymes

5. Magnetic resonance imaging (MRI)
6. Magnetic resonance angiography (MRA)

E. Tissue biopsies as indicated with cytologic studies
F. Laparoscopy, peritoneoscopy
G. Electrocardiogram (ECG) with follow-up evaluation as dictated by medical history and/or physical findings

## OPERATIVE PROCEDURES

Surgical intervention is usually indicated when a medical regimen or conservative therapy is no longer sufficient to alleviate or control the underlying gastrointestinal pathophysiologic condition. Some of the more frequently encountered surgical procedures will be briefly defined.

**I. Esophageal Procedures**

A. Cervical esophagostomy
  1. Purpose: often done as part of first-stage repair for tracheoesophageal fistula or esophageal atresia repair in infants
  2. Description: surgical formation of opening into esophagus at cervical level

B. Colon or gastric tube interposition
  1. Purpose: used in presence of esophageal atresia or after severe distal esophageal damage
  2. Description: usually a piece of colon is used to establish continuity between esophagus and stomach

C. Esophageal dilation
  1. Purpose: to allow freer passage of food and fluids into stomach; used to correct achalasia, esophageal spasms, and strictures
  2. Description: dilating instruments (bougies) passed in increasingly larger sizes to enlarge lumen of esophagus

D. Pneumatic or balloon dilation
  1. Purpose: to relieve or reduce esophageal obstruction caused by strictures
  2. Description: inflatable dilators inserted through instrument channel of endoscope and then passed into stricture, where balloon is gradually inflated

E. Esophagomyotomy (Heller procedure)
  1. Purpose: to allow food to pass from esophagus to stomach when a segment of esophagus is narrowed, causing functional obstruction
  2. Description: surgical division or anatomic dissection of muscles at distal esophagogastric junction, leaving mucosa intact

F. Herniations: surgical repair of hiatal, esophageal, or diaphragmatic hernias accomplished through either an abdominal or a thoracic approach; herniation is part of stomach protruding through an opening, or hiatus, in diaphragm
  1. Purposes
     a. To restore herniated part below diaphragm
     b. To narrow esophageal hiatus
     c. To recreate esophagogastric angle to enhance lower esophageal sphincter (LES) function
     d. To stop reflux of gastric contents
  2. Description
     a. Collis-Belsey and Collis-Nissen repairs: esophageal lengthening with antireflux wrap of distal esophagus
     b. Hill repair: abdominal approach that narrows esophageal orifice and fixes esophagogastric junction in intraabdominal position; includes 180-degree wrap of stomach around esophagus

c. Belsey Mark IV repair: performed through incision in left side of chest; consists of 240-degree wrap of distal portion of esophagus with fundus of stomach; this partial fundoplication is technically difficult, and risk of leakage or diverticulum developing in esophagus is higher because sutures are required in esophageal wall; newer procedure: modified thoracoscopic Belsey repair
d. Nissen fundoplication: transabdominal or laparoscopic (similar to open approach) treatment for sliding esophageal hiatal hernia; a portion of fundus of stomach is mobilized and completely wrapped around (360 degrees) distal portion of esophagus to prevent stomach displacement into posterior portion of mediastinum through diaphragmatic defect
e. Toupet partial fundoplication: alternative antireflux procedure; the fundal wrap is reduced to 180 to 200 degrees

G. Sclerotherapy of esophageal varices
1. Purpose: to obliterate esophageal varices to reduce risk of bleeding or hemorrhage
2. Description: endoscopic procedure involving injection of a sclerosing agent (e.g., sodium morrhuate) into or around varices in esophagus

## II. Gastric Procedures

A. Gastrectomy
1. Purpose: to remove all or a portion of diseased organ
2. Description: surgical removal of whole or a part of stomach
a. Antrectomy: involves almost a 50% distal gastrectomy; antral mucosa (site of gastrin formation) is removed, usually in conjunction with truncal vagotomy; remaining portion of stomach is anastomosed to duodenum; may be combined with pyloroplasty
b. Billroth I (gastroduodenostomy): removal of pylorus of stomach and duodenum with anastomosis of stomach to proximal jejunum
c. Billroth II (gastrojejunostomy): removal of pylorus of stomach and duodenum with anastomosis of upper portion of stomach and proximal portion of jejunum
d. Total gastrectomy: usually done for cancer of stomach or abdominal esophagus; reconstruction after total gastrectomy is usually by esophagojejunostomy
e. Near total gastrectomy: may be done for treatment of gastroparesis
f. Roux-en-Y gastrojejunostomy: bypass procedure indicated for cancer of pancreas

B. Gastric bypass operation
1. Purpose: performed for morbid obesity
2. Description: lower 90% to 95% of stomach is stapled off, allowing only upper 5% to 10% of stomach to receive food; upper stomach is anastomosed by an approximately 1 cm opening to jejunum to allow intestinal absorption and elimination of food

C. Gastric stapling or partitioning operation
1. Purpose: performed for morbid obesity
2. Description: stomach is divided with staples into larger lower section (90% to 95% of stomach) and small upper section; 1 cm opening is left in staple line, usually at edge of stomach, to allow food to pass slowly from upper section into lower section
3. May have to later convert to gastric bypass for failed staple lines

D. Vertical-banded (Mason) gastroplasty
1. Purpose: performed for morbid obesity
2. Description: window is made with staples near lesser curve of stomach and a row of staples is placed vertically from this window to greater curved side of esophagogastric junction; Marlex band is placed around stomach from lesser curve to window to control gastric outlet size

E. Gastroenterostomy
1. Purpose: to create an artificial passage between stomach and small intestine
2. Description: surgical anastomosis between stomach and small intestine, usually jejunum

F. Gastrostomy
   1. Purpose: used for long-term stomach decompression or to introduce food into gastrointestinal system
   2. Description: creation of gastric fistula or opening through abdominal wall

G. Percutaneous endoscopic gastrostomy
   1. Purpose: endoscopic procedure performed with local anesthesia for patients who are poor risks for laparotomy or general anesthesia (e.g., patients with closed head injuries, stroke, or head or neck cancers) for feeding or decompression
   2. Description: insertion of gastrostomy tube through incision made at point where anterior portion of stomach wall is tented with endoscope, making contact with parietal peritoneum; traction on tube maintains contact between stomach and abdominal wall

H. Pyloromyotomy
   1. Purpose: to widen pyloric opening
   2. Description: muscle fibers of outlet of stomach are cut without severing mucosa

I. Pyloroplasty
   1. Purpose: to increase size of pyloric opening in presence of pyloric stenosis or scarring caused by ulcer disease; usually performed in conjunction with vagotomy when done for latter
   2. Description: repair of pylorus used to establish opening in presence of pyloric or prepyloric obstruction

J. Vagotomy
   1. Purpose: to reduce amount of gastric acid secreted and lessen chance of recurrence of gastric ulcer
   2. Description: sectioning of vagus nerve or its branches; choices of vagotomy include truncal, selective, superselective, or parietal cell vagotomy; may be accomplished by laparoscopic approach

### III. Biliary, Hepatic, and Pancreatic Procedures

A. Surgical correction of biliary atresia (condition in which extrahepatic bile ducts are nonpatent, seen primarily in infants)
   1. Roux-en-Y procedure
      a. Purpose: used when proximal extrahepatic bile ducts are patent and distal ducts are occluded; for bypass in cancer of bile duct and pancreatitis
      b. Description: distal end of divided jejunum is anastomosed to patent remnant of proximal bile duct
   2. Hepatic portoenterostomy (Kasai procedure)
      a. Purpose: used when proximal extrahepatic ducts are totally occluded
      b. Description: removal of entire extrahepatic biliary tree; bile drainage is established by anastomosis of intestinal conduit to transected ducts at liver hilus

B. Cholecystectomy
   1. Purpose: to treat cholelithiasis and cholecystitis
   2. Description: removal of gallbladder and its cystic duct; may be through traditional "open" approach or by laparoscopy; laparoscopic approach may use laser, electrosurgical cautery or harmonic scalpel to remove gallbladder from liver bed and ligate vessels and ducts

C. Cholecystostomy
   1. Purpose: to decompress gallbladder of debilitated patient with acute cholecystitis or cholelithiasis unable to tolerate cholecystectomy at that time
   2. Description: formation of opening into gallbladder through abdominal wall; if stones are present, approach may be by angiography with lithotripsy to break up stones

D. Choledochotomy
   1. Purpose: usually for removal of stones
   2. Description: incision of common bile duct

E. Common bile duct exploration
   1. Purpose: to check for stones and/or strictures; frequently performed at time of cholecystectomy
   2. Description: exploration of common bile duct; T-tube drain is left in place for a period of time postoperatively to ensure patency of common bile duct; can use laparoscopic approach

F. Hepaticojejunostomy
   1. Purpose: to repair stricture of common bile duct after laparoscopic or open cholecystectomy; may also be done for patients with bile duct cancer
   2. Description: creation of anastomosis between hepatic duct and jejunum

G. Portal systemic shunt
   1. Purpose: primarily used for treatment of portal hypertension and decompression of esophagogastric varices; increasing use of transjugular intrahepatic portosystemic shunt procedures reducing the number of older shunt procedures
   2. Description: shunts divert, either partially or totally, venous blood flow to liver; types of shunts include end-to-side, side-to-side, interposition, Sarfeh portacaval; interposition (adult) or direct (pediatric) mesocaval; distal splenorenal, mesoatrial (Budd-Chiari syndrome management). Occasionally, Sugiura procedures (combines esophageal transection, extensive esophagogastric devascularization, and splenectomy, while para-esophageal collateral vessels are preserved) are done for varices in patients who are not candidates for other types of shunt procedures

H. ERCP with sphincterotomy
   1. Purpose: to remove retained common duct stones after biliary tract surgery, for patients with multisystem disease who are poor risks for surgery, or as an emergency measure in patients with common bile duct obstruction (single or multiple stones) resulting in cholangitis; may be done preoperatively to explore common bile duct in patients needing laparoscopic cholecystectomies
   2. Description: by use of side-viewing fiberoptic endoscope, pancreatic, biliary, and hepatic ducts are cannulated through ampulla of Vater and visualized fluoroscopically after retrograde injection of radiopaque contrast medium

I. Hepatectomy: excision of all or part of liver; increasing use of segmentectomies and wedge resections for patients with liver metastases; cryotherapy also used to treat liver cancer

J. Hepatic lobectomy: surgical removal of one of four lobes of liver; may be accomplished with total vascular occlusion intraoperatively

K. Hepatoduodenostomy (hepaticoduodenostomy): establishment of opening from liver into duodenum

L. Peritoneovenous shunts (e.g., LeVeen or Denver)
   1. Purpose: used in an attempt to control ascites by reinfusing peritoneal fluid into venous system; patients with limited hepatic reserve who may not tolerate blood being shunted away from liver are candidates
   2. Description: unidirectional silicone elastomer valve and catheter are inserted into peritoneum; other end is tunneled subcutaneously up to neck and inserted into internal jugular vein and then threaded into superior vena cava or right atrium

M. Liver transplant
   1. Purpose: replacement of diseased liver with donor liver
   2. Description: effective approach for treatment of liver failure of various causes because of development of improved surgical techniques, venous bypass method, and newer antirejection agents

N. Pancreatectomy
   1. Purpose: to treat necrosis, abscess, pseudocysts, or intractable pain from injury or pancreatitis
   2. Description: partial resection or total removal of pancreas; total removal results in diabetes and other metabolic difficulties; may use jejunal loop to drain

O. Pancreaticoduodenectomy (Whipple's procedure)
   1. Purpose: to treat cancer of head of pancreas and for resectable localized cancers of ampulla, distal common bile duct, or duodenum
   2. Description: removal of proximal portion of pancreas, adjoining duodenum, lower portion of stomach, gallbladder, and common bile duct
P. Cystogastrostomy, cystoduodenostomy, cystojejunostomy
   1. Purpose: to treat pancreatic pseudocysts that do not disappear spontaneously
   2. Description: decompressive procedures for internally draining pseudocysts that are fixed to retrogastric area or duodenum or not in proximity to either stomach or duodenum
Q. Pancreas transplant
   1. Purpose: to treat diabetes mellitus
   2. Description: donor pancreatic tissue transplanted into recipient, achieved through various techniques: whole organ or segmental graft, with duct management either occluded or drained into a hollow viscus
R. Splenectomy or splenorrhaphy
   1. Purpose: to treat traumatic injuries to spleen, thrombocytopenic purpura refractory to other treatment, anemias, and myeloproliferative disorders (e.g., leukemia)
   2. Description: excision or repair of spleen, either by open or by laparoscopic approach
S. Transjugular intrahepatic portosystemic shunt (TIPS)
   1. Purpose: definitive treatment for patients who bleed from portal hypertension; major limitation: up to 50% have shunt stenosis or shunt thrombosis within the first year; may be ideal therapy for patients needing short-term portal decompression (those awaiting liver transplantation who fail sclerotherapy)
   2. Description:
      a. Nonoperative, functions like a side-to-side portosystemic shunt (effective in treating ascites), adverse side effects include total portal diversion and encephalopathy
      b. Procedure: a needle is advanced from a hepatic vein to a major portal branch and a guide wire is placed; a hepatic parenchymal tract is created by balloon dilation and an expandable metal stent is placed, creating the shunt

## IV. Small Intestine

A. Duodenojejunostomy: creation of opening or passage from obstructed or stenosed duodenum into jejunum
B. Feeding jejunostomy
   1. Purpose: to allow access for alimentation in presence of functioning gastrointestinal tract
   2. Description: permanent opening or fistula into jejunum through abdominal wall
C. Ileostomy
   1. Purpose: created after total proctocolectomy for Crohn's disease or ulcerative colitis or less frequently for multiple colorectal carcinomas, familial polyposis coli, ischemia, trauma, and congenital anomalies where colon remains intact
   2. Description: creation of passage through abdominal wall into ileum
D. Continent ileostomy (Kock's pouch or Barnett continent intestinal reservoir)
   1. Purpose: to create a reservoir for feces after total proctocolectomy
   2. Description: construction of an intestinal reservoir created by joining a loop of terminal ileum and forming a nipple valve; after healing is complete, patient controls expulsion of feces and gas by emptying reservoir/pouch with catheter
E. Roux-en-Y anastomosis: diverting procedure where two anastomoses are constructed, creating Y shape in intestines
   1. Biliary Roux-en Y: choledochojejunostomy and jejunojejunostomy
   2. Gastric Roux-en-Y: gastrojejunostomy and jejunojejunostomy

F. Small bowel resection
   1. Purpose: to treat trauma, mesenteric thrombosis, regional enteritis, radiation enteropathy, strangulated small bowel obstruction, neoplasm, congenital atresia, or enterocutaneous fistulas
   2. Description: excision of varying lengths of small intestine; profound consequences with resection of more than 75% of small intestine (e.g., "short gut" syndrome)

## V. Colon or Large Intestine

A. Abdominoperineal resection
   1. Purpose: generally performed for cancer of rectum
   2. Description: two-step surgical procedure in which anus, rectum, and sigmoid colon are removed en bloc; through incision extending from pubis to above umbilicus, a segment of lower bowel is mobilized and divided; proximal end is exteriorized through separate stab wound as a single-barreled colostomy or ileostomy; distal end is pushed into hollow of sacrum and rectum is removed through perianal route
B. Appendectomy
   1. Purpose: to remove inflamed or perforated appendix or as prophylactic measure at time of other abdominal surgery
   2. Description: excision of vermiform appendix normally performed through incision in right lower quadrant of abdomen; may also be performed by laparoscopic technique
C. Cecostomy
   1. Purpose: temporary measure to relieve obstruction distal to cecum
   2. Description: construction of opening into cecum
D. Colectomy
   1. Purpose: to treat tumors, bleeding, inflammation, or trauma of large intestine
   2. Description: surgical removal of all or part of colon
E. Restorative proctocolectomy (total proctocolectomy with ileal reservoir and anal anastomosis)
   1. Purpose: to provide nearly normal bowel function while removing need for abdominal stoma; used for selected patients with ulcerative colitis or familial polyposis coli
   2. Description: pouch made from terminal ileum is created and then anastomosed to rectum at or just above dentate line; J-shaped ileoanal or larger W-shaped reservoir is most common, also S-shaped
F. Colostomy
   1. Purpose: incision of colon to create fistula between bowel and abdominal wall
   2. Description: either temporary or permanent; placement of ostomy site is individualized; location depends on pathologic condition involved (e.g., transverse colostomy, sigmoid colostomy) and patient's anatomy and lifestyle; mucous fistula may also be created for decompression of cancer-caused obstruction of lower colon
G. Herniorrhaphy
   1. Purpose: to reduce or repair hernias; may be inguinal, femoral, umbilical, incisional, or ventral in origin
   2. Description: approach may be open or laparoscopic; prosthesis of polypropylene mesh or fabric (Marlex) may cover weakened area to secure and prevent recurrence, especially for larger incisional, ventral, and inguinal hernias; incarcerated or irreducible hernias may become strangulated, necessitating emergent repair
H. Omphalocele (excision): rare defect of periumbilical abdominal wall seen primarily in premature infants; omphalocele sac may contain small and/or large bowel, liver, or spleen
   1. Primary closure
      a. Purpose: used for omphaloceles with small abdominal defects
      b. Description: omphalocele sac is excised and abdominal wall muscles and skin edges are reapproximated
   2. Staged repair
      a. Purpose: used for large omphaloceles

b. Description: omphalocele is encased in silicone elastomer mesh sack that is sutured in place around defect; viscera are gradually moved into abdominal cavity in stages

I. Polypectomy
1. Purpose: to remove isolated colonic polyps
2. Description: using snare and electrocautery, polyps are removed endoscopically; large polyps may require open colectomy

**VI. Rectal and Anal Procedures**

A. Low anterior resection
1. Purpose: to treat malignancies of rectosigmoid area
2. Description: rectum-containing tumor is excised; rectal stump and proximal bowel are anastomosed either with suture or with staples; drains are generally placed and exit through abdomen

B. Transanal excision of polyps or masses
1. Purpose: to remove polyps or masses from the anal or rectal areas
2. Description: excision of polyps or masses using an anal approach

C. Anal fissurectomy
1. Purpose: to treat chronic anal fissures not responding to medical treatment or anal dilation
2. Description: scarred anal tissue that originates from rectal tear that was infected or ulcerated is excised; concomitant anal sphincterotomy and/or hemorrhoidectomy may be done

D. Anal sphincterotomy
1. Purpose: to treat severe anal stenosis
2. Description: cutting of anal sphincter; anoplasty normally is required to reestablish anal tissue and mucosal integrity

E. Anal fistulotomy or fistulectomy
1. Purpose: to treat, by either incision or excision, fistulous tracts in anal canal
2. Description: infection of anal duct gland creates fistula in ano, which may be incised and drained or excised and packed to heal by granulation

F. Hemorrhoidectomy
1. Purpose: excision of hemorrhoids usually done to relieve severe pain or chronic bleeding that does not respond to cortisone suppository treatment or for repeated thrombosis
2. Description: hemorrhoids may be ligated by use of rubber band slipped over varicosity, causing tissue necrosis and sloughing of hemorrhoid in approximately 1 week; usually little or no anesthesia is required; surgical treatment consists of clamping and excision by scalpel, cautery, or laser; anesthesia may be local, regional, or general

G. Duhamel and Soave procedures
1. Purpose: to treat Hirschsprung's disease in children
2. Description: in both Duhamel and Soave procedures, aganglionic bowel is resected and proximal, healthy colon is pulled through and anastomosed to anus

H. Pilonidal cystectomy
1. Purpose: to prevent recurrence of infection and abscess formation in pilonidal sinus
2. Description: excision of entire cyst wall and sinus tracts, removing necrotic tissue, debris, hair, etc.; wound may be packed open, closed, or closed with tissue flaps

## INTRAOPERATIVE CONCERNS

**I. Proper Positioning**

A. Maintain neurovascular integrity
1. Padding and support of all body parts with particular attention given to vulnerable areas (e.g., elbows, sacrum, heels, occiput)

2. For comfort
3. To maintain proper alignment in presence of arthritis, lumbar disorders, and contractures
4. To preserve integrity of popliteal nerve and/or ulnar/brachial nerve plexi when lithotomy or exaggerated arm abduction is used

B. Prevent complications
1. Proper application of electrosurgical grounding pads to prevent cautery burns; avoid contact with metal or hard surfaces
2. Careful positioning changes of anesthetized patient (to and from Trendelenburg's or lithotomy position) to prevent adverse alterations in tidal volume and cardiac output; position of padding and support rechecked after each change
3. Protect skin from shearing while positioning and moving

**II. Cardiovascular Stability**

A. Factors influencing altered fluid volume, electrolyte, and nutritional status
1. Chronic bleeding
2. Diarrhea
3. Vomiting
4. Increased secretions
5. Fluid loss: nasogastric suctioning, fistula drainage, bowel preparation, and length of operative procedure

B. Problems with preceding factors if not corrected preoperatively
1. Hypotension: caused by deficits in circulating volume
   a. Poorly tolerated in pediatric, elderly, and debilitated patients vulnerable to adverse effects of hypotension as result of decreased body reserve necessary to handle crises
   b. Rapid fluid (blood) loss is potential problem as result of rich intestinal blood supply and its proximity to aorta and vena cava
   c. Rapid fluid resuscitation with crystalloid or colloid solution can result in overhydration, leading to pulmonary edema and congestive heart failure in compromised patient
2. Altered electrolyte balance: cardiac dysrhythmias can occur with abnormal potassium or calcium levels
3. Clotting abnormalities caused by poor nutritional status or hemodilution or in presence of liver disease
   a. Decreased vitamin K, leading to decreased levels of factors V, VII, IX, and X
   b. Prolonged prothrombin times

**III. Thermal Regulation**

A. Hyperthermia
1. Elevated temperature on arrival in the operating room, possibly as a result of infection, peritonitis, or other inflammatory process
2. Anesthesia care provider must observe for signs and symptoms of possible adverse reaction to anesthetic agents and muscle relaxants, which may lead to malignant hyperthermia, either in operating room or in postanesthesia care unit (PACU) (see Chapter 17)

B. Hypothermia
1. Prolonged exposure of abdominal viscera causes loss of body heat leading to hypothermia
   a. Procedures of 3 or more hours
   b. Extensive gastrointestinal resection
2. Temperature-control methods
   a. Room temperature control
   b. Use of warming mattresses, convective warming devices, and protective coverings
   c. Warming of IV and irrigating fluids

**IV. Drug Interactions and Other Concerns**

A. Nondepolarizing muscle relaxants (see Chapter 9)
1. Antagonized by hypothermia
2. Patients may "re-curarize" with postoperative warming
3. May have slowed return of neuromuscular function because of hypothermia and decreased elimination of some relaxants (those eliminated by Hoffman elimination [ester hydrolysis])
4. Potentiated by broad-spectrum antibiotics (mycins, aminoglycosides)

B. Metabolism and excretion of medications impaired in presence of liver dysfunction, renal failure, and obesity

C. Avoidance of use of histamine-releasing agents such as morphine sulfate and curare is important consideration in certain patients
1. Histamine release can cause hypotension in hypovolemic patient
2. Morphine sulfate can cause spasm of sphincter of Oddi, producing severe right upper quadrant or substernal pain in patient with biliary obstruction or disease
   a. Especially noticeable when administered preoperatively
   b. Severity of symptoms (pain, nausea, diaphoresis, hypotension) require that myocardial infarction be ruled out
   c. Symptoms usually abate with administration of naloxone (Narcan) to reverse morphine sulfate

D. Rapid sequence induction ("crash" induction): possible indications
1. History of gastroesophageal reflux
2. Stricture of gastroesophageal sphincter
3. History of recent eating before emergency surgery
4. Bowel obstruction
5. History of gastroparesis

E. Spillage of feces or bile into peritoneal cavity is potential cause of chemical or bacterial peritonitis and should be documented

## POSTANESTHESIA CARE

### NURSING DIAGNOSIS

Examples of related nursing diagnostic categories include:
- Altered peripheral tissue perfusion
- Altered gastrointestinal tissue perfusion
- Urinary retention
- Altered nutrition: less than body requirements
- Ineffective airway clearance
- Ineffective breathing pattern
- Pain
- Fluid volume deficit related to surgical procedure
- Altered health maintenance related to lack of knowledge of surgical procedure and postoperative care

**I. Assessment and Patient History to Determine Nursing Priorities**

A. Preliminary ABCs
1. Airway
2. Breathing
3. Circulation

B. Patient record and report from perioperative nurse and anesthesia care provider
   1. Demographic data on patient
   2. Preoperative hematocrit, other blood values
   3. Preoperative vital signs: blood pressure, pulse, respirations, oximetry saturation, and temperature
   4. Preoperative medication history
   5. Operative procedure
   6. Anesthetic agents, narcotics, and sedatives administered preoperatively and intraoperatively
   7. Neuromuscular blocking agents administered
   8. Reversal agents administered
   9. Intake and output: estimated blood loss, colloid/crystalloid plasma expanders, blood products received, urine output, other measurable fluid losses (peritoneal, gastric, etc.)
   10. Other intraoperative medications (antibiotics, digoxin, lidocaine, diuretics, etc., with times given)
   11. Types of drains in place
   12. American Society of Anesthesiologists (ASA) classification of patient
   13. Allergies and sensitivities (medications, physical agents)
   14. Brief history, physical limitations, sensory and communication barriers
   15. Pain assessment scale appropriate for patient (developmental stage and level of education)

**II. Observation and Care***

A. Cardiovascular system
   1. Monitor vital signs per unit routine; check perfusion to extremities
      a. Risk for radical shifts in body fluids as result of inadequate fluid replacement, excessive replacement, preoperative status, presence of fistula, vomiting, diarrhea, intestinal obstruction, third spacing, nasogastric drains and tubes
      b. Sequestered fluid in gastrointestinal tract (resulting from tumor, stricture, adhesions, paralytic ileus, or surgical manipulation) is lost to circulating volume of body; it is in a potential or "third" space; in general, third-space fluid does not begin to mobilize until second or third postoperative day
      c. Stress responses resulting in hormonal alterations can lead to retention of fluids and potential for fluid overload postoperatively
   2. Observe for hemostasis; observe for and document coagulation deficiencies (oozing, bruising, and petechiae)
      a. In a patient with a history of coagulation problems or one who has received massive transfusions, coagulation difficulties can occur; malabsorption, impaired digestion, or altered liver function will affect clotting
   3. Leg exercises, range of motion (ROM) at least every hour as part of "stir-up" regimen; antiembolism stockings, sequential compression devices or low-dose anticoagulation as ordered
      a. Deep vein thrombosis (DVT) formation is potential complication of immobility; laparoscopic procedures increase risk of emboli as result of air insufflation; active ROM exercises stimulate venous return from extremities

B. Genitourinary system
   1. Monitor intake and output every hour and specific gravity every 4 hours
      a. Potential for decreased urine output as result of fluid shifts (see information on cardiovascular system)
   2. Assess bladder distension if no indwelling catheter in place
      a. Bladder distension is common postoperative problem

---

*Rationale(s) given for each intervention

3. Note color of urine
   a. Retraction or pressure placed on bladder or kidney during surgery can traumatize bladder or kidney

C. Endocrine system
   1. Document blood glucose levels, urine glucose, and ketones as appropriate
      a. Surgical intervention and operative stress on body systems alter pancreatic enzymes and insulin production
         (1) Diabetic patients are observed for same reasons
         (2) Blood glucose can be monitored with blood glucose monitor (Chemstix or glucometer) at bedside

D. Respiratory system
   1. Document routine postanesthesia nursing interventions ("stir-up" or "wake-up" regimens) and their results concerning lung auscultation, deep breathing, incentive spirometry, coughing to mobilize and expectorate secretions, turning, and ROM exercises
      a. Prevention of decreased lung expansion leading to atelectasis, congestion, and hypostatic pneumonia resulting from oversedation or lack of sedation, hypoxia, fluid overload, decreased ventilatory excursion
   2. If central line (CVP or pulmonary artery catheter) is placed intraoperatively or in PACU, obtain chest film
      a. Demonstration of correct catheter placement and confirmation of presence or absence of pneumothorax
   3. Document chest drainage and chest tube function
      a. Follow PACU routine for care of chest tubes for patients undergoing pulmonary approach for upper gastrointestinal surgery (esophageal resection, hiatal herniorrhaphy)

E. Gastrointestinal system
   1. NPO (nothing by mouth)
      a. Nausea and vomiting may be present because of effects of anesthesia, decreased intestinal motility, malfunctioning nasogastric tube, and disease process
   2. Nasogastric tube assessment
      a. Check for proper tube placement by auscultating with stethoscope over gastric area while inserting 20 to 50 cc air into tube
         (1) If nasogastric tube was placed intraoperatively under direct visualization, check with surgeon before irrigating or repositioning; if tube is properly placed, rush of air should be heard
      b. Secure tube to nares with correct taping technique
         (1) Taping or securing tube properly decreases risk of necrosis or damage of nares and inadvertent dislodgment of tube
   3. Maintain patency of nasogastric or gastrostomy tube
      a. To decrease tension on gastric suture line
      b. Notify surgeon of excessive drainage from tubes or drains so that IV fluid and rates can be adjusted; initial 24-hour drainage is bloody changing to dark serosanguineous to bile colored over the next 24 to 72 hours
   4. Irrigation or manipulation of nasogastric tubes
      a. Do not irrigate or manipulate nasogastric tube unless specifically ordered
         (1) Nasogastric tube lies close to anastomosis (gastric resection, some pancreatic procedures involving stomach)
      b. Check, if nasogastric tube to dependent drainage, for proper securing of tube to eliminate manipulation
         (1) Nasogastric tube may be used as stent anastomosis in esophageal procedures
      c. Notify surgeon if nasogastric tube is accidentally removed or becomes displaced
         (1) Attempts to replace tube can result in esophageal perforation

5. Assess abdominal girth (abdominal distension) and auscultate bowel sounds
   a. Anastomotic leak, hemorrhage, malfunctioning nasogastric tube, ileus, and mechanical obstruction may cause abdominal distension, nausea, and vomiting
6. Observe and document status of stoma color and drainage from stoma and position of stoma to skin; notify surgeon of any sudden or progressive change in stoma color
   a. Altered color may indicate increasing edema leading to decreased circulation or generalized poor circulation to bowel
   b. Maintain patency of decompression tube after creation of continent ileostomy; gently irrigate pouch with normal saline solution (30 ml every 3 hours is commonly ordered)
      (1) Surgically created pouch is fragile because of many anastomoses until healed and matured

F. Dressings and drains
1. Document dressing status every hour or as needed
   a. Keeping dressing dry promotes wound healing by minimizing potential breeding ground for bacterial contamination
2. Reinforce or change dressing per preferred routine or as ordered
   a. Dry dressings are more comfortable for patient
3. Monitor amount of drainage on dressings and from drains; establish expected drainage amounts with surgeon when patient arrives in PACU; notify surgeon of excessive or questionable quantities of drainage
   a. Significant blood or fluid losses can occur from incisions or drain sites that may require replacement or exploration of site
4. Document both abdominal and perineal dressings after abdominoperineal resection
   a. Sump or Penrose (cigarette or tube) drains may be present in perineal incision, a likely area for copious serosanguineous drainage

G. Positioning
1. Lateral recumbent position
   a. Side-lying position is usually more comfortable for patients who have had rectal or perineal procedures
2. Elevate head of the bed (reverse Trendelenburg; not head up and hips flexed)
   a. Elevating head decreases weight against diaphragm to promote improved respiratory excursion and facilitate gas exchange

H. Temperature (see information on hyperthermia and hypothermia under Intraoperative Concerns)
1. Monitor temperature on admission to PACU; warm or cool patient as indicated with warming lights, hypothermia or hyperthermia blankets, convective warming devices
   a. Vital signs should include temperature monitoring on PACU admission and every 1 to 2 hours until discharge
2. Take axillary, oral, or tympanic temperatures on patients with permanent colostomies, ileostomies, or rectal/anal incisions or following pull-through or stapled low anterior resections
   a. Perforation of suture or staple lines is possible if rectal/anal incision exists or if rectum has been totally removed

I. Pain control
1. Assess location, pattern, intensity, and duration of pain; if possible, use pain assessment tool, requiring patient to identify quality of pain or discomfort; initiate pain relief measures; medicate patients according to PACU routine and Agency for Health Care Policy and Research (AHCPR) guidelines
   a. Pain management will vary from institution to institution; pain is subjective; patient complaining of pain should be believed and comfort measures initiated
2. Observe for incisional splinting
   a. Splinting can lead to increased $P_{CO_2}$ level because of inadequate gas exchange

3. IV route preferred for narcotic administration
   a. Absorption time and onset of action are less predictable when intramuscular injections are administered in cold patient
4. Patient-controlled analgesia, epidural analgesia, incisional or field blocks may provide significant pain relief in selected patients
   a. Adequate pain control may improve ventilation, promote deep breathing and coughing, and allow patient to move more easily, especially after procedures with large or upper abdominal incisions
   b. Gastric surgical procedures are generally considered the most painful postoperatively; aggressive and appropriate pain management is desirable

**III. Postoperative Complications**

A. General complications (not in order of occurrence or severity)
   1. Atelectasis and respiratory problems
   2. Bladder distension
   3. Paralytic (adynamic) ileus
   4. Hemorrhage or shock
   5. Wound infection
   6. Dehiscence or evisceration
   7. Peritonitis
   8. Hiccups (singultus)
   9. Anastomotic leak
   10. Anastomotic stomal obstruction
   11. External fistulas
   12. Electrolyte and fluid imbalances
   13. Stress ulceration
   14. Pulmonary embolus
   15. Pancreatitis
   16. Toxic shock syndrome

B. Specific system complications
   1. Pulmonary
      a. Hypoventilation: most frequent and dangerous pulmonary complication after surgery; various causes
         (1) Preoperative medication
         (2) Anesthetic agents
         (3) Narcotic administration preoperatively, intraoperatively, and postoperatively
         (4) Pain
         (5) Patient position
      b. Atelectasis constitutes 90% of all pulmonary complications
         (1) Acute gastric dilation or ascites in advanced cancer can cause elevation of diaphragm, leading to decreased size of chest cavity and atelectasis (can also lead to shock)
   2. Cardiovascular
      a. Venous thrombosis
      b. Hypotension
      c. Shock
         (1) Hypovolemic
         (2) Bacterial or septic
      d. Myocardial infarction
      e. Cerebrovascular accident

## ACKNOWLEDGEMENT

I thank Patricia Helzerman, BSN, RN, and Beverly J. Schmid, BS, RN, CNOR, RNFA, for their assistance in preparing this chapter.

## BIBLIOGRAPHY


Acute Pain Management Guideline Panel. *Acute Pain Management: Operative or Medical Procedures and Trauma. Clinical Practice Guideline.* AHCPR Pub. No. 92-0032. Rockville, MD, Agency for Health Care Policy and Research, Public Health Service, U.S. Department of Health and Human Services, Feb. 1992.

Alspach JG (ed): *Core Curriculum for Critical Care Nursing,* 5th Ed. Philadelphia, WB Saunders, 1998.

Amato EJ: A nursing reference: Gastrointestinal tubes and drains. *Crit Care Nurs* 2:50–57, 1982.

Amato EJ: A nursing reference: Gastrointestinal tubes and drains. II. Esophageal tubes. *Crit Care Nurs* 3:46–48, 1983.

Ashcraft KW, Holder TM (eds): *Pediatric Surgery,* 2nd Ed. Philadelphia, WB Saunders, 1993.

Ball KA: *Endoscopic Surgery.* Mosby's Perioperative Nursing Series. St Louis, Mosby–Year Book, 1997.

Black JM, Matassarin-Jacobs E: *Medical-Surgical Nursing: Clinical Management for Continuity of Care,* 5th Ed. Philadelphia, WB Saunders, 1997.

Boggs RL, Wooldridge-King M (eds): *AACN Procedure Manual for Critical Care,* 3rd Ed. Philadelphia, WB Saunders, 1993.

Brozenec SA: Caring for the postoperative patient with an abdominal drain. *Nurs 85* 15:55–57, 1985.

Cason CL, Seidel SL, Bushmiaer M: Recovery from laparoscopic cholecystectomy procedures. *AORN J* 63(6):1099–1116, 1996.

Clark GJ, Onders RP, Knudson JD: Laparoscopic distal pancreatectomy procedures in a rural hospital. *AORN J* 65(2):334–343, 1997.

Clochesy JM, Breu C, Cardin S, et al (eds): *Critical Care Nursing,* 2nd Ed. Philadelphia, WB Saunders, 1996.

Collins LG: Laparoscopic extraperitoneal herniorrhaphy. *AORN J* 63(6): 1089–1098, 1996.

Coventry DM: Anaesthesia for laparoscopic surgery. *J R Coll Surg Edinb* 40:151–160, 1995.

Fairchild SS: *Perioperative Nursing: Principles and Practice,* 2nd Ed. Boston, Jones and Bartlett, 1996.

Gray H, Pick TP, Howden R (eds): *Gray's Anatomy: Descriptive and Surgical.* Philadelphia, Running Press, 1991.

Greenberger ND: *Gastrointestinal Disorders: A Pathophysiologic Approach,* 4th Ed. Chicago, Year Book Medical Publishers, 1989.

Guyton AC: *Human Physiology and Mechanisms of Disease,* 6th Ed. Philadelphia, WB Saunders, 1997.

Hulka JF, Reich H: *Textbook of Laparoscopy,* 3rd Ed. Philadelphia, WB Saunders, 1998.

Moody FG et al (eds): *Surgical Treatment of Digestive Disease,* 2nd Ed. Chicago, Year Book Medical Publishers, 1990.

Nora PF (ed): *Operative Surgery: Principles and Techniques,* 3rd Ed. Philadelphia, WB Saunders, 1990.

O'Brien DD, Burden N: The ASC as a special procedures unit. In Burden N: *Ambulatory Surgical Nursing.* Philadelphia, WB Saunders, 1993.

O'Hanlon-Nichols T: Book assessment series: Gastrointestinal system. *Am J Nurs* 98(4):48–52, 1998.

O'Toole MT: Advanced assessment of the abdomen and gastrointestinal problems. *Nurs Clin North Am* 25(4):771–776, 1990.

Pilcher CJ, Wesolowski MS, Jawad MA: Laparoscopic applications for abdominal trauma injuries. *AORN J* 64(3):366–375, 1996.

Rogers MA, Cox JA: Laparoscopic paraesophageal hernia repair with Nissen fundoplication. *AORN J* 67(3):536–551, 1998.

Sabiston DC (ed): *Textbook of Surgery,* 15th Ed. Philadelphia, WB Saunders, 1997.

Stengel JM, Dirado R: Laparoscopic Nissen fundoplication to treat gastroesophageal reflux. *AORN J* 61(3):483–489, 1995.

Thibodeau GA: *Anthony's Textbook of Anatomy and Physiology,* 14th Ed. St Louis, Mosby, 1994.

Thompson J, McFarland G, Hirsch J, et al: *Mosby's Manual of Clinical Nursing,* 4th Ed. St Louis, Mosby, 1997.

Tilkian SM, Conover MH, Tilkian AG: *Clinical and Nursing Implications of Laboratory Tests,* 5th Ed. St Louis, Mosby, 1995.

Vander AJ et al: *Human Physiology: The Mechanisms of Body Function,* 6th Ed. New York, McGraw-Hill, 1994.


## REVIEW QUESTIONS

**1. Which gastric procedure involves removal of the pylorus of the stomach and the duodenum?**

A. Antrectomy
B. Billroth II
C. Gastrectomy
D. Gastroplasty

**2. For what purpose would a Duhamel or Soave procedure be performed?**
   A. Treatment of cancer of the head of the pancreas
   B. Treatment of diabetes mellitus
   C. Open an obstructed or stenosed duodenum
   D. Treatment of Hirschsprung's disease

**3. Why is proper positioning important intraoperatively?**
   A. Prevention of cautery burns
   B. Prevention of hypothermia
   C. Maintenance of neurovascular integrity
   D. Maintenance of fluid status

**4. What problems may be encountered if altered fluid, electrolyte, and nutritional status is not corrected preoperatively?**
   A. Altered electrolyte balance
   B. Hypotension
   C. Clotting abnormalities
   D. All of the above

**5. Prolonged exposure of abdominal viscera and/or extensive gastrointestinal resection may cause what problem?**
   A. Electrolyte imbalance
   B. Hypothermia
   C. Decreased cardiac output
   D. Hyperthermia

**6. What are the potential problems with the cardiovascular system in the patient who has undergone a gastrointestinal procedure?**
   A. Third spacing, fluid overload, hypovolemia
   B. Increased bladder distension, glucose intolerance, tachycardia
   C. Lung collapse, hypothermia, abdominal distension
   D. Hyperthermia, bradycardia, pain

**7. What is the most frequent and dangerous pulmonary complication after surgery?**
   A. Hiccups
   B. Pulmonary embolus
   C. Hypoventilation
   D. Pneumonia

**8. What postoperative complication is characterized by decreased tissue perfusion and increased peripheral vasoconstriction?**
   A. Deep vein thrombosis
   B. Renal failure
   C. Peritonitis
   D. Shock

**9. What are some of the nursing interventions for the patient after gastrointestinal surgery?**
   A. Maintain oxygenation
   B. Monitor fluid status
   C. Maintain patency of tubes and/or drains
   D. All of the above

**ANSWERS:** 1. B, 2. D, 3. C, 4. D, 5. B, 6. A, 7. C, 8. D, 9. D

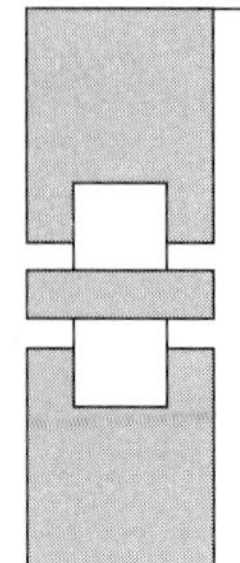

CHAPTER 24

# *The Gynecologic Surgical Patient*

Gwen Lynn Nelson, MSN, RN, CNOR

## OBJECTIVES

**Study of the information represented by this outline will enable the learner to:**

1. Identify the anatomy and physiology of the gynecologic system.
2. Discuss gynecologic pathophysiology as it relates to surgical intervention.
3. Define assessment parameters of the surgical gynecologic patient.
4. Identify major and minor gynecologic operative procedures.
5. Prioritize important elements of postanesthesia care unit (PACU) care specific to the gynecologic patient, including positioning, hemorrhagic complications, airway management, fluid and electrolyte balance, and pain control.
6. Discuss potential perioperative complications of the gynecologic patient.

Patients undergo gynecologic surgery for acute or chronic, elective or emergent reasons. Surgical intervention may be required for a variety of indications ranging from simple diagnostic procedures to radical excisions for malignancy.

This chapter defines and discusses major and minor gynecologic procedures and perioperative concerns. Nursing management strategies are discussed as they relate to specific complications.

## ANATOMY AND PHYSIOLOGY

I. **Normal Anatomy and Physiology** (Figs. 24–1 and 24–2)
   A. Vulva
      1. Consists of numerous structures referred to collectively as external genitalia
      2. Main structures
         a. Mons veneris
         b. Labia majora
         c. Labia minora
         d. Clitoris
         e. Urinary meatus
         f. Vaginal orifice
         g. Bartholin's glands
         h. Skene's glands
   B. Vagina
      1. Located between rectum and urethra
      2. Collapsible tube
         a. Composed mainly of smooth muscle lined with mucous membrane
         b. Cervix protrudes into uppermost portion of anterior wall
         c. External outlet protected by fold of mucous membrane called hymen

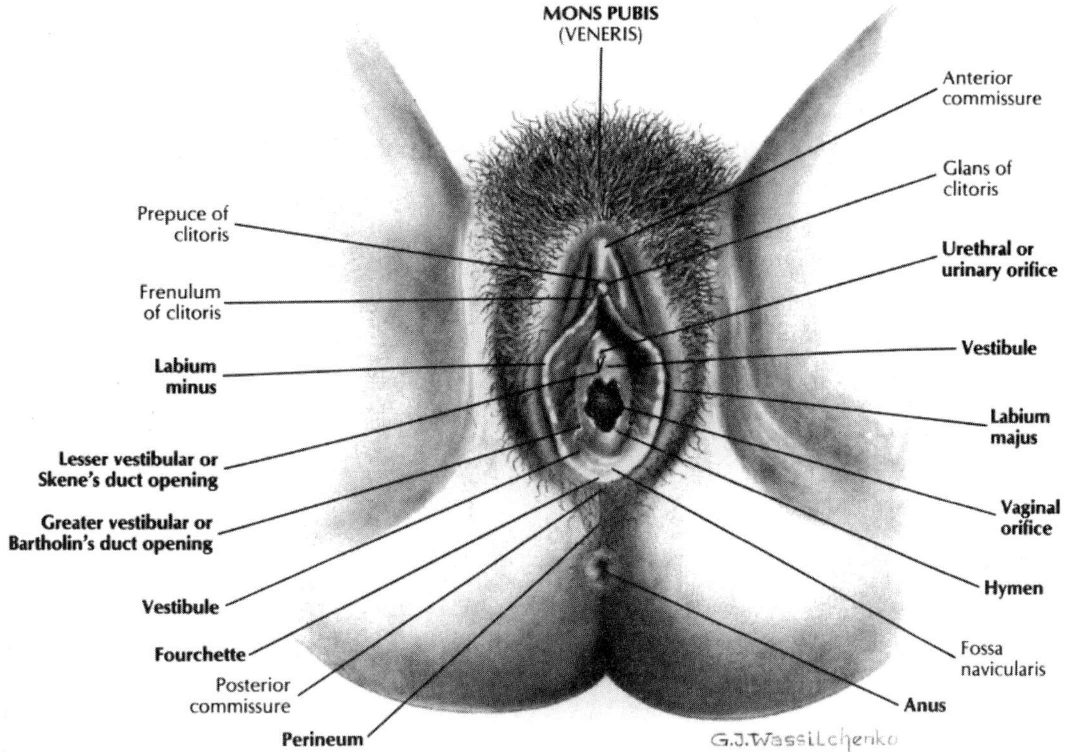


**FIGURE 24–1** External female genitalia. (From Bobak IM, Jensen MD, Lowdermilk DL: *Maternity and Gynecologic Care,* 5th Ed. St Louis, Mosby, 1993.)

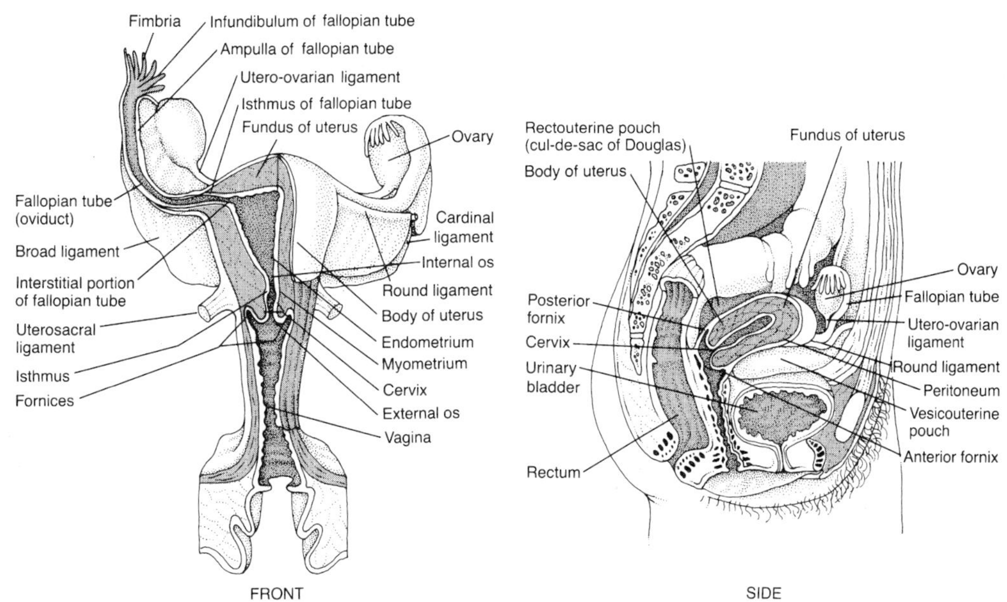


**FIGURE 24–2** Internal female genitalia. (From Ignatavicius DD, Bayne MV: *Medical-Surgical Nursing* [p 1629]. Philadelphia, WB Saunders, 1991.)

3. Physiology
   a. Excretory duct for uterine secretions and menstrual flow
   b. Lower portion of birth canal
   c. Receives seminal fluid
   d. Coital organ

C. Uterus
1. Located in pelvic cavity between bladder and rectum
   a. Anchored in place by eight ligaments
      (1) Broad ligaments
      (2) Round ligaments
      (3) Cardinal ligaments
      (4) Uterosacral ligaments
   b. Capable of considerable mobility
      (1) Often in abnormal positions
         (a) Retroflexion
         (b) Anteflexion
2. Consists of body and cervix
   a. Fundus: bulging upper surface of body of uterus
3. Wall of uterus has three layers
   a. Endometrium
   b. Myometrium
   c. Peritoneum
4. Blood supply
   a. Uterine arteries
   b. Branches of internal iliac arteries
5. Physiology
   a. Menstruation
   b. Pregnancy
   c. Labor

D. Fallopian tubes
1. Attached to uterus at upper, outer angles
2. Has same three layers as uterus; endometrial layer ciliated
3. Mucosa and peritoneum in direct contact at distal ends
4. Physiology
   a. Serve as ducts for ova to reach uterus
   b. Fertilization of ova normally occurs here

E. Ovaries
1. Located behind and below fallopian tubes; situated on both sides of uterus
2. Anchored to uterus and broad ligament
3. Consist of graafian follicles
   a. Embedded in connective tissue base
   b. Follicles are in all stages of development; usually one each month is expelled into abdominal cavity
4. Physiology
   a. Formation of ova
   b. Secretion of estrogen and progesterone

## PATHOPHYSIOLOGY

**I. Congenital and Anatomic Abnormalities**

A. Imperforate hymen

B. Herniations
1. Cystocele: herniation of bladder that causes anterior vaginal wall to bulge downward

2. Rectocele: formed by protrusion of anterior rectal wall (posterior vaginal wall) into vagina
3. Enterocele: herniation of cul-de-sac of Douglas, which almost always contains loops of small intestine
4. Urethrocele: pouchlike protrusion of urethral wall and thickening of connective tissue around urethra

C. Uterine displacement
D. Prolapsed uterus
E. Bicornuate uterus
F. Septate uterus
G. Tubal incompetency

## II. Endocrine (Hormonal) Dysfunction

A. Endometriosis
B. Dysfunctional uterine bleeding
C. Stein-Leventhal syndrome (polycystic ovary syndrome)

## III. Growths and Neoplasms

A. Cysts: closed sack or pouch with definite wall that contains fluid, semifluid, or solid material
   1. Bartholin's (gland)
   2. Ovarian
B. Uterine fibroids or myomatas: tumor containing muscle tissue
C. Carcinomas: malignant tumor growth in epithelial tissue
   1. Vulvar
   2. Cervical
   3. Uterine
   4. Ovarian
D. Polyps: benign tumor with pedicle; usually removed if there is a possibility that it will become malignant; prone to bleed
   1. Cervical
   2. Uterine
E. Condylomata: wartlike growths of the skin; usually seen on external genitalia or in anal region

## IV. Infections and Inflammatory Processes

A. Pelvic inflammatory disease (PID)
   1. Affects abdominal organs
   2. May result in infertility
B. Abscesses
   1. Perineal region
   2. Abdominal organs
C. Fistulas
   1. Urethrovaginal
   2. Rectovaginal

## V. Pregnancy Related

A. Abortion
   1. Incomplete: abortion in which parts of products of conception have been retained in uterus
   2. Missed: abortion in which fetus has died before twentieth completed week of gestation, but products of conception are retained in uterus for 8 weeks or longer
   3. Therapeutic: abortion performed when mental or physical health of mother is endangered by continuation of pregnancy
B. Incompetent cervix

C. Ectopic pregnancy: pregnancy occurring outside uterine cavity
   1. Commonly occurs in fallopian tube
   2. Life threatening if ruptured; may result in hemorrhage or loss of tube or ovary
D. Hydatidiform mole: degenerative process in chorionic villi that gives rise to multiple cysts and rapid growth of uterus with possible hemorrhage; usually surgically removed by laparotomy

## PREOPERATIVE ASSESSMENT

**I. Laboratory Values**
   A. Hematology values
      1. Complete blood cell count
      2. Type and screen
   B. Chemistry values
      1. Serum electrolytes
      2. Serum glucose
      3. Serum pregnancy test
   C. Urinalysis
      1. Bacteria
      2. Glucose
      3. Protein
      4. Ketones
      5. Red blood cells
   D. Cytologic studies
      1. Papanicolaou (Pap) smears
      2. Previous cryotherapy
      3. Biopsy reports

**II. Radiologic Studies**
   A. Chest film: cardiopulmonary problems
   B. Ultrasonography

## OPERATIVE PROCEDURES

**I. Diagnostic**
   A. Laparoscopy
      1. Direct visualization of pelvic organs through endoscope
      2. Scope passed through small abdominal wound (additional puncture sites made for major and minor laparoscopic procedures that require additional instrumentation)
      3. Minor procedures accomplished through endoscope
         a. Lysis of adhesions
         b. Tubal lavage: ascertains fallopian tube patency
         c. Tubal ligation
         d. Biopsy of tissue
         e. Aspiration of cysts
         f. Aspiration of peritoneal fluid for cytologic study
         g. Oocyte retrieval for in vitro fertilization procedure (IVF)
      4. Major procedures accomplished through endoscope
         a. Enucleation of intramural myomata
         b. Ovarian cystectomy
         c. Oophorectomy

- d. Adnexectomy
- e. Tuboplasty
- f. Fimbrioplasty
- g. Removal of ectopic tubal pregnancy
- h. Lymphadenectomy

B. Laparotomy
1. Incision of abdominal wall
2. Allows for exploration of abdominal cavity

C. Culdoscopy
1. Direct visualization of uterus and adnexa through endoscope
2. Passed through posterior vaginal wall

D. Culdocentesis
1. Aspiration through vaginal wall of blood or pus through cul-de-sac
   - a. Good diagnostic tool to rule out ruptured ectopic pregnancy
   - b. Used to detect intraperitoneal bleeding or cul-de-sac hematoma

E. Dilatation and curettage (D and C)
1. Dilation of cervical os
2. Curettage of endometrial lining
3. Performed for tissue assay, cervical biopsy, or correction of bleeding

F. Hysteroscopy
1. Dilatation of cervical os
2. Passed through cervical os into uterus
3. Direct visualization of uterine lining

G. Cervical biopsy
1. Excision of cervical tissues
2. Performed for tissue assay

H. Uterine aspiration (dilatation and evacuation)
1. Introduction of suction into uterus
2. Vaginal approach
3. Removal of uterine contents
4. Termination of pregnancy or remaining products of conception

I. Hydrotubation
1. Insufflation of fallopian tubes
2. Ascertains fallopian tube patency

## II. Removal of Growths and Organs

A. Bartholinectomy: excision of Bartholin's gland

B. Marsupialization of Bartholin's cyst
1. Creation of open pouch around excised Bartholin's gland and cyst
2. Facilitates drainage and healing

C. Laser therapy (carbon dioxide, Nd:Yag, argon)
1. Condylomata
2. Cervical cancer in situ
3. Endometriosis
4. Lysis of adhesions; surgical approaches
   - a. Laparotomy
   - b. Laparoscopy

D. Oophorectomy: excision of ovary; surgical approaches
1. Laparotomy
2. Laparoscopy

E. Oophorocystectomy: excision of ovarian cyst; surgical approaches
1. Laparotomy
2. Laparoscopy

F. Salpingectomy: excision of all or portion of fallopian tube; surgical approaches
   1. Laparotomy
   2. Laparoscopy
G. Hysterectomy: excision of uterus; surgical approaches
   1. Vaginally
   2. Abdominally
   3. Laparoscopic-assisted vaginal hysterectomy (LAVH)
H. Hysterosalpingo-oophorectomy: removal of uterus, fallopian tubes, and ovaries
I. Radical hysterectomy and lymphadenectomy
   1. Laparotomy to remove uterus, tubes, ovaries, upper vagina, supporting ligaments, and pelvic lymph nodes; extensive dissection of ureters and bladder also involved
   2. Portions of this procedure may be performed by laparoscopy (e.g., pelvic lymph node dissection)
   3. Treatment for malignancy
J. Vulvectomy
   1. Excision of labia majora, labia minora, and surrounding structures
   2. Treatment for premalignancy or malignancy
   3. Usually requires skin graft
K. Salpingo-oophorectomy: removal of fallopian tube and all or part of associated ovary; surgical approaches
   1. Laparotomy
   2. Laparoscopy

## III. Anatomic Corrections

A. Hymenotomy
   1. Incision of hymen membrane
   2. Opens vaginal orifice
B. Hymenectomy
   1. Excision of hymen membrane
   2. Enlarges vaginal opening
C. Anterior colporrhaphy
   1. Removal of excess anterior vaginal tissue
   2. Tightens vaginal wall
   3. Prevents or corrects bladder herniation into vagina
D. Posterior colporrhaphy
   1. Removal of excess posterior vaginal tissue
   2. Tightens vaginal wall
   3. Prevents or corrects rectal herniation into vagina
E. Salpingoplasty (tuboplasty)
   1. Microscopic reconstructive surgery of the fallopian tube.
   2. Procedure to restore patency of fallopian tube—obstructed portion of fallopian tube may be removed and the tube reconstructed to create patency to promote fertilization
      a. Reversal of tubal ligation
      b. PID
      c. Adhesions
      d. Ectopic pregnancy
F. Salpingostomy
   1. Surgical incision of fallopian tube
   2. Performed to remove ectopic pregnancy before rupture of fallopian tube
G. Ovarian wedge resection
   1. Removal of ovarian cortex segment
   2. Removal of ovarian cyst
   3. Treatment for infertility

H. Marshall-Marchetti or Stamey procedure and other suspension procedures
   1. Repair of fascial support and pubococcygeal muscle
   2. Restores bladder and urethral support

**IV. Other Common Procedures**

A. Tubal ligation
   1. Ligation or cauterization of fallopian tubes
   2. Prevents pregnancy
   3. Surgical approaches
      a. Laparoscopy
      b. Minilaparotomy
      c. Vaginal (posterior colpotomy)

B. Dilatation and evacuation
   1. Dilatation of cervical os
   2. Evacuation of retained tissue in uterus

C. Removal of hematoma

D. Suturing of vaginal or cervical lacerations

E. Shirodkar/cerclage: surgical placement of nonabsorbable suture around the incompetent internal cervical os to prevent premature cervical dilation during pregnancy

F. In vitro fertilization (IVF) and embryo transfer: retrieval of oocytes from ovary, followed by in vitro fertilization with sperm and implantation of fertilized oocytes (embryos) into uterine cavity
   1. Treatment for long-standing infertility
   2. Other approaches to IVF
      a. Gamete intrafallopian transfer (Gift): requires one patent fallopian tube. Prepared semen with retrieved oocytes inserted into fallopian tube through laparoscope. Fertilization occurs within patient
      b. Zygote intrafallopian transfer (Zift): placement of fertilized eggs into the right and left fallopian tubes
   3. Surgical approaches
      a. Laparoscopy
      b. Minilaparotomy
      c. Vaginal aspiration with ultrasonographic guidance
   4. Complications: ectopic pregnancy, spontaneous abortion

G. Endometrial ablation
   1. Laser or electrosurgical technology used to treat dysfunctional uterine bleeding
   2. Surgical approach: hysteroscopy
   3. Monitor intake and output of irrigating fluid to avoid fluid overload

## INTRAOPERATIVE CONCERNS

### NURSING DIAGNOSIS

Examples of related nursing diagnostic categories include:

- High risk for injury related to surgical position
- High risk for impaired skin integrity
- Fluid volume deficit
- Fluid volume overload
- Potential infection

**I. Positioning**
- A. Affecting considerations
  1. Loss of pain sensation
  2. Disturbances of neurovascular systems
  3. Skeletal deformities
- B. Lithotomy position
  1. Peroneal nerve damage
  2. Vascular compromise
  3. Check pedal pulses before and after positioning

**II. Skin Integrity**
- A. Chemical burns (prepping solutions)
- B. Prevent prepping solutions from pooling under patients
- C. Allergic reactions
- D. Placement of electrosurgical dispersive pad on healthy muscular tissue
- E. Pad bony prominences or pressure points

**III. Fluid Volume Deficit**
- A. Blood loss
- B. Surgical manipulation
  1. Visceral traction: intraoperative tissue irritation or injury
  2. Rapid decompression of abdomen during removal of ovarian and uterine tumors
- C. Positional changes altering blood pressure
  1. Lithotomy
  2. Trendelenburg's

**IV. Infection**
- A. Exogenous microorganisms
  1. Break in surgical aseptic technique
  2. Microorganisms on surgical field or surgical wound
- B. Endogenous microorganisms
  1. Hematoma or tissue fragments left in pelvis become source for abscess formation
  2. Rupture of infected cyst

## POSTANESTHESIA CONCERNS

### NURSING DIAGNOSIS

Examples of related nursing diagnostic categories include:
- Potential for infection
- Alteration in comfort
- Ineffective airway clearance
- Fluid volume deficit
- Fluid volume overload
- Potential for urinary retention

**I. Drainage Systems**
- A. Wound drains: facilitate fluid evacuation from surgical site
  1. Hemovac
  2. Jackson-Pratt
  3. Hystero-vac
  4. Penrose

B. Nasogastric tube: used when excessive gastric or bowel manipulation is anticipated or has occurred
C. Indwelling catheter: prevents bladder distension and tension on new suture lines
  1. Foley catheter
  2. Suprapubic cystostomy tube: vaginal approach to surgical interruption
  3. Nursing concerns
    a. Avoid traction on all catheters; may secure with tape or catheter strap
    b. Avoid occlusion of small-lumen cystostomy tubes
    c. Avoid contamination of drainage system(s)

**II. Vaginal Drainage**
A. Assess presence of vaginal packing or cervical drains
B. Record amount and characteristics of vaginal drainage

**III. Pain Control**
A. Assess pain location
  1. Operative site
  2. Shoulder pain: laparoscopy (pneumoperitoneum); referred pain from $CO_2$ under diaphragm through phrenic nerve
  3. Surgical positioning
B. Encourage changes of position for comfort
C. Apply warm blankets as needed
D. Use ice packs as ordered
E. Administer analgesics per PACU policy or physician order

**IV. Antiembolic Care Related to Lithotomy Position, Obesity, Smoking**
A. Assess signs of thrombus formation
B. Encourage active leg movement frequently
C. Apply antiembolic stockings as ordered
D. Apply venous compression device as ordered
E. Administer anticoagulants as ordered

**V. Gynecologic Complications**
A. Hemorrhage
  1. Types
    a. Intraperitoneal hemorrhage
      (1) Occurs in first few hours
      (2) Usually arterial in origin
      (3) Accompanied by inability to clot: decreased fibrinogen
    b. Retroperitoneal hemorrhage
      (1) Occurs early to late in postoperative period
      (2) Can be arterial, venous, or capillary
      (3) Usually less severe than intraperitoneal hemorrhage
    c. Wound: localized at incision site
  2. Symptoms and signs
    a. Internal bleeding
      (1) Decreasing blood pressure
      (2) Increasing rate and weakening pulse
      (3) Decreasing sensorium
      (4) Evidence of bleeding
        (a) Frank, bloody vaginal drainage
        (b) Increasing abdominal pain, rigidity, and girth
    b. Wound bleeding
      (1) Swelling
      (2) Ecchymosis
      (3) Oozing suture line

3. Nursing actions
   a. Internal bleeding
      (1) Obtain laboratory blood samples
      (2) Administer blood and fluids as ordered
      (3) Obtain vital signs as indicated
      (4) Administer supplemental oxygen
      (5) Place patient in Trendelenburg's position or raise legs if indicated
      (6) Administer oxytocic agents (Ergotrate) or oxytocin (Pitocin) IM or IV per physician's order; used in prevention and treatment of postabortal hemorrhage as a result of uterine atony
      (7) Monitor blood pressure, pulse, and uterine response
      (8) Prepare to return patient to surgery; maintain NPO
         (a) Exploration
         (b) Cautery or ligation of bleeding vessel(s)
         (c) Evacuation of hematoma
   b. Wound bleeding
      (1) Record amount and characteristics of wound bleeding
      (2) Application of pressure dressing
      (3) Application of ice packs
      (4) Cautery or ligation of bleeding vessel(s)

B. Pulmonary embolism
   1. Cause: embolism of pulmonary artery
      a. Blood clot
      b. Fat globule
      c. Air bubble
   2. Symptoms of major obstruction
      a. Sudden onset of chest pain
      b. Anxiety
      c. Productive cough with hemoptysis
      d. Tachypnea
      e. Tachycardia
      f. Cyanosis
      g. Shock
   3. Nursing actions
      a. Supplemental oxygen
      b. Ventilatory support
      c. Narcotic administration
      d. Bronchodilators: aminophylline
      e. Anticoagulation therapy
      f. Cardiovascular support: dopamine

C. Fluid and electrolyte imbalance
   1. Cause
      a. Underestimation of fluid and blood loss during surgery
      b. Intravascular fluid shifting into interstitium
      c. Overhydration
      d. Correction of fluid imbalance without correction of electrolyte imbalance
   2. Symptoms
      a. Hypovolemia (fluid volume deficit)
         (1) Hypotension
         (2) Tachycardia
         (3) Tachypnea
         (4) Oliguria
         (5) Dryness of skin, mucosa

b. Hypervolemia (fluid volume excess)
   (1) Hypertension
   (2) Tachycardia
   (3) Chest rales or rhonchi
   (4) Dyspnea
   (5) Scleral edema
c. Electrolyte imbalance
   (1) Cardiac dysrhythmia
   (2) Confusion
   (3) Disorientation
   (4) Vomiting

3. Nursing actions
   a. Obtain appropriate laboratory samples
      (1) Hemoglobin and hematocrit
      (2) Electrolytes
      (3) Urine
         (a) Specific gravity
         (b) Osmolality
   b. Administer fluid and blood components as ordered
   c. Administer supplemental oxygen
   d. Monitor urinary output as indicated
   e. Monitor for dysrhythmia
   f. Monitor vital signs as indicated
   g. Administer appropriate medications
      (1) Diuretics
      (2) Hypovolemia to assess renal function and protect renal tubules
      (3) Hypervolemia to reduce total body fluid
      (4) Electrolytes, especially potassium
      (5) Sodium bicarbonate to correct metabolic acidosis
      (6) Vasopressors for temporary maintenance of blood pressure

## BIBLIOGRAPHY

Atkinson LJ, Fortunato N: *Berry & Kohn's Operating Room Technique,* 8th Ed. St Louis, Mosby–Year Book, 1996.

Berger PH, Saul HM: Radical hysterectomy treatment for advanced cervical carcinoma. *AORN J* 52:1212, 1990.

Bobak IM, Jensen MD, Lowdermilk DL: *Maternity and Gynecologic Care: The Nurse and the Family,* 5th Ed. St Louis, Mosby–Year Book, 1993.

Dickinson SP, Bury GM: Pulmonary embolism: Anatomy of a crisis. *Nursing* 19(4):34–42, 1989.

Drain CB: *The Post Anesthesia Care Unit: A Critical Care Approach to Post Anesthesia Nursing,* 3rd Ed. Philadelphia, WB Saunders, 1994.

Haspel-Siegal A: Fallopian tube anastomosis procedures to restore fertility. *AORN J* 65(1):75–86, 1997.

Hawkins JW, Higgins LP: *Maternity and Gynecologic Nursing: Women's Health Care.* Philadelphia, JB Lippincott, 1989.

Herbst A, Mishell D, Stencheuer M, Droegenmueller W: *Comprehensive Gynecology,* 2nd Ed. St Louis, Mosby–Year Book, 1992.

Hunt RB: *Atlas of Female Infertility Surgery,* 2nd Ed. St Louis, Mosby–Year Book, 1992.

Jones HW, Wentz AC, Burnett LS: *Novak's Textbook of Gynecology,* 11th Ed. Baltimore, Williams & Wilkins, 1988.

Levine RL: Pelviscopic surgery in women over 40. *J Reprod Med* 35:597, 1990.

Martin J: *Positioning in Anesthesia and Surgery,* 2nd Ed. Philadelphia, WB Saunders, 1987.

Meeker MH, Rothrock JC: *Alexander's Care of the Patient in Surgery,* 9th Ed. St Louis, Mosby–Year Book, 1991.

Minelli L et al: Laparoscopically assisted vaginal hysterectomy. *Endoscopy* 23:64, 1991.

Mishell DR, Kirschbaum TH: *Yearbook of Obstetrics and Gynecology.* St Louis, Mosby–Year Book, 1997.

*Physician's Desk Reference,* 51st Ed. Montvale, NJ, Medical Economics, 1997.

Robinson BJ: The perioperative nurse's role in assisted-fertility procedures. *AORN J* 65(1):87–93, 1997.

Rothrock JC: *Perioperative Care Planning.* St Louis, Mosby–Year Book, 1990.

Thibodeau GA, Patton KT: *Anatomy and Physiology,* 2nd Ed. St Louis, Mosby–Year Book, 1992.

Ulmer B: Cervical intraepithelial neoplasia. *AORN J* 59(4):851–860, 1994.

Vasilev SA, Liming PR: Ectopic pregnancy: Etiology, diagnosis, treatment. *AORN J* 54:1030, 1991.

Wynn RM: *Obstetrics and Gynecology: The Clinical Core,* 4th Ed. Philadelphia, Lea & Febiger, 1988.

## REVIEW QUESTIONS

**1. For what purpose is a dilatation and evacuation performed?**
   A. Removal of uterine contents
   B. Ascertain patency
   C. Facilitation of drainage and healing
   D. Specimen testing

**2. Which procedure restores patency of a fallopian tube?**
   A. Salpingectomy
   B. Salpingostomy
   C. Oophorocystectomy
   D. Salpingoplasty

**3. What chemistry values are useful as preoperative assessment parameters?**
   A. Glucose
   B. Serum pregnancy test
   C. Electrolytes
   D. All of the above

**4. What potential problem should be assessed after a patient has been in the lithotomy position?**
   A. Femoral artery damage
   B. Brachial plexus damage
   C. Peroneal nerve damage
   D. Achilles tendon damage

**5. Which of the following causes arterial hypotension?**
   A. Surgical manipulation
   B. Positional changes
   C. Blood loss
   D. All of the above

**6. Which one of the following is not characteristic of intraperitoneal hemorrhage?**
   A. Occurs early to late in the postoperative period
   B. Is accompanied by an inability to clot
   C. Is usually arterial in origin
   D. None of the above

**7. What is the cause of a pulmonary embolism?**
   A. Dislodging of a clot from the lungs to the legs
   B. Abnormal clotting of blood in the pulmonary vein
   C. Lodging of a blood clot or air bubble in a pulmonary artery
   D. Electrolyte imbalance causing an abnormal flow of blood through the lungs

**8. What drug therapy may be used in treatment of pulmonary embolism?**
   A. Sodium nitroprusside (Nipride), vitamin K
   B. Anticoagulant, dopamine
   C. $K^+$ supplement, nitroglycerin
   D. Reversal agents, antiemetics

**9. What are the signs and symptoms of an electrolyte imbalance?**
   A. ECG abnormalities, confusion, vomiting
   B. Hypertension, bradycardia, vomiting
   C. Somnolence, scleral edema, dyspnea
   D. None of the above

**10. What are the appropriate nursing actions for fluid or electrolyte imbalance?**
   A. Administer oxygen
   B. Monitor for dysrhythmia
   C. Monitor urinary output every hour
   D. All of the above

**ANSWERS:** 1. A, 2. D, 3. D, 4. C, 5. D, 6. A, 7. C, 8. B, 9. A, 10. D

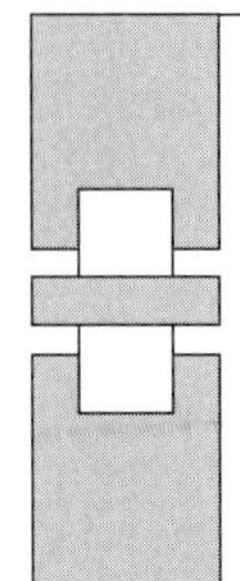

CHAPTER 25

# The Obstetric Surgical Patient

Judith H. Poole, MN, RNC, FACCE
Denise White, MSN, RNC

## OBJECTIVES

**Study of the information represented by this outline will enable the learner to:**

1. Discuss the physiologic changes of pregnancy.
2. Describe the pathophysiology, potential problems, assessment parameters, and nursing implications for common complications of pregnancy.
3. Describe commonly used obstetric anesthesia techniques and their impact on pregnancy.
4. Identify various assessment techniques to ascertain fetal well-being.
5. List appropriate nursing interventions in the care of the postanesthesia obstetric patient after low-risk and high-risk vaginal and surgical delivery.
6. Describe the pathophysiology, potential problems, assessment parameters, and nursing implications for various postpartum complications.
7. Explain the pharmacology, indications for use, and potential complications of commonly used obstetric medications.

## PHYSIOLOGIC CHANGES OF PREGNANCY

### I. Cardiovascular System

A. Maternal myocardial hypertrophy due to increased circulatory volume load of pregnancy
B. Enhanced myocardial contractility
C. Third heart sound by 20 weeks' gestation (90% of women)
D. Systolic ejection murmur (95% of women)
   1. Caused by systemic vasodilation and augmented cardiac ejection
E. Cardiac output (CO) progressively increases 30% to 50% to 6 to 7 L/min at rest
   1. Before 20 weeks' gestation, increase is due to maternal tachycardia and increased blood volume
   2. After 20 weeks' gestation, increase is due to significant increased stroke volume and is associated with reversible myocardial hypertrophy
   3. Increases further with labor and certain disease states; highest immediately post partum
   4. CO profoundly affected by maternal position; best in lateral or semi-Fowler's with uterine displacement and lowest in supine and standing
F. Heart rate increased 10% to 20% because of blood volume overload and hormonal changes
   1. Heart rate is positional: standing > sitting > supine
G. Stroke volume increases 30% to 40%
H. Exacerbation of preexisting cardiac disease with critical period for decompensation occurring between 24 to 32 weeks' gestation and in immediate postpartum period
I. Elevation of the diaphragm causes the heart to shift anteriorly and to the left
J. Electrocardiography (ECG) changes during pregnancy
   1. Sinus tachycardia with shortening of PR and uncorrected QT intervals

2. QRS axis shifts to the right during the first trimester but may shift left during the third trimester
3. T-wave axis shifted left
4. Depressed ST segments and isoelectric or low-voltage T waves in left-side precordial and limb leads

K. Circulatory blood volume progressively increases 40% to 50%
1. Women with preeclampsia do not expand their vascular volume to the extent that nonpreeclamptic women do; hemoconcentrated
2. Pregnancy hypervolemia acts as protective mechanism against excessive peripartum blood loss
3. Pregnancy should be considered a natural hypervolemic state with primary renal sodium and water retention

L. Plasma volume progressively increases 45% to 50%
1. Responsible for dilutional anemia during pregnancy and spontaneous autotransfusion at delivery
2. Albumin binding of drugs and local anesthetic less in pregnant state

M. Red blood cell (RBC) volume increases 25% to 30%
1. Plasma volume > RBC mass results in physiologic anemia of pregnancy
2. Expansion related to increased hematopoiesis in bone marrow and liver
3. Physiologic anemia, increased hematopoiesis, and associated transfer of approximately 300 mg of maternal iron to fetus during gestation creates iron deficit of approximately 800 mg by midpregnancy
4. 2,3-DPG concentration increased during pregnancy and affinity of maternal hemoglobin for oxygen decreased, enhancing oxygen transfer to fetus

N. White blood cell (WBC) volume increases 40% to 50%
1. Highest immediately post partum

O. Coagulation
1. Pregnancy is hypercoagulable state related to enhanced potential for coagulation and thrombosis; increase in late pregnancy and immediately post partum
2. Plasma fibrinolytic activity decreased as result of placental inhibitors but can return to normal within 1 hour after delivery
3. Tissue thromboplastin released into circulation with placental separation; increases chance of thrombosis
4. Platelet counts appear to remain in normal range

P. Hemodynamic changes (Table 25–1)

## II. Pulmonary System

A. Diaphragm elevated because of compression of enlarging uterus

B. Anteroposterior and transverse diameters increase, resulting in decreased residual volume

**TABLE 25–1 Normal Hemodynamics During Pregnancy**

| PARAMETER | NORMAL VALUE |
|---|---|
| Central venous pressure (CVP) | 1–7 mm Hg |
| Pulmonary artery pressure (PAP) | Systolic, 18–30 mm Hg<br>Diastolic, 6–10 mm Hg<br>Mean, 11–15 mm Hg |
| Pulmonary artery occlusion pressure (PAOP) | 6–10 mm Hg |
| Systemic vascular resistance (SVR) | 1210 ± 266 |
| Pulmonary vascular resistance (PVR) | 78 ± 22 |
| Cardiac output (CO) | 6–7 L/min (at rest) |
| Cardiac index (CI) | 3.2 ± 0.7 |
| Left ventricular stroke work index (LVSWI) | 45 ± 9 |

C. Weight gain, edema, and mucosal hypervascularity may change anatomy significantly
   1. Internal diameter of trachea reduced
   2. If endotracheal intubation required, a small-caliber endotracheal tube should be used (e.g., a 6.5 mm endotracheal tube)
      a. Facilitates intubation
      b. Prevents mucosal trauma
   3. Should avoid nasotracheal intubation

D. Nasal and respiratory tract mucosa become edematous and hyperemic

E. Nasal congestion and epistaxis common and may obstruct nasal airway

F. $O_2$ consumption increases to accommodate fetus and maternal hyperdynamic function
   1. $O_2$ consumption increases progressively by 10% to 20% and may increase by 100% during labor

G. Respiratory rate increases ≈15%

H. Lung volumes
   1. Tidal volume increases 40%
   2. Inspiratory reserve volume no change or slight increase
   3. Expiratory reserve volume decreases 20%
   4. Residual volume decreases 20%

I. Lung capacities
   1. Inspiratory capacity increases 5% to 10%
   2. Vital capacity no change
   3. Expiratory capacity decreases 20%
   4. Functional residual capacity decreases 20%
   5. Total lung capacity no change or slight decrease

J. Acid-base balance
   1. Maternal oxyhemoglobin dissociation curve shifted to right during pregnancy
   2. Arterial blood gas values (ABGs) (see Table 25–2)
   3. Pregnancy is state of compensatory respiratory alkalemia

## III. Gastrointestinal System

A. Anatomic and physiologic changes in gastrointestinal tract predispose pregnant woman to silent regurgitation, active vomiting, and pulmonary aspiration, especially during impaired consciousness

## IV. Renal System

A. Renal calyces, pelves, and ureters dilate progressively beginning at twelfth week because of mechanical compression at pelvic inlet
   1. Increased risk of urinary tract infection (UTI) due to urinary stasis

B. Glomerular filtration rate (GFR) and renal plasma flow (RPF) increase 40% to 50% by twentieth week of gestation

C. Blood urea nitrogen (BUN) and creatinine decrease 40% by midpregnancy because of increased GFR and RPF

D. Renal tubular function
   1. Tubular reabsorption of electrolytes and water increases in proportion to GFR

**TABLE 25–2 Arterial Blood Gas Values**

| | NONPREGNANT | PREGNANT |
|---|---|---|
| pH | 7.35–7.45 | 7.40–7.44 |
| $Pao_2$ | 80–100 | 104–108 |
| $Paco_2$ | 35–45 | 27–32 |
| $HCO_3^-$ | 22–26 | 18–22 |

2. Glycosuria common in pregnancy related to augmented GFR, which results in filtered load of glucose that exceeds tubular reabsorption capacity
   a. Increased concentrations of aldosterone, estrogens, cortisol, human placental lactogen (HPL), and prolactin
   b. Aortocaval compression by gravid uterus
3. Renin-angiotensin-aldosterone system
   a. All components increase during pregnancy because of their increased regulatory roles in circulatory volume and sodium balance

## V. Hepatic System

A. No change in hepatic size or blood flow; metabolism changes in pregnancy lead to liver storage and conversion changes

B. Lactic dehydrogenase (LDH), alkaline phosphatase, and leukocyte alkaline phosphatase slightly increase

C. Aspartate aminotransferase (AST, serum glutamic oxaloacetic transaminase [SGOT]) and alanine aminotransferase (ALT, serum glutamic pyruvic transaminase [SGPT]) unchanged

D. Serum albumin decreases

E. Cholesterol increases 40% to 50% and free fatty acids increase 60%

## VI. Endocrine System

A. Pituitary gland enlarges as result of its function as master of all glandular function

B. Thyroid gland enlarges in response to need for increased basal metabolism rate (BMR); $T_4$ uptake increases; $T_3$ uptake decreases

C. Increased cortisol and catecholamine production raise maternal heart rate and BMR

D. Increased levels of HPL, an insulin antagonist, lead to diabetogenic state; insulin requirements increase in type I diabetic patients during pregnancy

## VII. Neurologic System

A. During pregnancy, neurologic and sensory systems are influenced by altered hormonal levels and alterations in other systems

B. Eye shows mild corneal edema and thickening; intraocular pressure decreases; progressive decrease in blood flow to conjunctiva

C. Edema and erythema of vocal cords accompanied by vascular dilation, and small submucosal hemorrhage may occur

D. Pain response during intrapartum period
1. Perception of pain influenced by physiologic, psychologic, and cultural factors
2. Specific role of β-endorphins in pregnancy is unknown
   a. Pain during intrapartum period may be modulated by endorphins that alter release of neurotransmitters from afferent nerves and interfere with efferent pathways
   b. Endorphins may increase pain threshold
   c. Lower doses of analgesics and anesthetics during labor may be used because of increased endorphins

E. Musculoskeletal changes
1. Mobility of sacroiliac joints and symphysis pubis increased due to relaxin and progesterone effects
2. Distension of abdomen tilts pelvis forward, shifting center of gravity, changing posture and gait

## VIII. Reproductive System

A. Changes in reproductive system are result of increased vascularity and hormone production

B. Vulva and vagina become more vascular and elastic because of increased estrogen levels

C. Cervix becomes softer and shorter and appears cyanotic (Goodell's sign) because of prostaglandins.

D. Ovaries may be enlarged for up to 14 to 16 weeks because of corpus luteum production of progesterone and estrogen to maintain endometrium.
E. Breast tissue becomes more vascular because of elevated progesterone and estrogen levels

## PREGNANCY COMPLICATIONS

**I. Ectopic Pregnancy**
  A. Definition
    1. Pregnancy implanted outside uterus
    2. 90% occur in fallopian tube
    3. Ultrasonography or laparoscopy for diagnosis
    4. Laparotomy may be performed after diagnosis; may remove pregnancy by laparoscopic procedure
  B. Potential problems
    1. Shock from preoperative or intraoperative hemorrhage
    2. Pain control
    3. Rh-factor sensitization
    4. Aspiration during intubation and extubation
    5. Emotional crisis
  C. Nursing assessments and interventions
    1. Administer blood or blood products if indicated and as ordered
    2. Assess for trauma to bladder, ureters
    3. Assess and intervene for alteration in comfort
    4. Assess for postoperative complications related to abdominal surgery or laparoscopy
    5. Administer Rh immune globulin if woman is Rh negative
    6. Give emotional support

**II. Incompetent Cervix**
  A. Definition
    1. Painless dilation of cervix during second trimester
    2. Repeated second-trimester abortions in absence of uterine contractions
  B. Surgical intervention; cerclage
    1. McDonald's suture: Mersilene suture placed at cervicovaginal junction and removed for labor
    2. Shirodkar procedure: Mersilene tape encircles cervix, passed under mucosa
      a. May remove for labor
      b. If future childbearing desired, will remain intact and birth will be by elective cesarean
    3. Optimal timing for placement is after first trimester (≈14 to 18 weeks' gestation completed)
  C. Potential postoperative complications
    1. Uterine contractions
    2. Rupture of membranes
    3. Hemorrhage
    4. Fetal compromise because of anesthesia
    5. Aspiration
    6. UTI related to Foley catheter
  D. Nursing assessments and intervention
    1. Maintain lateral position or uterine displacement to increase uterine perfusion
    2. Administer $O_2$ through face mask at 8 to 12 L/min
    3. Maintain intravenous (IV) line for adequate hydration
    4. Assess Homan's sign (pain on dorsiflexion of foot)
    5. Monitor and interpret laboratory values, especially hemoglobin and hematocrit

6. Foley catheter care to prevent infection
7. Reproductive
   a. Position in slight Trendelenburg's position to decrease cervical pressure
   b. Maintain perineal pad count, monitoring amount, color, and consistency of vaginal discharge
   c. Assess fetal heart rate (FHR) through Doppler ultrasonography, fetoscope, or electronic fetal monitoring; normal range, 120 to 160 bpm
   d. Palpate fundus for uterine resting tone and uterine activity
   e. Assess for maternal perception of fetal movement if >18 to 20 completed weeks of gestation
   f. Administer tocolytic agent as indicated (see information on medications)
8. Assess for pain

## III. Nonobstetric Surgery During Pregnancy

A. Types of procedures
   1. Trauma most frequent indication for surgery in pregnant patient (see information on obstetric trauma)
   2. Acute appendicitis and ovarian tumors second most common indications
   3. Cholecystectomy
   4. Orthopedic injuries

B. Anesthesia
   1. Effects on altered maternal physiology must be considered
      a. Goal is to provide maternal anesthesia without stimulating uterine activity or precipitating preterm labor
      b. Surgical anesthesia designed to maintain uteroplacental perfusion and prevent preterm labor
      c. Fetal oxygenation directly dependent on maternal oxygen and carbon dioxide tensions
   2. Effects on developing fetus must be considered in timing of surgery and anesthesia
      a. Incidence of fetal loss increases during first and second trimesters
      b. If elective, procedure should be deferred until at least 6 weeks post partum
      c. Urgent surgical procedures that must be done, but that can be delayed, are best postponed until late second or early third trimester
      d. Regional anesthesia decreases teratogenic drug exposure to fetus

C. Potential problems same as for cervical cerclage

D. Nursing assessments and interventions same as for cervical cerclage

## IV. Preterm Labor

A. Definition: labor that occurs between 20 and 37 completed weeks of pregnancy; exact cause usually unknown

B. Risk factors
   1. Maternal
      a. Cardiopulmonary or renal disease
      b. Diabetes
      c. Hypertensive disease (preeclampsia-eclampsia, chronic hypertension)
      d. Abdominal surgery during pregnancy
      e. Abdominal trauma
      f. Uterine or cervical anomalies
      g. Maternal infection (systemic, intrauterine)
      h. Hypovolemia
   2. Fetal
      a. Multifetal gestation
      b. Polyhydramnios
      c. Fetal infection
      d. Placental abnormalities

C. Nursing assessments
  1. Maternal
    a. History
    b. Uterine activity
      (1) Uterine contractions ≥4/hr
      (2) Menstruation-like cramps, including thigh pain
      (3) Pelvic pressure
      (4) Low, dull backache
      (5) Change in vaginal discharge or leaking of fluid
      (6) Abdominal cramping with or without diarrhea
      (7) Thigh pain, cramping
    c. Cervical status
      (1) Effacement ≥80%
      (2) Dilatation ≥2 cm
      (3) Soft consistency
    d. Membrane status
    e. Confirm gestational age of fetus or length of pregnancy
  2. Laboratory test
    a. Complete blood count (CBC)
    b. Electrolytes
    c. Urinalysis or urine culture or both
    d. Cervical cultures
  3. Fetal
    a. Ultrasonography for fetal viability and to rule out anomalies incompatible with life
    b. Biophysical profile
    c. Nonstress test
    d. Electronic fetal monitor
D. Interventions
  1. Initial supportive measures
    a. Bed rest
    b. Hydration
    c. Empty bladder
    d. Lateral position
  2. Pharmacologic interventions (see information on medications)
    a. Magnesium sulfate ($MgSO_4$)
    b. β-sympathomimetics
      (1) Terbutaline (Brethine)
      (2) Ritodrine (Yutopar)
    c. Calcium channel blockers
    d. Prostaglandin synthetase inhibitors
    e. Oxytocin antagonists (atosiban [Antocin])
  3. Implement management protocol specific to each patient
    a. Baseline vital signs
      (1) Monitor for signs of intraamniotic infection (IAI)
      (2) Monitor for signs of pulmonary edema
    b. Continuous fetal monitor
    c. Thorough systems assessment
    d. Strict measurement of intake and output (I&O)
    e. Maintain lateral decubitus position or uterine displacement
  4. Assess for adverse effects of treatment
  5. Provide psychosocial and emotional support
  6. Administration of corticosteroids to enhance fetal lung maturation

## V. Hypertensive Disorders

A. Definitions
   1. Chronic hypertension: hypertension present before pregnancy or elevations of blood pressure (BP) more than 6 weeks after delivery
   2. Preeclampsia: hypertension with proteinuria after twentieth week of gestation
   3. Eclampsia: seizures or coma in woman with signs and symptoms of preeclampsia; no underlying neurologic history
   4. Chronic hypertension with superimposed preeclampsia-eclampsia
   5. Transient hypertension: development of hypertension during pregnancy or immediate postpartum period; no proteinuria

B. Risk factors
   1. Young primigravida or older multipara
   2. Maternal age <18 years or >35 years
   3. Weight <100 pounds or morbid obesity
   4. Diabetes mellitus
   5. Hydatidiform mole
   6. Multifetal gestation, large fetus, fetal hydrops, polyhydramnios
   7. Preeclampsia in previous pregnancy
   8. Familial history of renal, hypertensive, or vascular disease
   9. Presence of chronic renal disease, hypertension, vascular or autoimmune disease

C. Pathophysiology
   1. Early in disease process, increased CO or increased systemic vascular resistance (SVR) increases BP
      a. Increased CO with decreased SVR causes turbulent blood flow through vessels; predisposes to endothelium damage
      b. Endothelium damage activates hemostatic system
      c. Kidneys respond to hemodynamic changes by inducing vasospasms as protective mechanism initially; later in process, vasospasms cause signs and symptoms seen
   2. Multiorgan vasospasm
      a. Autoimmune or immune response occurs
      b. Increased vascular tone
      c. Increased thromboxane levels and decreased prostacyclin levels cause vasoconstriction
   3. Disease process produces state of decreased uteroplacental perfusion
      a. Decreased placental production of prostacyclin
      b. Activation of intravascular coagulation
      c. Decreased maternal vascular production of prostacyclin and other vasodilators causes vasoconstriction
      d. Increased vascular permeability further decreases colloid oncotic pressure (COP)

D. Nursing assessments
   1. Signs and symptoms
      a. Hypertension
         (1) BP 140/90 after twentieth week
         (2) Mean arterial pressure >105 mm Hg; mean arterial pressure ≥85 in second trimester associated with increased risk of poor perinatal outcome
      b. Edema
         (1) Not necessary for diagnosis
         (2) Intracellular and extracellular edema may be present
         (3) Window into organ integrity and oxygenation status
         (4) Significant finding when hypertension or proteinuria present
      c. Proteinuria
         (1) Ominous sign (doubles perinatal morbidity and mortality)
         (2) Late symptom caused by destruction of protein-sparing reticulum in kidney
         (3) Excretion of 1 g/L in random specimen or 0.3 g/L/24 hr

2. Clinical features of severe preeclampsia
   a. Systolic BP ≥160 mm Hg or diastolic BP ≥110 mm Hg
   b. Proteinuria >5 g/24 hr or 3+ or 4+ on dipstick
   c. Oliguria of <400 to 500 ml/24 hr (<30 ml/hr or 100 ml/4 hr)
   d. Cerebral or visual disturbances
   e. Hepatic, pulmonary, or cardiac involvement
   f. Thrombocytopenia
   g. Development of eclamptic seizures
   h. Development of HELLP (hemolysis, elevated liver enzymes, low platelets) syndrome (see p. 509)
3. Laboratory studies
   a. CBC shows elevated hemoglobin and hematocrit and thrombocytopenia
   b. Chemistries
      (1) Elevated serum creatinine, uric acid, and BUN
      (2) Reduced creatinine clearance, alkaline phosphatase
   c. Liver function
      (1) Increased LDH, ALT (SGOT), AST (SGPT)
      (2) Decreased serum glucose (severe hypoglycemia increases risk of maternal mortality)
   d. Coagulation studies
      (1) Decreased fibrinogen, angiotensin (AT) III, and platelets
      (2) Increased fibrin degradation products, factor VIII activity, and platelet aggregability
4. Obtain thorough maternal health history to include medical and obstetric information
5. Cardiovascular assessment
   a. Vital signs and BP; frequency of assessment dictated by condition of mother and fetus during the antepartum, intrapartum, and postpartum periods
   b. Edema increases or changes every shift
   c. Daily weight at same time on same scale
   d. Assess skin color, temperature, turgor
   e. Noninvasive assessments of cardiac output
   f. Capillary refill
   g. ECG and pulse oximetry as indicated by clinical condition
   h. Level of consciousness (LOC), behavior
6. Respiratory assessment
   a. Assess respiratory rate, quality, and pattern
   b. Auscultate breath sounds at least every shift
   c. Assess skin color and mucous membranes for cyanosis
   d. Monitor oxygenation status with pulse oximetry as indicated
   e. LOC, behavior
7. Renal assessment
   a. Assess urinary output every 1 to 4 hours
   b. Evaluate urine for protein every 1 to 4 hours
   c. Maintain 24-hour urine collection as indicated
   d. *Strict* I&O
8. Central nervous system (CNS) assessment
   a. Assess deep tendon reflexes (DTRs) and clonus hourly (absence of DTRs is earliest sign of magnesium toxicity)
   b. Assess LOC and changes in behavior
   c. Assess for headache or visual disturbances
   d. Assess for signs of increasing intracranial pressure and cerebral edema
9. Reproductive assessment
   a. Assess for uterine hypertonicity

b. Assess for postpartum hemorrhage
c. Fetal assessments for well-being or intolerance of intrauterine environment
10. Assess for signs of worsening disease
a. Headache
b. Blurred vision
c. Nausea and vomiting
d. Change in LOC
e. Epigastric pain
f. Developing coagulopathy
11. Keep calcium gluconate at bedside (antidote for magnesium sulfate)

E. Medical management
1. Delivery only cure
2. Magnesium sulfate for seizure prophylaxis (see information on medications); diazepam no longer used
3. Antihypertensive therapy if diastolic BP ≥110 mm Hg
4. Do not give diuretics
a. Will further deplete an already depleted intravascular bed
b. Indicated for cardiogenic pulmonary edema
5. Do not give heparin; will increase risk for intracranial hemorrhage
6. Administration of colloid solutions will increase risk of pulmonary edema

F. HELLP syndrome
1. Triad consists of hemolysis, elevated liver enzymes, and low platelets
a. Hemolysis
(1) Vasospasms cause endothelial damage, leading to platelet aggregation and fibrin network formation
(2) RBCs forced through fibrin network at increased pressure, causing hemolysis
(3) Hematocrit decreased, bilirubin and LDH levels increased
(4) Burr cells and schistocytes may be present on red blood cell morphology
b. Elevated liver enzymes
(1) Microemboli form in hepatic vasculature
(2) Hepatic blood flow decreases, resulting in ischemia
(3) Liver enzymes increase; LDH first to elevate
c. Low platelets
(1) Platelet consumption occurs
(2) Thrombocytopenia with platelets <50,000 associated with coagulopathies
(3) Patient on low-dose aspirin therapy will have impaired platelet function irrespective of platelet number
2. Signs and symptoms
a. Nausea and vomiting
b. Epigastric tenderness
c. Right upper quadrant pain or tenderness
d. Significant hypertension and proteinuria may not be present initially
e. May be present as early as second trimester
3. Is a form of severe preeclampsia; management same

G. Eclampsia
1. Complicates ≈5% of all pregnancies
2. Pathologic mechanisms implicated in development of eclampsia
a. Cerebral vasospasm and ischemia
b. Cerebral infarcts and hemorrhage
c. Cerebral edema
d. Disseminated intravascular coagulation (DIC)
e. Hypertensive encephalopathy
f. Metabolic encephalopathy

3. Management
   a. Prevent maternal injury
   b. Maintain adequate oxygenation
      (1) Control airway and ventilation
      (2) Mechanical ventilation may be required
   c. Minimize risk of aspiration
   d. Give adequate $MgSO_4$ (see information on medications)
      (1) Loading dose of 4 to 6 g IV over 20 minutes
      (2) Then 2 to 4 g/hr IV infusion
      (3) Always administer as secondary infusion
   e. Assess for and control elevated increased intracranial pressure (ICP)
4. Goals of therapy
   a. Control of seizures
      (1) Magnesium sulfate as stated above
      (2) If seizures persist, give additional 2 g IV bolus of $MgSO_4$ slowly at rate not to exceed 1 g/min
      (3) For seizures refractory to magnesium sulfate, give 250 mg sodium amobarbital slowly IV
      (4) For rare case of status epilepticus, diazepam, 10 mg, may be administered slowly IV
   b. Correction of hypoxia and acidosis
   c. Control of severe hypertension (diastolic BP >110 mm Hg)
      (1) Give antihypertensive agents cautiously because intravascular hypovolemia often accompanies preeclampsia-eclampsia; thus these patients are more sensitive to antihypertensive effects
      (2) Not necessary to acutely normalize BP; overcorrection may result in uteroplacental hypoperfusion and fetal compromise
      (3) Maintain diastolic BP of 90 to 100 mm Hg
      (4) Administer calcium channel blockers or β-blockers with caution in patient receiving $MgSO_4$ therapy (can lead to cardiopulmonary collapse)
   d. Deliver products of conception
      (1) During acute eclamptic episode, fetal bradycardia common
      (2) If fetal bradycardia persists beyond 10 minutes, preparation should be made for cesarean delivery, and abruption should be considered cause for bradycardia
      (3) Often advantageous to fetus to allow intrauterine recovery from maternal seizure, hypoxia, and hypercapnia
   e. Monitor fluid I&O
5. Nursing responsibilities
   a. Note onset of seizures, progress of seizure, body involvement, and length of convulsion
   b. Maintain and protect airway
   c. Administer oxygen by tight face mask at 10 to 12 L/min
   d. Administer anticonvulsant
   e. Suction secretions
   f. Evaluate lungs for aspiration
   g. Evaluate cardiac status
   h. Evaluate fetus
   i. Evaluate uterine activity; placental abruption or precipitous birth possible
   j. Evaluation for timing and route of birth
6. Postpartum management
   a. Assessment and intervention continue with same intensity for minimum of 24 hours

   b. Additional assessments for recurrent eclampsia, postpartum hemorrhage, development of DIC, development of HELLP syndrome, development of acute renal failure

## VI. Hemorrhage

A. Hemorrhagic disorders in pregnancy are medical emergencies
   1. Hemorrhage remains major cause of maternal death
   2. Blood loss may reach 35% before hypovolemic shock occurs

B. Placenta previa
   1. Definition: improper implantation of placenta in lower uterine segment; either partial or complete
   2. Risk factors
      a. Endometrial scarring
      b. Early or late ovulation leading to immature or delayed development of decidua at time of implantation
      c. Impeded endometrial vascularization
      d. Increased placental mass
   3. Pathophysiology
      a. Normally, blastocyst implants into upper portion of uterus, where blood supply is rich
      b. With previa, blastocyst implants itself in lower uterine segment, over or near internal os
   4. Signs and symptoms and diagnosis
      a. Painless continuous or intermittent uterine bleeding, especially during third trimester
      b. Onset while woman at rest or in midst of activity without pain
      c. Normal uterine tone
      d. The earlier in gestation the bleeding, the worse the outcome; fetal effect depends on total blood loss, not number of bleeding episodes
      e. Preterm labor develops in 30% of pregnancies complicated by placenta previa
   5. Management depends on gestational age, amount of bleeding, and placental location
      a. Diagnosis by ultrasonography 95% to 99% accurate
      b. Gestational age <37 weeks: manage expectantly if bleeding stops, no labor, and fetal well-being established; home care appropriate for stable patient
      c. Gestational age >37 weeks: deliver
      d. Evidence of maternal or fetal compromise despite gestational age of fetus: deliver

C. Abruptio placentae
   1. Definition: premature separation, either partial or total, of normally implanted placenta from decidual lining of uterus after 20 weeks' gestation
   2. Bleeding may be concealed or apparent with any classification of abruption
   3. Risk factors
      a. Hypertensive disorders (chronic or preeclampsia-eclampsia)
      b. Multiparity
      c. Previous abruption
      d. Trauma, especially blunt abdominal
      e. Uterine anomaly
      f. Folic acid deficiency
      g. Smoking
      h. Cocaine use
      i. Premature rupture of membranes or sudden decompression of uterus
   4. Pathophysiology
      a. Degeneration of spiral arterioles that nourish endometrium and supply blood to placenta

b. Process leads to rupture of blood vessels and bleeding quickly occurs
c. Separation of placenta takes place in area of hemorrhage
5. Signs and symptoms and diagnosis
a. Signs and symptoms related to amount of concealed blood trapped behind placenta and degree of separation
(1) Sudden and stormy onset
(2) External or concealed dark venous bleeding
(3) Shock greater than apparent blood loss
(4) Severe and steady pain
(5) Uterine tenderness and hypertonicity (early finding)
(6) Firm to boardlike uterine fundus (late finding)
(7) Uterus may enlarge and change shape
(8) Fetal heart tones may or may not be present
b. Diagnosis made on basis of presenting symptoms and physical assessment
(1) Severe and moderate abruptions are more easily diagnosed, whereas mild abruptions may be more difficult to diagnose because vaginal bleeding may be only presenting symptom
(2) Ultrasonographic examination ordered to rule out placenta previa; abruptio placentae may not be diagnosed by ultrasonography
6. Management depends on degree of abruption suspected, fetal status, and maternal status
a. Expectant management: emphasis placed on maintaining cardiovascular status of mother and developing plan for birth of fetus
b. Emergency management
(1) Restore blood loss quickly
(2) Maintain vital organ function
(3) Continuous electronic fetal monitor
(4) Correct coagulation defect or defects if present
(5) Expedite delivery
c. Vaginal delivery if woman hemodynamically stable, fetus stable, or fetal death
d. Cesarean birth in presence of fetal distress, profuse bleeding, coagulopathy, or increasing uterine resting tone

D. Nursing assessments and interventions for placenta previa and abruptio placentae
1. Fundamental areas of concern
a. Mother's condition as primarily evidenced by degree of obstetric hemorrhage
b. Fetal condition, including gestational age
2. Nursing assessment plays vital role in this evaluation process
3. Intensive observation and monitoring
a. Vital signs and noninvasive assessments of cardiovascular status and organ perfusion
b. Strict I&O
c. Record amount of bleeding
4. Fluid resuscitation
a. Stable IV site with large-bore catheter (two IV lines possible)
b. IV fluid replacement
c. Blood replacement therapy
5. Assessment of renal function
a. Strict I&O
b. Foley catheter
c. Urinary output of at least 30 ml/hr
6. Hemodynamic monitoring
a. Pulmonary artery catheter more reflective of intravascular volume status
b. Consider use of pulmonary artery catheter if aggressive fluid resuscitation required

7. Fetal evaluation as indicated
8. Verify maternal Rh status; administer RhoGAM as indicated

E. Adherent retained placenta
   1. Risks
      a. Associated with increased maternal morbidity and mortality because of hemorrhage leading to hypovolemic shock
      b. No sure signs of abnormally adherent placenta during pregnancy
   2. Types
      a. Placenta accreta: slight penetration of myometrium by placental trophoblast; most common; may be removed manually
      b. Placenta increta: deep penetration of myometrium by placental trophoblast; requires surgical intervention
      c. Placenta percreta: perforation of uterus by placenta; requires surgical intervention
   3. Unusual placental adherence may be partial or complete

F. Uterine inversion
   1. Partial or complete inversion of uterus (turning inside out) after delivery is potentially life-threatening complication
   2. Signs and symptoms
      a. Primary presenting sign is hemorrhage
      b. Pelvic mass noted on vaginal examination
      c. No fundus palpable when attempting fundal massage
      d. Patient expresses feeling of fullness in vagina
      e. Patient symptomatic for hypovolemic shock
   3. Management involves all of the following interventions
      a. Combat shock
      b. Replace uterus after woman has received tocolysis or deep anesthesia
         (1) Give oxytocic as ordered; only after uterus has been replaced
         (2) Uterus may be packed if inversion seems to recur
      c. Abdominal or vaginal surgery may be necessary to reposition uterus if successful manual replacement fails
      d. Give blood replacement therapy as indicated
      e. Initiate broad-spectrum antibiotic therapy
      f. Nasogastric tube to minimize paralytic ileus
   4. After replacement of uterus do not massage fundus because inversion may recur

G. Hydatidiform mole
   1. One of three types of gestational trophoblastic neoplasms
      a. Most often seen in women who have had ovulation stimulation with clomiphene (Clomid), in women of lower socioeconomic groups, and in women at both ends of reproductive spectrum
      b. Increased risk for development of choriocarcinoma
   2. Signs and symptoms
      a. Vaginal bleeding may be dark brown (resembling prune juice) or bright red, either scant or profuse
      b. Uterine size greater than expected gestational size
      c. Anemia from blood loss, excessive nausea and vomiting (hyperemesis gravidarum), and abdominal cramps caused by uterine distension relatively common findings
      d. Preeclampsia occurs in about 15% of cases, usually between 9 and 12 weeks' gestation
   3. Management
      a. May abort spontaneously
      b. Suction curettage offers safe, rapid, and effective method of evacuation of hydatidiform mole in almost all women

c. If woman does not desire preservation of reproductive function, may benefit from primary hysterectomy as method of choice for evacuation of hydatidiform mole and concurrent sterilization
d. Induction of labor with oxytocic agents or prostaglandins not recommended because of increased risk of hemorrhage
e. Will require effective contraception for 12 months

## VII. Multiple Gestation

A. Perinatal morbidity and mortality increase with multifetal gestation because of
  1. Birth weight
  2. Gestational age
  3. Presentation of each fetus
  4. Mode of delivery
  5. Interval of time between deliveries
B. Diagnosis
  1. Most important factor in successful outcome is early diagnosis
  2. Most important clinical finding suggestive of multifetal gestation is fundal height or uterine size disproportionately greater than date
  3. Ultrasonography for confirmation of diagnosis
C. Maternal complications
  1. Hypertension complicates 14% to 20% of twin pregnancies vs. 6% to 8% of singleton pregnancies
  2. Sepsis with premature rupture of membranes three times more frequent
  3. Postpartum hemorrhage occurs in approximately 20% of all multifetal pregnancies
  4. Anemia occurs two times more frequently
D. Fetal and neonatal complications
  1. Preterm labor and birth
  2. Congenital anomalies
  3. Discordant growth
E. Nursing implications
  1. Assess for anemia, polyhydramnios, preeclampsia, preterm labor
  2. At risk for placenta previa
  3. After delivery, assess for postpartum hemorrhage

## VIII. Obstetric Trauma

A. Leading cause of nonobstetric maternal death in women of childbearing age
  1. Motor vehicle accidents currently leading cause of injury
  2. Physical abuse may become leading cause (≈15% to 20% of all pregnant women are battered)
  3. Physiologic changes of pregnancy may contribute to injury severity and treatment
  4. Maternal mortality most often from injuries sustained from motor vehicle accidents: head injuries; followed by multiple internal injuries, which lead to hypovolemic shock and exsanguination
B. Abdominal trauma
  1. Significance
    a. First-trimester fetus protected by bony pelvis and amniotic fluid buffer
    b. Second-trimester pregnancy has become abdominal with minimum protection to fetus from pelvis
    c. Third trimester
      (1) With fetal engagement, increased risk for fetal skull fractures, intracranial bleeding
      (2) Increased risk for placental abruption; usually within first 48 hours
      (3) Complications unique to pregnancy
        (a) Uterine trauma or rupture
        (b) Bladder trauma or rupture

(c) Amniotic fluid embolus
(d) Placental abruption

d. Significant trauma statistics in general population can be used to anticipate complications in pregnant trauma victim

2. Blunt abdominal trauma
   a. Motor vehicle accidents most common cause
   b. Head injury and exsanguination from vessel rupture most common cause of maternal death
   c. Leading cause of fetal death is maternal death
   d. Leading cause of fetal death when mother survives is abruptio placentae
3. Penetrating abdominal trauma
   a. Morbidity related to point of entry and number of organs penetrated
   b. As pregnancy advances, abdominal organs are displaced upward and laterally
   c. Growing uterus may afford protection to abdominal organs located posterior to uterus, but fetus may be placed in position of greater risk
   d. All penetrating abdominal wounds may require laparotomy for full surgical exploration
   e. Gunshot wounds
      (1) Most common
      (2) Prognosis worse in that bullet path unpredictable and multiorgan involvement may occur
      (3) Greater damage to abdominal organs because of pregnancy displacement if bullet leaves uterine cavity
      (4) If bullet path limited to uterus, can have fetal, umbilical cord, or placenta damage
   f. Stab wounds
      (1) Second most common
      (2) Prognosis better than with gunshot wounds
      (3) Upper abdomen wounds may be complicated by damage to placenta, abdominal organs, lungs, heart; fetus usually protected
      (4) Lower abdomen wounds may be complicated by damage to fetus, bladder

C. Thermal trauma
   1. Skin integrity affected = body systems compromised
   2. Prognosis depends on extent and depth of burn
   3. Especially vulnerable to intravascular volume deficit and hypoxia
   4. Increased risk for preterm labor resulting from maternal hypoxemia (maternal $PaO_2$ <60 mm Hg increases fetal compromise)
   5. Fetal survival depends on maternal stabilization and survival

D. Pelvic trauma
   1. Bony ring fracture may cause fetal skull fracture or maternal bladder trauma or rupture
   2. Retroperitoneal bleeding risk increases because of engorgement of pelvic veins
   3. Genitourinary trauma results in greater blood loss related to increased vascularity
   4. Bowel (small and large) trauma possible

E. Modifications of care for pregnant trauma victim related to pregnancy physiology
   1. Cardiovascular system
      a. Blood volume increase means greater blood loss needed to show signs and symptoms of shock
      b. Plasma volume expansion >red blood cell mass increase so there is physiologic anemia during pregnancy
      c. Resting heart rate increases by 15 to 20 bpm during pregnancy
      d. Decreased SVR and increased CO may delay development of cool, clammy skin with hypovolemic shock
   2. Respiratory system
      a. Normally in compensated respiratory alkalemia during pregnancy

b. Decreased oxygen reserve and less tolerant of hypoxia as a result of increased metabolic rate and oxygen consumption
c. Because chest wall is broadened and diaphragm elevated, thoracostomy will be performed above normal site
d. Peripheral edema, dyspnea, and third heart sound normal for pregnancy but may clinically mimic congestive ventricular failure

3. Gastrointestinal system
a. Because abdominal viscera displaced and compressed, risk of liver or splenic rupture is increased; abdominal injury may be masked or mimicked; altered patterns for referred pain; rebound tenderness may be present or absent
b. Decreased gastric motility, prolonged gastric emptying time, and incompetent esophageal sphincter: increased risk for aspiration
c. Increased pelvic venous congestion: increased risk for hemorrhage
d. Protruding uterus or bladder: increased risk for trauma

4. Hematologic system in hypercoagulable state: increased risk for thrombosis

F. Nursing assessments and implications
1. Must remember that normal physiologic and anatomic changes of pregnancy will mask serious alterations in maternal status
2. Primary survey assessment
a. Airway
b. Breathing
c. Circulation
d. Neurologic status
e. Interventions
(1) Establish and maintain airway; nasal airway inappropriate because of increased vascularity of pregnancy
(2) Administer oxygen at 10 to 15 L/min through tight nonrebreather mask
(3) Place nasogastric tube to decrease risk of aspiration
(4) Anticipate need for mechanical ventilation if respiratory rate <12 or >25; obtain ABGs and avoid exacerbation of acidosis by keeping $P_{CO_2}$ to normal pregnancy values
(5) Initiate cardiopulmonary resuscitation (CPR) as indicated, maintaining uterine displacement
(6) Establish venous access
(7) Pneumatic antishock garment (MAST) may be indicated; abdominal compartment may be left uninflated once pregnancy becomes abdominal organ
(8) Control hemorrhage
3. Secondary survey assessment
a. Reassess neurologic status
(1) A: alert, oriented
(2) V: responds to verbal stimulus
(3) P: responds to pain only
(4) U: unresponsive
b. Examine for head injuries
c. Reassess chest and circulation
d. Anticipate laboratory and x-ray studies
(1) Kleihauer-Betke: maternal blood test to diagnose fetomaternal hemorrhage; indirect Coombs' test to detect maternal Rh sensitization
(2) APT test: blood test to determine whether specimen is maternal or fetal blood
e. Assess abdomen, noting pain, tenderness, distension
f. Assess musculoskeletal status
g. Reproductive assessment
(1) Contraction frequency, duration, intensity, resting tone
(2) Assess fundal height for approximate gestational age assessment

(3) Inspect perineum for bleeding, rupture of membranes
(4) If no bleeding, assess for cervical dilation
(5) Assess for signs and symptoms of abruptio placentae
h. Assess for fetal status
4. Circulatory support essential; however, vasopressors should not be routinely used
a. Peripheral vasoconstrictors will increase maternal mean arterial pressure but decrease uterine blood flow
b. Central vasoconstrictors will concomitantly increase uterine blood flow and mean arterial pressure
c. Assessment and treatment priorities for pregnant burn victim same as any other
(1) Airway patency
(2) Maintain normal intravascular volume
(3) Provide maximum oxygenation

**IX. Cardiac Disease**

A. Normal pregnancy physiology can have an impact on preexisting cardiac disease
1. Pregnancy is high-flow, low-resistance state
2. Increased CO causes patient to report signs and symptoms that mimic cardiac disease; diagnosis during pregnancy therefore complicated or missed
3. Increased CO and blood volume in presence of decreased SVR and COP will predispose to peripheral edema, especially of lower extremities
4. Accentuated jugular pulse may be normal
5. Slight enlargement occurs because of upward and leftward displacement of heart; alters chest x-ray and ECG findings
6. Benign dysrhythmias occur
7. Hemodynamic values altered (see information on normal physiology)

B. Pregnancy counseling should be done before conception; pregnancy outcome depends on
1. Functional capacity of heart
2. Underlying lesion
3. Likelihood of other complications that increase cardiac load during pregnancy and puerperium
4. Quality of medical care available
5. Psychosocial and economic capabilities of patient, her family, and community

C. Significance of cardiac disease during pregnancy
1. Maternal mortality based on NYHA functional classification
a. Class I = <1% mortality
b. Class II = 5% to 15% mortality
c. Class III = 25% to 50% mortality
d. Class IV = >50% mortality
e. Pregnancy increases NYHA class by at least one class; 40% of women with overt failure were class I early in pregnancy
2. Risk of maternal death by type of heart disease
a. Group 1 consist of the following diagnoses: atrial septal defect, ventricular septal defect, patent ductus arteriosus, pulmonic or tricuspid disease, corrected tetralogy of Fallot, bioprosthetic valve, NYHA class I and II mitral stenosis; mortality risk <1%
b. Group 2 consist of the following diagnoses: NYHA class III and IV mitral stenosis, aortic stenosis, aortic coarctation without valvar involvement, uncorrected tetralogy of Fallot, previous myocardial infarction, Marfan syndrome with normal aorta; mortality risk 5% to 15%
c. Group 3 consists of the following diagnoses: pulmonary hypertension, aortic coarctation with valvar involvement, Marfan syndrome with aortic involvement; mortality risk 25% to 50%

D. General management of woman with cardiac disease during pregnancy
   1. Collaborative effort of obstetrician, cardiologist, anesthesiologist, nursing, and other needed disciplines
   2. Goals
      a. To prevent congestive heart failure (CHF)
      b. To react promptly to early signs of CHF
      c. To aggressively assess for and react to early signs of pregnancy complications (preeclampsia, diabetes, infection)
      d. To prevent recurrence of acute rheumatic fever
      e. To prevent infective endocarditis
   3. Avoid causes of tachycardia; treat when sustained heart rate >100 bpm

E. Management principles
   1. Intrapartum
      a. First stage
         (1) Labor and deliver in same room
         (2) Monitor pulse, BP, respiratory status, lung bases, and I&O
         (3) Keep heart rate <100 bpm
         (4) Prophylactic antibiotics for ventricular septal defect, aortic and mitral disease
         (5) Examine and reevaluate cardiac status of patient in labor
         (6) Semi-Fowler's position or best position as determined with invasive or non-invasive monitoring for CO and oxygenation status
         (7) Never place in lithotomy position, even for delivery
         (8) Adequate analgesia (narcotic epidural appropriate)
         (9) Digitalis if needed
         (10) Drugs and equipment to treat pulmonary edema
         (11) Oxygen therapy and pulse oximetry
         (12) ECG monitoring as indicated
         (13) Cesarean birth for obstetric reasons only
         (14) Prevent fluid overload; use infusion pumps for all IVs and keep accurate I&O
      b. Second stage of labor (delivery)
         (1) Recognize signs of decompensating heart
         (2) Shorten second stage (episiotomy and forceps)
         (3) Avoid Valsalva's maneuver
         (4) Cesarean birth for obstetric reasons only
         (5) Atraumatic delivery
         (6) Do not put patient in lithotomy position
      c. Third stage of labor (delivery of placenta)
         (1) Avoid postpartum hemorrhage
         (2) Strict I&O
         (3) Beware of antidiuretic effect and cardiovascular effects of oxytocin
         (4) Beware of cardiovascular effects of prostaglandin preparations; avoid methergine
   2. Fourth stage (postpartum)
      a. Observe in postanesthesia care unit (PACU) or labor and delivery (L&D) for at least 24 hours after delivery
      b. Invasive hemodynamic monitoring as indicated
      c. At least one third of maternal deaths occur in first 24 hours after delivery

**X. Pulmonary Disease**

A. Pregnancy causes dramatic, predictable alterations in pulmonary function
   1. $Pao_2$ must remain >60 mm Hg for adequate fetal oxygenation, providing all other factors influencing oxygen transfer across intervillous spaces remain optimum

2. Increased oxygen consumption associated with corresponding increase in $CO_2$ excretion

B. Pulmonary edema
   1. Obstetric causes
      a. Noncardiogenic pulmonary edema: aspiration of gastric contents, sepsis, blood transfusion reactions, DIC, pregnancy-induced hypertension, amniotic fluid embolism
      b. Cardiogenic pulmonary edema: fluid overload, magnesium sulfate or β-mimetic tocolytic agents, decreased contractility
   2. Predisposing conditions
      a. Frequent complication of preeclampsia-eclampsia
      b. β-mimetic therapy for preterm labor
      c. Preexisting cardiac disease
      d. Altered pulmonary capillary permeability
   3. Treatment same as any patient with pulmonary edema taking fetal status into consideration

C. Pulmonary embolism
   1. Incidence
      a. ≈1:2000 pregnancies
      b. Untreated deep venous thrombosis (DVT) correlates with 15% to 24% incidence of pulmonary embolism
      c. Mortality 12% to 15%
   2. Predisposing conditions
      a. Pregnancy
      b. Prior history of DVT or pulmonary embolism
      c. Surgical procedures, immobility
      d. Obstetric complications
      e. Inherited coagulopathies
      f. Antiphospholipid antibody syndrome
      g. Age, race
      h. Greatest risk is in immediate postpartum period
   3. Treatment
      a. Anticoagulation with heparin
      b. Antepartum management includes prophylactic anticoagulation
      c. If anticoagulation given during antepartum period, maintain full anticoagulation during labor
      d. Low-molecular-weight heparin preparations appropriate for use during pregnancy

D. Pneumonia
   1. Associated with several maternal and fetal complications
   2. Pregnancy predisposes to aspiration; immune system altered during pregnancy
   3. Varicella very dangerous to mother and fetus
   4. *Mycoplasma* common in pregnancy and is difficult to diagnose
   5. Bacterial infection often occurs as a secondary infection
   6. Treatment
      a. Prompt diagnosis
      b. Supportive therapy
      c. Oxygen
      d. Antibiotics

E. Asthma
   1. Incidence
      a. Relatively common
      b. Prognosis during pregnancy depends on severity before pregnancy, season of year, presence of other respiratory infections, and patient's emotional state

2. Effects of asthma during pregnancy
   a. No consistent effect
   b. Slightly higher risk for prematurity, intrauterine growth restriction (IUGR) because of decreased oxygenation
   c. Must consider fetal risks of drug therapy
   d. Exacerbations rare during labor
   e. If severe, may require pregnancy termination
   f. If prostaglandins used, should use prostaglandin $E_2$, a bronchodilator, instead of prostaglandin $F_2\alpha$, a bronchoconstrictor
3. Treatment
   a. Supportive therapy
   b. Oxygen therapy
   c. Bronchodilators
   d. Antibiotics

F. Amniotic fluid embolism
1. Incidence
   a. Rare phenomenon, unique to pregnancy
   b. From National Registry, mortality >60%; of those women that survive insult most sustain neurologic sequelae
2. Etiology; see Fig. 25–1.
3. Presentation
   a. Acute onset of respiratory distress
   b. Shock out of proportion to blood loss
   c. Sudden, unexplained onset of DIC
   d. Seizures
   e. Acute-onset pulmonary edema
   f. Chest pain rare
   g. Acute cardiovascular collapse
4. Treatment
   a. Maintain oxygenation
   b. Maintain CO and BP

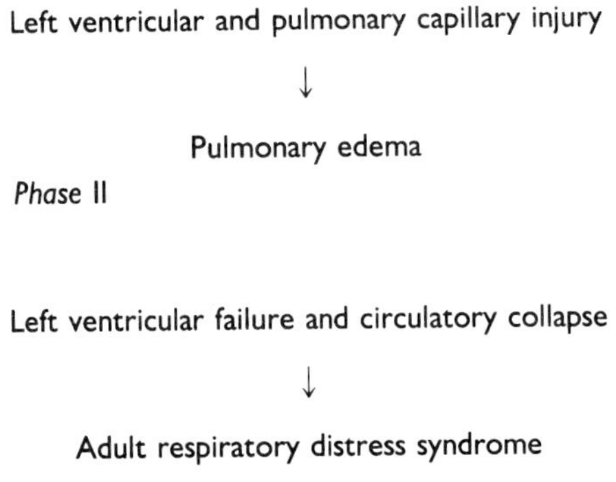

Release of amniotic fluid

↓

Transient pulmonary artery spasm

*Phase I* Hypoxia

↓

Left ventricular and pulmonary capillary injury

↓

Pulmonary edema

*Phase II*

Left ventricular failure and circulatory collapse

↓

Adult respiratory distress syndrome

**FIGURE 25–1** Etiology of amniotic fluid embolism.

c. Treat coagulopathy
d. Initiate CPR

G. Nursing implications for pulmonary disease during pregnancy
1. Multifaceted care
2. Maintenance of adequate ventilatory function
3. Optimize oxygen exchange
4. Arterial blood gas measurement
5. Monitor patient's response to therapy
6. Emotional support
7. Avoid hypoxemia during suctioning or ventilatory tubing changes
8. Hemodynamic monitoring as indicated
9. Adjust mechanical ventilation setting to reflect normal pregnancy pulmonary parameters and arterial blood gas values

**XI. Maternal Resuscitation**

A. Causes of cardiopulmonary arrest in pregnancy
1. Maternal cardiac disease
2. Severe preeclampsia, HELLP syndrome, eclampsia
3. Preexisting medical conditions
4. Acute complications
   a. Pulmonary embolism or amniotic fluid embolism
   b. Aspiration pneumonia
   c. Hypermagnesemia
   d. Anaphylaxis, laryngeal edema, bronchospasms
   e. Anesthesia
   f. Trauma
   g. Sepsis

B. CPR during pregnancy
1. Pregnancy is high-flow (CO), low-resistance (SVR) state
2. Thorax is less compliant, making mouth-to-mouth ventilation and chest compressions more difficult and less effective
3. Decreased chest compliance impedes success of standard closed-chest cardiopulmonary resuscitation
4. Before 24 weeks' gestation, objective is maternal conservation; after 24 weeks' gestation, fetal well-being may influence management decisions
5. Prompt emergent delivery increases maternal survival; if no maternal response within 4 minutes, bedside cesarean delivery or open-chest massage recommended
6. After 12 weeks, uterus is abdominal organ
   a. Decreased thoracic compliance
   b. Decreased venous return
   c. Causes aortic or vena caval compression
   d. Decreased forward flow of blood with compressions
   e. Causes respiratory impedance
7. If fetus of viable gestational age (>24 weeks)
   a. Maternal hypoxia shunts blood from uteroplacental unit
   b. Fetal $Paco_2$ increases as maternal $Paco_2$ increases, resulting in fetal metabolic acidosis

C. Modifications required during pregnancy when doing CPR
1. Uterine displacement
2. Correction of acidosis; rapid correction of maternal metabolic acidosis with sodium bicarbonate increases fetal $Paco_2$ levels
3. Rapid initiation of endotracheal intubation for ventilation with 100% oxygen a must
4. Defibrillation as indicated for appropriate cardiac dysrhythmias

5. Resuscitation drug therapy as indicated
6. Do not forget pulseless electrical activity, also known as electromechanical dissociation; common cause of pulseless rhythms during pregnancy is hypovolemia
7. Be prepared to initiate neonatal resuscitation

D. If delivery fails to facilitate successful maternal resuscitation
1. Consider thoracotomy and open-chest cardiac massage
2. Consider use of cardiopulmonary bypass in the following situations
   a. Method of rewarming hypothermic patients; especially if result of rapid, massive volume infusion
   b. Bupivacaine-induced cardiac toxicity (bupivacaine is slowly dissociated from the myocardial sodium channels)
   c. Pulmonary embolectomy in presence of massive pulmonary embolus

**XII. Infectious Diseases**

A. Significance
1. Infections during pregnancy responsible for significant morbidity and mortality
2. Pregnancy generally regarded as an immunosuppressed condition

B. Sexually transmitted diseases
1. *Chlamydia*
2. Gonorrhea
3. Syphilis
4. Human immune deficiency virus (AIDS)
5. Toxoplasmosis
6. Hepatitis
7. Cytomegalovirus
8. Herpes simplex virus
9. Human papillomavirus

C. Treatment per identified infectious process

## OBSTETRIC ANESTHESIA

**I. General Anesthesia**

A. Indications
1. Rapid induction required for maternal or fetal compromise
2. Failed regional anesthesia

B. Anesthetic implications
1. Decreased anesthesia required because of physiologic, anatomic, and hormonal changes of pregnancy
2. More rapid loss of consciousness and protective airway reflexes at lower inspired concentrations of inhaled and IV anesthetics
3. Airway changes may lead to difficulty in intubation
4. Magnesium sulfate therapy may cause prolonged neuromuscular blockade

C. Maternal effects
1. Complications of endotracheal intubation and extubation
   a. Increased risk of gastric regurgitation and aspiration
   b. Failed intubation a leading cause of anesthesia-related maternal death
2. Uterine activity
   a. Ketamine increases uterine resting tone and muscular activity
   b. Nitrous oxide has no significant effect on uterine tone
   c. Halogenated gases decrease uterine resting tone, uterine muscle tension, and spontaneous uterine activity

3. Uterine blood flow
   a. Decreased with ultra-short-acting barbiturate induction agents
   b. Deep anesthesia leading to significant decrease in maternal CO and BP leads to decreased uterine blood flow
   c. Endogenous catecholamine release from inadequate general anesthesia or airway manipulation can decrease uterine blood flow

D. Fetal effects
1. Neonatal depression can result from placental transmission of depressant IV drugs or inhalation agents
2. Effects depend on length of time of exposure and agent used

E. Nursing implications
1. Premedicate obstetric patients with Bicitra or $H_2$-receptor antagonist to decrease gastric acidity
2. Judicious use of narcotic analgesia before delivery of fetus and during immediate PACU period
3. Maintain uterine displacement with hip wedge at all times if undelivered
   a. Aortocaval compression in supine position may cause profound hypotension
4. Hyperventilation should be avoided; hypocarbia and positive pressure ventilation decrease uterine blood flow
5. Be aware of potential for postpartum hemorrhage

## II. Regional Anesthesia

A. Subarachnoid block (spinal)
1. Anesthetic implications
   a. Increased blood volume and inferior vena caval compression by uterus during pregnancy lead to engorgement of epidural veins
      (1) Increased risk of intravascular injections
      (2) Increased risk of catheter migration into epidural veins
   b. Epidural and subarachnoid spaces decrease in size and diameter
   c. Higher levels of sensorimotor blockade achieved during spinal anesthesia in pregnancy
   d. Ability to generate expiratory airway pressure (cough) decreases by 50% with spinal; 10% with epidural
   e. Contraindications same as general population
2. Maternal effects
   a. Easier to perform than lumbar epidural
   b. Rapid onset of action
   c. Provides a solid sensory block and profound motor block
   d. Intense blockade of sympathetic fibers results in higher incidence of hypotension
   e. Spinal headache may occur (<5%)
   f. Total spinal is rare but can lead to paralysis of respiratory muscles
   g. Side effects may include nausea, vomiting, shivering, and urinary retention
   h. Uterine hypertonicity or hypercontractility and uterine artery vasoconstriction may occur from unintentional IV administration of the "caine" drug
3. Fetal effects
   a. Maternal hypotension may lead to decreased uteroplacental blood flow
   b. Hypoxia can occur because of decreased uteroplacental perfusion
   c. Fetal bradycardia (heart rate <100 bpm) may occur
4. Nursing implications
   a. Before administration, hydrate with minimum IV bolus of 500 to 1000 ml to compensate for vasodilation caused by sympathetic blockade
   b. Assist with positioning and provide emotional support during procedure
   c. Maintain uterine displacement intrapartum or intraoperatively

d. Monitor maternal vital signs frequently
e. Promptly treat hypotension (systolic BP <100 mm Hg) with lateral positioning, increase IV fluids, and/or administer IV ephedrine to maintain uteroplacental perfusion
   (1) Slight Trendelenburg's position with lateral tilt prevents cranial spread of intrathecal anesthesia
   (2) Elevating legs increases preload
   (3) Mean arterial pressure more reflective of hypotension status than systolic and diastolic BP
f. Assess dermatome levels bilaterally
g. Assess for urinary retention
h. Monitor fetal heart tones; fetal bradycardia precedes maternal hypotension
i. Be alert for total spinal
j. Physician's order may include lying flat after administration to avoid headache; however, this is controversial

B. Lumbar epidural and caudal anesthesia
1. Epidural catheter frequently used as continuous technique to provide analgesia and anesthesia
2. Anesthetic implications
   a. Epidural space decreased in diameter and size because of increased blood volume
   b. Pain relief is slower and a higher volume of anesthetic agent is required than for spinal
   c. Continuous infusion of low concentrations of local anesthetics into epidural space vs. intermittent epidural injections offers the following advantages
      (1) Total volume of anesthetic less
      (2) Degree of motor blockade minimized; pelvic muscle tone maintained
      (3) Fewer hypotensive episodes
   d. With continuous infusion a potential complication is intravascular or subarachnoid migration of catheter during infusion or progressively increasing levels of anesthesia with resulting hypotension and respiratory distress
   e. Contraindications same as spinal
3. Maternal effects
   a. Produces good analgesia, which alters maternal physiologic responses to pain and lowers maternal catecholamine levels
   b. Hypotension may occur because of sympathetic blockade
   c. Woman awake and active participant in birth
   d. Systemic toxic reactions after epidural are rare but may be caused by
      (1) Unintentional placement of drug in subarachnoid space
      (2) Excessive amount of drug in epidural space
      (3) Accidental IV injection
4. Fetal effects same as spinal
5. Epidural narcotics
   a. Use of intrathecal and epidural routes for opiate-type agents
   b. Common agents
      (1) Morphine (Duramorph)
      (2) Fentanyl (Sublimaze)
      (3) Meperidine (Demerol)
      (4) Hydromorphone (Dilaudid)
   c. Mechanism of action involves specific opiate receptors in spinal cord
   d. Advantages
      (1) Decreased potential for toxic reaction
      (2) Long-lasting pain relief with minimal effects on voluntary muscle function or cardiovascular status
      (3) Minimal effects on fetus

e. Disadvantages
   (1) Pruritus
   (2) Nausea and vomiting
   (3) Urinary retention
   (4) Respiratory depression

6. Nursing implications
   a. Same as spinal (1 to 8)
   b. With epidural narcotics, pruritus most common side effect; can be treated with antihistamines, naloxone, or narcotic agonist-antagonist
   c. Sedation sometimes seen; not always accompanied by respiratory depression
   d. Respiratory depression can occur up to 24 hours after initial administration of narcotic anesthesia
   e. Platelet count <100,000 or bleeding times >10 minutes require anesthesia consultation before removing epidural catheter
   f. Monitor for progression of profound block
   g. Observe for intravascular infusion
      (1) Tinnitus
      (2) Light-headedness
      (3) Circumoral tingling or numbness
      (4) Metallic taste in mouth
      (5) Convulsions
      (6) Urinary retention

## III. Local Anesthesia and Nerve Blocks

A. Indications and actions
   1. Pudendal block
      a. Provides perineal anesthesia for second stage, delivery, episiotomy or laceration repair, forceps or vacuum extractor delivery
      b. Relatively simple procedure but requires thorough knowledge of pelvic anatomy
   2. Local infiltration
      a. Accomplished by injection of anesthetic agent into intracutaneous, subcutaneous, and intramuscular area of perineum
      b. Used at time of delivery for episiotomy
   3. Paracervical block
      a. Anesthetizes inferior hypogastric plexus and ganglia to provide relief of pain from cervical dilation
      b. Given during active labor
      c. Does not give perineal pain relief

B. Anesthetic implications
   1. Increased vascularity of perineal area, vagina, and cervix increases possibility of rapid absorption of agent, resulting in systemic toxic reactions
   2. Relatively simple to administer

C. Maternal effects
   1. Rapid onset of analgesia
   2. Hematomas may occur as result of vessel damage
   3. Maternal hypotension rare
   4. No relief of uterine contractions
   5. Systemic toxic reaction can occur from IV injection

D. Fetal effects
   1. Fetal bradycardia frequently follows paracervical block because of systemic absorption of drug or accidental injection into fetal scalp
   2. Usually few fetal effects with local infiltration

E. Nursing implications
   1. Local anesthesia and nerve blocks usually do not alter maternal vital signs
   2. After paracervical block, carefully monitor FHR for bradycardia; if <110 bpm, increase IV infusion rate, displace uterus, administer supplemental oxygen
   3. Observe for vaginal hematoma

**IV. Psychologic and Alternative Techniques for Pain Relief**

A. Psychoprophylaxis
   1. Combines positive conditioning of mother with education on process of childbirth
   2. Basis is belief that pain of labor and birth can be suppressed by reorganization of cerebral cortical activity
      a. Conditioned pain responses replaced by newly created "positive" conditioned reflexes
      b. Pain with purpose of delivering baby

B. Hypnosis
   1. Hypnoidal trance provides maternal analgesia with no maternal or fetal compromise
   2. Use not widespread

C. Acupuncture or acupressure

D. Therapeutic touch

## ASSESSMENT OF FETAL WELL-BEING

**I. Uterine Activity**

A. Assessment of uterine activity
   1. Frequency
   2. Duration
   3. Intensity

B. Resting tone (uterus at rest) is the time during which fetus receives most of its oxygen and nutrients and eliminates most of excess carbon dioxide

**II. FHR Characteristics**

A. FHR tracing reflects complex physiologic processes that occur in fetus and mother

B. Mechanisms
   1. FHR is result of interaction between central and autonomic nervous systems and heart
   2. Primary intrinsic factors
      a. Autonomic nervous system
         (1) Parasympathetic = cholinergic
         (2) Sympathetic = adrenergic
      b. Chemoreceptors
         (1) Respond to chemical changes in blood and compensate accordingly
         (2) Decreased $O_2$ = increased heart rate
      c. Baroreceptors
         (1) Maintain constant pressure
         (2) Increase heart rate with decreased BP to increase CO
   3. Secondary intrinsic factors
      a. Cerebral cortex
      b. Hypothalamus
      c. Medulla oblongata
      d. Adrenal medulla
      e. Adrenal cortex

4. Extrinsic factors
    a. Placental physiology
    b. Umbilical blood flow
    c. Uterine blood flow
    d. Contractions
    e. Fetal reserve
    f. Maternal cardiopulmonary function
    g. Maternal environment
    h. Fetal-maternal response to drugs

C. Baseline FHR
1. Approximate mean FHR during a 10-minute period excluding periodic or episodic changes, periods of increased FHR variability, or segments of the baseline that differ by 25 bpm or more; minimum baseline duration must be at least 2 minutes
2. Normal = 110 to 160 bpm
    a. Tachycardia
        (1) Rate >160 bpm for >10 minutes
        (2) Causes
            (a) Fetal hypoxia (early sign)
            (b) Maternal fever
            (c) Drugs
            (d) Maternal hyperthyroidism
            (e) Fetal anemia
            (f) Fetal cardiac dysrhythmias
            (g) Maternal hypovolemia
    b. Bradycardia
        (1) Rate <110 bpm for >10 minutes
        (2) Causes
            (a) Hypoxia (late sign)
            (b) Fetal cardiac dysrhythmias
            (c) Drugs
            (d) Hypothermia
            (e) Reflex

D. Periodic FHR patterns
1. Accelerations
    a. Sign of fetal well-being
    b. An abrupt (onset to peak in less than 30 seconds) increase in FHR over baseline of at least 15 bpm
        (1) Duration is at least 15 seconds from the onset to return to baseline and no longer than 2 minutes
        (2) Before 32 weeks' gestation an acceleration will have a peak ≥10 bpm above the baseline and will last ≥10 seconds
    c. Presence of accelerations rules out metabolic acidosis
    d. No intervention required
2. Early decelerations
    a. A visually apparent gradual decrease (onset of deceleration to nadir of at least 30 seconds) and return to baseline FHR associated with a uterine contraction
        (1) Coincident in timing; nadir of deceleration coincident with peak of contraction
        (2) Most cases the onset, nadir, and recovery are coincident with beginning, peak, and ending of contraction, respectively
    b. Benign pattern
    c. Vagal response to head compression
    d. No intervention required

3. Variable decelerations
   a. A visually apparent abrupt decrease (onset of deceleration to beginning of nadir <30 seconds) in FHR from baseline
      (1) Decrease below baseline is at least 15 bpm, lasting (from baseline to baseline) at least 15 seconds
      (2) Onset, depth, and duration commonly vary with successive uterine contractions
   b. Result of cord compression
   c. Reflects diminished blood flow to fetal heart and fetal hypoxia, hypotension, or hypertension
   d. Treat with maternal position change; obtain obstetric consultation
4. Late decelerations
   a. A visually apparent gradual decrease (onset of deceleration to nadir lasts 30 seconds or more) and return to baseline FHR associated with a uterine contraction
      (1) Delay in timing, with nadir of deceleration late in relation to peak of contraction
      (2) Onset, nadir, and recovery are late in relation to the beginning, peak, and ending of the contraction, respectively
   b. Response to fetal hypoxia secondary to uteroplacental insufficiency
   c. In presence of abnormal baseline rate, may be ominous
   d. Treat with measures to improve uteroplacental perfusion; obtain obstetric consultation

## POST PARTUM

**I. Vaginal Birth Without Complications**

A. Anesthesia: see previous section

B. Postpartum observations

1. Vital signs
   a. Blood pressure consistent with baseline during pregnancy
      (1) Orthostatic hypotension may be present for 24 hours
      (2) Increased BP may be caused by preeclampsia, anxiety, essential hypertension
      (3) BP not reliable indicator of hypovolemia or shock
   b. Temperature >100.4° F (38° C) after 24 hours may indicate infection
   c. Tachycardia (>100 bpm) may indicate hemorrhage, pain, fever, dehydration
   d. Tachypnea (>24) may indicate respiratory disease
   e. Lungs should be clear to auscultation
2. Condition of uterine fundus
   a. Firm, midline, at level of umbilicus first 24 hours
   b. Involution occurs at rate of 1 cm/d
   c. Boggy or higher than suggested normal level may indicate uterine atony related to overdistended uterus, structural anomalies, or overdistended bladder
   d. Overdistended bladder may cause lateral deviation of uterus
3. Lochia
   a. Rubra
      (1) Bright red, bloody, may have small clots
      (2) Characteristic fleshy odor
      (3) 1 to 3 days post partum
      (4) Heavy to moderate flow
   b. Serosa
      (1) Pink to pink brown, serous, no clots
      (2) Usually no odor
      (3) 5 to 7 days after delivery
      (4) Decrease in flow

c. Alba
(1) Cream to yellowish, may be brownish
(2) Usually no odor
(3) 1 to 3 weeks after delivery
(4) Scant flow
d. Excessive lochia may be caused by uterine atony, laceration, hematoma, retained placental fragments, infection
e. Malodorous lochia indicative of infection
4. Perineum
a. Slight edema normal
b. Assessment of episiotomy
(1) Redness
(2) Edema
(3) Ecchymosis
(4) Discharge
(5) Approximation
c. Rectal area free of hemorrhoids, hematoma
5. Urinary system
a. Output up to 3000 ml/d
b. Distended bladder may cause uterine atony
c. Burning on urination or inability to void may suggest infection
d. Bladder atony may occur after instrument delivery or regional anesthesia
6. Intestinal elimination
a. Bowel movement by day 2 or 3 after delivery
b. Constipation may indicate sluggish bowel or pain (fear of pain also possible)
c. Diarrhea may be from multiple factors
7. Breasts
a. Assess feeding method
b. Soft to palpation
c. Colostrum may be present; milk in 2 to 4 days
d. Nipples intact, erect
e. Swollen, painful breasts may indicate infection
8. Rh status: Is RhoGAM indicated?
C. Personal care and comfort
1. Ambulation
2. Shower or bathing
3. Perineal care
4. Sitz bath
5. Breast support and comfort
6. Rest and exercise
7. Nutrition
8. Emotional adjustment
D. Family relations
1. Visitors
2. Children at home
3. Sexuality and birth control
4. Role transitions
5. Adaptation of family routines
E. Infant care

## II. Cesarean Birth Without Complications

A. Anesthesia: see previous section
B. Potential complications same as for any patient undergoing abdominal surgery

C. Postoperative assessments same as for any patient undergoing abdominal surgery
D. Postpartum assessments same as for vaginal delivery

**III. High-Risk vs. Critical Care**
A. About 1% of obstetric population requires critical care management
B. Pregnant-specific diseases and medical complications of pregnancy that often require critical care management
1. Preeclampsia
2. Cardiac disease
3. Septic shock
4. Adult respiratory distress syndrome
5. Diabetic ketoacidosis
6. Thyroid storm
C. Care multidisciplinary approach with collaboration between obstetric and critical care units

**IV. Emergency Hysterectomy**
A. Cesarean hysterectomy usually emergency procedure
1. Emergency indications requiring hysterectomy
a. Uterine atony (43%)
b. Placenta accreta (30%)
c. Uterine rupture (13%)
d. Extension (unplanned) of low transverse incision (10%)
2. Complications
a. Increased blood loss
b. Occasional injury to either bladder or ureters
c. Increased anesthesia exposure
3. Nursing assessments and interventions same as for nonobstetric abdominal hysterectomy

## POSTPARTUM COMPLICATIONS

**I. Hemorrhage**
A. Remains major cause of maternal death
B. Causes
1. Early pregnancy
a. Spontaneous abortion
(1) Termination of pregnancy before viability of fetus
(2) ≈15% of all clinically apparent pregnancies end in spontaneous abortion
(3) Caused by abnormal embryonic development, chromosomal defects, inheritable disorders; many early losses from unknown origin
(4) Signs and symptoms depend on duration of pregnancy; bleeding, with varying degrees of pain
b. Incompetent cervix (see information on pregnancy complications)
c. Ectopic pregnancy (see information on pregnancy complications)
d. Hydatidiform mole (see information on pregnancy complications)
2. Nursing implications for early pregnancy bleeding
a. Obtain history of woman's chief complaint, pain, bleeding, and last menstrual period
b. Initial database includes vital signs, previous pregnancies, previous pregnancy outcomes, type and location of pain, quantity and nature of bleeding, allergies, and emotional status

c. Possibility of ectopic pregnancy suspected in woman with history of missed menstrual period, spotting, and pelvic pain, in addition to a history of pelvic infection, intrauterine device (IUD) use, or tubal surgery
d. If internal bleeding present, assessment will reveal vertigo, shoulder pain, hypotension, and tachycardia
e. Obtain ordered diagnostic and laboratory tests: pregnancy test; complete blood count (CBC); blood typing for group, Rh factor, and crossmatching; ultrasonography; chest x-ray film; or ECG if needed
f. Immediate nursing care focuses on stabilization
g. Correct fluid and electrolyte imbalances
h. Analgesics as appropriate
i. IV oxytocin, 10 U in 500 ml of infusate, may be needed to induce or augment abortion; ergot products contraindicated until uterus is emptied
j. Antibiotics as necessary
k. Blood volume replacement; transfusion may be required
l. RhoGAM should be given within 72 hours of pregnancy loss if patient is Rh negative
m. Prepare for surgical procedure if appropriate
n. Grief support and anticipatory guidance

3. Late pregnancy bleeding
   a. Placenta previa (see information on pregnancy complications)
   b. Abruptio placentae (see information on pregnancy complications)
4. Postpartum hemorrhage
   a. Most common and most serious type of excessive obstetric blood loss
      (1) Leading cause of maternal morbidity and mortality
      (2) Accounts for ≈10% of nonabortive maternal deaths
      (3) ≈8% of all deliveries complicated by postpartum hemorrhage
   b. Definition
      (1) Traditionally, loss of ≥500 ml of blood after delivery
      (2) More meaningful definition is loss of 1% or more of body weight; 1 ml of blood weighs 1 g
   c. Pathophysiology
      (1) Control of bleeding from placental site accomplished by prolonged contraction and retraction of interlacing strands of myometrium
      (2) Most common causes of postpartum hemorrhage, in approximate order of frequency, are mismanagement of third stage of labor, uterine atony, lacerations of birth canal, hematologic disorders, medical complications, infection
      (3) Uterine atony is marked hypotonia of uterus
         (a) Occurs with grand multipara, hydramnios, fetal macrosomia, or multifetus gestation
         (b) Other causes include traumatic delivery, halogenated anesthesia, magnesium sulfate, rapid or prolonged labor, chorioamnionitis, and use of oxytocin for induction or augmentation of labor; postpartum filling of urinary bladder
         (c) Management goal is to eliminate cause, administer oxytoxic agent, and maintain contraction of uterine muscle
      (4) Lacerations of birth canal
         (a) Second only to uterine atony as major cause of postpartum hemorrhage
         (b) Continued bleeding despite efficient postpartum uterine contractions demands inspection or reinspection of birth passage (labia, perineum, vagina, cervix)
         (c) Causative factors: operative delivery (forceps or vacuum extraction),

aseptic or uncontrolled spontaneous delivery, congenital abnormalities of maternal soft tissue, contracted pelvis, fetal size or position, prior scarring, varices
(d) Management depends on identification of source of bleeding and repair of laceration

5. Summary of diagnosis and management of hemorrhage
   a. Identify source of bleeding early
   b. ORDER
      (1) O = oxygenation
      (2) R = replace intravascular volume
      (3) D = drug therapy as needed to maintain hemodynamic status
      (4) E = evaluate patient status and effectiveness of treatment
      (5) R = remedy underlying cause
   c. REACT
      (1) Resuscitation = assessments, stabilization, venous access
      (2) Evaluate = did initial actions improve patient status?
      (3) Arrest hemorrhage = eliminate cause of hemorrhage, including traditional pharmacologic management or surgical intervention
      (4) Consultation = care may require collaboration with medicine or anesthesia, transfer to critical care unit
      (5) Treat complications = anticipate complications that occur because of hypovolemia, hypotension, and shock
   d. Treat cause
      (1) Atony
         (a) Fundal compression
         (b) IV solution of oxytocin; never given as undiluted IV push bolus
         (c) Methylergonovine (Methergine), 0.2 mg IM; *contraindicated in patient with history of hypertension*
         (d) Alprostadil (Prostin/15 M), 0.25 to 1.5 mg IM; use with caution in women with history of reactive airway disease or asthma, cardiac disease, hepatic disease, or systemic lupus erythematosus
      (2) Hematoma
         (a) Evacuate
         (b) Ligate areas of bleeding
      (3) If patient is unresponsive
         (a) Arterial ligation or embolization
         (b) Hysterectomy
         (c) Umbrella pack
         (d) Military antishock trousers

## II. Shock

A. Because of expanded blood volume in pregnancy, early signs and symptoms of hemorrhagic shock may be masked
   1. Earliest sign will be mild tachycardia with no change in blood pressure
   2. COP reduced during pregnancy; will be further reduced with fluid resuscitation, increased risk for pulmonary edema
B. Must be suspicious if excessive bleeding present; do not forget hidden sources of bleeding
   1. Placenta previa, abruptio placentae, placenta accreta
   2. Severe preeclampsia, HELLP syndrome, or eclampsia
   3. Coagulopathies (chronic DIC)
   4. Abdominal trauma
   5. Amniotic fluid embolism

C. Shock is an emergency situation in which perfusion of body organs may become severely compromised and death may ensue
D. Aggressive treatment necessary to prevent adverse sequelae
   1. Initiate standing orders: start IV fluids and obtain CBC and coagulation studies, maintain airway
   2. If patient is still pregnant, maintain uterine displacement
   3. Trendelenburg's position may interfere with cardiopulmonary functioning
   4. Anticipate need for invasive hemodynamic monitoring
E. Nursing implications
   1. Assess and record respiratory rate, quality, and pattern
   2. Assess and record pulse rate and quality
      a. Rate increases and becomes irregular as shock progresses
      b. Immediate postpartum period: physiologic bradycardia; may further mask mild tachycardia
   3. Assess and record blood pressure, capillary refill, pulse oximetry, skin color, and temperature
   4. Assess and record LOC and mentation
   5. Evaluate hemodynamic parameters if pulmonary artery catheter used

## III. Pulmonary Embolism; Deep Vein Thrombosis (DVT)

A. Leading cause of maternal morbidity and mortality during pregnancy and puerperium is thromboembolic disease caused by hypercoagulable state
B. DVT
   1. Venous stasis in presence of hypercoagulability leads to development of DVT
   2. DVT predisposes to development of pulmonary embolism
   3. First sign of DVT may be pulmonary embolism
C. Women with DVT or pulmonary embolism in association with pregnancy may have no significant medical risk factors or problems
   1. Conditions with increased associated risk include prior history of DVT or pulmonary embolism, surgical procedures, immobility, obstetric complications, and hereditary deficiency of AT III, protein C, or protein S
   2. Time of greatest risk is immediate postpartum period, especially after cesarean birth
D. Nursing implications
   1. Primary goal is maintenance of pulmonary function
   2. Frequent assessments of respiratory status
   3. Oxygen exchange should be facilitated by positioning and supplemental oxygen administration
   4. Pulse oximetry should be used to monitor oxygen saturation in conjunction with ABGs
   5. Administer heparin to maintain an aPTT of 1.5 to 2 times that of control levels or a plasma heparin level of 0.2 to 0.3 IU/ml antepartum (0.1 to 0.2 IU/ml intrapartum)
   6. Anticipate need for protamine sulfate to reverse heparin effects (1 mg of protamine sulfate neutralizes 100 U of heparin; maximal single dose, 50 mg)
   7. Assess for signs of preterm labor if patient has not delivered (see information on preterm labor)

## IV. Disseminated Intravascular Coagulation (DIC)

A. Pathophysiology
   1. Pathologic form of clotting that is diffuse and consumes large amounts of clotting factors

2. All aspects of coagulation system involved
3. Pregnancy predisposes to DIC because of changes in coagulation system
4. Pregnancy conditions that increase risk for DIC
   a. Abruptio placentae
   b. Preeclampsia, HELLP syndrome, eclampsia
   c. Retained dead fetus syndrome
   d. Sepsis
   e. Amniotic fluid embolism
   f. Saline induction of abortions
   g. Excessive hemorrhage

B. Nursing implications
   1. Be aware of maternal predisposing conditions
   2. Cardiovascular assessment
   3. Respiratory assessment

## COMMONLY USED OBSTETRIC MEDICATIONS

| CLASS | ACTION | INDICATIONS |
|---|---|---|
| **Oxytocins**<br>Pitocin<br>Methylergonovine maleate (Methergine) | Increased uterine contractions stimulate milk ejection | Stimulate labor<br>Incomplete abortion<br>Postpartum bleeding |
| **Alprostadil** (Prostin) | Increases uterine contractions | Second-trimester abortion<br>Postpartum uterine atony unresponsive to oxytocin |
| **Magnesium sulfate** ($MgSO_4$) | Decreases neuromuscular irritability and CNS irritability | Prevents seizures in preeclampsia-eclampsia<br>Inhibits preterm contractions |
| **Tocolytics**<br>Terbutaline | Relaxes smooth muscle<br>β-agonist | Bronchospasm<br>Inhibits preterm labor |
| Ritodrine (Yutopar) | Decreased uterine contractions<br>β-agonist | Preterm labor |
| **RhoGam** | Decreases immune response | Rh-negative woman after exposure to Rh-positive blood |
| **Bromocriptine** (Parlodel) | Inhibits prolactin | Prevents lactation<br>Parkinson's disease<br>Female infertility |
| **Antihypertensives** | | |
| Hydralazine | Arteriolar dilator<br>Decreases pulmonary vascular resistance | Essential hypertension, preeclampsia with diastolic BP >110 mm Hg |
| Labetolol | Adrenergic antagonist<br>Increases BP | Essential hypertension<br>Hypertensive crisis |

4. Renal assessment
5. CNS assessment
6. Fetal assessment
   a. Assess whether FHR baseline is appropriate for gestational age
   b. Assess for changes in baseline rate
   c. Assess for late decelerations
7. Monitor laboratory assessments for worsening condition or for signs of improvement
8. Assess for preterm labor
9. Institute supportive measures to correct acidosis, hypotension, and hypoperfusion
10. Initiate vigorous volume replacement
11. Initiate blood component replacement

| POTENTIAL COMPLICATIONS | SPECIAL NOTES |
|---|---|
| Transient dysrhythmias<br>Uterine tetany<br>Water intoxication | Hypertensive crisis possible if methergine given when patient is hypertensive<br>Undiluted IV oxytocin produces hypotension; administer as undiluted infusion |
| Fever<br>Chills<br>Nausea and vomiting<br>Diarrhea | Given IM or into myometrium |
| Toxicity<br>Loss of DTRs<br>Respiratory depression<br>Cardiovascular collapse | Toxicity reversible with calcium gluconate<br>Careful administration of narcotics, CNS depressants, calcium channel blockers, β-blockers |
| Tremors<br>Anxiety<br>Dysrhythmias<br>Nausea and vomiting<br>Pulmonary edema | May be given IV, SQ, or PO |
| Tachycardia<br>Hypotension<br>Dysrhythmias<br>Restlessness and tremors<br>Hyperglycemia or hypoglycemia<br>Pulmonary edema | Contraindicated in abruptio placentae, intrauterine infection, severe preeclampsia, and diabetes |
| Irritation at site<br>Myalgias<br>Lethargy | Must be given within 72 hours of delivery or abortion |
| Headache<br>Nausea and vomiting<br>Rash<br>Orthostatic hypotension<br>Reflex tachycardia<br>Headache<br>Nausea and vomiting | With hypotensive agents can produce significant hypotension<br>May potentiate hypertension |
| Bradycardia<br>Dysrhythmias<br>Nausea and vomiting | α-, β-blocker |

## BIBLIOGRAPHY


American Academy of Pediatrics, American College of Obstetricians and Gynecologists: *Guidelines for Perinatal Care,* 4th Ed., Elk Grove, Ill, The Academy, 1997.

American College of Obstetricians and Gynecologists. ACOG Educational Bulletin No. 175. *Invasive Hemodynamic Monitoring in Obstetrics and Gynecology.* December 1992.

American College of Obstetricians and Gynecologists. ACOG Educational Bulletin No. 199. *Blood Component Therapy.* November 1994.

American College of Obstetricians and Gynecologists. ACOG Educational Bulletin No. 143. *Diagnosis and Management of Postpartum Hemorrhage.* July 1990.

American College of Obstetricians and Gynecologists. ACOG Educational Bulletin No. 219. *Hypertension in Pregnancy.* January 1996.

American College of Obstetricians and Gynecologists. ACOG Educational Bulletin No. 224. *Pulmonary Disease in Pregnancy.* June, 1996.

American College of Obstetricians and Gynecologists. ACOG Educational Bulletin No. 225. *Obstetric Analgesia and Anesthesia.* July 1996.

Bonica JJ, McDonald JS (eds): *Principles and Practice of Obstetric Analgesia and Anesthesia,* 2nd Ed. Baltimore, Williams & Wilkins, 1995.

Briggs GG, Freeman RK, Yaffee SJ: *Drugs in Pregnancy and Lactation,* 4th Ed. Baltimore, Williams & Wilkins, 1994.

Burke ME, Poole JH: Common perinatal complications. In Simpson KR, Creehan PA (eds): *AWHONN Perinatal Nursing.* Philadelphia, Lippincott-Raven, 1996.

Chestnut DH (ed): *Obstetric Anesthesia: Principles and Practice.* St. Louis, Mosby, 1994.

Clark SL, Cotton DB, Hankins GDV, Phelan JP: *Handbook of Critical Care Obstetrics.* Boston: Blackwell Scientific Publications, 1994.

Clark SL: New concepts of amniotic fluid embolism: A review. *Obstet Gynecol Surv* 45:360, 1990.

Clark SL, Hankins GDV, Dudley D, Dildy G, Porter T: Amniotic fluid embolus: Analysis of the National Registry. *Am J Obstet Gynecol* 172:1159, 1995.

Creasy RK, Resnik R (eds): *Maternal-fetal Medicine: Principles and Practice,* 3rd Ed. Philadelphia, WB Saunders, 1994.

Cunningham FG, MacDonald PC, Gant NF, Leveno KJ, Gilstrap LC, Hankins GDV, Clark SL: *Williams Obstetrics,* 20th Ed. Stamford, Conn, Appleton & Lange, 1997.

Daddario JB, Johnson G: Trauma in pregnancy. In Mandeville LK, Troiano NH (eds): *High-Risk Intrapartum Nursing* (pp 255–282). Philadelphia, JB Lippincott, 1992.

Dantzker DR: Effects of pulmonary embolism on the lung. *Anesthesiol Clin North Am* 10:781, 1992.

Datta S (ed): *Anesthetic and Obstetric Management of High-Risk Pregnancy,* 2nd Ed. St Louis, Mosby, 1996.

Dehring DJ: Pulmonary thromboembolism. *Anesthesiol Clin North Am* 10:869, 1992.

Dunn PA, Poole JH: Critically-ill pregnant or postpartum woman: General principles for care. In Dunn PA (ed): *Maternal and Newborn Nursing.* Philadelphia, Little, Brown, 1996.

Frederickson HL, Wilkins-Haug L (eds): *OB/GYN Secrets.* St Louis, Mosby, 1997.

Gabbe SG, Niebyl JR, Simpson JL (eds): *Obstetrics: Normal and Problem Pregnancies,* 3rd Ed. New York, Churchill Livingstone, 1997.

Gillie MH, Hughes SC: Amniotic fluid embolism. *Anesthesiol Clin North Am* 10:55, 1993.

Hankins GDV, Synder R, Clark SL, Schwartz L, Patterson W, Butzin C: Acute hemodynamic and respiratory effects of amniotic fluid embolism in the pregnant goal model. *Am J Obstet Gynecol* 168: 1113, 1993.

Harvey C, Hankins GDV, Clark SL: Amniotic fluid embolism and oxygen transport patterns. *Am J Obstet Gynecol* 174:304, 1996.

Hayashi R: Obstetric hemorrhage and hypovolemic shock. In Clark SL, Cotton DB, Hankins GDV, Phelan JP (eds): *Critical Care Obstetrics* (pp 199–211) Boston: Blackwell Scientific Publications, 1991.

Higby K, Xenakis E, Pauerstein C: Do tocolytic agents stop preterm labor? A critical and comprehensive review of efficacy and safety. *Am J Obstet Gynecol* 168:1247, 1993.

James DK, Steer PJ, Weiner CP, Gonik G (eds): *High Risk Pregnancy: Management Options.* Philadelphia, WB Saunders, 1994.

Johnson MD, Luppi CJ, Over D: Cardiopulmonary resuscitation in pregnancy. In Gambling, D (ed): *Obstetric Anesthesia and Uncommon Disorders.* Philadelphia, WB Saunders, 1998.

Katz RL (ed): Obstetrical anesthesia. I. *Semin Anesthesia* 10:221, 1991.

Katz RL (ed): Obstetrical anesthesia. II. *Semin Anesthesia* 11:1, 1992.

Kaufmann BS, Young CC: Deep vein thrombosis. *Anesthesiol Clin North Am* 10:823, 1992.

Knuppel RA, Drukker JE (eds): *High-risk Pregnancy: A Team Approach,* 2nd Ed. Philadelphia, WB Saunders, 1993.

Knuppel RA, Hatangadi SB: Acute hypotension related to hemorrhage in the obstetric patient. *Obstet Gynecol Clin North Am* 22:111, 1995.

Mandeville LK, Troiano NH (eds): *NAACOG High-risk Intrapartum Nursing.* Philadelphia, JB Lippincott, 1992.

May KA, Mahlmeister LR: *Comprehensive Maternity Nursing: Nursing Process and the Childbearing Family,* 3rd Ed. Philadelphia, JB Lippincott, 1994.

Merkatz PD, Goldenberg RL: *New Perspectives on Prenatal Care.* New York, Elsevier, 1990.

Parer JT: *Handbook of Fetal Heart Rate Monitoring,* 2nd Ed. Philadelphia, WB Saunders, 1997.

Poole JH: Getting perspective on HELLP syndrome. *Am J Matern Child Nurs* 13:432, 1988.

Poole JH: Legal and professional issues in critical care obstetrics. *Crit Care Nurs Clin North Am* 4:687, 1992.

Poole JH: Pulmonary embolism. *NAACOG's Clin Issues Perinatal Women's Health Nurs* 3:461, 1992.

Poole JH: HELLP syndrome and coagulopathies of pregnancy. *Crit Care Nurs Clin North Am* 5:475, 1993.

Poole JH: Hypertensive states, hemorrhagic disorders, and infectious disease. In Bobak IM, Lowdermilk D (eds): *Essentials of Maternity Nursing,* 4th Ed. St Louis, Mosby–Year Book, 1995.

Poole JH, White D, Hall SP: *Crisis OB: The Video Series. Part I: Emergency and Complicated Deliveries.* St. Louis, Mosby, 1995.

Poole JH, White D, Hall SP: *Crisis OB: The Video Series. Part II: Hypertension in Pregnancy.* St. Louis, Mosby, 1995.

Poole JH, White D, Hall SP: *Crisis OB: The Video Series. Part III: Hemorrhagic Disorders in Pregnancy.* St. Louis, Mosby, 1995.

Poole JH: Hematological/vascular disorders. In Dunn PA (ed): *Maternal and Newborn Nursing.* Philadelphia, Little, Brown, 1996.

Poole JH: Hypertensive disease in pregnancy. In Dunn PA (ed): *Maternal and Newborn Nursing.* Philadelphia, Little, Brown. 1996.

Poole JH: Sepsis. In Dunn PA (ed): *Maternal and Newborn Nursing.* Philadelphia, Little, Brown, 1996.

Poole JH: Trauma. In Dunn PA (ed): *Maternal and Newborn Nursing.* Philadelphia, Little, Brown, 1996.

Poole JH: Maternal hemorrhagic disorders. In Bobak IM (ed): *Maternity and Gynecologic Care,* 6th Ed. St. Louis, Mosby, 1997.

Poole JH: *Hypertensive Disorders of Pregnancy.* March of Dimes. In press.

Poole JH: HELLP syndrome and eclampsia: Aggressive management of preeclampsia. *Crit Care Nurs Clin North Am.* In Press.

Poole JH: Pregnancy following liver transplant. *J Perinatal Neonatal Nurs.* In Press.

Repke JT: *Intrapartum Obstetrics.* New York, Churchill Livingstone, 1996.

Scott JR, DiSaia PH, Hammond CB, Spellacy WN (eds): *Danforth's Obstetrics and Gynecology,* 7th Ed. Philadelphia, JB Lippincott, 1994.

Shnider SM, Levison G (eds): *Anesthesia for Obstetrics,* 3rd Ed. Baltimore, Williams & Wilkins, 1993.

Simpson KR, Creehan PA (eds): *AWHONN Perinatal Nursing.* Philadelphia, JB Lippincott, 1996.

White D, Poole JH: *Obstetrical Emergencies for the Perinatal Nurse.* March of Dimes, 1996.


## REVIEW QUESTIONS

**1. Oxygen consumption increases by what percentage in the obstetric patient?**

A. 10% to 20%
B. 45% to 50%
C. 100%
D. No change

**2. Nursing interventions for the preeclamptic-eclamptic patient would include:**

A. Administration of magnesium sulfate
B. Continuous ECG monitoring
C. NPO
D. Pad count

**3. What is the antidote for magnesium sulfate toxicity?**

A. Calcium gluconate
B. Diazepam (Valium)
C. Naloxone (Narcan)
D. Ephedrine

**4. The best position in which to place the obstetric patient to prevent vena caval compression is:**
A. Lateral decubitus
B. Prone
C. Supine
D. Trendelenburg's

**5. The first-line drug to restore uterine tone and decrease uterine bleeding is:**
A. Oxytocin (Pitocin)
B. Bromocriptine mesylate (Parlodel)
C. Ergonovine maleate (Ergotrate)
D. Methylergonovine maleate (Methergine)

**6. Which drug is contraindicated when these symptoms are present: abruptio placentae, severe preeclampsia, intrauterine infection, and diabetes?**
A. Diazepam (Valium)
B. Hydralazine hydrochloride (Apresoline)
C. Magnesium sulfate
D. Ritodrine hydrochloride (Yutopar)

**7. What is the most common adverse reaction when regional anesthesia is used?**
A. Tachycardia
B. Numbness
C. Hypotension
D. Nausea and vomiting

**8. Dilutional anemia of pregnancy is due to:**
A. Increase in plasma volume
B. Increase in heart rate
C. Decrease in albumin/globulin ratio
D. Decrease in red cell mass

**9. The most common cause of postpartum hemorrhage is:**
A. Placenta previa
B. Abruptio placentae
C. Uterine atony
D. Retained placenta

**10. The acid-base disturbance seen most commonly in pregnancy is:**
A. Compensatory respiratory alkalemia
B. Metabolic alkalosis
C. Mixed respiratory and metabolic alkalosis
D. Partially compensated metabolic alkalosis

**11. Preeclampsia is characterized by:**
A. Hypotension, dehydration, glycosuria
B. Hypertension, edema, proteinuria
C. Seizures, oliguria, thrombocytopenia
D. Weight gain, polyuria, tachycardia

**12. Normal FHR baseline is:**
A. 80 to 110 bpm
B. 90 to 120 bpm
C. 120 to 160 bpm
D. 160 to 200 bpm

**13. Symptoms of magnesium sulfate toxicity include:**
   A. Loss of airway reflexes, tachycardia, seizures
   B. Hiccups, premature contractions, hypertension
   C. Fever, agitation, tachypnea
   D. Loss of deep tendon reflexes, respiratory depression, cardiovascular collapse

**14. The oxytocic agent contraindicated in the hypertensive patient is:**
   A. Pitocin
   B. Syntocinon
   C. Methergine
   D. Prostin/15 M

**ANSWERS:** 1. A, 2. A, 3. A, 4. A, 5. A, 6. D, 7. C, 8. A, 9. C, 10. A, 11. B, 12. C

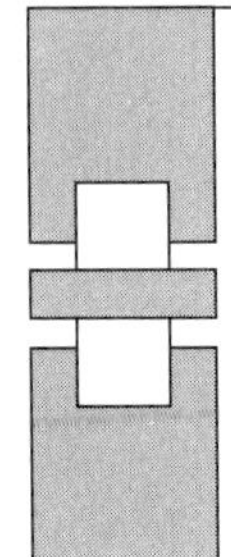

CHAPTER 26

# The Orthopedic Surgical Patient

Laura Kull Quigley, MS, RN, ONC

## OBJECTIVES

**Study of the information represented by this outline will enable the learner to:**

1. Identify nursing diagnoses specific to the orthopedic surgical patient.
2. Detail the components of an orthopedic neurovascular assessment.
3. Discuss the assessment and management of compartment syndrome.
4. Describe the pathophysiology and management of arthritic disorders.
5. Detail nursing care priorities for patients with casts.
6. Discuss the various types of traction and the nursing care priorities for patients in traction.
7. Discuss the treatment and nursing management of the patient with a fracture.
8. Describe common orthopedic surgical procedures and their associated nursing priorities.

NOTE: Spine surgery is covered in Chapter 21.

## ANATOMY AND PHYSIOLOGY

I. **Skeletal System**
   A. System of living connective tissue, high in mineral content
      1. Haversian system
         a. Nourishes bone tissue
         b. Made up of blood vessels and lymphatics
      2. Types of bone
         a. Cortical (compact) bone
            (1) Dense, hard outer layer of bone
            (2) Found in shafts of long bones
            (3) Poor blood supply
         b. Trabecular (cancellous) bone
            (1) Spongy, porous bone
            (2) Found at the ends of long bones and in vertebrae
            (3) Rich blood supply
      3. Types of cells
         a. Osteoblasts: form new bone
         b. Osteocytes: mature bone cell
         c. Osteoclast: resorb bone
   B. Functions of the skeleton
      1. Provides framework for the body
      2. Provides attachment and leverage for muscles, facilitating movement
      3. Protects vital organs and soft tissue
      4. Manufactures red blood cells
      5. Provides storage for minerals

C. Divisions of skeleton
  1. Axial: framework of head and trunk
  2. Appendicular: framework of arms and legs
D. Classification of bones
  1. Long bones
    a. Diaphysis: shaft of bone
    b. Epiphysis: ends of bone
    c. Metaphysis: flared portion between diaphysis and epiphysis
    d. Physis or epiphyseal plate: growth plate between epiphysis and metaphysis of immature bone
    e. Periosteum: covering of bone
  2. Short bones
    a. Sesamoid or accessory bones: carpals, tarsals, patella
  3. Flat bones
    a. Skull
    b. Ribs
    c. Pelvic girdle
  4. Irregular bones
    a. Ossicles of ear
    b. Vertebrae

**II. Articular System or Joints**

A. Point of union of two bones
  1. Cartilage
    a. Hyaline
      (1) Found at the end of long bones
      (2) Avascular, aneural, relatively elastic tissue
      (3) Nourished by diffusion of synovial fluid
    b. Fibrocartilage
      (1) Found at musculotendinous insertions and in the wrist, knee, acromioclavicular joint, and intervertebral discs
      (2) Higher tensile strength than hyaline
    c. Synovium
      (1) Lines bones of freely moving joints
      (2) Vascular tissue
      (3) Produces synovial fluid
B. Classification of joints according to movement
  1. Synarthroses
    a. No movement
      (1) Sutures of mature skull
  2. Amphiarthroses
    a. Slight movement
      (1) Symphysis pubis
      (2) Sutures of immature skull
  3. Diarthrosis or synovial joints
    a. Freely moveable
    b. Supported by ligamentous attachment of bone to bone

**III. Muscular System**

A. Made up of muscle cell bundles
B. Possess rich vascular supply
C. Covered by fascia
D. Attached to bone by tendons
E. Produces bodily movement by contraction
F. Controlled by complex interaction with the central nervous system

## PATHOPHYSIOLOGY OF THE MUSCULOSKELETAL SYSTEM

**I. Common Congenital and Developmental Abnormalities**

A. Joint dysplasia
  1. Incomplete formation of diarthrodial joint
  2. May lead to chronic subluxation or dislocation of joint
  3. Developmental dysplastic hip (DDH), including congenital dislocated hip, may lead to early secondary osteoarthritis

B. Torsional problems of the long bones
  1. Deformity related to abnormal development of bone
     a. Metatarsal adductus: metatarsal deviated medially
     b. Tibial torsion: tibia rotated externally or internally
     c. Femoral anteversion: leads to intoeing with internal or external rotation of leg
  2. In extreme cases may require surgical intervention

C. Clubfoot
  1. Anomaly characterized by inversion of foot and forefoot, adduction, and equinus
  2. Classified as fixed or rigid

D. Osteogenesis imperfecta ("brittle bone disease")
  1. Genetic disease characterized by a defect in collagen synthesis, generalized osteopenia and metabolic abnormalities
  2. Classified according to severity: types I to III

E. Legg-Calvé-Perthes disease
  1. Idiopathic avascular necrosis of femoral head
  2. Seen in school-aged children
  3. May lead to residual deformity of femoral head, fracture, or early secondary osteoarthritis

F. Slipped capital femoral epiphysis
  1. Disruption of the growth plate leading to posterior displacement of the femoral head on the femoral neck
  2. Seen in preteen and teenage children
  3. May lead to avascular necrosis of the femoral head, limb shortening, or early secondary osteoarthritis

G. Scoliosis
  1. Lateral curvature of spine with vertebral rotation
  2. Classified according to causative factors
     a. Idiopathic
        (1) Unknown origin: accounts for 90% of cases
        (2) Most frequent in children 10 to 12 years of age
        (3) Occurs 10 times more frequently in females
        (4) Familial pattern may be present
     b. Congenital
        (1) Develops in early embryonic life (6 to 8 weeks)
        (2) Malformation of spine occurs, resulting in hemivertebrae or failure of segmentation of vertebrae
     c. Neuromuscular
        (1) Neuropathic (paralytic): associated with spina bifida, poliomyelitis, or cerebral palsy
        (2) Myopathic: associated with muscular dystrophy
     d. Additional types of scoliosis
        (1) Acquired: seen in rheumatoid arthritis, rickets, spinal cord tumors, and neurofibromatosis
        (2) Traumatic: resulting from vertebral fracture after radiation

**II. Metabolic Bone Disease**

A. Osteoporosis
   1. Common disorder characterized by a generalized reduction in the mass and strength of bone leading to high risk for fracture
   2. Rate of bone resorption is greater than rate of bone formation
   3. Risk factors are multiple and include Caucasian or Asian race, small skeletal frame, estrogen deficiency or postmenopausal condition, inactivity or immobility, high caffeine or alcohol consumption, low-calcium or high-protein diet
      a. Fractures of wrists, femoral head, vertebrae, and pelvis common and may be induced by minor trauma

B. Paget's disease (osteitis deformans)
   1. Slow, progressive disease caused by initial bone resorption, followed by period of reactive bone formation
   2. New bone has reduced strength and is highly vascular

C. Rickets
   1. An abnormal calcification of bone seen in childhood, leading to soft and deformed bones
   2. Related to deficiency in vitamin D caused by nutritional deficit or inability to absorb or use vitamin D

D. Osteomalacia
   1. Demineralization of bone in the adult leading to soft, deformed bones ("adult rickets")
   2. Related to inadequate supply of calcium or phosphorus caused by nutritional deficit or absorptive problem

**III. Neoplastic disorders**

A. Primary bone or soft tissue tumors
   1. Benign or malignant tumors of the bone, cartilage, connective tissue, or vascular tissue near bone
   2. May lead to local bone destruction and weakening of the tissue
   3. Relatively uncommon

B. Bone metastasis
   1. Spread of malignancy from a primary site of origin to bone
   2. Lytic or blastic lesions may lead to bone destruction, weakening, and impending or actual fracture
   3. Frequent sequelae of common malignancies of the breast, prostate, lung, kidney, thyroid, and bladder

**IV. Infection**

A. Bone or joint tuberculosis
   1. Infection of the bone or joint by *Mycobacterium tuberculosis,* leading to cartilage or bone destruction
   2. Weight-bearing joints and vertebral bodies most common sites
   3. May require surgical drainage of abscesses in addition to aggressive pharmacologic treatment

B. Osteomyelitis
   1. Microbial invasion of bone leading to acute or chronic infection
   2. Classified according to method of microbial invasion
      a. Hematologic: acute or chronic infection spread to the bone through circulatory system
         (1) More common in children
         (2) More easily treated in children because of higher vascularity of their bone and supportive tissue

b. Contiguous: infection of the bone by direct extension of bacteria from infected soft tissue or surgical site
   (1) More common in adults older than 50 years of age
   (2) Risk factors include orthopedic surgeries or soft tissue trauma
c. Traumatic: infection of the bone by direct contamination with environmental or bodily microbes
   (1) More common in young males and children
   (2) Risk factors include penetrating wounds, intramedullary rods, and open fractures

C. Septic arthritis
1. Microbial invasion of the synovial membrane, commonly bacterial in origin, leading to joint infection
2. Joint infection usually accompanied by signs and symptoms of systemic infection
3. May lead to destruction of articular cartilage and early secondary osteoarthritis

## V. Arthritic Disorders

A. Osteoarthritis (degenerative joint disease or osteoarthrosis)
1. Progressive noninflammatory disorder of diarthrodial joints characterized by loss of articular cartilage, marginal osteophytes (spurs), subchondral cysts, and sclerotic changes
   a. Most common form of arthritis
   b. Primarily affect weight-bearing joints: hips, knees, spine, shoulders, interphalanges
2. Classified by causative factor
   a. Primary osteoarthritis
      (1) Cause unknown
      (2) Increased with obesity, history of repetitive trauma to joint, and age
   b. Secondary osteoarthritis
      (1) Related to preexisting factors
      (2) Seen after trauma to joint, dysplasia, or other pediatric or congenital disorders of the joint, sepsis, or as a result of a primary disease involving the joint such as hemophilia
3. Clinical findings
   a. Asymmetric distribution
   b. Pain or stiffness in joint, especially with weight-bearing activities
   c. Crepitation of joint
   d. Deformity of joint or decrease in range of motion
   e. Possible swelling and warmth of joint
   f. Gait disturbance (limp)
4. Conservative treatment
   a. Reduction of risk factors
      (1) Weight loss if needed
      (2) Decrease in weight-bearing activities
   b. Gait rest devices (cane, crutch)
   c. Local application of heat or cold
   d. Pharmacologic therapy
      (1) Oral nonsteroidal antiinflammatory drugs (NSAIDS)
      (2) Oral analgesics
      (3) Intraarticular injection of steroid or local anesthetic
      (4) Intraarticular injection of synovial fluid viscosupplement (hylagan products)
5. Surgical options
   a. Arthroscopy: diagnositic or for removal of loose bodies
   b. Joint fusion (arthrodesis)
   c. Osteotomy: option in early arthritis accompanied by deformity
   d. Resection arthroplasty

e. Hemiarthroplasty: common in hip (Austin-Moore type or bipolar prosthesis) and shoulder
f. Total joint replacement

B. Rheumatoid arthritis
1. Chronic systemic inflammatory disease potentially affecting multiple organs and joints, also considered an autoimmune disorder
   a. Extraarticular manifestations
      (1) Cardiovascular changes: fibrinous pericarditis, cardiac myopathy, vasculitis
      (2) Pulmonary changes: pulmonary nodules, pleuritis, pulmonary fibrosis, pleural effusion
      (3) Neurologic: peripheral neuropathy, carpal tunnel syndrome, nerve entrapment
      (4) Gastrointestinal: bowel and mesenteric vasculitis, malabsorption, enlarged spleen
      (5) Ocular: scleritis, episcleritis, Sjögren's syndrome
      (6) Integument: rheumatoid nodules, vasculitic skin lesions, purpura
      (7) Hematologic: anemia, thrombocytopenia, granulocytopenia, increased sedimentation rate
      (8) Constitutional: fatigue, malaise, fever
   b. Articular manifestations
      (1) Synovial proliferation
      (2) Pannus formation
      (3) Destruction of articular cartilage, with cartilage erosion, bone cysts, and osteophytes
      (4) Tendon and ligament scarring and shortening with ligamentous laxity, subluxation, and contracture
2. Causative factors
   a. Etiology unknown, multiple theories exist
      (1) Infectious
      (2) Traumatic
      (3) Stress related
   b. Genetic predisposition exists
   c. Seen in all ages, affecting females to males 3:1
3. Clinical manifestations (musculoskeletal)
   a. Polyarticular symmetric joint distribution
      (1) Can affect any synovial joint
      (2) Most severe changes in weight-bearing joints
   b. Joint swollen, erythematous, and warm to touch
   c. Joint pain, stiffness, and possible contracture
   d. Joint deformity, laxity, or subluxation
      (1) Deformities of knees, feet, phalanges possible
      (2) Subluxation of cervical vertebrae
   e. Muscle atrophy
4. Conservative treatment
   a. Joint protection techniques
      (1) Weight loss if needed
      (2) Decrease in weight-bearing activities
      (3) Use of large, more proximal joints in more activities
   b. Gait rest devices (cane, crutch)
   c. Program of rest and exercise
   d. Application of heat or cold
   e. Splinting or bracing of joint
   f. Pharmacologic therapy
      (1) Oral nonsteroidal antiinflammatory drugs (NSAIDS) or salicylates
      (2) Oral analgesics
      (3) Oral corticosteroids

            (4) Oral or parenteral gold therapy
            (5) Oral remittive agents: choloroquine phosphate
            (6) Oral immunosuppressives: methotrexate, cyclophosphamide, azathioprine
            (7) Intraarticular injection of steroid or local anesthetic
    5. Surgical options
        a. Fusion of cervical spine or small joints (e.g., wrist)
        b. Synovectomy
        c. Osteotomy
        d. Tendon repair or transfer
        e. Hemiarthroplasty
        f. Total joint replacement

**VI. Traumatic Disorders**

A. Strain
1. Musculotendinous injury caused by overstretching, repetitive stress, or misuse
2. Classified according to degree of injury to musculotendinous unit
    a. First degree: mild stretching or injury
    b. Second degree: moderate stretching or tearing
    c. Third degree: severe stretching, leading to rupture of the body or insertion site of the musculotendinous unit

B. Sprain
1. Ligamentous injury caused by overstretching or overuse
2. Classified according to degree of injury to ligament
    a. First degree: mild injury involving tear of few ligamentous fibers
    b. Second degree: moderate injury with tearing of up to one half of ligamentous fibers
    c. Third degree: severe injury leading to rupture of the body of the ligament or from its bony attachment

C. Dislocation or subluxation
1. Disruption of the contact of articulating surfaces of a joint caused by force to joint or development abnormality
    a. Dislocation: complete disruption of joint
    b. Subluxation: partial disruption of joint
2. Most common in shoulder joint
3. May be accompanied by soft tissue injury including nerve palsy
4. Recurrent dislocation may necessitate surgical repair of soft tissue or reconstruction of joint

D. Fracture
1. Disruption of the normal continuity of a bone, often accompanied by soft tissue trauma
2. Classification of fractures
    a. Severity of the fracture
        (1) Compound (open): bone is broken with communication of the fracture site with an external wound
        (2) Simple (closed): bone is broken with skin intact
        (3) Complete: continuous fracture line through entire section of bone
        (4) Incomplete: break in continuity of one side of cortex only, as in the "greenstick" fracture
        (5) Displaced: edges of fractured bone are not aligned, with higher risk for neurovascular damage
        (6) Nondisplaced: edges of fractured bone remain aligned
        (7) Impacted: fractured bone fragment forcibly driven into an adjacent bone ("telescoped")
        (8) Avulsion: separation of small fragment of bone at the site of a ligament or tendon attachment

b. Direction of the line of fracture
   (1) Longitudinal (linear): fracture line runs parallel to the axis of the bone
   (2) Oblique: fracture line runs at a 45-degree angle to the axis of the bone
   (3) Spiral: fracture line encircles bone shaft
   (4) Transverse: fracture line runs at a 90-degree angle to the longitudinal axis of the bone
   (5) Comminuted: multiple fracture lines divide the bone into multiple fragments
c. Etiology of the fracture
   (1) Stress (fatigue): fracture occurs as result of repetitive microtrauma or an excessive musculotendinous pull that exceeds the strength of the bone
   (2) Pathologic (spontaneous): fracture through an area of disease-weakened bone, usually related to minor trauma
   (3) Compression: fracture resulting from compressive force
d. Fractures by name
   (1) Pott's fracture: a fracture at distal fibula associated with severe tibiofibular disruption
   (2) Colles' fracture: a fracture of the distal radius within 1 inch of joint in a characteristic manner

3. Etiology of fractures: fractures occur when the bone is subjected to more stress than it can absorb
4. Predisposing factors for fractures: factors that reduce bone strength or forces that exceed bone strength
   a. Age: extremes in age
   b. Nutritional deficiency: diet low in calcium, low in vitamin D, or high in protein
   c. Metabolic diseases
   d. Inactivity or immobility: bone remains strongest under stress ("Wolff's Law")
   e. Physical abuse or trauma
5. Fracture healing: healing maximized when bone edges are approximated
   a. Hematoma forms at site of fracture (first 24 hours)
   b. Leukocytes infiltrate site, followed by macrophages
   c. Fibrous matrix of collagen proliferates at site
   d. Highly vascular "callus" forms
   e. Callus converts to loosely woven bone
   f. Callus calcifies and remodels (full fracture "union")
6. Goals of fracture management
   a. Reduce fracture to normal anatomic alignment
   b. Promote bone healing
   c. Maintain extremity function
7. Methods of fracture reduction
   a. Closed reduction: reduction achieved without surgical intervention
      (1) Continuous traction: skin or skeletal
      (2) Manual traction
      (3) Splints or casts
      (4) External fixation
   b. Open reduction and internal fixation (see page 558)

## ASSESSMENT PARAMETERS

**I. Vascular assessment**
   A. Pulses
      1. Note rate, rhythm, quality
      2. Compare distal to proximal pulses and side to side

B. Skin color
   1. Note pallor or blanching, suggestive of insufficient arterial blood flow
   2. Note duskiness or cyanosis, suggestive of insufficient venous return
   3. Compare side to side
C. Skin temperature
   1. Note increase or decrease in temperature
   2. Compare side to side
D. Capillary refill
   1. Compress nail bed and quickly release; expect return of color within 2 to 3 seconds
      a. Rapid refill suggests venous congestion
      b. Slow refill suggests arterial insufficiency
   2. Compare side to side
E. Edema
   1. Note location and severity of edema
   2. Note effect of elevating extremity above heart level on extent of edema
   3. Compare side to side

**II. Peripheral Nervous System Assessment**

A. Sensory component
   1. Note patient's ability to detect sensory stimulation (pain, light touch, deep touch, heat or cold, vibratory sense, proprioception, two-point discrimination)
   2. Note location and severity of any change
   3. Compare side to side
B. Motor component
   1. Note patient's ability to actively move extremity through range of motion (ROM)
   2. Grade strength of major muscle groups
      a. Grade 5: Active ROM against strong resistance (considered "normal" in well functioning adult)
      b. Grade 4: Active ROM against moderate resistance
      c. Grade 3: Active ROM against gravity only
      d. Grade 2: Weak, incomplete ROM against gravity
      e. Grade 1: No notable motion, but visible contractility of muscle group
      f. Grade 0: No motion or visible contractility
   3. Compare side to side

**III. Integrated Peripheral Nervous System Assessment of Extremities**

A. Upper extremity
   1. Radial nerve
      a. Sensory: touch web space between thumb and index finger
      b. Motor: extend wrist, hyperextend thumb
   2. Median nerve
      a. Sensory: touch tip of index finger
      b. Motor: oppose thumb to small finger
   3. Ulnar nerve
      a. Sensory: touch tip of small finger
      b. Motor: abduct fingers
B. Lower extremity
   1. Peroneal nerve
      a. Sensory: touch lateral side of great toe, medial side of second digit
      b. Motor: dorsiflex ankle, hyperextend great toe
   2. Tibial nerve
      a. Sensory: touch each lateral and medial aspect on sole of foot
      b. Motor: plantar flex ankle, flex great toe

## COMPLICATIONS COMMON TO ORTHOPEDICS

I. **Deep Vein Thrombosis (DVT)**
   A. Definition: obstruction of deep venous circulation by a blood clot, usually distal to the cusp of a venous valve
   B. Etiology: Virchow's triad
      1. Venous stasis: immobilization, peripheral edema
      2. Vascular wall damage: trauma, traction of vessel during limb manipulation (dislocation), surgery
      3. Hypercoagulable state: clotting disorder, dehydration
   C. Incidence and risk factors
      1. Seen in 40% to 60% of patients with lower extremity surgery or injury
      2. Factors increasing risk for DVT: increased age, surgery (especially orthopedic, abdominal, gynecologic), immobility, lower extremity trauma, previous DVT, obesity, use of oral contraceptives, and coexistence of peripheral vascular disease, malignancy, stroke, pregnancy, or cardiac disease
      3. Factors decreasing risk for DVT: high mobility, good hydration, use of epidural anesthesia, use of anticoagulants
   D. Postanesthesia care
      1. Assess for signs and symptoms of DVT: most common at least 48 to 72 hours after immobilization or surgery
         a. Unilateral edema of the lower extremity, unrelieved with elevation
         b. Warmth, redness, tenderness, "fullness" of lower extremity
      2. Monitor results of diagnostic tests
         a. Noninvasive: Doppler ultrasonography
         b. Invasive: ascending contrast venography (most diagnostic)
      3. Initiate interventions to prevent DVT
         a. Provide adequate hydration
         b. Encourage maximal mobility and early ambulation
         c. Apply mechanical devices per order: antiembolic hose, sequential compression devices to lower leg or calf, plantar "foot pumps"
            (1) Apply device to both extremities in operating room or PACU if possible to combat early DVT formation
            (2) Inconclusive data exist comparing device effectiveness with or without anticoagulation
         d. Administer anticoagulants per order
            (1) Oral warfarin: may be ordered day before, day of surgery, or in first 24 hours postoperatively
            (2) Low-molecular-weight heparin: generally begun at least 12 hours postoperatively
            (3) Antiplatelet aggregates: may be ordered in first 24 hours postoperatively
      4. Initiate early interventions to treat patient with known DVT
         a. Administer anticoagulation per order: bolus heparin, then adjust to achieve recommended international normalized ratio (INR)
         b. Decrease risk for clot embolization
            (1) Maintain patient on bedrest per order: common with large proximal DVT
            (2) Avoid aggressive massage of involved extremity
            (3) Administer thrombolytic agent: uncommon therapy
            (4) Prepare patient for surgical intervention: inferior vena cava filter inserted if multiple DVT

II. **Pulmonary Embolism (PE)**
   A. Definition: complete or partial obstruction of the pulmonary artery or one of its branches by a systemically mobile thrombus or foreign body

B. Causes: as listed for DVT

C. Incidence and risk factors

1. Seen clinically in 10% to 20% of patients undergoing major lower extremity surgery, fatal up to 10% of the time
2. Factors increasing the risk for PE: unrecognized DVT and all other risk factors for DVT

D. Postanesthesia care

1. Assess for signs and symptoms of PE: most common 48 to 72 hours after injury or surgery; vary with degree of vessel occlusion
   a. Dyspnea, tachypnea, restlessness
   b. Pleuritic chest pain, cough or hemoptysis, rales, pulmonary friction rub, hypoxemia
   c. Tachycardia
2. Monitor results of diagnostic tests
   a. Noninvasive
      (1) ECG: may show T wave inversion and ST depression
      (2) Chest x-ray film: may show wedge-shaped defect and accompanying diaphragmatic elevation
   b. Invasive
      (1) Arterial blood gases: may be normal or show hypoxemia
      (2) Lung scan (ventilation/perfusion studies): not reliable in absence of signs and symptoms
      (3) Pulmonary angiography: highly diagnostic; usually performed only if lung scan nondiagnostic because of risk of examination
3. Initiate interventions to prevent PE: see DVT
4. Initiate interventions to treat patient with known PE
   a. Promote adequate gas exchange
      (1) Position patient in high Fowler's
      (2) Instruct on slow deep breathing
      (3) Provide oxygen: nonrebreathing mask common
      (4) Prepare for intubation if necessary
   b. Administer anticoagulation per order: bolus heparin, then adjust to achieve recommended INR
   c. Decrease risk for clot embolization: see DVT

## III. Fat Embolism Syndrome (FES)

A. Definition: the mobilization of fat and free fatty acids that leads to acute pulmonary insufficiency

B. Causes

1. Mechanical theory: fat from the marrow of broken bones embolized to lung and occludes small pulmonary vessels
2. Biochemical theory: stress response leads to release of catecholamines; free fatty acids mobilize; chylomicrons coalesce in lung and increase capillary permeability within the alveoli

C. Incidence and risk factors

1. Seen clinically in 1% to 10% of patients with fractures; 5% to 10% of patients with multiple fractures or pelvic fractures; up to 50% of patients with fractures may have subclinical FES; seen rarely with insertion of intramedullary rods or stemmed prostheses
2. Factors that increase the risk for FES: invasion of the intramedually canal, sepsis, shock

D. Postanesthesia care

1. Assess for signs and symptoms of FES: often present 12 to 48 hours after causative event, often rapidly progressing
   a. Confusion, agitation, anxiety
   b. Tachypnea, dyspnea, pulmonary edema
   c. Hypoxemia, hypocarbia
   d. Tachycardia, dysrhythmias, substernal chest pain

e. Hypotension
f. Petechiae of trunk or conjunctiva: occur 50% of time
g. Pyrexia
2. Monitor results of diagnostic tests
a. Noninvasive
(1) ECG: may show atrial fibrillation
(2) Chest x-ray film: may show diffuse pulmonary infiltrate
b. Invasive
(1) Arterial blood gases: may be normal or show hypoxemia
(2) Central venous pressure: elevated
(3) Pulmonary wedge pressure: initially reduced because of decreased perfusion of left atrium, later may rise
(4) Lung scan: may be performed in stable patient to rule out pulmonary embolism
(5) Pulmonary angiography: may be performed in stable patient to rule out pulmonary embolism
(6) Laboratory findings: elevated serum lipase, sedimentation rate, triglycerides, and glomerular filtration rate, decreased hematocrit, increased fat in urine
3. Initiate interventions to prevent FES
a. Maintain stability of fractured limbs
b. Treat sepsis and shock aggressively
c. Provide adequate hydration
d. Administer methylprednisolone to maintain the integrity of the pulmonary vascular system: controversial
4. Initiate interventions to treat patient with known FES: early diagnosis and aggressive treatment critical
a. Promote adequate gas exchange
(1) Position patient in high Fowler's
(2) Instruct on slow deep breathing
(3) Provide oxygen: nonrebreathing mask common
(4) Prepare for intubation: common
b. Administer corticosteroids: creates antiadhesive effect on platelets, decreases inflammation of vascular membranes
c. Administer diuretics: reverses pulmonary edema
d. Support cardiovascular system
(1) Provide adequate fluid replacement
(2) Administer blood products
(3) Enhance blood pressure: dopamine
(4) Enhance pulmonary arterial pressure and right ventricle afterload: nitroglycerin drip

## IV. Compartment Syndrome

A. Definition: condition in which increased pressure within a muscle compartment may lead to severe neurovascular compromise; in cases of massive muscle destruction may also see myoglobinuric renal function
B. Cause: any event that leads to increased extracompartment or intracompartmental pressure, leading to ischemia and edema
C. Incidence and risk factors
1. Uncommon in general population; most commonly associated with fractures or injuries of the lower extremities
2. Factors that increase the risk for compartment syndrome
a. Fracture
b. Severe soft tissue injury (e.g., crush injury)
c. Prolonged limb compression
(1) Restrictive wraps, cast, brace, or apparatus

(2) Prolonged compression of limb: unconscious victim lying on own limb, prolonged pressure from positioning device during lengthy surgery
(3) Prolonged use of antishock trousers
(4) Tight fascial closure

d. Internal bleeding
e. Increased capillary permeability: related to histamine release
(1) Infiltrated intravenous fluids or medications
(2) Some poisonous snake bites
(3) Severe frostbite

3. Postanesthesia care
a. Assess for signs and symptoms of compartment syndrome: perform comprehensive neurovascular assessment noting deterioration as follows
(1) Pain: most universal symptom related to muscle ischemia; pain extreme, unrelieved, aggravated by passive flexion or extension of digit or limb, not well localized, involves entire compartment
(2) Pallor: seen in early stage related to compression of artery; later may be seen as cyanosis
(3) Paresthesias: commonly seen change related to compression of sensory nerve; burning, searing, electric sensations
(4) Pulselessness: in early stage pulse with decreased strength; later, pulse nonpalpable but audible on Doppler ultrasonography; in later stages no pulse found on Doppler ultrasonography
(5) Paralysis: in early stage may be motor weakness related to compression of motor nerve; in later stage may be complete paralysis
(6) Rigid or "tight" limb representing compartment engorgement
(7) Decreased urine output, with dark urine

b. Monitor results of diagnostic tests
(1) Direct measurement of compartment pressures: variety of methods in which catheter is inserted into the compartment; catheter is purged with normal saline; monitor intracompartmental pressure; pressures greater than 30 to 35 mm Hg considered diagnostic and warrant surgical intervention
(2) Laboratory findings of muscle destruction and renal insufficiency: elevated serum CPK-MM, potassium, phosphate, BUN, and creatinine; reduced serum calcium and pH; elevated urine myoglubin

c. Initiate interventions to prevent compartment syndrome
(1) Perform comprehensive neurovascular assessment on all patients at risk
(2) Provide early measures to decrease lower extremity edema: elevate limb above heart level, ice limb at site of injury or surgery
(3) Decrease potential for further injury: carefully handle injured part; maintain traction, brace, cast, etc.

d. Initiate interventions to treat patient with suspected or diagnosed compartment syndrome
(1) Perform comprehensive neurovascular assessment every 15 minutes with special attention to compartment at risk
(2) Maintain limb in neutral at level of heart: enhances arterial blood flow, reduces possible neurovascular impingement
(3) Remove ice: reduce vasoconstriction
(4) Release or remove restrictive wraps, splints, or casts
(5) Assess pain and administer analgesics
(6) Maintain accurate input and output (I & O) records
(7) Provide emotional support
(8) Assist with compartment pressure checks
(9) Prepare patient for fasciotomy per order: extensive surgical decompression of compartment; high risk for infection as a result of ischemic conditions

## KEY CONCEPTS IN ORTHOPEDIC CARE

**I. Goals of Care**
- A. Restore or improve function
- B. Reduce or eliminate pain
- C. Promote self-care

### NURSING DIAGNOSIS

- Pain
- Pain management deficit
- Impaired physical mobility
- Knowledge deficits regarding mobility skills
- Self-care deficits
- Activity intolerance
- High risk for skin breakdown
- Potential for infection
- High risk for ineffective coping
- Potential for neurovascular compromise

## COMMON THERAPEUTIC DEVICES

**I. Casts**
- A. Purpose
  1. Provide temporary immobilization
  2. Prevent or correct deformities
  3. Support bone and soft tissue during healing process
  4. Promote early weight bearing
- B. Types of casts
  1. Short extremity cast
     - a. Applied for stable fractures or tertiary sprains
     - b. May be weight bearing vs. nonweight bearing
  2. Long extremity cast
     - a. Applied for stable or unstable fractures
     - b. Immobilizes joint to protect soft tissue injuries: Achilles tendon rupture
  3. Cylinder cast
     - a. Applied to treat stable fractures of long bones
  4. Body cast
     - a. Immobilizes spine (e.g., postoperative spinal fusion)
     - b. Corrects deformities (e.g., scoliosis)
  5. Spica cast
     - a. Immobilizes complex joint: shoulder, hip, thumb
     - b. Prevents dislocation of complex joint while promoting soft tissue healing
- C. Materials
  1. Plaster of Paris
     - a. Applied by wrapping wet plaster strips
     - b. Easily molded
     - c. Heavier weight
  2. Fiberglass
     - a. Applied by wrapping wet plastic roll
     - b. More difficult to mold
     - c. Lightweight

- D. Early postcasting care
  - 1. Promote cast drying
    - a. Plaster of Paris: may take 24 hours or greater to dry
      - (1) Leave cast uncovered and open to air
      - (2) Use fans to aid drying of large casts
      - (3) Position casted part on pillow or smooth surface
      - (4) Move cast on pillow or with palms to avoid plaster indentation
      - (5) Advise patient to expect feeling of warmth as cast dries
    - b. Fiberglass: dry within 30 minutes
      - (1) Blot moisture from surface with paper towel
      - (2) Use blow dryer on cool or warm setting to aid drying of cast and skin
  - 2. Prevent complications related to ineffective breathing pattern with body or spica cast
    - a. Note rate and quality of respirations
    - b. Reposition patient in more upright position if possible
    - c. Teach relaxation techniques, deep controlled breathing
  - 3. Protect skin
    - a. Remove loose particles of plaster or plastic from cast edges and skin
    - b. Cover edges of cast to prevent skin irritation, especially important in peroneal area
      - (1) Turn edge of skin liner (stockinette) over cast edge and secure with tape
      - (2) If stockinette not used, "petal" edge with transpore tape or moleskin
      - (3) Insert diaper at buttocks to prevent soiling in children with body or spica cast
    - c. Instruct patient to avoid putting any object between cast and skin
  - 4. Reduce postoperative or postinjury swelling
    - a. Elevate extremity on pillow above level of heart
    - b. When cast dry, apply ice to area of injury or fracture
  - 5. Assess neurovascular status of extremity
    - a. Perform "Integrated Bedside Assessment of Extremity"
    - b. Note amount and change in bloody drainage on cast and in dependent areas

## II. Traction

- A. Definition: Application of pulling force in the presence of a counterforce
- B. Purpose
  - 1. Aligns fragments of displaced bones, preventing further soft tissue injury
  - 2. Reduces muscle spasm
  - 3. Maintains limb length
  - 4. Maintains alignment of limb, while resting soft tissue
  - 5. Reduces contracture/deformity
- C. Types of traction
  - 1. Skin traction
    - a. Traction force applied wraps, straps, or prefabricated boots secured to body (e.g., Russell's or Buck's traction)
    - b. Uses
      - (1) Short-term immobilization of stable fractures (e.g., Buck's traction for proximal femoral fractures)
      - (2) Intermittent traction (e.g., cervical neck traction)
    - c. Techniques of application
      - (1) Traction applied at bedside by trained individual
      - (2) "Customized" devices applied using webroll and moleskin
      - (3) Prefabricated devices (e.g., boots)
      - (4) Traction weight generally no more than 10 pounds (4.5 kg)
  - 2. Skeletal traction
    - a. Traction applied directly to bone through transcortical or pericortical wires or screws (e.g., Halo traction)

b. Uses
   (1) Long-term immobilization of fractures (commonly greater than 1 week)
   (2) Short to long-term immobilization of unstable fractures of long bones or pelvis
c. Techniques of application
   (1) Traction applied at bedside or in operative suite
   (2) Local anesthetic applied to skin and injected into periosteum
   (3) Conscious sedation also commonly used with pediatric patients
   (4) Amount of weight to traction according to patient's body weight and complexity of fracture, usually 15 to 40 pounds
   (5) Use of portable x-ray to confirm fracture reduction

3. Manual traction
   a. Temporary traction applied by manual pull on extremity
   b. Uses
      (1) Maintenance of alignment and position of extremity when skin or skeletal traction is being readjusted
      (2) Short transport of patient
      (3) Dislocation or relocation of joint, casting of extremity and reduction of fracture
   c. Techniques of application: firm manual pull placed on extremity while taking care to avoid pressure on bony prominences

D. Nursing care of the patient in traction
   1. Maintain traction apparatus to ensure proper alignment of body
      a. Reposition patient in neutral alignment, usually supine
      b. Obtain specific orders for amount of traction pull, position of extremity in bed, and head of bed (elevating head of bed decreases counterforce of body)
      c. Readjust skin traction if device dislodged
      d. Apply manual traction to extremity whenever skeletal traction interrupted
      e. Avoid heavy coverings (blankets) over extremities, which may disrupt traction
      f. Inspect traction apparatus carefully every shift to ensure that bolts are tight on frame, knots are tight, and weights are free hanging
   2. Assess skin integrity
      a. Inspect pressure points between skin and apparatus
      b. Inspect bony prominences of body in bed
      c. Note redness, swelling, abrasion, pain caused by pressure
   3. Assess for neurovascular compromise
      a. Perform "Integrated Bedside Assessment of Extremity"
      b. Compare affected to nonaffected side
      c. Note potential problems caused by disrupted traction or inappropriately sized devices (e.g., boots)
   4. Assess for complications related to skeletal pin
      a. Note redness, purulent drainage, "tenting" of skin surrounding pin, or pain at insertion of skeletal pin
      b. Note signs and symptoms of infection in patient with long-standing traction

## III. External Fixator

A. Definition: method of rigid fixation applied using percutaneous pins/wire in bone that attach to a portable external frame

B. Purpose
   1. Reduces fractures, especially complex or open fractures
   2. Permits care of soft tissue wounds associated with fractures
   3. Corrects bony deformity
   4. Stabilizes fractures with delayed union or nonunion
   5. Stabilizes arthrodesis (fusion) of a joint

C. Types of external fixators
  1. Simple
    a. One or two bars on side(s) of limb (e.g., unilateral or bilateral frame)
    b. Used to treat less complex fractures
  2. Complex
    a. Multiple bars or semicircular rings placed in 3-D configuration around limb (e.g., triangular, quadrilateral, semicircular, or circular frame)
    b. Used to treat more complex fractures, often accompanied by soft tissue trauma

D. Nursing care of the patient with an external fixator
  1. Maintain external fixator
    a. Inspect device carefully every shift to ensure that bolts are tight on frame, with no movement of fixator pieces
    b. Move device and limb using pillow beneath extremity or by grasping longitudinal bars on each side of limb
  2. Assess for neurovascular compromise
    a. Perform "Integrated Bedside Assessment of Extremity"
    b. Compare affected to nonaffected side
  3. Assess for complications related to skeletal pin
    a. Note redness, purulent drainage, or pain at pin site
    b. Note signs and symptoms of infection in patient with long-standing device
    c. Note changes in sensory-motor status

**IV. Assistive Devices**

A. Definition: devices prescribed to assist in mobility by providing support to an injured or weakened lower extremity by redistributing weight to the upper extremities

B. Purpose
  1. Promote healing of traumatically fractured bones
  2. Promote healing of surgically osteotomized bones
  3. Support weakened or injured soft tissue

C. Weight-bearing prescription
  1. Non-weight-bearing (NWB): affected extremity should not touch floor
  2. Touch-down weight bearing (TDWB): foot rest on floor with no weight
  3. Partial weight bearing (PWB): 30% to 50% of body weight placed on affected extremity
  4. Weight bearing as tolerated (WBAT): as much weight as patient can tolerate without extreme pain
  5. Full weight bearing (FWB): full weight should be placed on affected extremity

D. General instructions for patients
  1. Take small, controlled steps at all times
  2. Wear sturdy, walking shoes with nonskid soles
  3. Avoid wet or snowy areas
  4. Remove throw rugs, electrical cords, excess furniture, and other obstructions from path of walking
  5. Stand erect, looking forward when walking
  6. Lead with strong, unaffected leg

E. Types of assistive devices
  1. Crutches
    a. Selection criteria: prescribed for persons with good coordination, balance, and upper body strength
    b. Types of crutches
      (1) Axillary: most commonly crutch where weight is born on wrist and by tricep contraction; consists of a central post, handgrip, and axillary pad

(2) Platform: crutch used to distribute weight to forearm; consists of a central post and forearm platform; reduces stress on arthritic wrist or fingers
(3) Canadian or Loftstrand: crutch used to distribute weight to wrist and hand; consists of a central post with a band that fits around the forearm

c. Proper fit of axillary crutches
(1) Instruct patient to stand erect while wearing comfortable walking shoes
(2) Raise or lower central post so that two or three fingers can be inserted between the axilla and axillary pad
(3) Raise or lower handgrips so that elbows are bent 20 to 30 degrees

d. Crutch gaits
(1) Two-point gait: patient advances one crutch at the same time as the contralateral leg, in alternating fashion (common with PWB)
(2) Three-point gait: patient advances both crutches along with affected leg (common in PWB, TDWB and NWB)
(3) Four-point gait: patient advances right crutch, left foot, left crutch, right foot, with three "points" on ground at all times (used only in patient with high disability)

e. Stair climbing
(1) Climbing up stairs: patient holds banister on affected side and both crutches in contralateral hand; patient steps up with unaffected leg and follows with crutches and affected leg to same stair
(2) Climbing down stairs: patient holds banister on affected side and both crutches in contralateral hand; with weight on "good leg," patient steps down with affected leg and crutches; patient brings unaffected leg down to same stair

2. Walkers
a. Selection criteria: prescribed for persons who require more stability than crutches, such as those with impaired balance or coordination
b. Types of walkers
(1) Simple walker: most common type of walker; consists of sturdy frame with handgrips
(2) Platform walker: walker used to distribute weight to forearm; consists of a sturdy frame with forearm platform; reduces stress on arthritic wrist/fingers
c. Proper fit of simple walker
(1) Instruct patient to stand erect while wearing comfortable walking shoes, heels even with back of walker
(2) Raise or lower all four legs of walker equally so that elbows are bent 20 to 30 degrees
d. Walker gait
(1) Patient advances walker a short arm length forward, planting walker firmly on all four legs
(2) Patient advances affected foot, then advances body forward while supporting weight on arms
e. Stairs: performed with folded walker in manner similar to stair climbing with crutches

3. Canes
a. Selection criteria: prescribed for patients with minor disability and good balance, often after use of crutches or walker
b. Types of canes
(1) Simple cane: central post with curved handle
(2) Quad cane: central post with four distal legs and curved handle
c. Proper fit of cane
(1) Instruct patient to stand erect while wearing comfortable walking shoes, cane 2 inches (5 cm) in front and 6 inches (15 cm) to the side of unaffected leg
(2) Raise or lower central post so that elbow is bent 20 to 30 degrees

d. Cane gait
   (1) Instruct patient to hold cane in hand opposite affected side
   (2) Patient puts weight on "good leg," advancing affected leg and cane a comfortable distance
   (3) Patient supports weight on both cane and affected leg, stepping through with "good leg"

e. Stairs: performed with cane hand opposite affected leg in manner similar to stair climbing with crutches

## COMMON OPERATIVE PROCEDURES

**I. Open Reduction Internal Fixation (ORIF) of Femoral Fracture**

A. Procedure: operative reduction of a fracture of the femur and stabilization with hardware

B. Purpose
   1. Attains and maintains reduction of fracture
   2. Enhances fracture healing through stability
   3. Allows for early mobilization of patient

C. Types of femoral fractures
   1. Femoral neck fracture
      a. Basillar: fracture at the distal neck of the femur
      b. Subcapital: fracture directly under the femoral head
   2. Intertrochanteric fracture: fracture on a line through the greater and lesser trochanter
   3. Subtrochanteric fracture: transverse fracture between the lesser trochanter and a site an inch or more below the greater trochanter
   4. Femoral shaft fracture: fracture between the greater trochanter and the knee

D. Commonly used fixation devices
   1. Wires and pins
   2. Bone screws
   3. Plates with screws
   4. Compression (sliding) hip screw
   5. Intramedullary rods/nails

E. Postanesthesia care
   1. Assess neurovascular status: perform comprehensive neurovascular assessment (see page 548)
   2. Maintain proper positioning
      a. Place extremities in neutral position
      b. Use trochanter roll (rolled sheet or blanket) or sandbag to prevent rotation of lower extremities
      c. Turn patient on physician order only
         (1) Usually approved to turn to unaffected side only
         (2) Maintain anatomic positioning by using pillows between legs and back for support
      d. Prevent dislocation after ORIF for femoral neck fracture (less stable because capsule of hip is interrupted)
         (1) Avoid hip flexion greater than 90 degrees
         (2) Avoid hip adduction by placing abduction devices between legs
         (3) Avoid extremes in rotation with trochanter roll
         (4) Provide overhead trapeze to aid patient movement
   3. Prevent extremity edema
      a. Elevate extremity above level of heart using pillows
      b. Avoid direct pressure in popliteal fossa

4. Monitor wound drainage
   a. Maintain patency of drainage device if present
   b. Expect pattern of decreasing drainage after first 2 to 4 hours postoperatively
   c. Assess for dependent drainage underneath operative site and for drainage on dressing or cast
   d. Maintain occlusive compression dressing, reinforcing if needed
5. Monitor for complications after femoral fracture (see also Common Orthopedic Complications)
   a. Infection
      (1) Most common with open fracture
      (2) Assess for systemic signs or symptoms of infection
      (3) Assess for local signs of infection (visibly reddened incision line)
      (4) Identify high-risk patient: malnourished or infirm patient, incontinent patient, patient with urinary tract infection or tooth abscess
   b. Deep vein thrombosis (DVT): High risk in patients who are elderly, dehydrated, immobile, or have history of DVT
   c. Pulmonary embolism (PE): High risk as for DVT
   d. Compartment syndrome: High risk in patients with prolonged limb compression, extensive soft tissue, vascular trauma, and sepsis
   e. Fat emboli syndrome (FES): High risk in patients with fracture of midshaft femur, fractures associated with sepsis or shock

## II. Arthroscopy

A. Procedure: examination of the interior of a joint with a small fiberoptic tube in effort to accurately visualize or treat the joint cavity
B. Purpose
   1. Diagnosis of pathologic condition
      a. Direct visualization of the articular surfaces, the synovium, supportive tissue, and foreign tissue
      b. Biopsy of synovium
   2. Treatment of pathologic condition
      a. Repair or resection of torn menisci
      b. Debridement of cartilage
      c. Removal of foreign body
      d. Arthroscopic-assisted ligament repair
      e. Fixation of minor damage to cartilage
C. Joints amenable to arthroscopy
   1. Knee: Most common
   2. Hip
   3. Ankle
   4. Shoulder
   5. Elbow
   6. Temporomandibular joint
D. Postanesthesia care
   1. Assess neurovascular status: perform comprehensive neurovascular assessment (page 548)
   2. Assess multiple portal sites
      a. Monitor dressing for drainage
      b. Maintain original dressing, reinforce with additional bulky dressing and Ace wrap if needed
   3. Prevent extremity edema
      a. Elevate extremity above level of heart with pillows
      b. Avoid direct pressure in popliteal fossa

4. Monitor for postarthroscopy complications (see also Common Orthopedic Complications)
   a. Infection
      (1) Monitor portal sites for redness, swelling, pain, erythema: most common complication is superficial infection
      (2) Instruct patient in manifestation of signs and symptoms of systemic and deep infection: uncommon, occurring more than 24 hours postoperatively
   b. Major complications: rare but may include DVT, PE, and compartment syndrome
5. Instruct patient regarding use of crutches
6. Provide for pain control
   a. Oral opioids commonly used postoperatively
   b. Parenteral patient-controlled analgesia (PCA) may be used for 24 hours when more extensive joint repair is performed (e.g., anterior cruciate ligament repair)
7. Position joint and allow for movement per order
   a. Avoid direct pressure under joint and on bony prominences
   b. Encourage active range of motion to all unaffected joints
   c. Provide continuous passive motion machine per order
   d. Provide for joint support with hinged brace or other device per order

**III. Arthroplasty (Joint Reconstruction)**

A. Procedure: reconstruction of articulating surfaces of joint
B. Purpose
   1. Relief of chronic disabling pain
   2. Improvement in joint function and activities of daily living
   3. Correction of deformity
   4. Prevention of further bone destruction
   5. Stabilization of joint
C. Joints replaced
   1. Most common arthroplasties
      a. Hip
      b. Knee
      c. Shoulder
   2. Other joints replaced
      a. Elbows
      b. Fingers (proximal interphalangeal joint [PIP], metacarpophalangeal joint [MCP])
      c. Wrist/thumb
      d. Ankle
      e. Temporomandibular joint
D. Common diagnosis prearthroplasty
   1. Degenerative arthritis (osteoarthritis or osteoarthrosis)
   2. Rheumatoid arthritis
   3. Avascular necrosis (osteonecrosis or ischemic necrosis)
   4. Posttraumatic arthritis
E. Types of arthroplasties
   1. Hemiarthroplasty (one joint surface reconstructed with artificial part)
      a. Cup arthroplasty: placement of metal cup over femoral head (uncommon in modern arthroplasties)
      b. Endoprosthesis: replacement of femoral head with stemmed prosthesis stabilized in proximal medullary canal
         (1) Austin Moore prosthesis: prosthetic femoral head articulates with natural acetabulum

(2) Bipolar prosthesis: prosthetic femoral head articulates with plastic liner of large metal "shell" placed against acetabulum (greatest motion is within prosthetic device)

2. Total joint arthroplasty: both joint surfaces reconstructed with artificial parts

F. Materials commonly used
   1. Metals
      a. Cobalt chromium
      b. Titanium or titanium alloys
   2. Ceramics
   3. Plastics (high-molecular-weight polymers)
   4. Polymethyl methacrylate ("bone cement")

G. Methods of component fixation in bone
   1. Cement
      a. "Gold standard" of fixation
      b. Cement injected under pressure
      c. Cement hardens in minutes, emits heat in process
      d. Allows for immediate full weight bearing on extremity
   2. Biologic ingrowth
      a. Microtextured surface of prosthesis allows bone to "grow into" and stabilize component
      b. Bone ingrowth optimized with tight fit of prosthesis into bone, healthy dense bone, and reduction of prosthetic motion in early stages of bone incorporation
      c. Attempts at "tight fit" can cause intraoperative fracture
      d. Postoperative weight-bearing restrictions generally continue for average 2 months
   3. Press fit
      a. Used for stemmed components only
      b. Stem impacted snugly into canal of bone with cement, stem mechanically supported by cortical bone

H. Potential complications common to arthroplasties (see also "Common Orthopedic Complications")
   1. Deep vein thrombosis
      a. Single most common complication with lower extremity joint arthroplasty
      b. Prophylaxis generally given to all patients
   2. Pulmonary embolism
   3. Fat embolism: rare, possible during insertion of stemmed devices or in situations of acute traumatic injury
   4. Compartment syndrome: rare, may occur as a result of compression of contralateral limb during surgery or with large wound hematoma
   5. Peripheral neurovascular impairment
   6. Infection
      a. Superficial wound infection
         (1) Generally limited
         (2) May be related to stitch abscess
         (3) Treated with topical or oral antibiotics or both
      b. Deep wound infection
         (1) Acute: attributed to perioperative event
         (2) Late: attributed to hematologic spread of infection in body from remote site (e.g., urinary tract infection or abscessed tooth)
         (3) Acute deep infection requires open irrigation of joint and possible exchange of liner and long-term antibiotics
         (4) Late deep infection often requires removal of prosthesis, debridement of bone or tissue, and long-term antibiotics

I. Postanesthesia care of the hip arthroplasty patient
   1. Assess neurovascular status
      a. Perform comprehensive neurovascular assessment at least every hour for first 4 hours
      b. Note signs of peroneal nerve palsy: possibly resulting from stretch injury caused by intraoperative hip dislocation, limb lengthening, or hematoma
         (1) Weak or absent dorsiflexion of foot and ankle against examiner resistance
         (2) Decrease or loss of sensation to lateral aspect of great toe, medial aspect of second toe
   2. Assess for signs of wound drainage: blood loss should not exceed 500 ml in first 8 hours
      a. Note dependent drainage on dressing and bed
      b. Note formation and extent of hematoma
         (1) May suggest active hemorrhage
         (2) May require surgical evacuation
      c. Maintain occlusive compression dressing to operative site, reinforcing if necessary
      d. Maintain drainage device if present
         (1) Closed suction device such as a Hemovac: most common suction device used
         (2) Gravity device: uncommon
         (3) Autotransfusion device: used to collect and reinfuse blood according to hospital guidelines
   3. Position lower extremity to reduce risk of dislocation
      a. Maintain operative extremity in neutral alignment
      b. Avoid hip adduction
         (1) Place pillow or abduction device between legs at all times
         (2) Turn patient carefully to unaffected side, maintaining abduction, if allowed
      c. Avoid hip flexion greater than 90 degrees
         (1) Avoid raising head of bed and foot of bed at same time
         (2) Encourage use of overhead trapeze for support during position changes
      d. Avoid extremes in hip rotation using trochanteric roll to side(s) of affected leg, considering surgical approach
         (1) Avoid internal rotation if posterior approach
         (2) Avoid external rotation if anterolateral approach
   4. Provide aids to enhance patient compliance to position restrictions (e.g., long handled reacher, long shoe horn, sock aid)
   5. Provide for pain control
      a. Instruct patient regarding use of parenteral patient–controlled analgesia
      b. Expect intravenous or epidural opioids postoperatively
   6. Prevent infection
      a. Use strict aseptic technique for all invasive procedures
      b. Insert Foley catheter if signs of bladder distension
      c. Instruct patient in aggressive pulmonary hygiene

J. Postanesthesia care of the knee arthroplasty patient
   1. Assess neurovascular status
      a. Perform comprehensive neurovascular assessment at least every hour for first 4 hours
      b. Note signs of tibial nerve palsy: possibly due to stretch injury caused by intraoperative knee dislocation, extensive swelling or hematoma
   2. Assess for signs of wound drainage: blood loss should not exceed 500 ml in first 8 hours (see interventions for hip arthroplasty, section I-2)
   3. Position extremity to reduce edema and prevent contracture
      a. Maintain operated extremity in neutral alignment
      b. Elevate extremity on pillow above level of heart
      c. Avoid placement of pillow beneath popliteal fossa
      d. Avoid prolonged side-lying with knee flexed
   4. Provide assistive devices to enhance patient's independence (e.g., long handled reacher, long shoe horn, sock aid)

5. Encourage aggressive range of motion of knee
   a. Activate continuous passive motion machine as ordered
      (1) Supplied and adjusted by trained personnel
      (2) Degrees of flexion and extension ordered by physician
      (3) Gradually increase knee flexion and extension per order according to patient tolerance
6. Provide for pain control (see interventions for hip arthroplasty, section I-5)
7. Prevent infection (see intervention for hip arthroplasty, section I-6)

K. Postanesthesia care of the shoulder arthroplasty patient
1. Assess neurovascular status
   a. Perform comprehensive assessment at least every hour for first 4 hours
   b. Note deficit in medial, radial, or ulnar nerve
2. Assess for wound drainage: blood loss should not exceed 150 ml in first 24 hours
   a. Note dependent drainage on dressing and bed
   b. Note formation and extent of hematoma
   c. Maintain occlusive compression dressing to operative site
   d. Maintain drainage device if present
      (1) Suction device: most common
      (2) Gravity device: uncommon
3. Positioning to reduce risk of dislocation
   a. Maintain postoperative extremity positioning
      (1) Shoulder adduction and internal rotation using sling and swathe dressing with affected arm at side: most common
      (2) Shoulder abduction with abduction frame or airplane splint: less common
4. Assist with measures to reduce edema
   a. Encourage range of motion to distal upper extremity joints distal to shoulder
      (1) Range of motion of fingers and wrist commonly encouraged at least every hour
      (2) Range of motion of elbow often allowed: patient lightly stabilizes upper arm with unaffected hand during elbow range of motion
5. Provide overhead trapeze and assistive devices to enhance patient ability to perform activities of daily living
6. Encourage range of motion of shoulder as soon as possible
   a. Activate continuous passive motion machine as ordered
      (1) Supplied and adjusted by trained personnel
      (2) Used in supine position or in chair-sitting position
      (3) Degrees and direction of movement ordered by physician
      (4) Increase shoulder motion per order and according to patient tolerance
7. Provide for pain control (see interventions for hip arthroplasty, section I-5)
8. Prevent infection (see intervention for hip arthroplasty, section I-6)

## IV. Spinal Fusion/Stabilization (Thoracolumbar Spine)

A. Procedure: surgical stabilization of the spine using mechanical instrumentation with or without bone graft augmentation

B. Purpose
1. Prevent progression of spinal deformity
2. Correct spinal deformity: lateral curves greater than 40 degrees
3. Reduce actual or potential neurologic or cardiopulmonary deficits

C. Methods of spinal fusion
1. Posterior spinal fusion with instrumentation
   a. Cotrel-Dubousset instrumentation: most common
   b. Harrington distraction rods or spinous process wiring
   c. Luque rods: most common for paralytic scoliosis

2. Anterior spinal fusion
   a. Zielke instrumentation
   b. Harms instrumentation
3. Combined anterior and posterior surgery
   a. Recommended for adults or children with severe deformities
   b. Anterior approach performed first, posterior approach commonly staged 5 days or more later
4. Bone graft
   a. Autograft harvested from iliac crest
   b. Graft placed on decorticated spine to encourage osteoinduction

D. Postanesthesia care
1. Assess neurovascular status: perform comprehensive neurovascular assessment every 15 minutes for the first 2 hours, then hourly
   a. Note bowel and bladder dysfunction
   b. Assist with somatosensory evoked potential (SEP) monitoring as ordered
2. Assess for headache, possibly related to spinal fluid leak
3. Assess for wound drainage
   a. Note dependent drainage on dressing and bed
   b. Note formation and extent of hematoma
   c. Maintain occlusive compression dressing to operative site
   d. Maintain drainage device if present
4. Position patient for safety
   a. Patient commonly positioned supine in regular hard bed: Stryker frame and Circo-electric bed not common
   b. Maintain patient in neutral body alignment
   c. Log roll patient side to side with physician order
   d. Assist patient's movement with draw sheet
   e. Discourage patient use of trapeze or pulling under patient's axilla (to avoid rod displacement)
5. Monitor for complications after spinal fusion (see also Common Orthopedic Complications)
   a. Reduced gas exchange and ineffective breathing patterns
      (1) Encourage coughing and deep breathing hourly
      (2) Assess equality and clarity of breath sounds
      (3) Obtain chest x-ray film after anterior fusion to determine lung expansion
      (4) Monitor arterial blood gases
      (5) Turn patient side to side every hour
   b. Gastric distension and decreased peristalsis
      (1) Auscultate for bowel sounds hourly in PAR
      (2) Insert nasogastric tube if necessary
      (3) Administer stool softener as needed

## V. Amputation

A. Procedure: surgical (or traumatic) removal of a body part

B. Purpose
1. Reduce risk of systemic sepsis
2. Control pain of ischemia
3. Maximize mobility

C. Types of amputation
1. Traumatic: results in extreme destruction of soft tissue and bone in the presence of infectious microorganisms

2. Elective
   a. Closed (flap): performed in the absence of infection
   b. Open (guillotine): performed in presence of infection, allowing drainage of infectious material

D. Indications for elective amputation
   1. Peripheral vascular disease: most frequent indication for lower extremity amputation, often associated with diabetes mellitus
   2. Severe trauma: most frequent indication for upper extremity amputation
   3. Other indications (in order of frequency)
      a. Acute or chronic infection: osteomyelitis or gas gangrene
      b. Trophic ulcers
      c. Severe crushing injuries
      d. Malignancies
      e. Frostbite
      f. Congenital deformities

E. Postanesthesia care of the patient after amputation
   1. Assess neurovascular status: perform comprehensive neurovascular assessment (page 548)
   2. Assess for signs of wound drainage
      a. Note dependent drainage on dressing and bed
      b. Note unusual odors or color of drainage (important in presence of infection)
   3. Maintain stump dressing
      a. Plaster cast: rigid dressing
         (1) Prevents swelling of stump
         (2) Protects stump from trauma
         (3) Used when patient will be fitted for immediate prosthesis (usually Pylon type)
      b. Soft dressing: gauze with elastic wrap
         (1) Prevents swelling of stump
         (2) Used when use of prosthesis unlikely
   4. Position extremity to minimize complications
      a. Elevate stump to facilitate venous return first 24 to 48 hours
      b. After 48 hours, position to prevent hip flexion contractures
         (1) Avoid stump elevation
         (2) Instruct patient to lie intermittently prone (encourages hip extension)
   5. Provide for pain control
      a. Administer parenteral opioids as ordered for postoperative surgical pain
      b. Assess for phantom limb pain
         (1) Pain sensation in area of absent, amputated limb
         (2) Common in first 24 to 48 hours postoperatively in traumatic amputation
         (3) Treated with narcotics and phenytoin
         (4) Adequate treatment important to reduce risk of chronic phantom pain syndrome
   6. Instruct patient regarding phantom limb sensation: sensation that amputated limb is present
      a. Inform patient that phenomenon is common in early postoperative period
      b. Instruct patient that sensation is normal phenomenon
      c. Treat with nonpharmacologic methods
   7. Provide emotional support

## VI. Replantation of Amputated Digits or Limbs

A. Procedure: reattachment of totally or partially amputated part involving restoration of vascular, nervous, bony, and soft tissue structures

B. Possible sites for replantation
   1. Upper extremity
      a. Digits
         (1) Most common traumatic amputation
         (2) Replantation attempted in proximal digit amputations, amputation of multiple digits, amputation of index finger or thumb
         (3) Viability after replantation 80% to 90%
         (4) Functional return after replantation 65%
      b. Arms: less successful result
   2. Lower extremity
      a. Digits: great toe
      b. Leg
         (1) Amputation through tibia or fibula shows unfavorable results with high infection rate
         (2) Leg length discrepancies common
C. Factors influencing prognosis
   1. Positive factors
      a. Clean-cut (guillotine) amputation
      b. Young patient
      c. Hemodynamically stable patient
      d. Absence of systemic disease
      e. No history of smoking, alcohol, or drug abuse
      f. Absence of gross contamination of wound
      g. Amputated part wrapped in gauze and placed in cool environment
      h. Replantation attempted within 24 hours
   2. Negative factors
      a. Crushing injury
      b. Extremes of age
      c. History of peripheral vascular disease, hypertension, or other chronic illness
      d. History of smoking, alcohol, or drug abuse
      e. Grossly contaminated wound
      f. Delay in retrieval and care of amputated part
      g. Delay in replantation
D. Postanesthesia care of the patient postreplantation
   1. Assess neurovascular status at least every 15 minutes
      a. Perform comprehensive bedside assessment
      b. Perform technical monitoring as ordered
         (1) Doppler ultrasonography
         (2) Temperature probes
         (3) Muscle contraction monitoring (evoked M wave)
         (4) Furometry readings (determines venous return)
      c. Promptly notify physician if negative change occurs
   2. Promote circulation and prevent vasoconstriction
      a. Elevate extremity above heart level
      b. Administer thrombolytic agents to decrease clotting in peripheral vessels
      c. Maintain room temperature at 78° to 90° F (26° to 30° C)
      d. Prevent patient exposure to nicotine and caffeine
      e. Maintain patient hydration
   3. Prevent infection
      a. Administer antibiotics as ordered
      b. Assess for signs and symptoms of infection
      c. Provide for nutritional needs necessary for wound healing (high-protein diet)

4. Provide for pain control
   a. Provide oral opioids as needed
   b. Assess pain carefully, noting changes in pain pattern suggestive of ischemia
5. Provide emotional support

## BIBLIOGRAPHY


Altman GT, Rogers VP: Is salvage reinfusion necessary in primary total knee replacement? *Contemporary Orthop* 11:30–38, 1995.

Altizer L: Total hip arthroplasty. *Orthop Nurs* 14(4): 7–18, 1995.

Bright LD, Georgi SD: How to protect your patient from DVT. *Am J Nurs* 94(12):28–32, 1994.

Brown C, Henderson S, Moore S: Surgical treatment of patients with open tibial fracture. *AORN J* 63(5): 873–878, 1996.

Buck M, Paice JA: Pharmacologic management of acute pain in the orthopaedic patient. *Orthop Nurs* 14(6): 14–23, 1994.

Cardona VD, Hurn PD, Mason PJB et al (eds.): *Trauma Nursing: From Resuscitation Through Rehabilitation,* 3rd Ed. Philadelphia, WB Saunders, 1998.

Davis LA: Pulmonary embolism: Early recognition and management in the postanesthesia unit. *J Post Anesth Nurs* 8(5):338–343, 1993.

Gallegos SJ, Michalec DL: Neurologic assessment of the orthopaedic patient. *Orthop Nurs* 15(5):23–29, 1996.

Genge ML: Epidural analgesia in the orthopaedic patient. *Orthop Nurs* 7(4):11–18, 1988.

Hansell MJ: Fractures and the healing process. *Orthop Nurs* 7(1):43–50, 1988.

Hefti D: Complications of trauma: The nurse's role in prevention. *Orthop Nurs* 14(6):9–16, 1995.

Hoppenfeld S: *A Guide to the Examination of the Spine and Extremities.* Norwalk, Conn, Appleton-Century-Crofts, 1982.

Magee DJ: *Orthopedic Physical Assessment,* 3rd Ed. St Louis, Mosby, 1997.

Maher AB, Salmond SW, Pellino TA (eds): *Orthopaedic Nursing,* 2nd Ed. Philadelphia, WB Saunders, 1998.

Moloney WJ, Schurman DJ, Hangen D et al: The influence of continuous passive motion on outcome in total knee arthroplasty. *Clin Orthop* 256:162–168, 1990.

National Association of Orthopaedic Nurses: *Orthopaedic Nursing Practice: Process and Outcome Criteria for Selected Diagnosis.* Pitman, NJ, Anthony J Janetti, 1986.

Osborne L, DiGicoma I: Traction: A review with nursing diagnosis and intervention. *Orthop Nurs* 6(4): 13–19, 1987.

Pellino TA, Mooney NE, Salmond SW, Verdisco LA (eds): *Core Curriculum for Orthopaedic Nursing,* 3rd Ed. Pitman, NJ, Anthony J Janetti, 1996.

Ross D: Acute compartment syndrome. *Orthop Nurs* 10(2):33–38, 1991.

Rounseville C: Phantom limb pain: The ghost that haunts the amputee. *Orthop Nurs* 11(2):67–71, 1992.

Schmalzried TP, Amstutz HC, Dorey FJ: Nerve palsy associated with total hip replacement: Risk factors and prognosis. *J Bone Joint Surg* 73A(7):1074–1080, 1991.

Slye DA: Orthopedic complications. *Nurs Clin North Am* 26(1):113–132, 1991.

Williamson VC: Amputation of the lower extremity: An overview. *Orthop Nurs* 11(2):55–65, 1992.


## REVIEW QUESTIONS

**1. The nursing management of patients with arthritic disorders usually includes which of the following conservative measures?**

A. Frequent neurovascular assessments
B. Application of electrical stimulation
C. Instruction on the use of nonsteroidal antiinflammatory medications and exercise
D. Application of abduction devices

**2. Which of the following interventions would not be used in caring for the patient with a plaster cast?**

A. Placement of additional padding between cast and extremity
B. Application of ice bag near the injury site
C. Avoidance of covering cast with heavy blanket
D. Elevation of extremity

**3. Indications for traction include which of the following?**
A. Alignment of fractured bones
B. Reduction of muscle spasms associated with fractures
C. Maintenance of limb length
D. All of the above

**4. What is an oblique fracture?**
A. Fracture parallel to the axis of a long bone
B. Fracture at a 45-degree angle to the axis of a long bone
C. Fracture that forms a spiral that encircles the bone
D. Fracture that creates a number of separate bone fragments

**5. During what time period does a fat embolus generally occur?**
A. 12 to 48 hours after trauma
B. 48 to 72 hours after trauma
C. 6 to 24 hours after trauma
D. 36 to 72 hours after trauma

**6. Postoperative care of the total hip replacement patient includes which of the following interventions?**
A. Maintenance of drainage device and application of Milwaukee brace
B. Positioning of operative hip in abduction and thrombosis prophylaxis
C. Use of continuous passive motion and spica hip wrap
D. Oral anticoagulants and volume expanders

**7. What is the most frequent indication for amputation of the lower extremity?**
A. Osteomyelitis
B. Trauma
C. Trophic ulcers
D. Peripheral vascular disease

**8. Postoperative care of the patient with shoulder replacement may include all of the following interventions except:**
A. Assessment of radial and ulnar nerve function
B. Maintenance of shoulder in adduction with internal rotation
C. Active range of motion of the shoulder to decrease upper extremity edema
D. Promotion of self-care with assistive devices

**9. Surgical correction of scoliosis in the adult is performed under what circumstances?**
A. Severe deformity of 40 degrees or more leading to changes in neurologic or cardiopulmonary status
B. Deformity necessitating at least intermittent use of lumbar support
C. Lateral intercostal angle changes progressing greater than 10 degrees
D. Physical examination revealing positive cross straight leg raise

**10. Methods to promote circulation and reduce vasoconstriction after digit replantation include which of the following interventions?**
A. Administration of antipyretic agents
B. Maintenance of room temperature between 78° and 90° F
C. IV infusion of caffeinelike compound
D. Compression dressing to wrist and forearm

**ANSWERS:** 1. C, 2. A, 3. D, 4. B, 5. A, 6. B, 7. D, 8. C, 9. A, 10. B

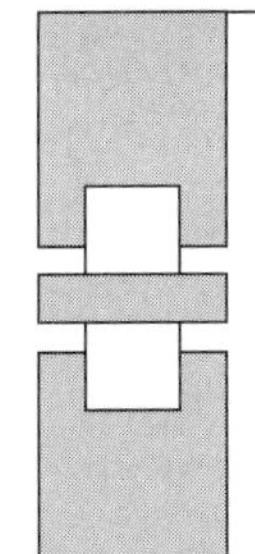

CHAPTER 27

# The Endocrine Surgical Patient

Barbara A. Gervasio, BSN, RN, CNOR

## OBJECTIVES

**Study of the information represented by this outline will enable the learner to:**

1. List the hormones produced by the thyroid, parathyroid, pituitary, and adrenal glands.
2. Identify the symptoms and diagnostic testing used to assess abnormal endocrine gland function.
3. Identify the surgical procedure and perioperative concerns of the patient having surgical treatment for Graves' disease, hypothyroidism, pheochromocytoma, hypersecretion of the pituitary gland, hyperaldosteronism, and hyperparathyroidism.
4. Develop a postanesthesia nursing care plan for the patient having subtotal thyroidectomy, bilateral adrenalectomy, hypophysectomy, and parathyroidectomy.
5. Discuss the postanesthesia concerns of the patient with Addison's disease.
6. Discuss the postanesthesia care of the patient with endocrine conditions, thyrotoxicosis, tetany, hypoglycemia in the insulin-dependent diabetic patient, diabetes insipidus, Addisonian crisis, and hyperparathyroid crisis.
7. Discuss the postanesthesia care of the diabetic patient.

Endocrine dysfunction may be the primary reason for surgery, as with hyperthyroidism, or it may be a chronic condition coexisting with the patient's primary diagnosis, as with diabetes mellitus. Understanding endocrine dysfunction both as a primary reason for surgical intervention and as a complicating factor with other disorders is essential for the postanesthesia care unit (PACU) nurse to provide appropriate care.

## THE THYROID GLAND: HYPERTHYROIDISM (See also Chapter 28)

The thyroid gland, in response to thyroid-stimulating hormone (TSH, released by the pituitary gland in response to thyrotropin-releasing hormone), produces thyroxine ($T_4$) and triiodothyronine ($T_3$) each day. $T_3$ has a short half-life, and $T_4$ has a half-life of 5 to 7 days. Peripheral tissue converts $T_4$ to $T_3$. $T_3$ is considered by some as the true tissue thyroid hormone, whereas $T_4$ is considered a plasma prohormone. Control of these hormones exists in the hypothalamus and pituitary gland on a negative-feedback cycle. Most patients seen in the postanesthesia care unit (PACU) are in a euthyroid state; patients who are commonly hyperthyroid are those with large airway thyroid glands or pregnant women in their first trimester.

I. **Causes of Thyroid Disorders**
   A. Multinodular toxic diffuse enlargement; Graves' disease
   B. Adenomas
   C. Malignancy
   D. Thyroiditis
      1. Viral, autoimmune, or unknown etiology
      2. Immunoglobulins found in serum of hyperthyroid patients mimic thyrotropin (also called thyroid-stimulating hormone, or TSH)

## II. Description: Hypermetabolic Condition Resulting in Excessive Secretion of Thyroid Hormone

## III. Signs and Symptoms

A. Cardiopulmonary
  1. Hypertension
  2. Tachycardia: 150 to 200 beats per minute (bpm) demonstrated as palpitations
  3. Increased cardiac output
  4. Systolic murmurs
  5. Tachypnea
  6. Atrial fibrillation

B. Gastrointestinal
  1. Weight loss
  2. Increased peristalsis
  3. Diarrhea and abdominal pain

C. Integumentary
  1. Fine, silky hair
  2. Hair loss
  3. Fever

D. Musculoskeletal
  1. Body thinness
  2. Muscle atrophy
  3. Muscle weakness

E. Nervous system
  1. Fine tremors
  2. Diaphoresis
  3. Hyperactive emotional state

F. Miscellaneous
  1. Enlarged thyroid gland
  2. Exophthalmos
  3. Menstrual cycle changes
  4. Heat intolerance

## IV. Diagnostic Laboratory Values—See Table 27–1

A. $T_3$ and $T_4$ levels; $T_3$ proportionately higher
B. Radioactive iodine (RAI) uptake elevated in Graves' disease
C. TSH level decreased in Graves' disease
D. Thyroid scan: demonstrates iodide-concentrating capacity of the thyroid gland
E. Ultrasonography: distinguishes between cystic and solid tumors
F. Antibodies to thyroid gland distinguish left thyroiditis and cancer

## V. Operative Procedures

A. Subtotal thyroid lobectomy: unilateral or bilateral excision of portion of lobe(s)
B. Thyroid lobectomy: removal of one lobe
C. Total thyroidectomy: removal of entire gland

**TABLE 27–1 Tests to Determine Thyroid Dysfunction**

| | THYROXINE $T_4$ | TRIIODOTHYRONINE $T_3$ | TSH |
|---|---|---|---|
| Hyperthyroidism | Elevated | Elevated | Normal |
| Hypothyroidism Primary | Low | Low/Normal | Elevated |
| Hypothyroidism | Low | Low | Low |
| Pregnancy | Elevated | Normal | Normal |

## VI. Preoperative Objectives

- A. Promote euthyroid state with antithyroid drugs; several weeks required to promote euthyroid state
  1. Propylthiouracil
     - a. 300 to 900 mg daily in divided doses given 6 to 12 weeks preoperatively
     - b. Blocks peripheral conversion of $T_4$ and $T_3$
  2. Methimazole
     - a. 30 to 60 mg daily in divided doses
     - b. May take 1 to 3 months to produce euthyroid state
     - c. Blocks uptake of iodine
  3. Sodium iodide and potassium iodide (Lugol's solution)
     - a. Emergently, iodide, 1 to 2 g of sodium salt intravenously (IV)
     - b. Less acutely, SSKI, 2 to 10 drops per day, or 10 to 20 drops of Lugol's solution daily
     - c. Decreases vascularity of gland
     - d. Inhibits release of thyroxine
  4. Propranolol
     - a. 40 to 640 mg/d in divided doses
     - b. Best single pharmacologic agent to control thyroid function
- B. Control hyperdynamic cardiovascular state
  1. Sodium restriction
  2. Digitalization
  3. Diuretics
  4. Propranolol (Inderal)
     - a. Drug of choice for severe tachycardia
     - b. Does not reduce oxygen demand
     - c. Blocks $T_4$ transformation to $T_3$
  5. Antihypertensive: reserpine; also causes bradycardia
- C. Increased preoperative sedation for already hyperactive patient
  1. Anticholinergics such as atropine may be omitted because of their tachycardic effect
- D. Preoperative instruction: emphasis on head and neck support when turning

## VII. Intraoperative and Anesthesia Concerns

- A. Agents
  1. Thiopental: succinylcholine is paralyzing induction agent of choice because it does not induce a hyperdynamic cardiovascular effect
  2. Propofol: short acting without cardiotonic properties
  3. Ketamine: may cause cardiovascular problems in euthyroid patients with a history of thyrotoxicosis
     - a. Increased cardiac output
     - b. Hypertension
     - c. Dysrhythmias
- B. Increased oxygen requirements due to
  1. Hypermetabolic state
  2. Increased temperature
  3. Tracheal deviation from retrosternal goiter compressing trachea
- C. Corneal drying or abrasions of exophthalmic eyes
- D. Vocal cord visualization for injury to recurrent laryngeal nerves
- E. Monitor for signs of thyroid storm: increased temperature, increased heart rate; esmolol 100 to 300 μg/kg/min to control tachydysrhythmia
- F. Avoidance of bucking (coughing) on endotracheal tube, which may stimulate hemorrhage
- G. Avoidance or treatment of hypotension

## VIII. Postanesthesia Nursing Concerns

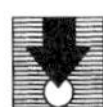

**NURSING DIAGNOSIS**

Examples of related nursing diagnostic categories include
- Ineffective airway clearance
- Ineffective breathing pattern
- Altered peripheral tissue perfusion
- Hyperthermia

A. Airway maintenance
  1. Supplementary humidified oxygen: aerosol or high-humidity face mask or tent
  2. Observation for respiratory distress
    a. Causes
      (1) Edema of glottis
      (2) Hematoma formation
    b. Signs
      (1) Dyspnea
      (2) Cyanosis
      (3) Crowing respirations or stridor
      (4) Retraction of neck muscles
      (5) Tracheal deviation
    c. Strategy
      (1) Immediate intubation if possible
      (2) Emergency tracheostomy

B. Suture line observation
  1. Wound hemorrhaging: usually an early complication
  2. Hematoma formation: can create respiratory difficulty
  3. Drainage devices: Penrose or Jackson-Pratt drains

C. Assessment of recurrent laryngeal nerve damage
  1. Assess and record quality of vocalization
  2. Assess and record any difficulty in swallowing

D. Positioning
  1. Semi-Fowler's position after reaction
  2. Neck support
  3. Avoidance of extremes in head flexion or extension

E. Avoidance of vigorous coughing; enhances hemorrhage

F. Protection of exophthalmic eyes
  1. Sterile artificial tears
  2. Lubricating ophthalmic ointment

G. Awareness of hormonal imbalances
  1. Tetany and hypocalcemia if parathyroid glands were removed (see information on parathyroidectomy)
  2. Thyrotoxic crisis (storm)
    a. Caused by sudden increase in circulating thyroid hormone
    b. May be confused with malignant hyperthermia
    c. 70% mortality if untreated
    d. Can occur up to 18 hours postoperatively
    e. Signs
      (1) Tachycardia
      (2) Profuse sweating
      (3) Hyperthermia
      (4) Severe dehydration

(5) Delirium, agitation, psychosis, convulsions, coma
(6) Pulmonary edema
(7) Atrial fibrillation
(8) Tachypnea
(9) Hypertension followed by hypotension
(10) Congestive heart failure

f. Treatment
(1) Adequate hydration with thiamine added because high output is causing this deficiency
(2) Cooling; aspirin is *not* recommended for treatment because it displaces $T_4$ from its carrier protein
(3) Sedation
(4) Medication
(a) Sodium potassium iodide, 1 to 5 g every 24 hours
(b) Propylthiouracil, 200 mg every 4 to 6 hours
(c) Cortisone: (100 to 200 mg) for persistent hypotension.
(5) Supplementary oxygen support
(6) Control of tachycardia: β-blockers to compete with catecholamines (propranolol)

## THE THYROID GLAND: HYPOTHYROIDISM

**I. Pathophysiology:** Hypothyroidism is a term that describes a decrease in circulatory $T_3$ and $T_4$. Development of hypothyroidism is usually gradual and insidious. Incidence is low in the general population: 0.5% to 0.8%.

**II. Causes**
A. Chronic thyroiditis (Hashimoto's thyroiditis), which progressively destroys thyroid function

**III. Signs and Symptoms**
A. Intolerance to cold
B. Bradycardia
C. Lethargy
D. Peripheral vasoconstriction
E. Decrease in cardiac output
F. Hyponatremia
G. Atrophy of adrenal cortex
H. Reduced platelet adhesiveness

**IV. Diagnostic Laboratory Values** (See Table 27–1)

**V. Anesthesia Concerns**
A. Sensitivity to opioids: no controlled studies exist to support the claim that hypothyroidism promotes sensitivity to inhaled anesthetic drugs or opioids. However, one should suspect sensitivity because exaggerated effects of depressants have been reported
B. Need for supplemental cortisone to correct adrenal insufficiency
C. Slow metabolism of drugs
D. Unresponsive baroreceptor reflexes
E. Impaired ventilatory response to arterial hypoxemia or hypercapnia
F. Hypovolemia
G. Delayed gastric emptying
H. Hyponatremia
I. Hypothermia
J. Anemia

K. Hypoglycemia
L. Adrenal insufficiency
M. Induction and maintenance of anesthesia
   1. Ketamine is commonly used for induction because it supports the cardiovascular system
   2. Succinylcholine used for paralysis of skeletal muscles
N. Early recognition of a decrease in cardiac dysfunction resulting in congestive heart failure

### VI. Postoperative Nursing

**NURSING DIAGNOSIS**

Examples of related nursing diagnostic categories include

- Decrease in cardiac output leading to CHF
- Decrease in circulating cortisone
- Fluid volume deficit
- Hypothermia
- Altered electrolytes
- Impaired respiration related to reduced sensitivity to hypoxemia
- Reduced sensitivity to opioids

## THE PARATHYROID GLAND: HYPERPARATHYROIDISM

Parathyroid hormone (PTH) mediates serum calcium levels. Decreased serum calcium levels result in bone resorption followed by increased renal resorption and gut uptake (with vitamin D) and release of PTH. The release of PTH is inhibited by rising serum calcium. Magnesium is necessary for PTH release and for its bone effect.

### I. Description

A. Primary hyperparathyroidism characterized by hypercalcemia and hyperphosphatemia
B. Disturbances in these two minerals result in major kidney and bone lesions
C. Secondary hyperparathyroidism results from parathyroid hyperplasia, producing decreased serum calcium levels
D. Bone lesions are primary outcomes
E. Overactivity of one or more parathyroid glands
F. Excessive secretion of PTH
G. Imbalance in calcium and phosphorus metabolism; increased calcium, 10.5 mg/dl (normal, 9 to 10.6 mg/dl)

### II. Cause of Disease Process

A. Secondary hyperparathyroidism
   1. Adenomas: 80%
   2. Hyperplasias: 10%
   3. Malignancies: 2%
   4. Previous head or neck radiation: therapy of choice during 1950s and 1960s for benign conditions of face and neck

## III. Assessment Parameters (Symptoms)

A. Cardiovascular
   1. Electrocardiogram (ECG) changes
      a. Prolonged PR intervals (rare)
      b. Shortened QT intervals (rare)
   2. Heart failure: tachydysrhythmias
B. Gastrointestinal: constipation
C. Musculoskeletal
   1. Muscle weakness
   2. Osteopenia
   3. Pathologic fractures
   4. Bone pain
D. Renal: chronic renal insufficiency, a late manifestation
   1. Polyuria
   2. Hypertension
      a. Renal impairment
      b. Calcium deposits in vessels
   3. Dehydration
E. Neurologic
   1. Somnolence
   2. Psychosis

## IV. Laboratory Clues

A. Hypercalcemia
   1. Serum level greater than 10.5 mg/dl
   2. Excessive bone resorption
B. Hypercalciuria
   1. Urine level greater than 300 mg/24 hours
   2. Leads to renal calculi and kidney damage
C. Hyperphosphaturia
D. Hypophosphatemia: less than 2.5 mg/dl
E. Elevated serum PTH level
F. Radiographic identification of bone demineralization

## V. Preoperative Objectives

A. Correct preexisting hypovolemia
B. Reduced elevated calcium levels
   1. Rehydration with normal saline, 6 to 10 L/24 hours
      a. Not Ringer's lactate (contains calcium chloride)
   2. Furosemide (Lasix): 80 mg/24 hours to enhance diuresis
C. Control dysrhythmias

## VI. Anesthesia Concerns

A. Hypotension: usually caused by hypovolemia
B. Bradycardia: occurs with manipulation near carotid sinus
C. Impaired renal function
   1. Volume overload possibility
   2. Monitoring for hyperkalemia
D. Pneumothorax possible during mediastinal exploration

## VII. Operative Procedures

A. Total parathyroidectomy: removal of all glands
B. Partial parathyroidectomy: removal of up to 3½ of the 4 glands, leaving metal clip in place to identify remaining glandular tissue

## VIII. Postanesthesia Nursing Concerns

**NURSING DIAGNOSIS**

Examples of related nursing diagnostic categories include:
- Ineffective airway clearance
- Ineffective breathing pattern
- Altered peripheral tissue perfusion
- Decreased cardiac output
- Pain
- Fluid volume deficit

A. Airway maintenance
B. Suture line observation (hematoma formation)
C. Assessment of recurrent laryngeal nerve damage
D. Positioning
E. Awareness of hormonal imbalances
  1. Within immediate postoperative period, calcium concentration begins to fall
  2. Uptake of calcium into bone may also deplete serum calcium
  3. Tetany: Decreased PTH secretion and acute hypocalcemia
    a. Signs
      (1) Laryngeal spasm
      (2) Apprehension
      (3) Tingling in toes, fingers, mouth
      (4) Positive Chvostek's sign: twitching of facial muscles if cheek is tapped over facial nerve
      (5) Positive Trousseau's sign: carpopedal spasm if circulation in arm is impeded with blood pressure cuff
    b. Treatment
      (1) Calcium chloride administered slowly IV (so as not to irritate veins)
      (2) Vitamin $D_2$ (calciferol) replaces PTH, increases serum calcium
      (3) Monitor for dysrhythmias, especially if patient is taking digitalis
  4. Hyperparathyroid crisis: increased circulating parathormone, calcium greater than 11 to 18 mg/dl
    a. Signs
      (1) Nausea and vomiting
      (2) Abdominal pain
      (3) Thirst, dehydration, hypovolemia
      (4) Dyspnea
    b. Treatment
      (1) Hydration
      (2) Calcitonin (parathormone antagonist)
      (3) Mithramycin for thrombocytopenia, renal problems
      (4) Prednisone to correct hypercalcemia
F. Psychologic support and reassurance; elevated calcium levels produce altered psychologic states
G. Hyperventilation: reduces calcium level

# THE PITUITARY GLAND: HYPOSECRETION OR HYPERSECRETION

## I. Pathophysiology
A. Causes of glandular dysfunction

1. Adenomas
2. Malignancies
3. Congenital abnormalities
4. Traumatic injuries causing increase in intracranial pressure
5. Infarction
6. Hypothalamic dysfunction

B. Hormonal influences
1. Anterior pituitary hypersecretion caused by adenomas
    a. Increases adrenocorticotropic hormone (ACTH) (Cushing's disease)
    b. Increases growth hormone (acromegaly)
    c. Increases prolactin
2. Anterior pituitary hyposecretion caused by adenomas or hypothalamic dysfunction
    a. Decreases growth hormone (dwarfism)
    b. Decreases TSH (hypothyroid)
    c. Decreases ACTH
3. Posterior pituitary deficiency or excess caused by intracranial tumors or infarctions
    a. Syndrome of inappropriate ADH secretion (SIADH)
        (1) Characterized by high levels of ADH
        (2) Clinical signs include serum hypoosmolality and hyponatremia
    b. Diabetes insipidus (DI)
        (1) Characterized by insufficiency in ADH
        (2) Clinical signs include polyuria, polydipsia, low urine specific gravity

**II. Assessment Parameters**

A. Anterior pituitary hypersecretion
1. Signs
    a. Acromegaly
        (1) Bone overgrowth of mandible, hands, feet
        (2) Soft tissue thickening
    b. Menstrual disturbances
    c. Headaches
    d. Visual disturbances
2. Diagnostic tests
    a. Radiographs of skull, hands, feet
    b. Radioactive plasma human growth hormone (HGH) levels

B. Anterior pituitary hyposecretion
1. Signs
    a. Hypothyroidism
    b. Obesity
    c. Decreased secondary sexual characteristics
    d. Dwarfism
    e. Headaches
2. Diagnostic tests
    a. Radiographs of skull
    b. Decreased radioactive iodine (RAI) uptake
    c. Decreased $T_4$
    d. Decreased urine ACTH level

C. Posterior pituitary hyposecretion: diabetes insipidus
1. Signs
    a. Polydipsia
    b. Polyuria
    c. Dehydration

2. Diagnostic test
   a. Hypoosmolar polyuria

## III. Operative Procedures

A. Hypophysectomy (removal of pituitary gland)
   1. For primary pituitary disease, tumors
   2. Palliative measure for treatment of breast and prostate cancer
B. Operative approaches
   1. Frontal craniotomy
   2. Transsphenoidal approach through nasal floor

## IV. Anesthesia Concerns

A. Anterior pituitary hypersecretion (increases ACTH, HGH)
   1. Acromegaly
      a. Overgrown mandible
      b. Jaw protrusion
      c. Soft tissue thickness, which may cause recurrent laryngeal nerve entrapment leading to paralysis
   2. Intubation problems: airway
      a. Mask fit may be a problem
      b. Long intubation blades may be indicated
   3. Retention of sodium and potassium may lead to cardiac dysfunction
   4. Inhibition of insulin leads to diabetes mellitus
   5. Cushing's disease–like symptoms (see information on adrenal gland: Cushing's disease)
   6. If a recent air pneumoencephalogram was performed, nitrous oxide is avoided to decrease risk of increased intracranial pressure
B. Anterior pituitary hyposecretion (decreases TSH, ACTH)
   1. Decreased anesthesia requirements as result of hypometabolism
   2. Intolerance to hypothermia
   3. Bradycardia
C. Posterior pituitary hyposecretion (decreases ADH): diabetes insipidus
   1. Tendency to dehydration with enormous urinary output
   2. Hypovolemia
   3. Hypotension

## V. Postanesthesia Nursing Concerns

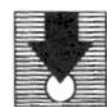

**NURSING DIAGNOSIS**

Examples of related nursing diagnostic categories include

- Potential for infection
- Fluid volume deficit or excess
- Hyperthermia
- Hypothermia
- Altered cerebral tissue perfusion

A. Decreased ACTH of greatest concern (see information on Addisonian crisis)
   1. Requires lifelong cortisone replacement
      a. Surgical stress increases cortisone requirements
      b. Persistent, unexplained hypotension; usually reversible with cortisone supplements
   2. Underlying diabetes mellitus (often unmasked with large doses of cortisone)
      a. Monitor blood sugar
      b. Observe for acidosis and diabetic coma

3. Decreased resistance to infection should the following complications occur
   a. Wound contamination
   b. Respiratory infection

B. Decreased ADH results in diabetes insipidus; deficiency state causes inability to conserve water
   1. Diabetes insipidus occurs immediately postoperatively (and for 24 hours after)
      a. Polyuria (6 to 24 L/d)
      b. Polydipsia
   2. Nursing intervention
      a. Observe for dehydration and hypotension
         (1) Monitor increased urinary output
         (2) Check specific gravity of urine
         (3) Monitor serum electrolytes; $Na^+$ important
      b. Administer as ordered
         (1) Vasopressin (Pitressin), 10 units subcutaneously every 6 hours
         (2) IV fluids at prescribed rates
      c. Observe for signs of fluid overload
         (1) Water intoxication: decreases serum sodium
         (2) Coma
         (3) Convulsions

C. Neurologic sequelae (because pituitary gland lies adjacent to hypothalamus)
   1. Hyperthermia
   2. Increased intracranial pressure
   3. Cerebrospinal fluid leakage
   4. Convulsions

D. Other concerns
   1. Temperature
      a. Hyperthermia from hypothalamic influence
      b. Hypothermia intolerance from decreased TSH, causing hypothyroid symptoms
   2. Suture line observation
      a. Hematoma formation
      b. Cerebrospinal fluid leakage

## THE ADRENAL GLAND (CORTEX): HYPERALDOSTERONISM

**I. Pathophysiology**

A. Primary aldosteronism
   1. Definition: syndrome caused by inappropriate increase in adrenal gland production of the mineralocorticoid aldosterone; normally, aldosterone produced in response to hyperkalemia and hypovolemia through renin-angiotensin system; aldosterone acts with kidney to increase potassium wasting and sodium retention
   2. Etiology
      a. Adenomas (Conn's syndrome): aldosterone producing
      b. Adrenocortical malignancies
      c. Adrenocortical hyperplasias
   3. Effects of increased aldosterone (most potent mineralocorticoid produced by adrenal glands)
      a. Sodium retention
      b. Water retention (hypervolemia)
      c. Hypertension
      d. Hypokalemia leads to alkalosis, dysrhythmias
      e. Generalized weakness

f. Paresthesia
g. Tetany
h. Hyperglycemia
i. Lowered plasma renins: renin-angiotensin system is primary regulator of aldosterone secretion

B. Secondary aldosteronism
1. Definition: aldosteronism caused by pathologic edematous condition and hypertension
2. Etiology
a. Ascites
b. Congestive heart failure
c. Obstructive renal artery disease
3. Resultant symptoms
a. Hypovolemia
b. Hyponatremia
c. Hypokalemia

## II. Diagnostic Parameters

A. Laboratory evaluation
1. Hypernatremia
2. Hypokalemia
3. Increased urinary aldosterone excretion
4. Hyperglycemia and glycosuria

B. Other diagnostic tests
1. Computed tomography (CT) scan for tumors
2. Electrocardiogram (ECG) changes reflecting hypokalemia
3. Changes in personality (hyperglycemia)
4. Adrenal vein serum aldosterone levels
a. Elevated values on side of tumor
b. Elevated values on both sides in secondary aldosteronism

## III. Operative Procedures

A. Unilateral adrenalectomy: removal of one adrenal gland
B. Bilateral adrenalectomy: removal of both adrenal glands

## IV. Preoperative Concerns

A. Preoperative correction of hypokalemia and hypertension
1. Spironolactone (Aldactone, Aldactazide): reverses physiologic effects of aldosterone
2. Potassium chloride supplements
3. Sodium restriction to promote potassium retention
4. Diuretics and digitalis for heart failure

B. Achieve highest possible state of stability before administration of anesthesia

## V. Anesthesia Concerns

A. Maintain normotensive blood pressure
1. Control of hypertension
a. Aggravated on induction and during tumor manipulation
b. Antihypertensive agents
(1) Vasodilators
(a) Nitroglycerin
(b) Sodium nitroprusside (Nipride)
(2) β-blockers (rarely used): phentolamine mesylate (Regitine)
2. Control of hypotension
a. Most likely occurrence after tumor removal (with decreased circulating aldosterone)
b. Management
(1) Increased volume administration
(2) Use of expanders (blood, albumin) may counter need for vasopressors

B. Deep muscle relaxation and anesthesia level
   1. Necessary for adequate exposure and manipulation of retroperitoneal tumors
   2. Aggravates hypotension after tumor removal
C. Maintain normal serum potassium
D. Monitor dysrhythmias
   1. Causes: hypokalemia, decreases catecholamine level
   2. Counteracting agents: digitalis, propranolol hydrochloride (Inderal)
E. Anesthetic agents and adjuncts
   1. Halothane: inhibits sympathetic responses but can sensitize myocardium to epinephrine, leading to dysrhythmias
   2. Enflurane: same effects as halothane with less myocardial stimulation
   3. Droperidol and fentanyl citrate (Innovar)
      a. Droperidol raises epinephrine threshold, reducing dysrhythmias
      b. Fentanyl has fewer histamine effects than other narcotics
   4. Nondepolarizing muscle relaxants (pancuronium, curare) increase histamine activity

## THE ADRENAL GLAND (CORTEX): CUSHING'S DISEASE

The anterior pituitary gland when stimulated by the hypothalamus will release ACTH. This release usually occurs early in the morning. In response to the ACTH, the adrenal cortex releases about 20 mg of cortisol daily. These hormones react on a negative-feedback basis. Cortisol has an anti-inflammatory effect, but its most important role is its response to stress.

### I. Etiology: Excess Output of Cortisol and Androgens from Adrenal Cortex

A. Hyperactivity of adrenal cortex resulting from adenoma or carcinoma
B. Overstimulation of adrenal cortices by increased ACTH from pituitary gland
C. Iatrogenic etiology: prolonged use of glucocorticoids
D. Congenital disorders

### II. Symptoms

A. Plethoric facies
B. Moon-shaped face
C. Hypertension
D. Ecchymosis and easy bruising
E. Thin skin
F. Buffalo hump
G. Hirsutism
H. Centripetal (truncal) obesity with muscle wasting
I. Poor wound healing
J. Osteoporosis

### III. Diagnostic Parameters

A. Laboratory indicators
   1. Elevated cortisol levels
   2. Decreased eosinophil levels
   3. Increased plasma ACTH if cause is pituitary gland
   4. Hypokalemia
B. Diagnostic indicators
   1. Skull films to identify pituitary tumors if increased ACTH level
   2. Adrenal scanning
      a. CT scan
      b. Radioactive cholesterol uptake
   3. Dexamethasone suppression test: failure to suppress cortisol secretion confirms diagnosis of Cushing's syndrome

**IV. Operative Procedures (Dependent on Etiology)**

A. Unilateral adrenalectomy: removal of one adrenal gland for localized adenoma
B. Bilateral adrenalectomy: removal of both adrenal glands; may be performed for pituitary tumors to decrease ACTH influence on adrenal glands
C. Hypophysectomy: removal of pituitary gland for microadenomas

**V. Operative Concerns**

A. Preoperative and intraoperative concerns
   1. Hypertension
   2. Hyperglycemia
   3. Hypokalemia
   4. Edema
B. Intraoperative and anesthesia concerns
   1. Compromised lung expansion
      a. Truncal obesity
      b. Awkward positioning for flank approach
   2. Positioning for exposure
      a. Abdominal approach; increases chance of splenic or pancreatic injury
      b. Flank approach
         (1) Pneumothorax possible if twelfth rib resected
         (2) Vena caval injury (rare)
   3. Cortisone supplement for surgical stress
   4. Electrolyte monitoring, especially of potassium
   5. Avoid hyperglycemia greater than 200 mg/dl
   6. Control hypertension resulting from blood volume increase
   7. Control hypotension resulting from loss of mineralocorticoids (aldosterone deficiency)

## THE ADRENAL GLAND (CORTEX): ADDISON'S DISEASE

**I. Pathophysiology**

A. Definition: adrenocortical insufficiency manifested by hyposecretion of cortisol and aldosterone
B. Etiology
   1. Autoimmune reaction
   2. Influence from other glandular conditions
   3. Congenital disorder
   4. Malignancy
   5. Infection
   6. Most common: glandular atrophy resulting from steroid therapy for other conditions (iatrogenic)

**II. Postanesthesia Significance**

A. Failure to recognize patients taking cortisone (for rheumatoid arthritis, asthma, colitis, etc.) or inadequately replacing cortisone during and after surgical procedures can result in acute addisonian crisis and death
B. Addisonian crisis is major complication after adrenal surgery

**III. Acute Addisonian Crisis**

A. Signs
   1. Prolonged hypotension and cardiac dysrhythmia (atrial fibrillation with rapid ventricular response)
      a. Decreased cardiac output

b. Decreased vascular resistance
c. Decreased wedge pressure
d. Lack of response to pressors; vessels respond poorly to dopamine or volume expanders
2. Fever
3. Nausea and vomiting
4. Electrolyte imbalance
a. Hypoglycemia
b. Hyponatremia
c. Hyperkalemia
5. Lethargy, somnolence lead to altered mental state and coma
B. Treatment
1. Hydrocortisone: up to 300 mg/70 kg/d
2. Symptomatic treatment of accompanying electrolyte imbalance

## THE ADRENAL GLAND (MEDULLA): PHEOCHROMOCYTOMA

Preganglionic fibers of the sympathetic nervous system end in the medullary portions of both adrenal glands. They stimulate the release of catecholamines and have very short half-lives, usually less than 1 minute. Catecholamines have both inotropic and chronotropic effects on the heart and blood vessels, inhibit the release of insulin, but stimulate liver glycogenesis. These effects are commonly seen in the "fight or flight" situation. Pheochromocytomas are catecholamine-producing tumors that typically cause hypertension; these tumors are rare and only 1 in 1000 cases of hypertension harbors a pheochromocytoma.

**I. Etiology**
A. Benign tumor of adrenal medulla: 90% of cases
B. Tumors in other locations
1. Thorax
2. Bladder
3. Brain
4. Along sympathetic chain
5. Aorta
6. Ovaries
7. Spleen
C. Tumors secrete catecholamines (norepinephrine, epinephrine)

**II. Effects of Increased Catecholamine Secretion**
A. Severe hypertension (paroxysmal or sustained)
B. Orthostatic hypotension
C. Cardiomegaly
D. Elevated blood sugar (from insulin suppression)
E. Elevated white blood cell count
F. Increased hematocrit (from decreased plasma volume)
G. Hypermetabolism

**III. Diagnostic Parameters**
A. Laboratory testing
1. 24-hour urine collection for catecholamines
a. Increase in both norepinephrine and epinephrine indicates adrenal pheochromocytoma
b. Increase in only norepinephrine indicates tumor may be of sympathetic origin
2. Vanillylmandelic acid (VMA), a by-product of catecholamine degradation, elevated in 80% of pheochromocytomas

3. Radioenzymatic: costly but measures plasma level
4. Clonidine: treat with single dose; decreases plasma norepinephrine

B. CT scan
1. Localizes tumor
2. 98% accurate

C. Symptoms
1. Cardiovascular (paroxysmal)
   a. Angina
   b. Palpitations
   c. Tachycardia
2. Gastrointestinal
   a. Abdominal pain
   b. Nausea
   c. Weight loss
3. Neuromuscular and vascular
   a. Headaches
   b. Diaphoresis
   c. Irritability
   d. Visual disturbances

## IV. Preoperative Management: Establish α-Adrenergic Blockage with Phenoxybenzamine Hydrochloride (Dibenzyline)

A. Beginning doses 20 to 30 mg daily, increasing to 60 to 250 mg daily until blood pressure controlled

B. Volume repletion

C. Control of tachycardia with β-blockers

## V. Operative Procedure: Radical Adrenalectomy Performed with Removal of Affected Gland and Adjacent Areolar Tissue

## VI. Operative Concerns with α- and β-Blocker Drugs

A. Avoidance of drugs causing histamine release or sympathetic stimulation
1. Narcotics
   a. Substitution of barbiturates for preoperative narcotic medication
   b. Use of fentanyl because of its decreased histamine release
2. Nondepolarizing muscle relaxants
3. Adrenergic drugs
4. Cholinergic blockers

B. Avoid sympathetic response during
1. Anesthesia induction
2. Tracheal intubation
3. Positioning
4. Manipulation of tumor
5. Ligation of venous drainage of tumor

C. Need for adequate $CO_2$ absorption to reduce increased catecholamine production

D. Continuous blood pressure monitoring
1. Electronic apparatus
2. Arterial monitoring

E. Have drugs readily available
1. Before tumor excision
   a. Phentolamine mesylate (Regitine)
   b. Sodium nitroprusside (Nipride)

2. After tumor excision if rebound hypotension occurs
   a. Norepinephrine
   b. Blood and volume expanders
3. Cortisone for replacement only if both adrenal glands excised

## POSTANESTHESIA NURSING CARE FOR PATIENTS WITH ADRENAL GLAND CONDITIONS

### NURSING DIAGNOSIS

Examples of related nursing diagnostic categories include
- Potential for infection
- Decreased cardiac output
- Ineffective airway clearance

**I. Hypotension**
A. More common than hypertension
B. Bleeding: adrenocorticoid insufficiency
C. Persistent, unexplained hypotension may precede adrenal crisis
D. Rebound epinephrine shock: complicated by receptors that have become insensitive and vascular reflexes that are slow to respond

**II. Hypertension**
A. Occasionally seen after excision of pheochromocytoma
B. Antihypertensive agents often more effective than when administered before tumor excision

**III. Electrolyte Values (Serum and Urine)**
A. Monitor
1. Decreases in serum $Na^+$
2. Increases in urine $Na^+$
3. Increases in serum $K^+$
   a. In unrecognized addisonian patient
   b. Transient with primary hyperaldosteronism
   c. When hypokalemia overcorrected
4. Serum glucose
   a. Hypoglycemia: unrecognized Addisonian patient
   b. Hyperglycemia: after excision of pheochromocytoma from related preoperative insulin suppression

**IV. Fluid Administration**
A. Hypertonic saline at prescribed rate
B. Blood, plasma, albumin for decreased hemoglobin, hematocrit, and volume
C. Sudden withdrawal of catecholamines postoperatively makes patient susceptible to rapid changes in blood pressure and fluid and electrolyte balance

**V. Wound Observation**
A. Increased infection susceptibility
B. Increased bleeding or hematoma formation
1. Resulting from easy bruisability and/or hypertension

2. Signal of internal hemorrhaging
3. Meticulous care necessary for dressing changes

## VI. Chest Film Confirmation

A. Bilateral lung expansion after adrenalectomy (if twelfth rib resection necessary)
B. Central venous pressure catheter placement

## VII. Complications

A. Shock
   1. Causes
      a. Addisonian crisis caused by decreased cortisol and aldosterone levels
         (1) After bilateral adrenalectomy
         (2) After any surgery on patients taking cortisone for chronic medical conditions
      b. Decreased circulating catecholamines after excision of pheochromocytoma
      c. Inadequate blood volume
   2. Treatment (specific to underlying causes)
      a. Hydrocortisone for Addisonian-related problems
      b. Norepinephrine (Levophed) drip for decreased catecholamine effects
      c. Blood, plasma, albumin for hypovolemia
B. Pneumothorax: atelectasis
   1. Occurs usually after rib resection
   2. Signaled by dyspnea, uneven chest expansion, chest pain, decreased to absent breath sounds
   3. Confirmed by chest film
   4. Treated with insertion of chest tube
C. Cerebrovascular accident
   1. Risk increases intraoperatively
      a. With inadequately controlled hypertension accompanying excision of pheochromocytoma
      b. With increased catecholamines and fluid overload
      c. With inappropriate aldosterone release, renal artery ligation
   2. Ascertained by postanesthesia evaluation
      a. Level of consciousness
      b. Ability to move all extremities
      c. Bilateral Babinski's sign present
      d. Pupillary changes
      e. Slurred speech
D. Cardiac dysrhythmias
   1. Causes
      a. Tachydysrhythmias: increased catecholamine circulating after excision of pheochromocytoma
      b. Uncorrected hypokalemia after hyperaldosteronism and Cushing's disease
   2. Treatment (specific to underlying cause)
      a. Propranolol (Inderal) for tachydysrhythmias
      b. Potassium supplements if decreased serum $K^+$
      c. Lidocaine for ventricular tachycardia and fibrillation
E. Infection
   1. Resulting from cortisone masking signs of infection
   2. Poor wound healing
F. Hypoglycemia
   1. Occurs from rebound hyperinsulinemia
   2. Results from removal of anti-insulin factor in tumor, enhanced glucoreceptor reactivity to insulin, or both

## DIABETES MELLITUS IN THE SURGICAL PATIENT

**I. Pathophysiology**

A. Etiology
   1. Syndrome characterized by glucose intolerance, large vessel disease, microvascular disease, and neuropathy
   2. Diabetic patient at higher risk for surgery and anesthetic complications than non-diabetic patient
   3. Cardiovascular complications responsible for 80% of diabetic deaths
   4. Amputation 20 times more likely in diabetic population

B. Types of diabetes mellitus
   1. Type I: insulin dependent (ketosis prone)
      a. Characteristics
         (1) Little or no endogenous insulin
         (2) Young
         (3) Lower than average body weight
      b. Causes
         (1) Genetic: human leukocyte antigen (HLA) immune antigen
         (2) Environmental: viruses
         (3) Autoimmunity: circulating islet cell antibodies
   2. Type II: maturity onset, (no longer referred to as non-insulin-dependent, NIDDM, as patients may require insulin as part of their disease management) nonketotic
      a. Characteristics
         (1) Overweight
         (2) Middle aged
         (3) Sometimes high levels of circulating insulin
         (4) Carbohydrate intolerance
      b. Causes
         (1) Problems at β-cell level
         (2) Insulin resistance or decrease in receptor sites
   3. Type III: impaired glucose tolerance (chemical or borderline diabetes); causes: receptor sites decreased or not receptive to insulin

**II. Incidence**

A. Estimated 14 million diabetic patients

B. 70% are 40 years old or older

C. Many surgical disorders such as cataracts, cholelithiasis, vascular disease have been identified in this group

D. Estimated that 50% of diabetic population experience at least one surgical intervention in their lifetime

**III. Special Effects of Diabetes on Surgical Problems**

A. Increased prevalence of macrovascular disease affecting coronary and cerebral arteries as well as peripheral arterial supply

B. Gastrointestinal and urinary bladder dysfunctions

C. Causes of occult infections
   1. Lowered resistance during periods of stress-induced hyperglycemia; glucose levels greater than 200 inhibit white blood cell activity
   2. Catabolic effect of insulin deficiency, which results in protein wastage and adversely affects wound healing
   3. Electrolyte and hormone deficiencies
      a. Potassium depletion causing decreased stroke volume, dysrhythmias
      b. Hyperkalemia may be result of renal impairment causing bradycardia, ventricular fibrillation
      c. Stress and trauma lead to hyperglycemia, may lead to ketoacidotic coma

## IV. General Adaptation Syndrome (GAS) Described by Selye

A. Sympathetic nervous system (adrenal medulla) stimulates production of catecholamines
   1. Increases heart rate
   2. Increases blood pressure
   3. Dilates bronchi

B. Blood glucose increases
   1. Catecholamines cause glycogen stores in liver to release glucose into blood system
   2. Glucocorticoids (primary cortisol) secreted by adrenal cortex cause liver to produce additional carbohydrates from fats, proteins
   3. Gluconeogenesis may elevate blood glucose levels 6 to 8 times normal

C. Along with increasing glucose levels, catecholamines inhibit pancreas from releasing insulin

D. Glucocorticoids decrease use of glucose in adipose tissue and stimulate formation of circulating insulin antagonist

E. Proclivity for infection
   1. Inadequate circulation to extremities
   2. Hyperglycemia; excellent culture media

## V. Operative Concerns

A. Preoperative evaluation
   1. Cardiovascular system
      a. One of most common causes of mortality in diabetic patients
      b. Painless angina occurs more often in diabetics than in general population
      c. For diabetics who have experienced a myocardial infarction, risk of reinfarction within 4 to 6 months is 11%
      d. Diagnostic tests
         (1) Serum lipid values
         (2) ECG
   2. Renal function
      a. Serum creatinine
      b. Blood urea nitrogen (BUN)
      c. Urinary output
   3. Serum values
      a. Glucose and acetone levels
      b. Glycosylated hemoglobin (hemoglobin A1C) to determine long-term (3 months) control of diabetes
      c. Electrolytes
         (1) Potassium
         (2) Sodium
         (3) Chloride
         (4) Bicarbonate

B. Drugs altering glucose levels
   1. Thiazides and loop diuretics
      a. Contribute to hyperglycemia
      b. Hyperglycemic effect may be outweighed by antihypertensive value
   2. Phenytoin (Dilantin): may cause mild hyperglycemia
   3. Propranolol
      a. Modified hypoglycemic reaction of insulin by blocking catecholamine release
      b. Possibly inhibits insulin release from pancreas
   4. Chlorpropamide (Diabinese): lengthy half-life necessitates discontinuance 24 to 36 hours preoperatively

C. Gastroparesis
   1. Caused by autonomic neuropathy

2. Results in weak or absent esophageal motility
    a. When diabetic patients lie flat, food and liquids pool in esophagus
    b. Delay in gastric emptying
    c. Risk of aspiration of gastric contents is intensified

D. Control of diabetes during surgery: both diabetic and nondiabetic patients are somewhat resistant to insulin during this stress period
    1. Goal: prevent hyperosmolar coma (usually in type II) and ketoacidosis without inducing hypoglycemia
        a. Maintain patient in well-hydrated anabolic state
        b. Avoid hypoglycemia or hyperglycemia by adequate preoperative preparation
        c. Frequent monitoring of blood glucose levels
    2. Operative strategy
        a. Schedule procedure as early in morning as possible
        b. Discontinue oral agents before surgery
            (1) Patients taking oral hypoglycemics may be given regular insulin before surgery
            (2) Titrated according to glucose levels
        c. Assess preoperative fasting blood glucose levels
        d. Begin IV fluids containing glucose at rate appropriate to keep patient well hydrated
    3. Insulin regimens
        a. Common method of insulin administration on day of surgery: ½ of patient's usual dose of intermediate-acting insulin subcutaneously on morning of surgery; absorption may be impeded if patient becomes too cold while exposed to low temperatures in operating suite
        b. More controlled method of insulin administration achieved with constant infusion of $D_5W$, 25 to 100 ml/hr piggyback with an insulin solution at 1 to 5 U/hr; most critical issue for maintaining insulin blood glucose levels is reliable blood glucose monitoring; rapid access crucial in monitoring these levels; many practitioners maintain intraarterial lines, a practical approach to access
        c. Glucose and insulin infusions may induce hypokalemia; potassium chloride may be added to infusion if renal function is satisfactory

## VI. Anesthesia Concerns

A. Type of anesthesia
    1. No "best" anesthetic for diabetic patients
    2. Inhalation agents cause less pronounced changes in blood glucose
    3. Stress and practice of rapid administration of glucose-containing IV fluids have more profound effect on blood glucose
    4. Regional blocks may be considered in some diabetic patients because they produce fewer metabolic disturbances

B. Avoidance of hypoglycemia and serious cerebral dysfunction
    1. Blood glucose level for diabetic patients commonly maintained between 120 and 220 mg/dl
        a. For protection against unexpected drop to hypoglycemia
        b. Elevations capable of causing significant glycosuria
    2. Subtle external signs
        a. Slight increase in pulse
        b. Decrease in urinary output

C. Avoidance of hyperglycemia
    1. Leads to glycosuria and significant polyuria, electrolyte imbalance, and dehydration of osmotic diuresis
    2. Diuresis and vasodilating drugs may render diabetic patient hemodynamically unstable during anesthesia

**TABLE 27–2 Insulin Profiles**

| INSULIN AGENT | ONSET (HOURS) | DURATION (HOURS) |
|---|---|---|
| Regular | 1 | 8 |
| Semilente | 1 | 14 |
| NPH | 2 | 24 |
| Lente | 2 | 24 |
| Protamine zinc | 4 | 36 |
| Ultralente | 4 | 36 |

3. Less resistance to infection
   a. Impaired phagocytosis
   b. Decrease in tissue strength and healing of wounds
   c. Increase in free fatty acids
4. Hypoglycemic agents (see Table 27–2)

D. Avoidance of hypoxemia, hypotension, impaired cardiac function
   1. Myocardial infarction
      a. Results from increased severity of large-vessel atherosclerosis
      b. One of leading causes of high mortality in diabetic patients
   2. Hypotension caused by persistent urinary losses will result in ketoacidosis
   3. Hypoxemia
      a. Influenced by long-term control of diabetic patients
      b. Increase in glycosylated hemoglobin will influence tissue oxygenation
      c. Increase in oxygen consumption in patient already borderline oxygenated as result of increased shunting (commonly seen in anesthetized patient) may result in pronounced hypoxemia

E. Avoidance of injury during anesthesia
   1. Patients with peripheral neuropathy vulnerable to positioning injuries
   2. Impaired gastric emptying should be anticipated

## VII. Postanesthesia Concerns

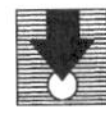

**NURSING DIAGNOSIS**

Examples of related nursing diagnostic categories include
- Potential for decreased cardiac output
- Potential for infection
- Potential for fluid volume deficit
- Potential for impaired respiratory function caused by aspiration

A. Assess levels of consciousness
   1. Persistent disorientation, unconsciousness may portend hypoglycemia
   2. Hyperglycemia (diabetic coma); occurs rarely immediately postoperatively

B. Monitor serum glucose on admission to PACU
   1. Serum levels are only accurate indication for insulin requirement
   2. Urinary glucose and acetone values reflect serum level of preceding few hours and lead to erratic control of hyperglycemia

C. Continue hydration
   1. Monitor urinary output
   2. Monitor vital signs

D. Monitor cardiac dysrhythmias
   1. Note hypokalemic change of ECG

   a. Depressed T wave and ST segment
   b. Prolonged QT interval
   c. U waves
2. Hypokalemia leads to increased premature ventricular contractions
3. Supplemental potassium for hypokalemia
4. Tachydysrhythmias; propranolol helpful
5. Persistent hypotension may require hydrocortisone

E. Prevention of infection: meticulous attention to sterile technique
1. Surgical dressings
2. Urinary catheter insertion
3. Invasive monitoring lines
4. Pulmonary hygiene

F. Complications
1. Sudden death from respiratory or cardiac arrest; respiratory arrests may be caused by severe autonomic neuropathy
   a. Avoid dehydration and electrolyte deficits
   b. Lactic acidosis
      (1) Associated with circulatory collapse, renal or hepatic failure, alcoholism
      (2) High mortality
2. Diabetic coma or acidosis caused by decreased insulin and increased insulin-antagonistic hormones (cortisol)
   a. Rarely seen in PACU
   b. Confirmation
      (1) Serum electrolytes
      (2) Increased potassium
      (3) Increased BUN
      (4) Increased serum osmolarity
      (5) Increased serum glucose and acetone level
      (6) Arterial blood gas pH decreases to 7.30; decreased bicarbonate levels
      (7) Tachypnea
      (8) Tachycardia
      (9) Polyuria
      (10) Hypotension
   c. Treatment
      (1) Fluid and electrolyte correction
      (2) Insulin administration
      (3) Bicarbonate for pH less than 7.20 (1 mEq/kg)
3. Hypoglycemic reaction
   a. Causes
      (1) Inadequate amount of glucose after insulin administration
      (2) Incorrect or overdosage of insulin
      (3) Hyperfunction of β-cells in pancreatic tumors
      (4) Brittle and juvenile diabetics eliciting undue response to insulin action
   b. Symptoms (sudden onset)
      (1) Weakness, dizziness
      (2) Moist, pale skin
      (3) Shallow breathing pattern
      (4) Confusion, incoherence
      (5) Combativeness
   c. Treatment (initiated before laboratory confirmation)
      (1) Obtain serum glucose for future confirmation
      (2) Immediate administration of dextrose 50% bolus (50 ml)
      (3) Observance of (often dramatic) return of orientation after dextrose bolus

## PANCREAS TRANSPLANTATION

I. **Overview:** At present, transplantation of the pancreas is the only treatment that can render type I diabetic patients euglycemic. In addition, secondary complications of diabetes are lessened and in some cases ameliorated. The incidence of success in whole organ pancreas transplant is 77% with the new antirejection agents. Higher morbidity exists with pancreas transplantation than in the more common simultaneous pancreas and kidney transplantation. Islet cell transplants are less common. Clinical trials for patients with diabetes and without kidney disease have not been performed in the number that would provide validity to the research. Less than 10% of a small sample of patients have achieved insulin independence.

II. **Preoperative Assessment**
   A. Pancreas transplants are *elective* procedures: hence the patient should have attained
      1. Absence of infection: diabetic patients should be screened for remote infection (i.e., UTI, respiratory, dental)
      2. Tight control of blood sugar
      3. Balance of electrolytes
   B. Systems review
      1. Nervous system: peripheral neuropathy and gastroparesis
      2. Cardiopulmonary hypervolemia, hyperkalemia, coronary artery disease (CAD)
      3. Musculoskeletal: joint immobilities or contracture osteopenia

III. **Preoperative Preparation**
   A. Medication
      1. Ranitidine, 50 mg, and metoclopramide, 10 mg
      2. Antibiotics: vancomycin or cefotaxime
   B. Blood availability
   C. Control hyperglycemia with regular insulin 25 U/250 ml 0.9% normal saline solution
   D. Arterial lines

IV. **Anesthesia Concerns**
   A. Rapid induction because of gastroparesis
   B. Muscle relaxants: succinylcholine used to induce if patient is eukalemic (3.5 to 5 mmol/nl)
   C. Atracurium for maintenance of blockade in patients with end-stage renal disease (ESRD)
      1. Glucose management: attempt to maintain serum glucose at 70 to 100 mg/dl
      2. After reperfusion of graft, slow the insulin infusion
   D. Control of $K^+$ levels: this is difficult to do because a high percentage of patients have wide fluctuations; treating variations in serum $K^+$ levels should be anticipated even with adequate glucose control
   E. Administration of immunosuppressive agents before graft reperfusion

V. **Postanesthesia Concerns**
   A. Pain management: incisional, joint, and neuropathic
   B. Hypovolemia if recently dialyzed; hyperkalemia and hypervolemia if not dialyzed
   C. Aspiration pneumonitis
   D. Control of glucose levels: usually an insulin infusion with 25 units of regular insulin in 250 ml 0.9% normal saline solution is used to maintain blood sugar at 70 to 100 mg/dl; hyperglycemia of 300 mg/dl is treated with boluses of regular insulin in addition to the insulin drip; it is important to control serum glucose by changing infusion rate rather than by bolus in patients who have glucose levels less than 250 mg/dl
   E. Noncardiogenic pulmonary edema associated with intraoperative immunosuppressives
   F. Protection of hemodialysis access sites
   G. Infection control: patients remain at high risk for infection
   H. Blood loss intraoperatively may require replacement in PACU

## BIBLIOGRAPHY


Barash PG, Cullen BF, Stoelting RK: *Handbook of Clinical Anesthesia.* Philadelphia, JB Lippincott, 1991.

Beahrs O: Complications in thyroid and parathyroid surgery. In Conley J (ed): *Complications of Head and Neck Surgery* (pp 239–245). Philadelphia, WB Saunders, 1989.

Firestone L, Lebowitz P, Cook C: *Clinical Anesthesia Procedures of Massachusetts General Hospital.* Boston, Little, Brown, 1988.

Goldman D: Surgery in patients with endocrine dysfunction. *Med Clin North Am* 71:499–509, 1987.

Hay I, Klee G: Thyroid dysfunction. *Endocrinol Metab Clin North Am* 17:473–509, 1988.

Kraft S, Mihm F, Feeley T: Postoperative endocrine problems. In Vender J, Spiess B (eds): *Post Anesthesia Care* (pp 216–232). Philadelphia, WB Saunders, 1992.

Roizen M: *Perioperative Management of the Diabetic Patient.* ASA Refresher Course Lectures (No. 164, p 1–5). Chicago, ASA, 1993.

Selye H: *Stress Without Distress.* Philadelphia, JB Lippincott, 1974.

Stoelting R, Dierdorf S: *Anesthesia and Co-Existing Disease,* 3rd Ed. New York, Churchill-Livingstone, 1993.

Stoelting R, Miller RD: *Basics of Anesthesia,* 3rd Ed. New York, Churchill Livingstone, 1994.

Wall R: *Anesthetic Challenges in the Patient with Endocrine Disease.* ASA Refresher Course Lectures (No. 143, p 1–7). Chicago, ASA, 1993.

Wall R: Anesthetic management of pheochromocytoma. *Prog Anesthesiol* 5:342–354, 1991.


## REVIEW QUESTIONS

**1. What describes hyperthyroidism?**

A. A state of hyperactivity caused by enlarged glands
B. An autoimmune disease of unknown cause
C. A hypermetabolic condition resulting in excessive secretion of thyroid hormone
D. A euthyroid state

**2. What characterizes hyperparathyroidism?**

A. Underactivity of one or more of the parathyroid glands
B. Excessive secretion of calcium
C. Allergy to iodine
D. Hypercalcemia and hyperphosphatemia

**3. What are signs of tetany?**

A. Apprehension, tingling in toes and fingers, positive Chvostek's sign
B. Impaired level of consciousness, muscle weakness, anxiety
C. Hypertension, hypoventilation, hypovolemia
D. Nausea, carpopedal spasm, generalized edema

**4. What are effects of anterior pituitary hyposecretion?**

A. Increases in circulating growth hormone
B. Increases in prolactin levels
C. Diabetes insipidus
D. Decreases in TSH

**5. What are effects of increased aldosterone?**

A. Sodium retention, hypotension, generalized weakness
B. Tetany, hyperglycemia, hypovolemia
C. Water retention, sodium retention, hypokalemia, tetany
D. Hypoglycemia, hypertension, hypotension

**6. Which symptoms characterize Cushing's disease?**

A. Moon face, hirsutism, buffalo hump
B. Obesity with muscle wasting, thick skin, hypotension
C. Ecchymosis, osteoporosis, muscle hypertrophy
D. Hyperkalemia, acne, truncal obesity

**7. Addisonian crisis is the major complication after adrenal surgery. What are signs of acute Addisonian crisis?**

A. Electrolyte imbalance, nausea and vomiting, hypotension
B. Cardiac dysrhythmias, hypertension, somnolence
C. Fever, exaggerated response to dopamine, coma
D. Hypernatremia, hyperglycemia, hypokalemia

**8. Pheochromocytomas are catecholamine-producing tumors that typically cause hypertension.**

A. False
B. True

**9. The diabetic patient having surgery may have a need for increased insulin as a result of what condition?**

A. Blood loss during surgery
B. Physical and emotional stress
C. Being NPO before surgery
D. Missing the usual dose of insulin the evening before surgery

**10. Hormonal responses to stress responsible for the increased need for insulin include which of the following?**

A. Release of glucagon from the pancreas
B. Pituitary hormones that suppress insulin production
C. Release of glucagon from the liver, secretion of catecholamines
D. Secretion of growth hormone from the pituitary and release of endorphins

**11. Thyrotoxic crisis (storm) resulting from a sudden increase in circulating thyroid hormone may be confused with malignant hyperthermia. Signs of thyroid storm include which of the following?**

A. Hyperthermia, tachycardia, profuse sweating, tachypnea
B. Dehydration, muscle rigidity
C. Pulmonary edema, atrial flutter, vomiting
D. Agitation, bradycardia, hypernatremia

**12. The general adaptation syndrome (GAS) described by Selye involves the body's response to stress, including which of the following?**

A. Glycogenolysis and decreases in blood glucose levels
B. Gluconeogenesis and inhibition of catecholamines
C. Increases in heart rate, blood pressure, and blood glucose
D. Weakness, incoherence, combativeness

**ANSWERS:** 1. C, 2. D, 3. A, 4. D, 5. C, 6. A, 7. A, 8. B, 9. B, 10. C, 11. A, 12. C

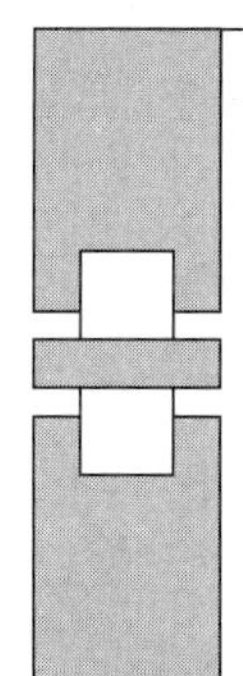

CHAPTER 28

# *The Otorhinolaryngologic and Head and Neck Surgical Patient*

Gwen Singleton, BSN, RN, CNOR, CORLN

Sue Silcox, AD, RN, CORLN

**OBJECTIVES**

**Study of the information represented by this outline will enable the learner to:**

1. Become familiar with the postanesthesia problems encountered in the ear, nose, throat, and head and neck patient and the nursing interventions required in the management of these problems.
2. Identify the pathophysiologic ear, nose, throat, and head and neck conditions requiring surgical interventions.
3. Understand the perioperative nursing concerns and rationale for the care of patients undergoing ear, nose, throat, and head and neck procedures.
4. Become familiar with the various surgical procedures performed in this specialty.
5. Know the methods and techniques necessary to maintain a patent airway after ear, nose, throat, and head and neck surgery.
6. Be aware of the possible complications that can arise after ear, nose, throat, and head and neck procedures and the nursing interventions required to correct these problems.

Patients having ear, nose, and throat (ENT), maxillofacial, and head and neck surgery present to postanesthesia care unit (PACU) nurses with specific physical and psychologic needs. The surgery performed on their upper airway creates feelings of discomfort, pressure, and suffocation with each breath. Communication with intubated, tracheostomy, and laryngectomy patients is difficult in the PACU. Frequent reassurance and explanations of what is happening are required.

The relatively minor nature and often short duration of many ENT procedures should not influence the PACU nurse to develop a false sense of security. Prevention and early detection of complications are primary objectives of nursing care with these patients.

## GENERAL NURSING CONCERNS FOR THE ENT AND HEAD AND NECK PATIENT

**I. Preoperative Concerns**

- A. Medical history assessment
- B. Nursing assessment
  - 1. Chief complaint
  - 2. Medications
    - a. Allergies
    - b. Current medications patient is taking
    - c. Use of aspirin, ibuprofen, or drugs containing aspirin (increased risk of bleeding)
    - d. Hormone therapy
    - e. Preoperative medications

3. Patient's understanding of surgical procedure and expected outcomes
4. Patient's psychosocial status

C. Laboratory and radiologic evaluations
1. Complete blood count (CBC)
2. Electrolytes based on patient history
3. Urinalysis
4. Coagulation studies
5. Availability of designated units, type, and crossmatch
6. Electrocardiogram (ECG)
7. Chest radiograph
8. Radiograph of sinuses, neck, mastoid
9. Computed tomography (CT)
10. Magnetic resonance imaging (MRI)

D. Preoperative instructions
1. Surgical procedure
2. Expected outcomes
3. Environment
4. Alterations in lifestyle
5. Self-care
6. Suctioning
7. Deep breathing
8. Pain management

**II. Intraoperative Concerns**

A. Nursing assessment
1. Assess respiratory status
2. Determine patient's comfort
3. Identify positioning needs
4. Establish priorities
5. Reinforce preoperative teaching, orient to operating room (OR) environment, instruct patient in postoperative dressings
6. Determine patient's anxiety or apprehension

B. Aseptic technique
C. Skin and tissue integrity
D. Correct counts
E. Medications given
F. Intake and output
G. Blood loss
H. Patient's condition at time of transfer to PACU

**III. Postoperative Concerns**

A. Nursing assessment
1. Respiratory status
2. Cardiovascular status
3. Neurologic status
4. Psychosocial status

B. Report from anesthesiologist or CRNA or OR nurse
1. Procedure, extent of surgery; complications
2. Anesthetic agents and medications administered
3. Blood loss and fluid replacement
4. Placement of drains, packing
5. Pertinent history, allergies

C. Pain status
D. Intake and output
E. Patient's position

F. Presence or absence of nausea
G. Patient's ability to communicate
H. Integrity of dressings and incision
I. Patient's temperature
J. Drainage from surgical site

## GENERAL CARE OF THE ENT, MAXILLOFACIAL, AND HEAD AND NECK SURGERY PATIENT

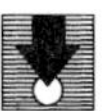

### NURSING DIAGNOSIS

Examples of related nursing diagnostic categories include:

- Potential for ineffective airway clearance
- Potential for infection
- Potential for impaired gas exchange
- Altered tissue perfusion
- Impaired communication

**I. Preparation**

A. Equipment
1. Oral and nasal airways
2. AMBU bag with various mask sizes
3. Laryngoscope with various blades (curved, straight, different sizes)
4. Endotracheal tubes and stylet
5. Adequate light source
6. Tracheostomy tray and tubes
7. Tracheal dilator
8. Suction apparatus
9. Wire cutters and scissors
10. Sponge forceps and tongue blades
11. Tonsil packs
12. Pillows for positioning
13. Tape
14. Fiberoptic bronchoscope readily available

B. PACU admission
1. Airway adequacy
2. Vital signs, including $Sao_2$
3. Level of consciousness
4. Intravenous (IV) site and patency
5. Application of humidified oxygen
6. Operative site: dressings, packing, drainage
7. Surgical and anesthesia reports
8. Report from OR nurse

**II. Maintaining Airway**

A. Positioning when no artificial airway is present
1. Unconscious or drowsy: use supine with head elevated or side-lying position; facilitates airway maintenance and drainage of secretions
2. Conscious: use semi-Fowler's position, which reduces venous and capillary bleeding and facilitates respiratory excursion

B. Indications of airway obstruction
1. Noisy breathing

2. Seesaw movement of chest and abdomen
3. Absent breath sounds
4. Decreased oxygen saturation

C. Nursing interventions to correct airway obstruction
1. Elevating head of bed
2. Repositioning of patient
3. Suctioning of patient secretions
4. Stimulating patient
5. Pulling mandible forward to relieve tongue obstruction
6. Inserting oral or nasal airway

D. When artificial airway (endotracheal tube or tracheostomy tube) is present
1. Administer oxygen with humidity through T piece or tracheal collar
2. Assessment of airway placement
   a. Auscultate for bilateral breath sounds
   b. Confirm placement of ET or tracheostomy tube by x-ray film
3. Assess need for suctioning
   a. Noisy respirations
   b. Restlessness
   c. Rising pulse and respiratory rates
   d. Decreasing oxygen saturation
   e. Cyanosis (late sign)

E. Suctioning technique
1. Prevent introduction of pathogens into lungs
   a. Use only sterile gloves and suction catheter
   b. Catheter used for oropharyngeal suctioning (nonsterile) is never used for tracheobronchial suctioning (sterile)
2. Prevent hypoxemia
   a. Preoxygenate with 100% oxygen before suctioning
   b. Suctioning should take less than 5 seconds
   c. Oxygenate between suction attempts
3. Catheters
   a. Should be long enough to reach bronchial mucosa
   b. Should have a diameter small enough to pass through ET tube without causing obstruction
4. Avoid mucosal damage
   a. After catheter touches bronchial mucosa, occlude air vent with gloved thumb
   b. Withdraw catheter with twisting motion

F. Complications of suctioning
1. Mucosal trauma (bleeding, edema)
2. Hypoxemia (causes)
   a. Catheter too large
   b. Excessive suction pressure
   c. Inadequate preoxygenation between suctioning periods
3. Asphyxia (inadequate oxygenation)
4. Dysrhythmias
   a. Multiple premature ventricular contractions (PVCs) from overstimulation or prolonged irritation of tracheal bifurcation
   b. Inadequate oxygenation

## III. Care of Intubated Patient

A. Advantages of ET tube over tracheostomy
1. Quicker insertion during emergency situations
2. No surgical trauma involved

B. Disadvantages of ET tube over tracheostomy
   1. Suctioning less effective
   2. Suctioning can cause airway trauma
   3. Friction against larynx can damage vocal cords
   4. Easier for patients to extubate themselves
C. Equipment necessary for intubation
   1. ET tubes in varied sizes
   2. Lubricant
   3. Laryngoscopes with functioning light and appropriate blade
   4. Syringe to inflate cuff
   5. Flexible stylet
   6. Suctioning apparatus
   7. Medications
      a. For topical vocal cord relaxation (lidocaine)
      b. For systemic muscle relaxation (e.g., succinylcholine)
   8. AMBU bag with oxygen
   9. Access to fiberoptic bronchoscope
D. Ascertaining correct tube positioning
   1. Observation of equal chest movement on inspiration
   2. Auscultation of bilateral breath sounds
   3. Confirmation by chest x-ray film
E. General considerations for nursing care
   1. Head elevation ideal for intubated ENT surgery patient
   2. Restrain arms lightly if patient is incoherent
   3. Relieve anxiety with frequent communication
      a. Provide pencil and paper for communication if patient is coherent
      b. Reassure patient of the need for the endotracheal tube
   4. Auscultate chest for breath sounds
   5. Suction only when necessary to avoid trauma
   6. Ascertain muscle strength periodically
   7. Provide sedation if indicated
F. Factors precipitating complications
   1. Airway trauma leading to soft tissue edema (causes)
      a. ET tube too large
      b. Cuff overinflated
      c. Excessive tube movement as result of inadequate securing
   2. Hypoxemia
      a. Tube displacement into esophagus (no breath sounds) or right main-stem bronchus (no breath sounds on left side)
      b. Prolonged suctioning
      c. Dislodging of oxygen source
      d. Obstruction of tube
         (1) Secretions
         (2) Tube kinking
         (3) Teeth clamping
G. Criteria for extubation
   1. Patient conscious
   2. Able to maintain airway
   3. Negative inspiratory force (NIF): −20 cm
   4. Adequate head lift, grip, muscle strength
   5. Stable cardiopulmonary system
   6. No active bleeding
   7. Arterial blood gas values (ABGs) or oxygen saturation levels remain within acceptable limits during spontaneous respirations

H. Procedure for extubation
   1. Keep equipment for reintubation close
   2. Suction endotracheal tube and mouth before deflating cuff to avoid aspiration of secretions
   3. Patient in sitting position if not contraindicated or supine with head elevated
   4. Administer humidified oxygen by face mask after extubation
   5. Watch patient closely for laryngospasm and respiratory insufficiency after extubation

**IV. Care of Patient with New Tracheostomy**

A. Bedside supplies
   1. Sterile suctioning equipment
   2. AMBU bag (bag valve mask)
   3. Humidified oxygen
   4. Sterile tracheostomy tubes
   5. Sterile forceps, tracheal hook, tracheal dilator (Trousseau)
   6. Supplies for cleaning tracheal tube or sterile disposable inner cannulas
   7. Supplies for changing dressings
   8. Syringe for inflating cuffed tubes (hemostat available if valve malfunctions)

B. General care
   1. Constant attendance by nursing personnel
   2. Monitoring of general condition
      a. Vital signs
      b. Oxygen perfusion (skin and mucosa color, percent saturation)
   3. Provision of adequate humidification with oxygen by tracheal collar or T piece (helps prevent mucous plugs)
   4. Periodic wound inspection
   5. Suctioning as necessary to maintain tube patency
   6. Maintenance of head elevation for comfort and ease of ventilation
   7. Sterile suctioning and cleaning of inner cannula or replacement of inner cannula with sterile, disposable inner cannula
   8. Providing patient with means of communication
      a. Pencil, paper on clipboard, magic slate, picture board, computer board

C. Possible complications
   1. Obstruction of tracheal tube
      a. Excessive secretions
      b. Mucosal edema
      c. Thickened mucoid plugs
   2. Expulsion of tracheal tube
      a. Causes
         (1) Poorly tied tube
         (2) Violent coughing
      b. Interventions
         (1) Hold incision open with hemostat or tracheal dilator
         (2) Never use force
         (3) Avoid pushing tube through soft tissue into mediastinum
   3. Hemorrhage
      a. Causes
         (1) Erosion of anterior wall of trachea from malpositioned cannula, loosened vessel ligature
         (2) Carotid "blow-out" after combined total laryngectomy with radical neck dissection (unique complication, not seen very often this decade)
      b. Indications
         (1) Heavy bleeding at incision site or over carotid
         (2) Bright red, bloody secretions

(3) Rapid pulse
(4) Increasing respiratory obstruction
(5) Restlessness

c. Interventions
(1) Direct pressure
(2) Reassurance
(3) Suctioning
(4) Tracheal cuff inflation
(5) Ventilation
(6) Ice packs
(7) Emergency equipment (gauze pads, vascular clips, suture ties, AMBU bag)

4. Other complications
a. Atelectasis
b. Mediastinal emphysema
c. Subcutaneous emphysema
d. Pneumothorax: unilateral (direct pleural injury) or bilateral (airway obstruction)
e. Potential for ventilation problems arising during emergency situations
(1) Total or partial laryngectomy
(2) Jaw immobilization devices
(3) Presence of packing

## V. Management of Nausea, Vomiting, and Aspiration

A. Causes
1. Irritation of gastric mucosa by swallowed blood
2. Problems with proprioception as result of middle or inner ear surgery
3. Intolerance of medications
4. Cerebral anoxia
5. Pain

B. Nursing interventions
1. Turn patient completely on one side in slight Trendelenburg's position to prevent aspiration should vomiting occur
2. Administer antiemetics
3. Administer analgesia as needed
4. Encourage deep breathing; administer oxygen for persistent nausea

C. Management of vomiting when jaws are wired in occlusion
1. Keep wire cutters, scissors, suction equipment at bedside at all times
2. Suction nares gently
3. Suction orally along molars (Yankauer preferred)
4. Turn patient completely on side with no pressure on operative site
5. Cut wires to permit thorough suctioning of oropharynx
6. Should aspiration occur, depending on severity, anticipate other interventions
a. Reintubation and suctioning
b. Respiratory therapy, mechanical ventilation, serial ABGs
c. Administration of steroids, antibiotics
d. Chest x-ray film

## VI. Detection of Early Hemorrhage

A. Frequent inspection of packing, dressing, or suture line if no dressing
B. Visualization of back of throat with aid of flashlight and tongue blade
C. Observation for frequent swallowing and nausea
D. Monitoring of vital signs with attention to trends
1. Rising pulse rate
2. Decreased blood pressure
3. Cool, wet pale skin
4. Increasing restlessness and/or apprehension

**VII. Discharge from PACU (Criteria and Policies Vary Among Institutions)**

A. Patient
1. Is conscious and able to maintain airway
2. Is able to maintain oxygen saturation greater than 92% after 15 minutes on room air without being stimulated
3. Remains as above for 30 to 45 minutes after extubation or administration of narcotic or narcotic antagonist

B. No active bleeding from operative site or drains

**VIII. Pediatric ENT Patient**

A. Special considerations
1. Preoperative concerns
   a. Fear of separation, pain, injury, death: establish trust, reassure patient
   b. Child's feelings of "loss of control": allow child to choose flavoring for anesthetic induction mask
   c. Anxiety and fear of child and parents: prepare child and parents
2. Intraoperative concerns
   a. Airway management: increased risk of laryngospasm and vomiting if child is induced while crying
   b. Maintenance of body temperature (pediatric patient loses temperature faster than adult): warm OR, keep patient covered, use of warm blankets, insulated drapes, convection warming blanket to prevent loss of body heat
3. Postoperative concerns
   a. Maintenance of body temperature: use of warm blankets, insulated drapes, keep patient covered, warm PACU, etc. to prevent further heat loss and restore body temperature
   b. Increased risk for bleeding because of postoperative crying: administer pain medication as needed, provide reassurance to child and parents, involve parents as early postoperatively as possible
   c. Fluid balance (pediatric patient dehydrates easier than adult): encourage fluid intake postoperatively, monitor IV fluids and output

## EAR

**I. Structure and Function**

A. Anatomy of ear (organ of hearing and equilibrium; Fig. 28–1)
1. Outer ear
   a. Visible portion consists of skin-covered flap of cartilage known as auricle or pinna
   b. Auditory canal (opening) leads to tympanic membrane (eardrum)
2. Middle ear
   a. Tympanic membrane
   b. Three small ossicles (bones)
      (1) Malleus (hammer)
      (2) Incus (anvil)
      (3) Stapes (stirrup)
   c. Eustachian tube
      (1) Connects middle ear to throat
      (2) Means by which air reaches middle ear
3. Inner ear converts mechanical impulses into nerve impulses
   a. Vestibule
   b. Cochlea
   c. Semicircular canals

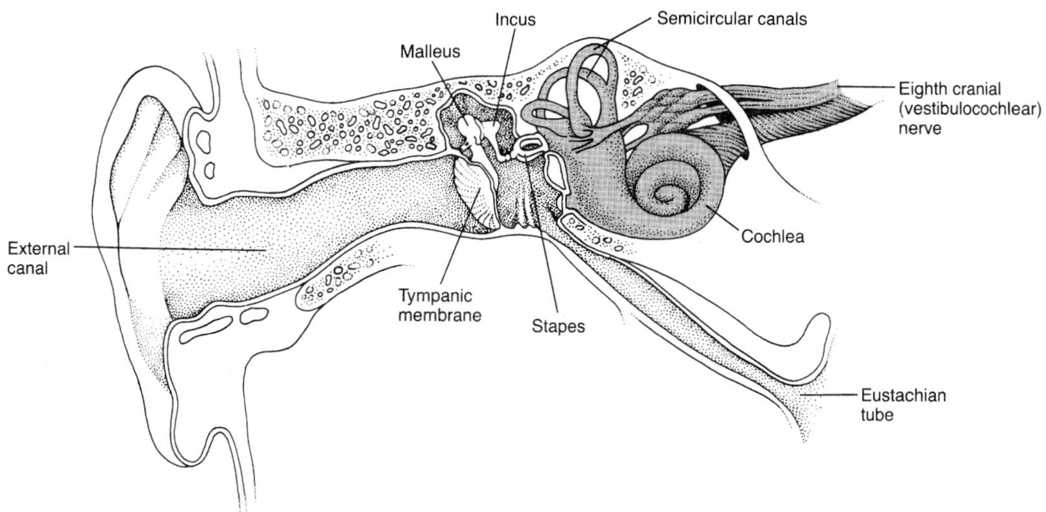


**FIGURE 28–1** Anatomic features of the internal ear. (From Ignatavicius DD, Bayne MV: *Medical-Surgical Nursing*. Philadelphia, WB Saunders, 1991, p 1077.)

B. Function of ear
   1. External ear receives sound waves
   2. Middle ear conducts sound waves received by external ear
   3. Inner ear serves as primary reception site for both hearing and balance
   4. Eustachian tube
      a. Ventilates middle ear to regulate its pressure
      b. Protects mastoid and middle ear from unwanted secretions
      c. Permits drainage of secretions from middle ear by mucociliary activity of its mucosal lining

## II. Surgical Procedures Performed on Ear

A. Myringotomy
   1. Description
      a. Small incision made into posteroinferior aspect of tympanic membrane to relieve pressure and to allow purulent drainage from middle ear
      b. Polyethylene tube can be inserted into eardrum
         (1) Makes long-term secretion drainage possible
         (2) Provides for aeration of middle ear
         (3) Relieves eustachian tube obstruction (thick, mucoid fluid)
   2. Indications
      a. Acute otitis media unresponsive to antibiotics
      b. Bulging tympanic membrane
      c. Multiple episodes of acute otitis media along with chronic otitis media
   3. Intraoperative concern: general anesthetic essential for children to ensure accurate incision of tympanic membrane and placement of tube

B. Tympanoplasty
   1. Description
      a. Refers to a variety of reconstructive surgical procedures performed on deformed or diseased middle ear components
      b. Involves use of microscope for work on minute, delicate structures
      c. Hearing may be maintained or improved by preserving middle ear conductive mechanisms

d. Postauricular (behind ear) or endaural (ear canal) approach used to expose middle ear
   (1) Extent of damage determined
   (2) Method of reconstruction determined
e. Materials used include grafts formed of
   (1) Cartilage
   (2) Bone
   (3) Fascia, skin (ear canal only)
   (4) Silicone, Teflon, hydroxyapatite
f. Some tympanoplasties carried out in two stages
   (1) First procedure performed to remove diseased tissue
   (2) Second stage involves reconstruction of hearing and middle ear function

2. Types
   a. Tympanoplasty, type I (myringoplasty): repair of tympanic membrane
   b. Tympanoplasty, type II: graft rests on incus
   c. Tympanoplasty, type III: graft attaches to head of stapes
   d. Tympanoplasty, type IV: graft attaches to foot plate of stapes
3. Indications
   a. Defects in tympanic membrane
   b. Necrotic destruction of ossicles
   c. Presence of cholesteatoma (a skin-lined sac that sheds debris into its center, thus enlarging the sac)
   d. Chronic drainage from ear canal
   e. Conductive hearing loss
   f. Trauma

C. Stapedectomy
   1. Description
      a. Procedure of choice for treatment of otosclerosis
      b. Various prostheses used with aid of microscope to replace stapes and reestablish normal sound pathway
   2. Indication: otosclerosis
   3. If chorda tympani is cut to expose stapes and foot plate, loss of taste to anterior two thirds of tongue will occur on affected side

D. Mastoidectomy
   1. Types
      a. Simple mastoidectomy
         (1) Postauricular incision most often used
         (2) All necrotic mastoid cells removed
         (3) Ossicles, tympanic membrane, and canal wall left intact
      b. Modified radical mastoidectomy
         (1) Removal of posterior and superior external bony canal walls
         (2) Mastoid and epitympanic spaces converted into common cavity
         (3) Tympanic membrane and functioning ossicles left intact
      c. Radical mastoidectomy
         (1) Removal of mastoid cells, posterior wall of external auditory canal, remnants of eardrum, ossicles (except stapes), and middle ear mucosa
         (2) Stapes left to protect entrance to inner ear
         (3) Middle ear orifice of eustachian tube cleaned of infected or diseased mucosa
         (4) Middle ear and mastoidal space converted into one cavity
   2. Indications
      a. Acute or chronic infection
      b. Extension of cholesteatoma into mastoid cells

E. Endolymphatic shunt
   1. Description
      a. Opening into endolymphatic sac, placement of shunt to allow excess endolymph to drain
      b. Shunt commercially prepared, or Silastic sheeting or tubing fashioned by surgeon
      c. Mastoidectomy performed to gain access into endolymphatic sac
   2. Indications
      a. Meniere's disease: persistent episodes of vertigo despite medical therapy
      b. Considered conservative therapy; alternative procedure: vestibular neurectomy
F. Vestibular neurectomy
   1. Description
      a. Vestibular branch of acoustic nerve (cranial nerve VIII) transected
      b. Craniotomy performed to gain access to nerve
   2. Indications
      a. Meniere's disease: endolymphatic shunt ineffective
      b. Hearing adequate: cochlear branch of cranial nerve VIII left intact
G. Labyrinthectomy
   1. Description
      a. Membranous labyrinth removed from horizontal semicircular canal
      b. Mastoidectomy performed to gain access
      c. Inner ear function destroyed
   2. Indication: Meniere's disease (endolymphatic shunt ineffective and hearing is poor)
H. Facial nerve decompression and exploration
   1. Description
      a. Compressed area of facial nerve (cranial nerve VII) is relieved
      b. Transected nerve repaired with nerve graft
      c. Performed through translabryrinthine or middle cranial fossa approach
   2. Indications
      a. Bell's palsy: idiopathic edema and inflammation of facial nerve (possibly viral in origin)
      b. Trauma (skull or mandibular fractures, gunshot wounds)
      c. Considered emergency procedure once nerve reaches certain stage of degeneration
I. Removal of acoustic tumor
   1. Description
      a. Removal of tumor arising from Schwann's cells of acoustic nerve (cranial nerve VIII)
      b. Performed by translabyrinthine or middle cranial approach (depending on size of tumor and degree of hearing loss)
J. Removal of glomus tumor
   1. Description
      a. Vascular tumor
      b. Locations
         (1) Middle ear
         (2) Intracranial

**III. Perioperative Nursing Concerns After Otologic or Neurotologic Surgery**

A. Preoperative concerns
   1. Nursing assessment
      a. Chief complaint
      b. Preoperative deficits: hearing, vertigo, tinnitus, facial nerve weakness
      c. Laboratory and radiologic evaluations
         (1) Coagulation studies, CBC

        (2) CT scans if ordered
        (3) Potassium level if patient is receiving diuretic therapy
    d. Physical limitations: arthritis, back problems
    e. Audiologic testing reports
  2. Preoperative instruction regarding postoperative course
    a. Nausea, vertigo
    b. Deep breathing, ambulation postoperatively (avoid coughing)
    c. Shampoo hair morning of surgery or night before surgery
    d. Lie on unaffected ear or back for first 24 hours
    e. Hearing may be diminished initially because of packing and dressing
  3. Other concerns
    a. Female during menstrual cycle: tendency toward bleeding intraoperatively (some surgeons will not consider a factor, yet should be noted preoperatively)
    b. Facial nerve function postoperatively

B. Intraoperative concerns
  1. Positioning: arthritis, lengthy neurotologic procedure, elderly patient
  2. Medications given
    a. Lidocaine with epinephrine for hemostasis
    b. Topical epinephrine for hemostasis
    c. Sedatives, if local anesthetic
  3. Local anesthetic
    a. Altered visual and hearing perception
    b. Positioning
    c. Anxiety
  4. Neurotologic procedures
    a. Intake and output
    b. Intraoperative facial nerve monitoring
    c. Safety
        (1) Neurologic status of upper extremities
        (2) Sponge and sharps count
        (3) Strict maintenance of sterile environment
    d. Neurologic status of patient before transport to PACU

C. Postoperative concerns
  1. Nausea, vomiting
  2. Vertigo
  3. Headache
  4. Complications
    a. Bleeding
    b. Nerve function
    c. Cerebrospinal fluid (CSF) leak
    d. Severe hearing loss
  5. Postoperative instructions
    a. Avoid bending and stooping
    b. Sit on side of bed, stand beside bed before ambulating
    c. Instruct patient to prevent prosthesis or graft dislodgement by avoiding
        (1) Nose blowing
        (2) Straining, especially during bowel movements
        (3) Lying on operative ear
        (4) Drinking through a straw
        (5) Smoking
        (6) Sneezing or coughing with mouth or nose closed; sneeze and cough with mouth and nose open
    d. Avoid getting ear wet

D. Key PACU concerns

**NURSING DIAGNOSIS**

Examples of related nursing diagnostic categories include:

- Potential for infection
- Altered mobility related to dizziness
- Impaired tissue integrity
- Knowledge deficit

1. Positioning
   a. Specific clarification from surgeon required for various positioning options
      (1) Operated ear positioned upward to prevent pressure and graft displacement
      (2) Head elevation (30 degrees or more) to minimize eustachian tube edema, especially after mastoid procedures
2. Dressings
   a. Middle ear packing must not be disturbed
      (1) Prevent contamination of operative site
      (2) Reinforce wet bandage with sterile dressing
3. Nausea, vertigo, vomiting
   a. Avoid excess motion
      (1) Transfer patient slowly and smoothly
      (2) Do not bump or jar bed
      (3) Keep side rails up
   b. Patient instructions
      (1) Avoid sudden turning; encourage slow, smooth motion
      (2) Encourage slow, deep breaths through open mouth to minimize nausea
      (3) Instruct patient to focus eyes and move slowly
   c. Administration of antiemetics
      (1) Often given intraoperatively
      (2) Given in PACU prophylactically
4. Potential for complications
   a. Nerve function assessment
      (1) Inability to smile, frown, close eyes, or purse lips is indicative of facial nerve deficit
      (2) To test functioning of facial nerve, ask patient to
         (a) Squeeze eyelids closed
         (b) Smile enough to show teeth
         (c) Pucker lips
         (d) Wrinkle forehead
         (e) Wrinkle nose
   b. CSF leak
      (1) Observe patient for clear nasal or ear drainage
   c. Pain
      (1) Notify surgeon of severe or unrelieved pain
   d. Severe hearing loss
      (1) Assess hearing loss immediately postoperatively, and report to surgeon if further loss occurs
      (2) Instruct patient of some hearing loss because of packing and ear dressing
   e. Report any of the following symptoms to surgeon
      (1) Drainage from ear or nose
      (2) Decreased hearing (from initially postoperatively)
      (3) Temperature elevation
      (4) Increased dizziness
      (5) Facial weakness

# THE NOSE AND MAXILLOFACIAL STRUCTURES

## I. Pathophysiology and Surgical Interventions

A. Nose
   1. Anatomy
      a. External nose made up of nasal bones, cartilages, and nasal septum
      b. Internal nose located between hard palate, cribiform plate, and nasopharynx
         (1) Nasal turbinates project from lateral walls of nose (resembling bony shelves)
            (a) Arranged one above the other
            (b) Separated by grooves or meatus
            (c) Act as drainage passages for sinuses
   2. Pathophysiology
      a. Deviated nasal septum caused by trauma or congenitally
      b. Erectile mucosa of septum and turbinates is chronically engorged because of inadequate airway on side of deviation
      c. Engorged mucosa affects sinus drainage through meatus
      d. Turbinates undergo degenerative changes
   3. Indications for surgery
      a. Septal deviation
      b. Nasal polyps
   4. Surgical procedures
      a. Septoplasty or submucous resection
         (1) Incision made intranasally in mucosa
         (2) Mucosa elevated from cartilage and bony septum
         (3) Deviated cartilage excised; thickened bone removed
         (4) Cartilage straightened; may be replaced
         (5) Mucosa resewn inside nares
         (6) Nose packed with impregnated gauze or commercially prepared splints or packs per surgeon's preference
   5. Perforated nasal septum
      a. Pathophysiology
         (1) Ulceration of nasal mucosa, with subsequent perforation of septal cartilage
         (2) Cartilage does not regenerate itself; thus surgery is usually advised
      b. Causes
         (1) Trauma
         (2) Foreign body
         (3) Previous septal surgery
         (4) Nose picking
         (5) Infection
         (6) Systemic diseases: tuberculosis, Wegener's midline granuloma, syphilis
         (7) Chemical irritation: cocaine sniffing, inhalation of arsenic and acids
      c. Surgical procedure: septoplasty
   6. Epistaxis
      a. Causes
         (1) Trauma
         (2) Tumor: juvenile nasopharyngeal angiofibroma (adolescent males)
      b. Surgical procedure
         (1) If vessel cannot be located, ligation of maxillary (and possibly ethmoid) artery
         (2) Sublabial incision used to ligate maxillary artery

B. Sinuses
   1. Anatomy
      a. Maxillary: paired sinuses in maxilla; superior wall is floor of orbit, medial wall is lateral wall of nose

   b. Ethmoid: honeycomb-like arrangement of cells in superior and lateral walls of nose and medial walls of orbits
   c. Sphenoid: paired sinuses located in sphenoid bone
   d. Frontal: paired sinuses located in frontal bone, with posterior wall adjacent to anterior cranial fossa
2. Pathophysiology
   a. Airfilled, mucosa-lined cavities
   b. Function of sinuses not known; speculated to decrease skull's weight or increase voice resonance
   c. Communicate with nose by meatus in nasal septum
      (1) Frontal, maxillary, and anterior ethmoid sinuses drain under middle turbinate
      (2) Posterior ethmoid and sphenoid sinuses drain under superior turbinate
   d. Fluid collects in sinuses during acute inflammation, or obstruction blocks their drainage
   e. Mucosa thickens because of chronic inflammation
   f. Ciliary action of mucosa cannot effectively clear fluid accumulation
   g. Chronic sinusitis may develop
3. Indications for surgery
   a. Acute or chronic sinusitis unresponsive to medical therapy
   b. Mucocele or polyps in sinus
   c. Tumor in sinus
4. Surgical procedures
   a. Endoscopic sinus surgery
      (1) Newest procedure designed to relieve obstruction at osteomeatal complex, reestablishing air flow from maxillary, ethmoid, and frontal sinuses
      (2) Procedure creates least disruption to normal function of nasal and sinus mucosa
      (3) Nasal cavity examined through telescope inserted into nares
      (4) Middle turbinate mucosa incised, excess mucosa and bony formations removed, to facilitate drainage
      (5) Sinuses may be entered to assess polyp, mucocele formation, or to drain fluid present
      (6) Nasal cavity packed with impregnated packing (resembling tampon) or impregnated gauze
   b. Nasal antrostomy or nasal antral window
      (1) Opening created in medial wall of maxillary sinus below inferior turbinate
      (2) Purulent secretions removed by suction
      (3) Nasal cavity packed with impregnated gauze or packing
      (4) Serves as additional drainage port for maxillary sinus
      (5) Usually closes within 1 to 2 years
   c. Caldwell Luc
      (1) Larger opening into maxillary sinus through sublabial incision
      (2) Performed to remove polyps, diseased tissue, or infection
      (3) Usually in combination with nasal antral window to ensure better drainage and aeration of maxillary sinus
      (4) Maxillary sinus and nasal cavity packed with impregnated gauze
      (5) Damage to maxillary division of trigeminal nerve (cranial nerve V) will cause permanent loss of sensation to upper lip
      (6) Procedure performed less frequently because of endoscopic sinus surgical procedure
   d. Ethmoidectomy
      (1) Performed by transantral (nasal) or external approach
         (a) Nasal approach
            (i) Ensures drainage and aeration

(ii) Removes bony formation between air cells
(iii) Also performed for orbital decompression in exophthalmos
(iv) May or may not be packed with impregnated gauze

(2) Complications
(a) Damage to optic nerve will result in impaired vision, blindness
(b) Damage to internal carotid artery will result in profuse blood loss, death

e. Sphenoidotomy
(1) Opening into sphenoid sinus to drain fluid, remove diseased mucosa
(2) Entrance may serve to remove tumor or as approach to removal of pituitary tumor (see Chapter 21)
(3) May be performed by nasal or external approach
(4) Complications may include injury to:
(a) Optic nerve
(b) Internal carotid artery
(c) Nasal septal artery
(d) Dura—possible CSF leak

f. Frontal sinus obliteration
(1) Approached either by eyebrow (brow) or scalp (bicoronal) incision
(2) Skin flap peeled toward face (if bicoronal is used) or toward apex of head (if brow is used) to expose entire frontal sinus
(3) Periosteum elevated; bone cut superiorly and laterally
(4) Sinus drained; diseased mucosa removed
(5) Abdominal incision may be made (left side) to remove fat to pack in sinus cavity
(6) Bone flap replaced; periosteum and skin closed
(7) Large pressure dressing (Kerlix, Kling) applied
(8) Postoperative edema includes face, especially around both eyes
(9) Possible complications
(a) Violation of posterior wall of sinus, communicating with dura (meningitis, brain abscess, etc.)
(b) Hematoma under scalp flap

C. Maxillofacial structures

1. Nasal bone fractures
a. Procedure: reduction
b. Usually accomplished through
(1) Closed digital manipulation
(2) Nasal packing, splinting, and taping
c. May have to use open reduction if further damage found
d. Will drain septal hematoma if present

2. Nasofrontal/ethmoidal
a. Procedure: open reduction with internal fixation
b. May need to repair lacrimal sac apparatus or medial canthal ligament

3. Orbital/zygomatic (cheek or malar bone) fracture: usually requires open exploration and manipulation
a. Orbital floor (blow-out)
(1) Orbital contents replaced; orbital floor restored
(2) May use Silastic, Teflon, or bone to support floor
(3) May use steel or titanium microplates and screws to align and hold bone fragments
b. Orbital rim: similar to orbital floor; repair rim
c. Trimalar
(1) Open reduction with internal fixation (wiring or fixation plates and screws)
(2) Floor of orbit may be explored

d. Zygomatic arch
   (1) Closed or intraoral reduction
4. Mandibular fractures
   a. Procedure: open reduction with internal fixation
      (1) Restore occlusion
      (2) Avoid nonunion of fracture with fixation
         (a) Fixation plates and screws
         (b) Interdental wiring
   b. Complications
      (1) May require tracheostomy if airway is compromised
      (2) Patient may aspirate vomitus if interdental wiring is used
5. Maxillary fractures
   a. Types
      (1) Le Fort I: toothbearing portion of maxilla is separated from upper maxilla
      (2) Le Fort II: fracture runs across orbital floor and nasal bridge
      (3) Le Fort III: craniofacial dysjunction (entire orbit and nasal bridge)
   b. Procedure
      (1) Open reduction with internal fixation
      (2) Performed when patient is stable and edema decreased
      (3) Fixation plates and screws; wiring used to stabilize fractured bones
      (4) Patient usually has other neurologic injuries

## II. Perioperative Nursing Concerns After Nasal, Sinus, and Maxillofacial Surgery

A. Preoperative concerns
   1. Nursing assessment
      a. Chief complaint
      b. History of infections
      c. History of trauma
      d. Laboratory and radiologic evaluations
         (1) Blood type and crossmatch if designated units are not available
         (2) Paranasal sinus films
         (3) CT of sinuses
      e. Structural involvement related to nasal problems
         (1) Impaired airway
         (2) Orbital edema
         (3) Hearing loss
         (4) Impaired swallowing
         (5) Altered taste
   2. Preoperative instruction
      a. Need to breathe through mouth
      b. Presence of nasal packing
      c. Difficulty in swallowing
      d. Dangers of nose blowing
      e. Soft diet, no straws
      f. Avoid straining, especially during bowel movements
B. Intraoperative concerns
   1. Blood loss (minimal to moderate)
   2. Anesthesia administered
      a. Method: local, standby, or general
   3. Medications
      a. Epinephrine, oxymetazoline HCl, cocaine (for vasoconstriction)
         (1) PACU cardiac considerations
            (a) Tachycardia

            (b) Dysrhythmias
            (c) Hypertension
        b. Muscle relaxants, narcotics: PACU airway problems
    4. Type of packing used: potential dislodgement
C. Postoperative concerns
    1. Airway
    2. Packing
    3. Position
    4. Reinforce preoperative teaching
    5. Pain management
D. Key PACU concerns

**NURSING DIAGNOSIS**

Examples of related nursing diagnostic categories include

- Ineffective airway clearance
- Altered tissue perfusion

1. Ensure and maintain patent airway
    a. Check patient's position
    b. Elevate head of bed
    c. Assess rate, quality of respirations
    d. Suction excess oral secretions
    e. Monitor vital signs
    f. Remind patient of nasal packing and need to mouth breathe
    g. Instruct patient to take slow, deep breaths
    h. Moisten oral mucosa as needed if applicable
    i. Moisten lips as needed
2. Prevention of aspiration
    a. Provide wire cutters at bedside to cut maxillary or mandibular fixation wires and suction vomitus
    b. Medicate patient for nausea
3. Position
    a. Progress from side-lying to semi-Fowler's
    b. Promotes nasal and sinus drainage
    c. Decreases edema
4. Packing dislodgement
    a. Provide equipment for reinsertion
        (1) Bayonet forceps
        (2) Nasal speculum
        (3) Scissors
        (4) Headlight
        (5) Tongue depressor
5. Drip pad changed approximately each hour for first 24 hours
6. Monitor for complications
    a. Inadequate airway
    b. Bleeding
    c. Visual, neurologic problems

## THE ORAL CAVITY, PHARYNX, AND LARYNX

**I. Pathophysiology and Surgical Interventions**

A. Anatomy
1. Oral cavity
   a. Extends from lips to anterior tonsillar pillars
   b. Contains teeth, hard and soft palates, anterior portion of tongue
2. Nasopharynx
   a. Extends from posterior opening of nose to soft palate
   b. Contains adenoid tissue and openings of eustachian tubes
3. Oropharynx
   a. Extends from soft palate to valleculae
   b. Portion of pharynx visible through mouth
   c. Contains tonsils, posterior portion of tongue
4. Hypopharynx
   a. Portion of pharynx from valleculae to larynx
   b. Contains posterior pharyngeal wall, epiglottis, and larynx
5. Larynx
   a. Extends from epiglottis to cricoid cartilage
   b. Contains hyoid bone; epiglottis; thyroid, cricoid, and arytenoid cartilages; false and true vocal cords
   c. Primarily serves for communication; plays vital role in respiration, coughing, and preventing aspiration

B. Pathophysiology
1. Primary functions are for speech, mastication of food, and airway
2. Indications for surgery
   a. Adenoid hypertrophy, serous otitis media
   b. Tonsillitis
   c. Peritonsillar abscess
   d. Ulcerations, lesions, masses
   e. Sleep apnea: redundant tissue of soft palate
   f. Foreign body ingestion
   g. Symptoms indicative of tumor

C. Surgical procedures
1. Adenoidectomy
   a. Methods
      (1) Sharp excision: control bleeding with cautery, pressure
      (2) Fulguration with cautery on high setting
2. Tonsillectomy: performed for tonsillitis and peritonsillar abscess (affected side only)
   a. Methods
      (1) Sharp or blunt dissections
         (a) Control of bleeding with ligatures, cautery, pressure, topical vasoconstrictor
      (2) Laser method: seldom used because of added cost
   b. Complications
      (1) Bleeding: critical during first 24 hours, then 7 to 10 days
      (2) Airway obstruction: primarily caused by laryngospasm
3. Intraoral excision
   a. May involve tongue, oral mucosa, floor of mouth, palate
   b. Methods (may require skin graft if mucosa is removed)
      (1) Sharp dissection
      (2) Laser excision
      (3) "Hot knife" excision

- c. Complications
  - (1) Airway obstruction from edema
  - (2) Hematoma under skin graft
4. Uvulopalatopharyngoplasty (UPP; UPPP)
   - a. Excision of uvula, excess tissue of soft palate
   - b. Tonsillectomy usually performed if tonsils present
   - c. Extensive excision of tissue may require tracheostomy during initial postoperative period
5. Endoscopic procedures by means of rigid or flexible scopes
   - a. Definition
     - (1) Laryngoscope: views oral cavity, oropharynx, hypopharynx, larynx through rigid metal scope
     - (2) Bronchoscopy: views trachea, bronchi by flexible or rigid scope
     - (3) Esophagoscopy: views epiglottis, esophagus by rigid or flexible scope
   - b. Complications
     - (1) Perforation of esophagus
     - (2) Airway obstruction
     - (3) Bleeding
     - (4) Integrity of teeth
   - c. Specific procedures
     - (1) Direct laryngoscopy; indications
       - (a) Hoarseness
       - (b) Tumor assessment
       - (c) Foreign body removal
       - (d) Laryngeal trauma: assess damage
       - (e) Infant stridor: congenital laryngomalacia
     - (2) Suspension laryngoscopy; indications
       - (a) Laryngeal polyps or cysts
       - (b) Laryngeal webs
       - (c) Vocal cord nodules
       - (d) Juvenile laryngeal papillomatosis
     - (3) Laser (*l*ight *a*mplification by *s*timulated *e*mission or *r*adiation) therapy during suspension laryngoscopy
       - (a) Carbon dioxide laser therapy
         - (i) Widely accepted form of removal of lesions
         - (ii) Beam is precise
         - (iii) Beam vaporizes undesirable tissue
       - (b) ET tubes must be metallic or wrapped with metallic tape to prevent accidental ignition with subsequent combustion
     - (4) Teflon injection of vocal cords
       - (a) Performed with direct laryngoscopy for some unilateral vocal cord paralyses
     - (5) Botulinum toxin injection
       - (a) Performed with suspension laryngoscopy for spastic dysphonia failing medical management
     - (6) Bronchoscopy
       - (a) Performed to evaluate respiratory tract and collect specimens for diagnosis of symptoms
         - (i) Persistent cough
         - (ii) Hemoptysis
         - (iii) Wheezing
         - (iv) Obstruction
         - (v) Neck nodes with unknown primary malignancy

(b) May use neodymium:yttrium-aluminum-garnet (Nd:YAG) laser to remove undesired tissue or achieve patent airway (palliation)
(c) Performed to remove foreign body
(7) Esophagoscopy
(a) Performed to evaluate esophagus and collect specimens for diagnosis of symptoms
(i) Esophageal carcinoma
(ii) Diverticula
(iii) Hiatal hernia
(iv) Stricture
(v) Varices
(b) Dilatation of strictures
(c) Evaluate dysphagia
(8) Triple endoscopy
(a) Combination of direct laryngoscopy, bronchoscopy, and esophagoscopy
(b) Performed for viewing location and extent of malignancy
(c) May be performed immediately before head and neck cancer surgery

## II. Perioperative Nursing Concerns After Oral Cavity, Pharyngeal, and Laryngeal Surgery

A. Preoperative concerns
1. Nursing assessment
a. Chief complaint
b. Respiratory status
c. Presence of sputum
d. Hoarseness
e. Dysphagia and odynophagia
f. Quality of voice
g. Allergies
2. Radiologic studies
a. Films of neck
b. Fluoroscopy
c. Barium swallow
d. CT or MRI of neck and chest
3. Medications
a. Preoperative medications
(1) Atropine sulfate to decrease production of secretions and depress vagal reflex occurring with stimulation of respiratory tract
(2) Metoclopramide (Reglan) to decrease gastric secretions
4. Psychosocial status
a. Emotional status: prepared for tracheostomy if airway is compromised
b. Prepare patient for voice rest if anticipated
B. Intraoperative concerns
1. Airway problems
a. Difficult intubation
b. Possible need for tracheostomy
c. Laryngeal trauma and edema
d. Laryngospasm
2. Dysrhythmias
a. Supraventricular tachycardia (SVT)
b. Premature ventricular contractions (PVCs)
c. Atrial dysrhythmias related to
(1) Hypoxemia
(2) Hypercarbia
(3) Increased circulating catecholamines (from sympathoadrenal response to stimuli)

3. Patient apprehension
    a. Must be reassured, especially in an airway crisis
    b. May be intubated awake
    c. Multiple procedures do not ensure patient is not apprehensive
4. Safety precautions if laser is used

C. Postoperative concerns
1. Respiratory status
2. Cardiovascular status
3. Reinforce voice rest; provide alternate means of communication

D. Key PACU concerns

**NURSING DIAGNOSIS**

Examples of related nursing diagnostic categories include:
- Ineffective airway clearance
- Decreased cardiac output
- Ineffective breathing pattern
- Pain

1. Respiratory care
    a. Cool, humidified oxygen
    b. Respiratory rate, quality
        (1) Stridor
        (2) Use of accessory muscles
        (3) Poor color
        (4) Anxiety
        (5) Tachycardia
2. Position
    a. Elevate head of bed as patient arouses
3. Medications
    a. Antibiotics
    b. Steroids
    c. Lidocaine (1.5 mg/kg)
        (1) Cough
        (2) Laryngospasm
4. Other concerns
    a. Integrity of teeth
    b. Presence of cough and bloody sputum
    c. Pain, soreness of tongue or throat
    d. Voice rest, avoidance of vocal cord irritation
    e. Ice collar for decreased swelling, increased comfort
    f. NPO until gag reflex returns

## SALIVARY GLANDS

**I. Pathophysiology and Surgical Interventions**

A. Anatomy
1. Primary glands and location
    a. Parotid: located on side of face
    b. Sublingual: located in floor of mouth, just below mucous membrane
    c. Submandibular: located below floor of mouth
2. Drainage ducts into floor of mouth
    a. Parotid: Stensen's duct (opposite upper second molar)

b. Submandibular: Wharton's duct (floor of mouth near frenula)
c. Sublingual: multiple ducts—some empty into floor of mouth, some empty into Wharton's duct

3. Major nerves
   a. Parotid: facial nerve (cranial nerve VII)
   b. Submandibular: marginal mandibular nerve
   c. Sublingual: hypoglossal nerve (cranial nerve XII) or lingual nerve

B. Pathophysiology
1. Conditions affecting production and flow of saliva
   a. Inflammation; pus present
   b. Chronic infection affecting duct
   c. Sialolithiasis causing partial or complete blockage of duct
   d. Trauma causing stenosis of duct
   e. Cysts
   f. Neoplasms
2. Surgical procedures
   a. Incision and drainage of pus
   b. Intraoral duct exploration with removal of stones
   c. Excision of salivary gland
      (1) Parotid gland excision: parotidectomy (superficial or total)
   d. Neck dissection: may be performed depending on type of malignant tumor
   e. Floor of mouth excision: may be performed for submandibular or sublingual malignancy depending on type

**II. Perioperative Nursing Concerns After Salivary Gland Surgery**

A. Preoperative concerns
1. Nursing assessment
   a. Chief complaint
   b. History of infections
   c. History of autoimmune diseases
2. Laboratory and radiologic evaluations
   a. Culture and sensitivity reports
   b. Blood type and crossmatch if malignancy is suspected, blood loss is anticipated, and designated donor units are not in storage
   c. CT or MRI of head and neck

B. Intraoperative concerns
1. Report stimulation of VII, manifested by facial movement, to surgeon
2. Location of graft site if anticipated
3. Patient must not be paralyzed as procedure begins

C. Postoperative concerns
1. Airway
2. Bleeding
3. Symptoms indicative of nerve deficit

D. Key PACU concerns

**NURSING DIAGNOSIS**

Examples of related nursing diagnostic categories include:
- Ineffective airway clearance
- Impaired tissue integrity
- Anxiety
- Pain

1. Effective airway
   a. Assess edema if intraoral procedure
   b. Assess edema and dressing if external incision
   c. Cool, humidified oxygen
   d. Tracheostomy care if performed
2. Bleeding
   a. Notify surgeon, especially after parotid surgery
3. Nerve deficit
   a. Assess function of facial nerve (cranial nerve VII): parotidectomy
   b. Assess function of marginal mandibular nerve: submandibular gland excision
   c. Assess function of hypoglossal nerve (cranial nerve XII): sublingual gland excision
4. Position
   a. Elevate head of bed 30 to 45 degrees
5. Suction
   a. If oral suction contraindicated, drain oral secretions from mouth
6. Closed wound drainage/nasogastric tube
   a. Attach to suction if ordered
   b. Assess drainage, report excess
   c. Assess proper location of nasogastric tube

## HEAD AND NECK

**I. Pathophysiology and Surgical Interventions**

A. Trachea and larynx
1. Tracheostomy
   a. Performed prophylactically with possibility of airway loss
      (1) Edema
      (2) Surgical interruption of upper airway
   b. Performed as emergency procedure if loss of airway imminent
   c. Performed for prevention of laryngeal stenosis or for pulmonary toilet in cases of prolonged oral intubation
2. Thyroplasty
   a. Performed to give a more permanent means of fixing paralyzed vocal cord
   b. Performed with anesthesia standby or general anesthesia
   c. Patients unable to tolerate procedure: Teflon vocal cord injection
3. Laryngectomy: performed to remove malignant growths of larynx, vocal cords, epiglottis
   a. Supraglottic laryngectomy: excision of laryngeal structures above true vocal cords
      (1) Normal airway remains
      (2) Voice remains normal
      (3) Aspiration a problem postoperatively
      (4) Contraindicated in patients with chronic obstructive pulmonary disease
      (5) May have to perform total laryngectomy if patient cannot manage aspiration
   b. Hemilaryngectomy: removal of part of larynx, usually one vocal cord, for superficial or confined lesion
      (1) Airway remains normal
      (2) Voice is hoarse
   c. Total laryngectomy: excision of larynx, vocal cords, and epiglottis
      (1) Airway now directly from trachea
      (2) Absence of voice or esophageal speech
      (3) Tracheoesophageal fistula may be established at time of laryngectomy to facilitate speech rehabilitation

4. Neck dissection
   a. Performed alone to remove malignant tumor, metastatic cervical lymph nodes, all nonvital neck structures
   b. Performed in combination with other cancer-removing procedures
      (1) Hemiglossectomy: removal of portion of tongue; may be reconstructed using radial forearm free flap
      (2) Partial mandibulectomy or hemimandibulectomy: removal of portion of mandible; may be reconstructed using iliac crest free flap
      (3) Partial esophagectomy: removal of portion of esophagus: may be reconstructed using jejunal free flap
      (4) Laryngectomy (see earlier discussion)
      (5) Tracheostomy (see earlier discussion)

## II. Perioperative Nursing Concerns for Tracheostomy and Laryngectomy Patient

A. Preoperative concerns
   1. Head and neck cancer patient
      a. Often an elderly person with degenerative diseases
         (1) Diabetes mellitus
         (2) Hepatic insufficiency, cirrhosis (alcohol abuse)
         (3) Renal disease
         (4) Cardiovascular disease
         (5) Pulmonary disease (usually a long history of smoking)
      b. Alcoholism not uncommon in head and neck cancer patients
         (1) Requires nutritional evaluation
         (2) May require sedation preoperatively and after surgery to counter delirium tremens
   2. Preoperative workup
      a. Pulmonary function testing
      b. Laboratory data
         (1) Type and crossmatch
         (2) Radiographs to rule out metastatic disease
         (3) Bone scan
   3. Preoperative instructions
      a. Presence of tracheostomy
      b. Description of tracheostomy care and suctioning
      c. Effect of surgery on voice quality and facial configuration
      d. Alternative means of communication
      e. Pain management

B. Intraoperative concerns
   1. Positioning: debilitated patient, patients with degenerative diseases, length of procedure, circulatory compromise
   2. Two surgical teams required if reconstructive microvascular flap used in reconstruction
   3. Patient safety: body, temperature; sponges and sharps count; primary surgery site is contaminated (trachea, esophagus, hypopharynx); intake and output

C. Postoperative concerns
   1. Need for exact understanding of existing airway should emergency ventilation be required
   2. Tracheal stoma becomes patient's only airway
      a. Oronasal passageway to lungs no longer exists
   3. Partial laryngectomy with tracheostomy
      a. Tracheostomy tube cuff must be inflated during emergency ventilation
      b. Oxygen can be lost through nose and mouth
   4. High humidity required when tracheal breathing takes place of nasal breathing
   5. Changed quality or absence of voice can be psychologically traumatic

6. Operative pain after neck surgery often light to moderate in severity
7. Dislodged nasogastric tube: do not reinsert (notify surgeon)
8. Maintain patency of wound drains
9. Complications
    a. Hemorrhage after combined laryngectomy with radical neck dissection; carotid blowout is an almost exclusive complication yet does not occur as often in this decade
    b. Airway obstruction
    c. Pneumothorax
    d. Impaired circulation to reconstructive flap; loss of flap
    e. Chyle leak (milky fluid in closed drainage)

D. Key PACU concerns

**NURSING DIAGNOSIS**

Examples of related nursing diagnostic categories include:

- Anxiety
- Knowledge deficit related to artificial airway
- Pain

## THYROID GLAND (See also Chapter 27)

**I. Pathophysiology and Surgical Interventions**

A. Anatomy
1. Thyroid gland located in anterior portion of neck
2. Consists of left and right lobes united by isthmus
3. Vascular supply: superior and inferior thyroid arteries
4. Nerves in proximity
    a. Recurrent laryngeal nerve
    b. Superior laryngeal nerve

B. Pathophysiology
1. Primary function: aid in metabolism (iodine)
2. Enlargement of gland may result in tracheal obstruction
3. Tumors
    a. Needle aspiration may be performed to determine type of tumor
    b. Lobectomy vs. total thyroidectomy (depending on pathologic condition)

C. Indications
1. Tumor
2. Hyperthyroidism (Graves' disease)
3. Hashimoto's thyroiditis

D. Complications
1. Recurrent laryngeal nerve injury
2. Hypoparathyroidism

**II. Perioperative Concerns for Thyroidectomy Patient**

A. Preoperative concerns
1. Nursing assessment
    a. Chief complaint
    b. Appearance of patient
    c. Current medications

2. Laboratory and radiologic evaluations
   a. Calcium, phosphorus levels
   b. Thyroid function tests; goal is euthyroid patient before surgery to decrease risk of postoperative thyroid storm
   c. Thyroid profile
3. Anxiety
   a. Potential diagnosis of malignancy
   b. Body image

B. Intraoperative concerns
1. Anesthetic induction if tracheal obstruction is present
2. Multiple specimens for pathologic examination; keep length of anesthetic and surgery to a minimum
3. Thyroid storm: see information on postoperative concerns

C. Postoperative concerns
1. Calcium level (thyroidectomy may result in intentional or accidental removal of parathyroid glands)
   a. Monitor by laboratory evaluation
   b. Observe patient for complaints of numbness surrounding lips; cramping, tingling of extremities
2. Signs and symptoms of bleeding or infection
   a. Temperature greater than 101° F
   b. Bleeding from incision
   c. Tachycardia
   d. Increased respirations
   e. Color, presence of drainage from incision site

D. Key PACU concerns

**NURSING DIAGNOSIS**

Examples of related nursing diagnostic categories include:
- Potential for ineffective airway clearance
- Anxiety
- Altered tissue perfusion
- Pain

1. Positioning
   a. Supine with head of bed elevated 30 degrees
2. Report from anesthesia personnel or OR nurse regarding parathyroid status
   a. Notify surgeon of
      (1) Low calcium level (calcium gluconate at bedside)
      (2) Cramping, tingling of extremities
      (3) Numbness around lips
   b. Administer calcium gluconate if ordered
3. Airway
   a. Report changes in respiratory rate or quality
   b. Assess quality of voice
   c. Obtain tracheostomy tray and tube at bedside if signs and symptoms indicate respiratory distress
4. Dressing
   a. Ensure dressing is not constrictive
   b. Monitor for bleeding or drainage

5. Thyroid storm
   a. Rare if patient is euthyroid (normal) before surgery
   b. Characterized by increased heart rate, increased blood pressure, heat intolerance, high oxygen consumption, sweating
   c. Treatment: (β-blocker, usually propranolol [Inderal])
   d. Differentiate thyroid storm from malignant hyperthermia (see Chapter 17)

## BIBLIOGRAPHY


Adams GL, Boies LR, Hilger PA: *Fundamentals of Otolaryngology*, 6th Ed. Philadelphia, WB Saunders, 1989.

Ballenger JJ: *Diseases of the Nose, Throat and Ear*, 14th Ed. Philadelphia, Lea & Febiger, 1991.

Baylor College of Medicine, Department of Otolaryngology: *Core Curriculum Syllabus*. Houston, The Author, 1997.

Bluestone CD, Stool SE, Kenna MA: *Pediatric Otolaryngology*, 3rd Ed. Philadelphia, WB Saunders, 1996.

Cummings CW, Fredrickson JM, Harker LA, Krause CJ, Richardson M, Schuller DE: *Otolaryngology—Head and Neck Surgery*, 3rd Ed. St Louis, Mosby–Year Book, 1997.

Davis RK: *Lasers in Otolaryngology: Head and Neck Surgery*. Philadelphia, WB Saunders, 1990.

English GM: *Otolaryngology*, Vols 1–3. Philadelphia, JB Lippincott, 1990.

Meeker MH, Rothrock JC: *Alexander's Care of the Patient in Surgery*, 10th Ed. St Louis, CV Mosby, 1995.

Sigler BA, Schuring LT: *Ear, Nose, and Throat Disorders*. St Louis, Mosby–Year Book, 1994.


## REVIEW QUESTIONS

**1. What is the treatment of choice for otosclerosis?**
   A. Myringotomy
   B. Tympanoplasty
   C. Mastoidectomy
   D. Stapedectomy

**2. Which of the following medication therapies should you report to the surgeon before otologic surgery?**
   A. Antibiotic
   B. Aspirin
   C. Acetaminophen (Tylenol)
   D. Antacid

**3. Which of the following measures should not be instituted for a patient immediately after a partial esophagectomy, radical neck dissection?**
   A. Elevate head of bed 30 to 45 degrees
   B. Place pillows under patient's knees for comfort
   C. Hyperextend the neck to facilitate airway clearance
   D. Verify proper location of nasogastric tube

**4. What is the rationale for providing highly humidified oxygen for a new tracheostomy patient?**
   A. Easier to provide than nonhumidified
   B. Involves use of respiratory therapy department
   C. Assists in prevention of mucous plugs
   D. Provides more comfort for the patient

**5. Which of the following supplies would you not want to provide for a total laryngectomy patient?**
   A. An additional tracheostomy tube of the same size
   B. Yankhauer and catheter for suctioning
   C. T-piece for oxygen delivery
   D. Face mask for oxygen delivery

**6. How often would you anticipate changing the drip pad of a patient who has just undergone a septoplasty?**

A. Every 2 hours
B. Immediately before discharge to patient care unit
C. Every 10 to 15 minutes
D. Approximately every half hour

**7. Identify a primary concern for the maxillofacial patient with interdental wiring:**

A. Provide a mirror to ensure patient is cosmetically acceptable
B. Patient will have pain
C. Patient may aspirate vomitus
D. Patient will be unable to communicate

**8. Which of the following laboratory reports will the PACU nurse be primarily concerned with in a patient after a total thyroidectomy?**

A. CBC
B. Potassium level
C. ABGs
D. Calcium level

**9. A patient with wired jaws begins to vomit. Your initial intervention should be:**

A. Cut the wires
B. Position the patient on operative side
C. Suction along molars gently
D. Administer antiemetic

**10. What complication, almost exclusively, is associated with a laryngectomy, radical neck dissection?**

A. Carotid blow-out
B. Pneumothorax
C. Laryngeal edema
D. Atelectasis

**11. Thyroid storm is characterized by:**

A. Hypocalcemia with acute symptoms
B. Bradycardia, hypotension, hypoxemia
C. Fever, diaphoresis, severe neck pain
D. Hypertension, tachycardia, heat intolerance

**ANSWERS:** 1. D, 2. B, 3. C, 4. C, 5. D, 6. A, 7. C, 8. D, 9. C, 10. A, 11. D

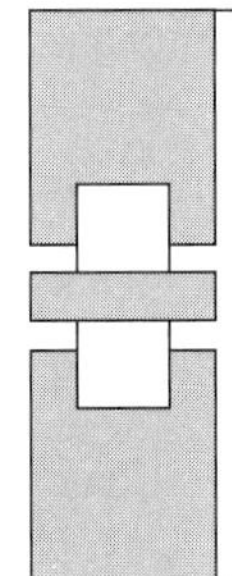

CHAPTER 29

# *The Ophthalmic Surgical Patient*

Kathleen S. Maes, BSN, RN, CRNO
Tracy Britton, BSN, RN, CRNO

## OBJECTIVES

**Study of the information represented by this outline will enable the learner to:**

1. Identify the important functions of the eye.
2. Detail the physiology of the eye.
3. Define the most common ophthalmic surgical procedures.
4. Discuss the nursing priorities specific to the ophthalmic surgical patient.
5. Describe the types of anesthesia that may be used for ophthalmic surgery.
6. Identify potential complications and their management for the ophthalmic surgical patient.

## I. Introduction

A. Eyeball as a whole is referred to as the globe; anteroposterior diameter is approximately 22 to 26 mm long, with the average being about 24 mm in the adult eye; circumference between 70 and 80 mm

B. Orbit of the average eye is approximately 40 cm in height, width, and depth; volume is approximately 30 cc; globe occupies about one fifth the total volume; orbit of the eye is basically spheric and of bony composition with a lining of muscle, connective tissue, and fat surrounding the globe for added protection

C. Ability to see well based on several properties
   1. Eyes must be healthy with all their structures intact
   2. Refractive mediums must be clear
   3. Eyes must also be in proper alignment to have binocular vision (ability for both eyes to fuse two images into one image; necessary for depth perception)

D. Eye movements
   1. Ability of eyes to look straight ahead continuously is called *fixation*
   2. Ability of eyes to move away from midline is called *divergence*
   3. Ability of eyes to draw together from midline, as when focusing on near objects, is called *convergence*
   4. Convergence, pupillary constriction, and accommodation taken together are referred to as the *accommodative reflex*
   5. *Accommodation* is the ability of the lens to become more convex to allow near vision
   6. *Constriction of pupil* allows a clearer image to be projected onto the retina
   7. *Dilation of the pupil* is a normal response to a decrease in the amount of light available

## II. Anatomy and Physiology of the Eye

A. Surface anatomy
   1. Eyelids: moveable folds of skin covering the eye externally; protect the eye from injury and excessive light; spread tear film over cornea by blinking
      a. Upper lid extends from lash line to eyebrow; kept open and elevated by levator palpebrae superioris muscle; orbicularis oculi muscle closes eye during winking, blinking, and forced closure

   b. Lower lid extends from lash line and moves without any line of demarcation to skin of cheek
2. Conjunctiva
   a. Mucous membrane covering sclera and inner lids
      (1) Lining upper and lower eyelids: palpebral conjunctiva
      (2) Extends over sclera to corneal margin: bulbar conjunctiva
   b. Provides mucus for lubrication
   c. Contains lymphoid tissue that provides for some immunologic protection
3. Canthi: triangular spaces formed by junction of lids in each corner of the eye
   a. Medial canthus: innermost angle; made up of two fleshy mounds
   b. Lateral canthus: outermost angle
4. Free margin of lid is approximately 2 mm wide; consists of
   a. Meibomian gland—largest sebaceous gland: located in lid
   b. Zeiss glands—small sebacous glands: open at hair follicles
   c. Moll's glands—sweat glands: open at border near lashes
   d. Lacrimal apparatus: produces and drains tears
      (1) Tear production
         (a) Lacrimal gland: produces up to 0.2 ml in 24 hours
         (b) Lacrimal duct: moves tears from glands to conjunctiva
      (2) Tear drainage
         (a) Lacrimal canaliculus: drains tears from eye
         (b) Lacrimal sac: collects tears
         (c) Nasolacrimal duct: drains tears from lacrimal sac to nose
5. Tear film
   a. Prevents evaporation: lipid layer (outermost layer) secreted by meibomian gland
   b. Nourishes the cornea: composed of water, salts, glucose, urea, proteins, lysozyme (antibacterial enzyme), immunoglobulins (middle layer): secreted by lacrimal gland
   c. Necessary for tear film stability and smooths corneal epithelial surface—mucus layer: secreted by goblet cells
6. Cornea: continuous with sclera and joins at limbus; greatest refractive structure of eye; clear because of lack of blood vessels and its dehydrated state; receives its nutrition from tears, aqueous, and capillaries in limbus
   a. Five layers
      (1) Epithelium: outermost layer, about five or six cells thick; heals rapidly without scarring and is extremely painful when traumatized
      (2) Bowman's layer: acellular and clear; heals with a scar
      (3) Stroma: consists of 90% of corneal thickness
      (4) Descemet's membrane: basement membrane of endothelium, transparent, elastic, no definite structure
      (5) Endothelium: one cell thick; regulates corneal dehydration through a sodium-potassium pump. Dehydration is necessary for cornea to remain clear; with hydration or corneal edema, corneal opacities result. Endothelial cells do not regenerate, causing the remaining cells to move together to compensate for cell loss
7. Aqueous humor: located between cornea and lens; produced by ciliary body's epithelial cells; clear, colorless, and of watery consistency; bathes and supplies nutrients to the cornea and lens
   a. Circulation
      (1) Aqueous constantly produced by ciliary process
      (2) Aqueous circulation flows as follows:
         (a) Produced by ciliary body
         (b) Posterior chamber: between anterior surface of lens and posterior surface of iris

   (c) Anterior chamber: between anterior surface of iris and endothelium of cornea
   (d) Trabecular meshwork: in anterior angle
   (e) Ultimate drainage site: canal of Schlemm

8. Uveal tract: three-part structure with various functions
   a. Iris: colored part of eye with an aperture in center (pupil)
      (1) Assists in regulating amount of light entering eye
         (a) Sphincter pupillae muscle: contracts to constrict pupil
         (b) Dilator pupillae muscle: dilates pupil
   b. Ciliary body: continuous with iris and adherent to sclera
      (1) Ciliary processes produce aqueous humor
      (2) Zonular fibers connect ciliary process to lens
   c. Choroid: continuous with iris and ciliary body; nourishes the retina
9. Angle structures: formed by angle that is posterior to cornea and anterior to the iris
   a. Assists in regulating intraocular pressure
10. Lens: transparent refractive structure of eye located between iris and vitreous body
   a. Lens capsule: bag surrounding lens
   b. Cortex: periphery of lens material
   c. Nucleus: central portion of lens; becomes harder and denser with age
11. Vitreous: clear, transparent, and avascular; occupies two thirds of volume of eye
   a. Thick, jellylike consistency; composition: 99% water and 1% collagen and hyaluronic acid
   b. Situated posteriorly to lens, surrounded by retina
   c. Assists in maintaining shape of eye
   d. Refractive medium
12. Retina: sensory receptor structure of eye
   a. Innermost lining of eye
   b. Thin, semitransparent neural layer consisting of light-sensitive receptor cells
      (1) Rods allow black, white, and gray vision; located in periphery
      (2) Cones allow color vision; located in macula
   c. Firmly attached at ora serrata, optic nerve, and choroid
   d. Records and processes images
13. Sclera: fibrous, white, opaque portion of eye
   a. Supporting structure
   b. Insertion site for all extraocular muscles
14. Optic nerve: approximately 25 to 30 mm in length
   a. Second cranial nerve; transmits impulses from retina to brain
   b. Optic disc is head of optic nerve; visible on ophthalmic examination
   c. Optic nerve leaves eye through muscle cone
15. Extraocular muscles
   a. Six extraocular muscles
      (1) Four rectus muscles: medial, lateral, superior, inferior
         (a) Medial: adducts eye (turns eye toward nose)
         (b) Lateral: abducts eye (turns eye away from nose)
         (c) Superior: elevates eye
         (d) Inferior: depresses eye
      (2) Two oblique muscles: superior, inferior
         (a) Superior oblique: turns eye down and in
         (b) Inferior oblique: turns eye up and out
   b. Four rectus muscles originate at apex of the orbit and form the muscle cone. They then diverge to their individual insertion sites: Fat surrounds muscle cone. Included in protective fat is the optic nerve, ophthalmic artery and vein, branches of oculomotor nerve, and ciliary ganglion

16. Intraocular muscles
    a. Sphincter pupillae muscle located at inner periphery iris
        (1) Constricts iris, making pupil smaller
        (2) Controlled by parasympathetic nervous system
    b. Dilator pupillae muscle is located in body of iris from root to sphincter muscle
    c. Ciliary muscle located within ciliary body
        (1) Ciliary muscle relieves or places tension on ciliary processes to change shape of lens for better focusing ability
        (2) Controlled by third cranial nerve (oculomotor)
17. Lid muscles
    a. Levator palpebrae superioris muscle elevates the eyelid
        (1) Innervated by third cranial nerve (oculomotor)
    b. Orbicularis oculi muscle responsible for closing the eyelid
        (1) Innervated by seventh cranial nerve (facial)
18. Parasympathetic nervous system
    a. Refers to craniosacral portion of autonomic nervous system; effects are typically specific instead of general (e.g., pupillary constriction)
        (1) Innervates ciliary muscle, sphincter pupillae muscle, and oculomotor nerve
19. Sympathetic nervous system
    a. Refers to thoracolumbar portion of autonomic nervous system
        (1) Activated by release of chemical transmitter norepinephrine
        (2) Innervates trabecular meshwork, dilator muscle, and uveal blood vessels
20. Cranial nerves
    a. Cranial nerve II: optic nerve; transmits impulses from retina to brain
    b. Cranial nerve III: oculomotor nerve; innervates levator palpebrae muscle; ciliary muscle; superior, inferior, and medial rectus muscles; and inferior oblique muscle
    c. Cranial nerve IV: trochlear nerve; innervates superior oblique muscle
    d. Cranial nerve V: trigeminal nerve; innervates cornea
    e. Cranial nerve VI: abducens nerve; innervates lateral rectus muscle
    f. Cranial nerve VII: facial nerve; innervates lacrimal glands and portions of face
21. Orbit: bones that make up orbit, consists of the following: frontal bone; lesser wing of sphenoid; greater wing of sphenoid; zygomatic bone; maxilla; palatine, lacrimal, and ethmoid bones
22. Circulation
    a. Two primary sources of arterial blood to the eye and orbit: ophthalmic artery and external carotid artery
    b. Venous drainage of orbit is mainly by superior and inferior ophthalmic veins

## III. Pathophysiology and Treatments

A. Orbit and globe
1. Fractures and trauma
    a. Orbital rim: requires surgical repair of fractures
    b. Blow-out fracture
        (1) Surgical repair with reconstruction of orbital floor (orbital floor implant)
    c. Ruptured globe
        (1) Surgical repair of lacerations
        (2) Evisceration: removal of contents of globe
        (3) Enucleation: removal of globe
2. Tumors
    a. Primary tumors: benign (hemangiomas, dermoid cysts, and lipomas)
        (1) Evisceration
        (2) Enucleation
        (3) Exenteration: removal of contents of orbit

b. Secondary tumors: malignant (melanomas, retinoblastomas, meningiomas, and optic nerve tumors)
(1) Radical surgical excision of tumor (enucleation or exenteration)
(2) Radiation plaque implants

B. Eyelids
1. Trauma
a. Laceration: surgical repair
2. Tumors
a. Primary or benign
(1) Excision of tumor
(2) Plastic reconstruction of lid
b. Secondary or malignant (basal cell and melanoma)
(1) Excision of tumor
(2) Plastic reconstruction of lid
3. Abnormal lid positions
a. Ectropion: outward turning of eyelid due to scar formation, loss of elasticity of lid tissue
(1) Surgical repair with wedge resection
b. Entropion: inversion of eyelid due to loss of tone of orbicularis muscle, loss of tissue elasticity, scarring, burns, trichoma
(1) Surgical repair with wedge resection
c. Ptosis: drooping of upper lid due to congenital malformation, neuromuscular disorders, trauma
(1) Surgical resection of levator muscle
(2) Traction suture to frontalis muscle
4. Inflammation (sty)
a. Hordeolum: typical causative agent is *Staphylococcus*
(1) Medical, pharmaceutical treatment
(2) May require incision and drainage
b. Chalazion: chronic inflammation of meibomian glands
(1) Surgical excision

C. Lacrimal apparatus
1. Dry eyes caused by insufficient tear production in lacrimal gland
a. Medical treatment: artificial tear eye drops
b. Punctal occlusion
2. Excessive tearing secondary to nasolacrimal duct obstruction
a. Lacrimal duct massage
b. Nasolacrimal probing
c. Nasolacrimal intubation
3. Inflammation (dacryocystitis)
a. Medical treatment
b. Surgical treatment: dacryocystorhinostomy (procedure to create an opening from lacrimal sac into nasal cavity, thereby relieving obstruction)

D. Conjunctiva
1. Inflammation (conjunctivitis)
a. Medical treatment
b. Pharmaceutical treatment
2. Neoplasm: pinguecula (benign) or pterygium (conjunctiva overgrows cornea)
a. Surgical excision with or without conjunctival graft

E. Muscles
1. Strabismus: deviation of eye(s) from normal parallel position due to lack of muscle coordination or congenital imbalance
a. Surgical treatment

(1) Resection: shortening of muscle to strengthen it
(2) Recession: lengthening of muscle to weaken it

F. Cornea
1. Ulceration or keratitis: ulcer or inflammation of cornea
   a. Exposure (lack of moisture or improper eyelid closure), e.g., Bell's palsy, exophthalmos, ectropion, loss of protective reflexes seen in anesthetized patient
      (1) Medical or pharmaceutical treatment
      (2) Tarsorrhaphy: surgical closure of eyelids
      (3) Corneal transplant
   b. Introduction of pathogens (bacterial, viral, fungal), e.g., herpes simplex or zoster, syphilis, *S. aureus*
      (1) Medical or pharmaceutical treatment
      (2) Corneal transplant
2. Edema: fluid in layers of cornea
   a. Disorders of corneal layer integrity (e.g., bullous keratopathy, corneal edema, Fuchs' dystrophy, complication of prior intraocular surgery, abuse of topical anesthetics)
      (1) Corneal transplant
3. Trauma: any injury to cornea (if superficial, involving only epithelial layer, no treatment will be necessary; however, if trauma results in scarring of deeper layers or involves center of vision, further treatment will be necessary)
   a. Abrasions
      (1) Patch
      (2) Ointment
   b. Lacerations
      (1) Patch
      (2) Ointment
      (3) Surgical repair
   c. Perforation
      (1) Surgical repair
   d. Foreign body
      (1) Removal
      (2) Surgical repair
   e. Chemical burns (acid, alkali, or thermal)
      (1) Irrigation
      (2) Corneal transplant
   f. Refractive error
      (1) Keratoconus: degenerative, cone-shaped deformity of cornea
         (a) Contact lenses
         (b) Corneal transplant
      (2) Myopia: focus of light rays in front of retina; nearsighted
         (a) Refractive correction (glasses or contact lenses)
         (b) Radial keratotomy (RK; cutting radial slices in cornea)
         (c) Automated lamellar keratoplasty (ALK): creating a surgical corneal flap, then surgically removing a disc of tissue from stroma and replacing the flap
         (d) Laser-assisted in-situ keratomileusis (LASIK): creating a surgical flap, then removing center portion of stromal layer with a laser, then replacing flap
      (3) Hyperopia: focus of light rays behind retina; farsighted
         (a) Refractive correction (glasses or contact lenses)
      (4) Astigmatism: light rays not refracted equally and therefore rays are not focused on retina
         (a) Refractive correction (glasses or contact lenses)
         (b) Astigmatic keratotomy (cutting arcs in periphery of cornea)

**IV. Anterior Segment**

A. Uveal tract
1. Uveitis: inflammation of all or part of uveal tract
   a. Allergies, irritants, infections, trauma, or associated with systemic disease can lead to glaucoma, corneal clouding, and lens degeneration
   b. Sympathetic ophthalmic uveitis: damage to uveal tract in one eye can result in blindness in fellow eye
      (1) Medical treatment
2. Glaucoma: sustained increase in intraocular pressure of the eye; resulting in vision loss and optic nerve damage, interference of aqueous fluid flow or increased production of aqueous fluid
   a. Open angle: opening of trabecular meshwork becomes narrowed, which increases resistance of fluid flow, with increase in intraocular pressure, chronic condition that leads to progressive optic nerve damage
      (1) Medical treatment: miotic drops (see drug section), topical β-blockers (decrease aqueous production) and epinephrine preparations (increase outflow)
      (2) Trabeculoplasty: laser surgical treatment
      (3) Surgical trabeculectomy: filter procedure
      (4) Pan ciliary photocoagulation: 270 degrees; ablation of ciliary processes
   b. Narrow angle (angle closure): angle is narrowed and, if these patients' eyes are dilated, may cause pupillary block that occludes outflow of aqueous and increases intraocular pressure; may constitute medical emergency
      (1) Medical treatment: osmotics and carbonic anhydrase inhibitors, miotics (see drug section)
      (2) Iridotomy: laser procedure to create opening for fluid flow
   c. Congenital: corneal haziness, infant eyes appear enlarged
      (1) Goniotomy: incision into trabecular meshwork; allows fluid to drain, decreasing pressure
   d. Secondary: uveal tract changes, infections, trauma, or lens changes; increase in intraocular pressure is result of specific disease
      (1) Treatment depends on whether glaucoma is open or closed angle

B. Iris
1. Iritis: inflammation of the iris
   a. Medical treatment (antibiotics and cycloplegics)
2. Congenital anomalies
   a. Aniridia: absence of iris
      (1) Medical treatment: colored contact lenses
   b. Coloboma: defect of iris; no treatment
3. Malignant melanoma
   a. Treatment depends on location
4. Trauma
   a. Contusion
      (1) Medical treatment: dilate pupil
   b. Laceration
      (1) Medical treatment: dilate pupil
      (2) Surgical treatment: surgical repair

C. Lens
1. Cataract: opacification of lens material; senile, congenital, traumatic, and other (resulting from other disease processes or pharmacologic treatments)
   a. Surgical treatment: cataract extraction with or without insertion of intraocular lens
      (1) Intracapsular: entire lens and capsule removed
      (2) Extracapsular: lens removed but capsule left in place and intraocular lens may be placed

(3) Phacoemulsification: ultrasonic frequency used to emulsify cataract; therefore a smaller incision used and capsule left intact for placement of intraocular lens
(a) Scleral tunnel: 3 to 5 mm incision with no stitches; incision seals self; hard plastic or foldable lens implants
(b) Clear cornea incision: 3 mm incision at corneal border; usually does not require stitches; foldable lens implant

b. Complications of surgical treatment
(1) Hyphema: blood in anterior chamber; no treatment required; will resolve by itself in time
(2) Ptosis: drooping of upper eyelid; surgical tightening of levator muscle required
(3) Increased intraocular pressure: pharmacologic treatment to lower pressure
(4) Ruptured posterior capsule resulting in need for vitrectomy (discussed below)
(5) Endophthalmitis: medical treatment; possible surgical intervention (vitrectomy)
(6) Retinal detachment
(7) Uveitis, corneal edema

D. Vitreous
1. Floaters: spots before eyes that may indicate pathophysiology; if caused by retinal tear, spots will remain
2. Flashes of light: caused by traction of vitreous pulling on retina
3. Vitreous hemorrhage: caused by leaking of retinal blood vessels
4. Vitreous membranes: scar tissue formed in vitreous resulting in traction on retina
5. Foreign body: introduction of any foreign body into the eye
6. Infection: postsurgical, traumatic, systemic introduction of any pathogen
7. Surgical intervention
   a. Vitrectomy: surgical removal of vitreous with replacement with intraocular salt solution
8. Surgical complications
   a. Retinal detachment: detachment of all or any part of the retina
   b. Endophthalmitis: infection of the vitreous

E. Retina
1. Central retinal artery occlusion: caused by embolus or arteriosclerosis; requires immediate treatment with global massage and anterior chamber paracentesis to lower intraocular pressure to dislodge clot
2. Central retinal vein occlusion: caused by hypertension, diabetes, or sluggish circulation; treated by cryotherapy or laser treatment or both
3. Retinal detachment: caused by trauma, vitreous traction, membranes, retinal degenerative disease processes or high myopes (myopic patients have anatomically longer eyes from anterior to posterior pole); may also be caused by holes, tears, or schisis (separation of retinal layers)
4. Surgical treatment: vitrectomy, cryopexy, scleral buckling, endophotocoagulation treatment (laser), membrane peeling, air-fluid exchange, injection of expandable gases or silicone oil or both

## V. Ophthalmic Anesthesia

A. Topical: used when performing tonometry, gonioscopy, suture removal, removal of superficial foreign bodies, and surgery on eye; in drops or ointment
1. Proparacaine hydrochloride (Ophthaine, Ophthetic), 0.5%: least irritating
2. Tetracaine hydrochloride (Pontocaine), 0.5% to 1%: stings on instillation
3. Cocaine, 2% to 5%: mostly used in 4% strength; may have some toxic effects on epithelium and may dilate pupil
4. Benoxinate hydrochloride (Dorsacaine), 0.4%: only topical anesthetic compatible with fluorescein and may be found in combined solution
5. Butacaine sulfate (Butyn), 2%

B. Injectable: used to provide anesthesia of globe and eyelids and paralysis of muscles responsible for movement of eye, eyelids, and facial muscles
   1. Drugs
      a. Procaine hydrochloride (Novocaine), 0.25% to 1%: less irritating to tissues
      b. Lidocaine hydrochloride (Xylocaine), 0.5% to 2%: most common agent used
      c. Etidocaine hydrochloride (Duranest), 0.5% to 1.5%: more rapid onset and longer acting than lidocaine
      d. Bupivacaine (Marcaine), 0.25% to 0.5%: rapid onset, may last several hours
      e. Mepivacaine hydrochloride (Carbocaine), 1% to 2%: least potent
   2. Adjunctive agents: may be combined with injectable anesthetics
      a. Epinephrine: 1:100,000: prolongs duration and reduces bleeding
      b. Hyaluronidase (Wydase): increases absorption of local anesthetic and reduces intraocular pressure
   3. Techniques
      a. Field nerve block: for surgery on eyelids
      b. Retrobulbar block: to anesthetize and immobilize the eye; anesthetic injected into muscle cone
         (1) Potential complications include trauma to optic nerve, retrobulbar hemorrhage, compression of globe, increased retrobulbar pressure
      c. Peribulbar block: to anesthetize and immobilize the eye; anesthetic injected into soft tissues of the globe, outside the muscle cone
      d. Local nerve block (Van Lint, Atkinson, O'Brien blocks): used to block facial nerve that supplies orbicularis muscle
         (1) Eye remains open (cannot close)

C. General anesthesia: indicated when surgery will be prolonged, when patient may be uncooperative, and for young children undergoing ophthalmic procedures

**VI. Drugs Commonly Used in Ophthalmic Surgery**

A. Mydriatics: dilate the pupil (sympathomimetic) by acting on dilator muscle of eye
   1. Phenylephrine hydrochloride (Neo-Synephrine hydrochloride), 2.5% to 10%
   2. Hydroxyamphetamine hydrobromide (Paredrine), 1%: mainly used in patients allergic to phenylephrine

B. Cycloplegics: dilate pupil and paralyze accommodation by action on ciliary muscles (parasymphatholytic)
   1. Atropine, 0.25% to 2%: in ointment or solution
   2. Homatropine hydrobromide, 1.2% and 5%: side effects rare and wears off faster than atropine
   3. Cyclopentolate hydrochloride (Cyclogyl), 0.5% and 1%: rapid onset and short duration
   4. Scopolamine (Hyoscine): fewer allergic responses than to atropine and can be used as a substitute; can precipitate acute-angle closure glaucoma
   5. Tropicamide (Mydriacyl), 0.5% to 1%: rapid onset, wears off in 1 hour

C. Miotics: constrict pupil by stimulating sphincter muscle of the iris
   1. Cholinergics: exert effect on iris sphincter, causing it to constrict and therefore constricting pupil; also work on zonules and open trabecula
      a. Pilocarpine hydrochloride, 0.5% to 6%: most commonly used in chronic management of angle-closure glaucoma
      b. Carbachol (Miostat), 0.75% to 3%: lasts longer than pilocarpine (may cause eye ache or headache)
      c. Acetylcholine chloride (Miochol), 10%: lasts only 10 minutes and mainly used intraoperatively
   2. Anticholinesterases: block release of cholinesterase, causing similar response to cholinergics; used for glaucoma
      a. Physostigmine salicylate (Eserine), 0.25% to 1%: most frequently used in ointment form; may cause allergic reactions and conjunctivitis

b. Isoflurophate (Floropryl): mainly used in ointment form and used to control intraocular pressure if other miotics fail
c. Demecarium bromide (Humorsol), 0.25%: action similar to isoflurophate
d. Echothiophate iodide (Phospholine iodide), 0.03% to 0.25%: long acting and may cause cataracts

D. Carbonic anhydrous inhibitors: block formation of aqueous and cause intraocular pressure to decrease; used for glaucoma
1. Acetazolamide (Diamox): oral and parenteral forms; 500 to 1000 mg daily
2. Methazolamide (Neptazane): oral doses of 50 to 100 mg daily
3. Ethoxzolamide (Cardrase): oral doses of up to 500 mg daily

E. Osmotics: used to lower intraocular pressure by drawing aqueous from eye
1. Mannitol, 20% solution given intravenously; known to cause hypovolemia because of its fluid reduction in other tissues
2. Urea (Ureaphil, Urevert), 30% solution given intravenously; may cause phlebitis and sloughing of skin if allowed to extravasate
3. Glycerin (Glyrol, Osmoglyn): thick, viscous liquid given orally to decrease intraocular pressure; sweetness may cause nausea and vomiting

F. Corticosteroids: used as anti-inflammatory agents
1. Prednisolone suspension (Pred Mild, Pred Forte)
2. Prednisolone solution (Hydeltrasol, Prednefrin S)
3. Hydrocortisone suspension, ointment, or solution
4. Dexamethasone 0.1% (Maxidex, Decadron) used in combination with neomycin and polymyxin (Maxitrol)

G. Topical antibiotics: anti-infectives in solutions or ointments
1. Chloramphenicol, 1.0% and 1.5% (Chloroptic ointment): broad spectrum
2. Gentamicin sulfate (Garamycin solution or ointment)
3. Bacitracin, neomycin, erythromycin, tetracycline, and sulfisoxazole (Gantrisin): ointment or solution
4. Neomycin with polymyxin or bacitracin (Neosporin, Statrol)

H. Diagnostic stains: for visualization of defects or corneal epithelium
1. Sodium fluorescein, 0.5%: stains defects bright green; used in retinal photography
2. Rose Bengal: used to dye degenerating epithelium red

I. Miscellaneous drugs used intraoperatively
1. α-Chymotrypsin (Chymar): enzyme that dissolves zonules; used mainly in intracapsular cataract surgery to facilitate extraction of lens
2. Sodium hyaluronate: viscoelastic substance used in cataract surgery to protect endothelium and to prevent adhesion formation
3. Flurbiprofen sodium (Ocufen), 0.03%: nonsteroidal anti-inflammatory used to inhibit miosis during cataract surgery
4. Alphagan: used to lower intraocular pressure

J. β-Blockers: used to decrease intraocular pressure
1. Timolol maleate (Timoptic), 0.25% to 0.5%: used to decrease intraocular pressure; contraindicated in patients with lung conditions (asthma)
a. May cause bronchospasm

## VII. Postanesthesia Care Unit (PACU) Considerations

A. Untoward complications listed in Table 29–1

B. Oculocardiac reflex: nervous response elicited by manipulation of extraocular muscles or any surrounding ocular tissue
1. Results in decreased heart rate, blood pressure, and level of consciousness
2. Any ophthalmic surgical patient susceptible
a. Risk increases with vitreoretinal and eye muscle surgery
3. Onset: immediate to 20 minutes postoperatively

**TABLE 29–1 Possible Complications of Ophthalmic Surgeries**

| SYMPTOMS | EXPECTED OUTCOMES | TREATMENT | POSSIBLE CAUSATIVE FACTORS |
|---|---|---|---|
| Pain | Minimal in most ophthalmic surgeries | Mild analgesic<br>Need for stronger medication may indicate possible complication | Increased intraocular pressure (IOP)<br>Surgical manipulation<br>Periorbital pressure from anesthesia<br>Pressure from dressing |
| Nausea and vomiting | Minimal after most ophthalmic procedures | Antiemetic | Oculocardiac reflex<br>Surgical manipulation<br>General anesthetic agents |
| Bleeding | Minimal in all ophthalmic procedures | Apply pressure<br>Reinforce dressing | Loose dressing |

NOTE: In all circumstances, notify physician of the following postoperative complications: extreme pain, unrelieved nausea and vomiting, and uncontrolled bleeding.

4. Injection of retrobulbar anesthesia may also stimulate response
5. Treatment: IV atropine

C. Positioning: postoperative positioning depends on procedure performed; no restriction on postoperative position necessary for most ophthalmic surgeries; patients receiving intraoperative injection of air, expandable gases (SF6 or C3F8), or silicone oil must be maintained in specific positions per physician order. Head of bed elevation is necessary for postoperative oculoplastic surgery patients; activities that should be avoided immediately after surgery: crying, bending, vomiting, and gagging

D. Presence of concomitant diseases or conditions
1. Cardiovascular: arteriosclerosis, hypertension
2. Endocrine: diabetes mellitus
    a. Leading cause of blindness worldwide
    b. Will need to consider preoperative and postoperative blood glucose monitoring
3. Vascular: atherosclerosis, renal disease
    a. May contribute to hypertension
4. Age: need for eye surgery can occur with any age patient
    a. Congenital problems corrected in infancy
    b. Degenerative changes most common in elderly
    c. Trauma can occur with any age

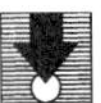

### NURSING DIAGNOSIS

Examples of related nursing diagnostic categories include

- Potential for injury due to visual impairment
- Alteration in comfort due to surgical manipulation (pain)
- Sensory-perceptual alteration due to instillation of eyedrops preoperatively or presence of eye patch postoperatively
- Anxiety due to unknown outcome of surgery

*The Future of Refractive Surgery*

Ophthalmologists are now able to correct a greater amount of myopia (1 to 14 diopters) than was previously possible with RK, ALK, or photorefractive keratectomy (PRK). The LASIK procedure is a method of reshaping the cornea (flattening the center of the cornea, thereby shortening the eye) so that light is focused on the retina.

A microkeratome makes a partial thickness incision across the top of the cornea to form a flap. A laser is then used to ablate a predetermined amount of corneal tissue. The corneal flap is then replaced and is held on the eye by the natural pump mechanism in the endothelium.

This procedure offers a high degree of accuracy with a low enhancement rate. Both eyes can be corrected during the procedure and the patients are reporting rapid visual recovery as well as minimal discomfort.

## BIBLIOGRAPHY


Cassin B, Soloman SA: *Dictionary of Eye Terminology,* 3rd Ed. Gainesville, Fla., Triad Publishing, 1997.

*Facts and Comparisons, October, 1997—Update* (p 478). St Louis, Wolters Kluwer, 1997.

Goldblum K (ed): *Core Curriculum for Ophthalmic Nursing.* Dubuque, Iowa, Kendell Hunt, 1997.

Litwack K: Practical points in the care of the patient having cataract surgery. *J Post Anesth Nurs* 8(2): 113–115, 1992.

Maloney W: Beveled blades have simplified clear corneal technique. *Ocular Surg News* 15(18):11, 1997.

*Physician's Desk Reference for Ophthalmology.* Oradell, NJ, Medical Economics, 1991.

Stein H, Slatt B, Stein R: *The Ophthalmic Assistant: A Guide for Ophthalmic Medical Personnel,* 6th Ed. St Louis, Mosby, 1994.

Thompson-Keith E: *Care of the Ophthalmic Patient.* Denver, Association of Operating Room Nurses, 1991.

Vaughn D, Asbury T, Riordan-Era P: *General Ophthalmology,* 14th Ed. Stamford, Conn, Appleton & Lange, 1995.


## REVIEW QUESTIONS

**1. Inflammation of the lacrimal sac is referred to as:**

A. Lacrimitis
B. Dacryocystitis
C. Conjunctivitis
D. Phlebitis

**2. The focusing portion of the eye is the:**

A. Aqueous
B. Vitreous
C. Lens
D. Cornea

**3. Hyaluronidase is frequently used in conjunction with injectable anesthetics because it:**

A. Increases absorption of the anesthetic
B. Decreases absorption of the anesthetic
C. Increases duration of the anesthetic
D. Decreases duration of the anesthetic

**4. Strabismus repair refers to correction of:**

A. An obstructed lacrimal duct
B. Defects of eye muscle coordination
C. Eversion of the eyelid
D. A cornea laceration

**5. Usual treatment for stimulation of the oculocardiac reflex is:**

A. IV lidocaine
B. Carotid massage
C. Ocular pressure
D. IV atropine

**6. Osmotics are frequently given to the patient having eye surgery. The purpose is to:**

A. Increase intraocular pressure
B. Decrease intraocular pressure
C. Stimulate renal function
D. Increase aqueous production

**7. "Dry eyes" indicate that there is a disorder in the:**
A. Lacrimal gland
B. Conjunctiva
C. Cornea
D. Sclera

**8. The surgical treatment for correction of congenital corneal haziness due to glaucoma is called:**
A. Enucleation
B. Trabeculoplasty
C. Radial keratotomy
D. Goniotomy

**9. Which of the following procedures is not a procedure for retinal disorders?**
A. Vitrectomy
B. Scleral buckling
C. Injection of expandable gases
D. Phacoemulsification

**10. Which type of medication dilates the pupil and paralyzes accommodation?**
A. Mydriatics
B. Miotics
C. Cycloplegics
D. Carbonic anhydrase inhibitors

**ANSWERS:** 1. B, 2. C, 3. A, 4. B, 5. D, 6. B, 7. A, 8. D, 9. D, 10. C

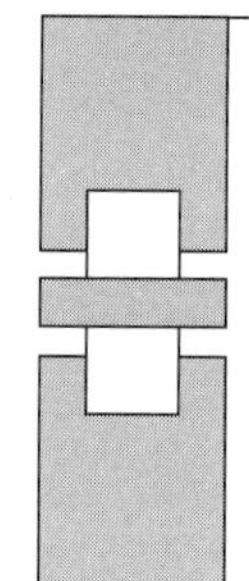

CHAPTER 30

# The Plastic Surgery and Burn Patient

Diane E. Fritsch, MSN, RN, CCRN, CS

## OBJECTIVES

**Study of the information represented by this outline will enable the learner to:**

1. Discuss the psychologic factors that affect the plastic surgery patient.
2. Describe common plastic surgery and burn procedures.
3. Discuss the pathophysiology of burn injury.
4. Identify anesthesia administration concerns for the plastic surgery patient.
5. Identify physiologic changes in the burn patient that have an impact on anesthetic administration.
6. Discuss postoperative management concerns for the burn patient, including airway management, temperature management, wound care, hypovolemia management, infection control, and pain management.
7. Discuss postoperative management concerns for the plastic surgery patient.

Plastic and reconstructive surgery may be performed for a variety of reasons. The procedures impact physical appearance as well as emotional well-being and body image. Plastic surgery may be elective and cosmetic, or it may be reconstructive, correcting congenital or acquired abnormalities. Anesthetic needs vary on the basis of the complexity of the procedure, from local anesthesia for simple lesion removal to prolonged general anesthesia for complex reconstruction.

This chapter discusses the perioperative needs of the plastic surgery and burn patient. Specific procedures will be reviewed and preoperative assessment and intraoperative and postoperative management discussed.

## ASSESSMENT

### I. Establish a Baseline Assessment in Which to Evaluate Postoperative Status

### II. Assess for Medical Conditions That May Affect Tolerance of Procedure or Healing

A. Pulmonary disease
   1. Prone positioning intraoperatively may affect ventilation
   2. Prolonged anesthesia increases pulmonary hygiene needs postoperatively

B. Cardiac disease
   1. Coronary insufficiency may affect tolerance of hypotensive anesthesia
   2. Cardiac function affects tolerance of prolonged reconstructive procedures

C. Diabetes mellitus affects wound healing

D. Medication history
   1. Use of steroids
   2. Use of aspirin products

E. History of bleeding disorders

F. Presence of infection
   1. Children with concurrent or recent upper respiratory infection are more likely to have laryngospasm or to cough during induction or emergence
G. Nutritional status
   1. Wound healing depends on adequate nutritional status particularly vitamin C, zinc, iron, and protein
   2. Poor nutritional status decreases ability to prevent infection

**III. Psychologic Readiness**
A. Determine patient's expectations of surgery
   1. Expectations realistic?
   2. Motivation for surgery?
   3. Reinforce that immediate results may not meet patient's expectations because of swelling, color changes, and suture lines
   4. Family expectations
   5. Reinforce that long-term results may not meet expectations
B. Impact of deformity on patient's self-perception
   1. How does patient view it as changing his or her life?
   2. How important is it to be attractive?
   3. Effect of others' reactions on patient
C. Psychologic evaluation may be suggested before procedure

**IV. Diagnostic Procedures** (vary by institution)
A. Local procedures
   1. Complete blood cell count
   2. Chemistry profile
B. General anesthesia
   1. Complete blood cell count
   2. Chemistry profile
   3. Electrocardiogram (ECG) in adults
   4. Pulmonary function testing if necessary
   5. Chest x-ray film (in adults or in children with pulmonary pathologic findings)
   6. Bleeding profile: prothrombin time/partial thromboplastin time (international normalized ratio [INR])

## COMMON PLASTIC SURGERY PROCEDURES

**I. Procedures for Facial Rejuvenation**
A. Rhytidectomy (facelift)
   1. Tightening of loose tissue in face
   2. May involve skin, fat, subcutaneous tissue, and muscle
   3. Standard incisions placed in the temporal area behind hairline
   4. Additional procedures may be performed in conjunction with rhytidectomy
      a. Tightening of underlying fascia in the superficial musculoapneurotic system (SMAS)
      b. Blepharoplasty, brow lifting, chemical peel, suction-assisted lipectomy or lipolysis (SAL)
B. Blepharoplasty
   1. Repair or reconstruction of upper or lower eyelid to correct "baggy" appearance
   2. Incisions placed in the crease of the upper lid and in the lower lid below lash margin
C. Mentoplasty (genioplasty)
   1. Surgical reshaping of chin

2. Modifications in mandible or insertion of prosthesis
3. Incisions placed inside mouth or beneath chin
4. May be performed in conjunction with rhinoplasty to provide a balanced facial profile

D. Rhinoplasty
1. Surgical reshaping of nose
2. May involve alteration or removal of bone, fat, cartilage
3. Incisions made inside the nose

E. Otoplasty
1. Surgical reshaping or repositioning of ears
2. May be performed on children after 6 years of age, when ears have reached most of their adult size

F. Dermabrasion
1. Removal of facial epidermis and part of superficial dermis to correct skin defects
   a. Acne or depressed scarring
   b. Wrinkles
   c. Irregular skin pigmentation
2. Use of sanding or rotating wire brushes on skin

G. Chemosurgery
1. Use of chemical agents to remove or destroy tissue
2. Chemical peel
   a. Use of chemicals to remove or destroy tissue
   b. Chemical peel
      (1) Phenol
      (2) Tricholoracetic acid
      (3) Alphahydroxy acid ("fruit peel")

## II. Dermapigmentation

A. Use of tattoos to add color or pigment to skin
B. May be used to camouflage scars or create areola after breast reconstruction

## III. Cleft Lip or Palate Repair

A. Repair of congenital lip or palate defects
B. Cleft lip repair
1. Obtain nostril symmetry and Cupid's bow of upper lip, and repair lip muscle
2. Commonly performed when child (rule of 10s):
   a. Is at least 10 weeks old
   b. Weighs at least 10 pounds (4500 g)
   c. Has a hemoglobin of 10 g/dl

## IV. Mammoplasty

A. Plastic surgery of breast
B. Augmentation mammoplasty
1. Increases size and modifies shape of breast to increase breast size or correct surgical defects
2. Insertion of prosthetic devices (e.g., tissue expanders that are inflated with normal saline)
   a. Submammary: beneath breast tissue on anterior surface of pectoralis muscle
   b. Submuscular: beneath pectoralis major and serratus anterior muscles

C. Reduction mammoplasty and mastopexy
1. Mammoplasty: excision of breast tissue with reconstruction of breast contour
2. Mastopexy: excision of redundant breast skin
3. Ideal candidate is adult past period of planned pregnancy within 10 to 15 pounds (6800 g) of ideal body weight

4. Incisions usually placed in the inferior pedicle maintaining nerve innervation to the nipple
5. Inform patient about potential for scarring

**V. Abdominoplasty**

A. Plastic repair of deformities of anterior abdominal wall
B. Removal of apron deformities (panniculus)
C. Repair of muscle wall from previous abdominal surgeries

**VI. Suction-Assisted Lipectomy**

A. Liposuction, lipolysis
B. Removal of subcutaneous fat tissue using blunt catheters and high-vacuum suction through small incisions in inconspicuous areas
C. May be performed in conjunction with other procedures
D. Ideal candidates have elastic skin with limited sun damage, pitting defects, cellulitis, or stretch marks and are within normal weight who have exercise- and diet-resistant fat deposits

**VII. Tissue Expansion**

A. Tissue stretched adjacent to defect to allow growth of tissue to use for repair
B. Silastic expanders placed under tissue to gradually stretch skin

**VIII. Skin Grafting** (see information on burn patient)

**IX. Flaps or Tissue Transfer**

A. Transplantation of skin, muscle, and blood supply from donor site to repair congenital or acquired tissue defects
   1. Breast reconstruction
   2. Repair of traumatic injury to extremities
   3. Repair of defects from cancer treatment
B. Types of flaps
   1. Delayed flap
      a. Donor tissue attached to recipient site without being separated from its blood supply
      b. Remains attached to donor site (by pedicle) until recipient circulation is established
   2. Local flaps
      a. Moved from location immediately adjacent to defect
      b. Maintains blood supply from original source
   3. Free flap
      a. Entire tissue and blood supply detached from donor site
      b. Requires prolonged microsurgery (6 to 12 hours)
C. Common sources of flaps
   1. Skin flaps
      a. Consists of skin and subcutaneous tissue
      b. May be placed to a remote area by means of pedicle
      c. May be advanced into a defect close to the donor site or moved at a pivotal point and rotated into the tissue defect
      d. Sources
         (1) Temporalis fascia: may be used to cover dorsum of hand or foot
         (2) Radial forearm: skin and fascia used for intraoral and extraoral defects
         (3) Lateral forearm: skin and fascia used to cover areas requiring a thicker coverage
         (4) Omentum: for areas that require pliable tissue (e.g., frontal sinuses)
   2. Muscle and myocutaneous flaps
      a. Movement of muscle with or without skin to cover defect
         (1) Local transfer
         (2) Free transfer

b. May require additional skin grafting at recipient site
c. Sources
(1) Latissimus dorsi
(2) Pectoralis major
(3) Tensor fascia lata
(4) Rectus abdominus
(5) Gluteus maximus
(6) Gracilis

**X. Z-plasty**
A. Use of Z-shaped incision to remove scar tissue
B. Requires tissue with elasticity

**XI. V-plasty**
A. Used to repair skin defects
B. Two triangular flaps of adjacent skin transposed

**XII. Repair of Congenital Craniofacial Deformities**
A. Repair of congenital defects from early closure of sutures (craniosynostosis)
B. Repair of congenital maxillofacial deformities
C. May require extensive skeletal reconstruction
D. May be performed in staged procedures

## INTRAOPERATIVE CONCERNS FOR THE PLASTIC SURGERY PATIENT

**I. Procedural Concerns**
A. Goals of plastic surgery procedures
1. Provide cosmetically acceptable result
2. Restore function
3. Promote healing with minimal scarring
4. Prevent infection
B. Procedures carefully planned before surgery
C. Patient positioning requirements
1. Provide comfortable access to surgical field
2. Prevent nerve decompression from improper positioning
a. Careful positioning
b. Padding of pressure points
3. Promote venous drainage
4. Provide for greatest hypotensive advantages (reduction of bleeding) if deliberate hypotensive technique is used
5. Positioned on table to allow for repositioning during procedure to evaluate results (e.g., mammoplasty)
D. Incision placement
1. Incisions placed so that scar lines lie parallel to existing skin lines or behind hair line
2. Skin lines represent areas with minimal tension
3. Cosmetic effect better if tension is minimized
4. Frequently found under long axis of muscle
E. Hemostasis
1. Muscle be obtained to promote good cosmetic effect
2. Bleeding under skin potentiates inflammation, infection, pressure, dehiscence
3. Achieved with ligation, electrocautery, pressure
F. Instrumentation
1. Microinstrumentation for nontraumatic repair

2. Use of operating microscope
   a. Provides three-dimensional view (stereoscopic) that must be clearly seen by surgeon and assistants
   b. Move carefully
3. May require separate instrument tables for donor and recipient sites
4. Lasers
   a. $CO_2$ laser, argon laser, Nd:YAG lasers may be used in aesthetic (cosmetic) surgery
   b. Uses
      (1) Removal of professional tattoos and traumatic tattoos caused by friction, scraping, or explosives
      (2) Alternative for skin resurfacing ($CO_2$ laser)
      (3) Laser blepharoplasty
5. Endoscopy
   a. Endoscope requires body cavity for insertion of scope and visualization
      (1) No natural cavities in plastic surgery operative areas
      (2) Cavity created by use of umbrella or balloonlike retractor on soft tissues
   b. Uses
      (1) Endoscopic forehead lift
      (2) Facelift
      (3) Augmentation or reduction mammoplasty
      (4) Abdominoplasty

G. Suction-assisted lipectomy
1. Patient marked in standing position before procedure
2. Small (1 to 2 cm) incisions used to minimize scarring
3. Adipose tissue aspirated using crisscross technique
4. Compression dressing applied to collapse tunnels created
5. Amount of volume loss must be evaluated to prevent hypovolemia and third spacing

H. Mammoplasty
1. Reduction mammoplasty
   a. Preoperative marking
   b. Areolar transplantation through free tissue transfer to pedicle
   c. Application of bra or compression dressing to maintain new breast contour and decrease fluid accumulation
2. Breast reconstruction
   a. May be performed at time of mastectomy if tumor size is small and no axillary involvement
   b. Materials used in reconstruction
      (1) Tissue expanders
      (2) Latissimus dorsi myocutaneous flap
      (3) Transverse rectus abdominal muscle flap
   c. Nipple reconstruction
      (1) Tattooing
      (2) Grafting
3. Positioning: patient is supine to allow sitting position when table is tilted to evaluate symmetry

I. Flaps
1. Time of procedure
   a. Absence of infection in recipient site
   b. Careful removal of devitalized tissue
2. Selection of donor flap
   a. Selection of muscle or skin that will appropriately fit defect
      (1) Should minimally impact patient's activity and function after removal
      (2) Muscle size will decrease at recipient site after denervation
   b. Selection of pedicle flap (delayed) flap that will comfortably reach defect

3. Preparation of recipient vessels
    a. Devitalized tissue carefully removed
    b. Selection of recipient blood vessels that have been minimally impacted by trauma of defect
4. Anastomosis of vessels
    a. Avoid twisting of vessels
    b. Vessels must be delicately handled
    c. Use of heparin-containing irrigating solutions
5. Maintenance of normal body temperature
    a. Warmed intravenous and irrigating fluids
    b. Room temperature regulation
    c. Warming blankets

## II. Anesthesia Concerns

A. Selection of anesthetic routes and agent
  1. Local anesthesia
      a. Suitable for minor plastic surgical procedures (e.g., skin lesions, rhinoplasty)
      b. May be used for outpatients or office patients
      c. Indicated for procedures that require patient participation (e.g., patients may need to open and close eyes during blepharoplasty)
      d. Selection of agent that lasts 50 to 100 minutes longer than anticipated length of surgery
  2. Regional anesthesia
      a. Suitable for procedures localized to extremity
          (1) Axillary, plexus blocks for upper extremities
          (2) Sciatic block for feet
          (3) Lumbar epidural or spinal for leg procedures
  3. General anesthesia
      a. Suitable for long procedures, pediatrics, and anxious patients
      b. Long plastic procedures generally require lighter general anesthesia
      c. Selection of inhalation agents
          (1) Agents that do not sensitize the heart to catecholamines because of large doses of epinephrine used in plastic procedures (e.g., isoflurane)
          (2) Agents that are less likely to precipitate coughing and laryngospasm, particularly in procedures of face and neck
          (3) Length of time required for elimination for short procedures (e.g., enflurane is rapidly eliminated if used in procedures that last less than 40 minutes)
          (4) Inducing deliberate hypotension
              (a) Selection of agents that induce hypotension
                  (i) Reduces blood loss
                  (ii) Improves visibility at surgical field
              (b) May be accomplished with volatile agents alone or in combination with ganglionic blocking agents, vasodilators, $\alpha$- or $\beta$-blockers
              (c) Used for reconstruction of head and neck
              (d) Hypotension onset and reversal performed slowly to prevent rapid blood pressure fluctuations (e.g., perfusion to organ is maintained)

B. Intraoperative management
  1. Airway management
      a. Method of intubation (oral or nasal) depends on access to surgical field
          (1) Nasal intubation for oral procedures
          (2) Use of oral or nasal RAE tube for cleft lip and palate repair (endotracheal tubes with sharp curves that promote access to field by surgeon)
          (3) Intubation may be difficult and require fiberoptic bronchoscope in patients, particularly children, with maxillofacial deformities

b. Ensure vigorous spontaneous breathing before extubation in patients with maxillofacial surgery
c. Esophageal or precordial stethoscope to assess ventilation
d. Monitor oxygenation
    (1) Transcutaneous oxygen measurement
    (2) Direct arterial blood gas measurement
    (3) Pulse oximetry
e. Carbon dioxide monitoring; end-tidal carbon dioxide
    (1) Elevated carbon dioxide levels result in vasodilation, which increases bleeding and intracranial pressure

2. Cardiovascular management
    a. ECG monitoring (including ST segment analysis) for patients at risk for coronary ischemia
        (1) From use of epinephrine
        (2) As result of deliberate hypotensive technique
    b. Direct or indirect blood pressure monitoring
        (1) Large blood loss common in plastic procedures
            (a) Crystalloids
            (b) Colloids
            (c) Blood products
        (2) Significant hypotension may result in graft or flap failure
    c. Positioning and position change
        (1) Anesthetic agents affect vascular homeostasis and reflect pressure control mechanisms
        (2) Position changes during procedure may be necessary
            (a) To access donor and recipient sites
            (b) To evaluate cosmetic result of procedure (e.g., mammoplasty)
        (3) Minimizing excessive hypotension
            (a) Slow, careful movement of patient
            (b) Maintain light anesthesia
3. Emergence from anesthesia
    a. Smooth emergence desired to prevent thrashing that may disrupt delicate suture lines
    b. Prevent excessive coughing, particularly in head and neck procedures
    c. Minimize nausea and vomiting

## POSTOPERATIVE CONCERNS FOR THE PLASTIC SURGERY PATIENT

### NURSING DIAGNOSIS

Examples of related nursing diagnostic categories include
- Pain
- Potential for infection
- Fluid volume deficit
- Alteration in tissue perfusion: peripheral
- Ineffective airway clearance
- Body image disturbance

**I. Airway Management**

A. Facial and neck surgery
1. Extubation may be delayed until patient is breathing vigorously and can protect airway with cough and gag reflex
    a. Avoid excessive coughing and straining because of increased facial blood pressure

b. Pressure of face mask may damage surgical procedure
c. Use of lidocaine endotracheally or intravenously may decrease coughing
2. Elevate head of bed to facilitate breathing
3. Monitor for increasing swelling and signs of obstruction
4. Monitor for signs of laryngospasm and bronchospasm
5. Assist patient with management of secretions
a. Position to facilitate drainage
b. Suction carefully as needed
6. Maintain airway equipment, including tracheostomy tray, in accessible location
7. Maintain suction and wire cutters at bedside if jaw is wired
B. Monitor oxygen saturation with pulse oximeter
C. Position patient to facilitate breathing, avoiding pressure to operative site

**II. Nausea and Vomiting**
A. Vomiting and retching should be avoided to minimize stress on suture lines
B. May be anticipated in patients
1. After oral or facial surgery because of blood in stomach
2. Who have received narcotic anesthesia
C. Medicate with antiemetics prophylactically and for treatment

**III. Wound Management**
A. Monitor operative site for pallor (arterial insufficiency) or bluish coloring (venous engorgement)
B. Monitor wounds for bleeding or hematomas
1. Bleeding: most common complication
2. Hematomas at operative site may damage operative site (especially rhytidectomy—may cause scarring along suture lines)
C. Minimal edema and ecchymosis may be expected
1. Elevate involved area above heart level
2. Evaluate for use of cool compresses (e.g., after blepharoplasty)
D. Avoid pressure or pulling on wounds
E. Assess integrity of dressings
1. Compression or pressure dressings may be used to control edema and maintain stability
a. After rhytidectomy
b. After mentoplasty
2. Supportive dressings and bras after mammoplasty to help maintain new breast contour
3. Assess for excessive pressure
4. Avoid manipulation of dressing
F. Avoid activities that would increase pressure to operative site
1. Vigorous coughing
2. Straining
3. Bending over in patients with procedures of head and neck
4. Positioning onto operative site
G. Monitor output from drains

**IV. Pain Control**
A. Evaluate need for analgesia
1. Narcotics
2. Nonnarcotics
3. Antiinflammatory agents
4. Avoid use of aspirin in patients where bleeding is a concern
B. Degree of discomfort may vary widely on the basis of type of procedure, anesthetic route, and patient's evaluation of pain

**V. Hypovolemia**

A. Large blood or fluid loss may have occurred intraoperatively
   1. Areas of face are highly vascular
   2. Blood loss may be significant after repair of cranial defects
   3. Liposuction may result in large fluid depletion

B. Evaluate for signs of hypovolemia
   1. Tachycardia
   2. Decreased blood pressure
   3. Delayed capillary refill
   4. Decreased urinary output

**VI. Positioning**

A. Patient should always be positioned to minimize pressure, sheer, and venous congestion

B. Mammoplasty
   1. Maintain arms adducted to minimize strain
   2. Elevate arm on side of mastectomy
   3. Minimize upper arm activity

C. Abdominoplasty
   1. Elevate head of bed, placing patient in V position
   2. Avoid excess stretch of abdominal wall

D. Face and neck surgery
   1. Elevate head of bed
   2. Prevent patient from lying on operative site

E. Myocutaneous flaps
   1. Prevent patient from lying on operative site
   2. Prevent compression of operative site by blankets

**VII. Specific Procedural Concerns**

A. Myocutaneous flaps
   1. Monitor for and prevent factors that promote vasospasm and thrombosis
      a. Hypothermia
         (1) Results in vasoconstriction
         (2) Arterial flow compromised
         (3) Use warming blankets, lights, warmed fluids, increased room temperature
      b. Hypotension
      c. Hypovolemia
         (1) Large blood loss may have occurred
         (2) Replacement with crystalloids and colloids
         (3) Excessive red cell replacement may raise hematocrit, causing sluggish capillary flow
      d. Agents that increase vasoconstriction and vasospasm (e.g., nicotine, caffeine)
   2. Assess condition of flap
      a. Skin temperature
         (1) Should be warm to touch
         (2) Coolness reflects reduced blood flow
      b. Capillary refill
         (1) Blanching within 2 seconds
         (2) Rapid blanching may indicate venous engorgement
         (3) Delayed blanching may indicate arterial insufficiency
         (4) Arterial and venous flow may be obtained by Doppler ultrasonography and are marked by surgeon with a marker or suture
         (5) Venous congestion frequently results in failure before arterial insufficiency
      c. Color
         (1) Normally white or gray immediately postoperatively

(2) Increasingly pale flaps suggest arterial insufficiency
(3) Bluish color suggests venous congestion
(4) Color of flap may be different from other skin in recipient area if obtained from tissue far removed

d. Edema
(1) Slight swelling is expected
(2) Significant swelling may indicate hematoma or venous congestion

3. Monitor drainage from drains every 30 to 60 minutes
   a. Gentle continuous suction
   b. Greater than 50 ml/hr is problematic
4. Monitor muscle donor site for bleeding
5. Antiplatelets or anticoagulants may be used to decrease platelet aggregation and thrombosis
   a. Low-molecular-weight dextran
   b. Heparin drip
   c. Aspirin
6. Flap failure is usually caused by inadequate circulation or infection

B. Repair of craniofacial deformities
1. Maintain elevation of head of bed to decrease intracranial pressure
2. Place on seizure precautions
3. Minimize activities that increase intracranial pressure
   a. Crying in children
   b. Straining
4. Medicate to provide comfort but not enough to mask neurologic symptoms

C. Cleft lip and palate repair
1. Position side to side, never prone
2. Avoid crying and restlessness that strain suture lines
3. Monitor for bleeding
   a. Swelling or hematoma at lip
   b. Excessive swallowing
4. Maintain in elbow extension splints
5. Gentle oral suctioning with soft-tip catheter

## VIII. Discharge for Ambulatory Surgical Patients

A. Ensure readiness for discharge
1. Alert and responsive
2. Pain controlled
3. Absence of bleeding and hematoma
4. Stable vital signs
5. Control of nausea and adequate oral intake
6. Urinary voiding
7. Ambulation

B. Ensure understanding of discharge instructions and follow-up care
1. Rhytidectomy
   a. Maintain elevation of head
   b. Apply cold compresses
   c. Maintain integrity of facial dressing
   d. Limit facial movement
   e. Normal sequelae
      (1) Temporary numbness of ears and cheeks
      (2) Mild pain
   f. Signs to report
      (1) Increased facial pain or unilateral numbness
      (2) Signs and symptoms of infection

2. Rhinoplasty
   a. Maintain nasal packing and avoid removal of clots from nose
   b. Change "drip pad" prn
   c. Use of antiemetics and analgesia
   d. Avoid pressure to nose, including glasses
   e. Sneeze through mouth
3. Blepharoplasty
   a. Minimize reading for 48 hours
   b. Elevate head
   c. Apply cool, moist compresses
   d. Expect periorbital ecchymosis and swelling
4. Mentoplasty
   a. Maintain dressing
   b. Liquid or soft diet
   c. Meticulous oral hygiene if oral incisions placed
5. Chemical face peel
   a. Avoid picking or scratching of skin
   b. Application of antibiotic or hydrocortisone ointments or powders
   c. Gentle facial cleansers
   d. Pain management
   e. Expectation of erythema
6. Dermabrasion
   a. Changing of antibiotic ointment and gauze per surgeon preference
   b. Expectation of weeping serous fluid
   c. Pain management

## OVERVIEW OF BURN INJURY

**I. Function of Skin**
- A. Protective barrier against trauma and infection
  1. Primary function
  2. First line of defense against infection
- B. Retention of body fluids
- C. Regulation of body temperature
  1. Vasoconstriction and vasodilation
  2. Evaporation of water
- D. Secretion and excretion
  1. Secretion of oil from sebaceous glands to lubricate skin, preventing cracks and organism invasion
  2. Excretion of water, sodium chloride, cholesterol, and urea from sweat glands
- E. Production of vitamin D
- F. Sensation
  1. Pressure, pain, touch, temperature
  2. Reaction to environmental stimuli
- G. Generates new skin
- H. Contributes to self-image

**II. Anatomy of Skin**
- A. Epidermis
  1. Outermost layer
  2. Made up of five layers
     a. Stratum corneum
     b. Stratum lucidum

c. Stratum granulosum
d. Stratum spinosum
e. Stratum germinativum
3. Surface and deepest layers of most importance in burn care
a. Stratum corneum
(1) Dead keratinized cells
(2) Provides vapor barrier and protects body from microorganisms and chemical irritants
b. Stratum germinativum
(1) Regenerates epithelial covering
(2) Necessary for spontaneous healing
4. Blood supplied by dermis
5. Lines skin appendages (e.g., sebaceous glands, sweat glands, and hair follicles)
a. New skin can be generated from lining of skin appendages even if epidermis is destroyed
6. Varies in thickness
a. Thickest at soles of feet, palms, scapula
b. Thinnest at eyelids

B. Dermis
1. True skin
2. Consists of collagen and fibrous connective tissue
3. Contains nerve endings, capillaries, lymph system
4. Skin appendages originate in dermis

C. Subcutaneous tissue (superficial fascia)
1. Attached to dermis by collagen
2. Contains adipose tissue and loose connective tissue
3. Holds burn tissue (eschar) tightly, making eschar removal difficult

D. Deep fascia
1. Surrounds muscle and blood vessel
2. Connects to periosteum of bone

**III. Determining Severity of Burn Injury**

A. Size of percent of body surface involved (TBSA, or total body surface area)
1. Rule of 9's (Fig. 30–1)
a. Body areas divided into equal multiples of 9
b. Head and each arm equal 9%
c. Chest, back, and leg equal 18% each
d. Perineum equals 1%
2. Berkow's method, or Lund and Browder chart
a. Used for children
b. Adjusts for differences in body part sizes between adults and children
(1) Head in child <2 years = 18%
(2) Each leg in child <2 years = 13%
3. 1% method
a. Used for quick assessment
b. Palmar surface of patient's hand equals approximately 1% TBSA
4. Major burn injury
a. Adults
(1) Greater than 25% TBSA partial-thickness burn, age <40 years
(2) Greater than 20% TBSA partial-thickness burn, age >40 years
(3) Greater than 10% TBSA full-thickness burn
b. Children
(1) Greater than 20% TBSA partial-thickness burn
(2) Greater than 10% TBSA full-thickness burn

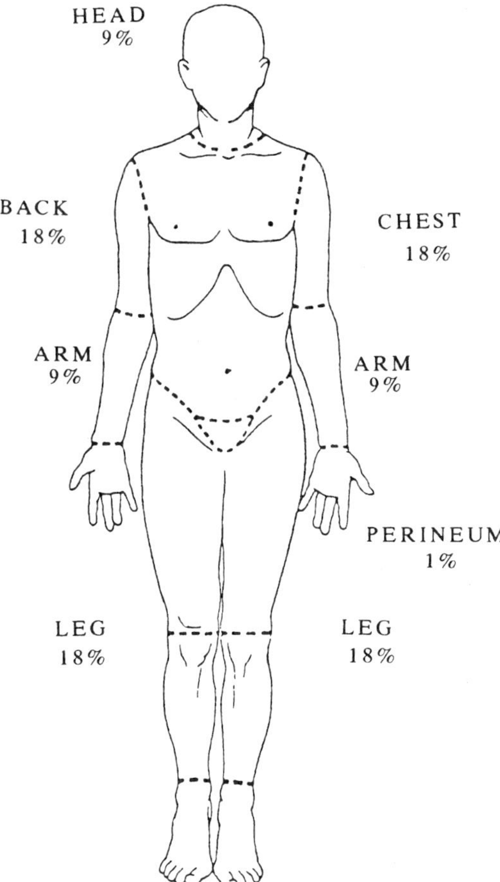


**FIGURE 30–1** The rule of nines.

c. Other factors
   (1) Burns of face, eyes, ears, hands, feet, and perineum
   (2) Electrical burns
   (3) Burns complicated by inhalation injury or major trauma
   (4) Patients with preexisting diseases may impact recovery (e.g., diabetes, congestive heart failure)

B. Depth of injury
1. Superficial injury (first degree)
   a. Affects epidermis only
   b. Appearance: skin intact, red, blanches
   c. Painful
   d. Healing time: 2 to 10 days
   e. Causes: flash burns, sunburn
2. Partial-thickness injury (second degree)
   a. Affects epidermis and part of dermis, leaving skin appendages intact
   b. Levels
      (1) Superficial partial-thickness: affects upper layers of dermis
      (2) Deep partial-thickness:
         (a) Affects lower layers of dermis
         (b) May convert to full-thickness injury
   c. Appearance
      (1) Superficial partial-thickness: red, moist, blistered, blanches

(2) Deep partial-thickness: deep red, moist, areas of white or yellow tissue, delayed capillary refill

d. Very painful

e. Healing time

(1) 5 to 21 days if affecting outer layers of dermis

(2) 21 to 35 days if affecting deeper layers of dermis

(a) May convert to full-thickness burn in first few days after burn

(b) May require skin grafting

f. Causes: scald, flame, chemicals

3. Full-thickness injury (third degree)

a. Affects epidermis and entire dermis and may extend to subcutaneous tissue, muscle, or bone

b. Appearance: hard, dry, leathery; color may be black, tan, white; nonblanching

c. Minimal to no pain

d. Healing time: requires excision and skin grafting

e. Causes: flame, scald, chemicals, electrical, contact with hot surfaces

C. Part of body involved

1. Specific areas of body have significant impact on healing, cosmetic appearance, and function

2. Head, face, and chest burns significantly related to respiratory function

3. Hand, face, and feet burns significantly related to cosmetics and function

4. Perineal burns significantly related to infection

5. Circumferential burns significant because of compromised circulation

D. Burning agent

1. Scald

a. Most common type of burn, especially in children

b. Caused by immersion, splash, or steam

2. Flame and flash burns

a. Second most common type of burn

b. Commonly associated with smoke inhalation

c. Frequently full thickness in nature

d. From house fires, kerosene or gasoline ignition

3. Contact burns

a. Area burned is well defined in appearance in shape of item contacted

b. May occur from hot metal, asphalt, or sand

4. Chemical burns

a. Less than 10% of all injuries

b. Acid or alkali

c. May be topical or ingested

d. More commonly from industrial accidents

5. Electrical

a. Least common

b. May cause significant internal or external damage

c. Direct current or alternating current

d. Alternating current more dangerous than direct current because of increased risk for cardiopulmonary arrest

e. Cataracts may occur 1 to 2 days to 3 years after burn

f. May require extensive reconstructive surgery (e.g., myocutaneous flaps)

E. Age of victim

1. Higher mortality in patients less than 2 years or older than 60 years

2. Thinness of skin in very young and very old makes injury more likely

3. Changes in immune status alter ability to heal

F. Preexisting medical conditions that impair healing process

1. Cardiovascular disease

2. Diabetes
3. Pulmonary disease: asthma, chronic obstructive pulmonary diseases (COPD)

G. Other associated injuries at time of burn that might affect healing
1. Smoke inhalation
2. Traumatic injury (e.g., fractures, closed head injury)
3. Need for tracheostomy significantly increases mortality risk

**IV. Physiologic Changes After Burn Injury**

A. Burn shock
1. Massive fluid and protein shifts from intravascular space to interstitium
a. Vasodilation, increased capillary permeability, and altered cell membrane at injury site
b. Hypovolemic shock occurs because of volume loss
c. Edema of tissues occurs from increased capillary permeability
2. Hypovolemia stage lasts for first 48 hours after injury
3. Sodium and protein lost from intravascular space into interstitium

B. Hypothermia
1. Loss of water and heat by evaporation
2. Loss of skin's ability to vasoconstrict or vasodilate in response to environmental temperature

C. Cardiovascular
1. Decreased cardiac output related to hypothermia, uncompensated hypovolemia, and release of myocardial depressant factor
2. Catecholamine release from stress response causes vasoconstriction and increases systemic vascular resistance
3. Potential for decreased organ perfusion exists

D. Pulmonary
1. Potential airway obstruction from edema of face and neck
2. Decreased chest wall compliance if chest expansion is impaired by chest burns
3. Bronchopulmonary mucosal damage from smoke inhalation

E. Metabolic
1. Hypermetabolic state occurs as result of stress response
2. Patient develops catabolic state

F. Immunologic
1. Postburn immunosuppression occurs from changes in humoral and cell-mediated immunity
2. Loss of skin as first line of defense

G. Hematologic
1. Potential red cell hemolysis from thermal injury
2. Decreased coagulation ability from loss of clotting factors into interstitium

H. Gastrointestinal
1. Development of paralytic ileus
2. Prone to stress ulcer development

I. Renal failure
1. Related to inadequate fluid resuscitation
2. Related to myoglobinuria from muscle damage in electrical and severe flame burns

## COMMON SURGICAL BURN PROCEDURES

**I. Escharotomy**

A. Indicated for circumferential full-thickness burns
1. Burn eschar acts as tourniquet
a. Decreases arterial flow
b. Causes venous congestion

2. Common sites are extremities or trunk

B. Linear incisions placed extending through burn eschar down to superficial fascia releasing constriction

C. May be performed with or without anesthesia
   1. Nerve endings in eschar are dead
   2. Premedication to relieve anxiety and discomfort

## II. Excision and Skin Grafting

A. Goal is to restore function and maximize cosmetic appearance
   1. Performed in burns with limited or inability to heal
   2. May require grafting months to years after injury to revise scar tissue
   3. Principles of grafting similar for burns and nonburn wounds requiring skin coverage

B. Nonviable tissue removed

C. Graft sources
   1. Autograft
      a. Patient's own skin used
      b. Permanent
   2. Cultured autologous human epithelium
      a. Biopsy of patient's skin obtained
      b. Skin grown in Petri dish and then grafted to patient
   3. Homograft (allograft)
      a. Skin obtained from another human
      b. Fresh cadaver
         (1) Provides a temporary covering to excised tissue awaiting permanent grafting
         (2) May be placed over a widely meshed autograft to promote graft take
         (3) Patient will eventually reject
      c. Processed human dermis (Alloderm)
         (1) Donated skin processed to remove components that cause rejection
            (a) Epidermis removed
            (b) Cells that contain antigen targets for rejection removed
            (c) Tissue (dermal matrix) freeze dried for storage
         (2) Procedure
            (a) Wound excised
            (b) Alloderm applied to wound bed
            (c) Thin autograft applied over Alloderm
   4. Skin substitutes
      a. Integra
         (1) Bilaminate skin substitute
            (a) Dermal analog of collagen fibers
            (b) Epidermal analog is Silastic membrane
         (2) Applied to excised wound
            (a) Dermal analog develops vasculature
            (b) Silastic membrane removed after dermal vascularity established (approximately 2 weeks)
            (c) Thin autograft applied after Silastic membrane is removed
         (3) Requires a two-step process
            (a) Excision and application of Integra
            (b) Removal of Silastic membrane and autograft
      b. Biobrane
         (1) Synthetic polymer dressing
         (2) Porcine collagen base with nylon covering
         (3) Placed over excised tissue
         (4) Patient's dermis binds with collagen base
         (5) Biobrane removed after dermal healing

(6) Patient must have capacity for dermal regeneration
(7) May be placed over donor sites
5. Heterograft (xenograft)
a. Tissue from another species, usually pigskin
b. Temporary covering over excised wounds

**III. Primary Closure**
A. May be used for small burns
B. Burn tissue is excised and closed primarily

## INTEROPERATIVE CONSIDERATIONS FOR THE BURN PATIENT

**I. Surgical Concerns**
A. Minimize physiologic stress experienced by patient
1. Limit operative time to 2- to 3-hour sessions
2. Limit excision to 20% of total body surface at any one operative session
B. Selection of donor sites
1. Preferred sites: thighs, buttock, abdomen, back, scalp
2. Best color match if skin is obtained from area near burn
C. Types of grafts
1. Split-thickness skin graft
a. Donor skin contains epidermis and part of dermis
b. 0.012-inch thickness
c. Graft "takes" as capillaries grow in from granulation bed into graft (begins to occur after 48 hours)
d. Donor site reepithelializes in 10 to 14 days and may be ready as donor site again in 21 days (scalp donor sites may heal in 7 days)
2. Full-thickness graft
a. Entire epidermis and dermis used as donor
b. Used to cover deep defects, tendons, bone
c. Requires split-thickness skin graft on donor area that full-thickness skin was removed from
d. Less hyperpigmentation and contracture than with split-thickness skin graft
3. Mesh graft
a. Split-thickness skin graft in which donor skin is passed through mesher to produce slits in skin
b. Allows for donor skin to be stretched to cover large area
(1) May be meshed 1.5 to 3 times original size
(2) Useful in large burns
c. Meshing helps prevent fluid or blood from accumulating under graft, which prevents "take"
d. Less cosmetically perfect than sheet graft
4. Sheet graft
a. Split-thickness skin graft placed on wound without meshing
b. Provides better cosmetic result, especially for hands, face, and neck
c. Fluid and blood can accumulate under graft, affecting "take"
D. Burn wound excision
1. Tangential (sequential) excision
a. Sequential removal of tissue until viable dermis is reached
b. Provides optimal functional and cosmetic result
c. Large blood loss may occur
d. May be difficult to determine end point of excision—too much or too little may be excised

2. Fascial excision
   a. Used in deep full-thickness burns that may extend into fat or underlying tissues
   b. Tissue is sharply dissected to fascia
   c. Blood loss is less than if tangentially excised
   d. Easier to determine end point of excision
   e. Risk of injury to nerves, joints, tendons
   f. Results in cosmetic defects

E. Control of bleeding
1. Patient may have considerable blood loss
2. Controlled with thrombin, epinephrine soaks, electrocautery
3. Hemostasis must be obtained before graft is placed

F. Factors promoting graft "take"
1. Hemostasis
2. Graft secured and immobilized
3. Prevention of infection
4. Good nutrition

## II. Anesthesia Concerns

A. Anesthetic agents
1. Pharmacokinetics may be altered because of physiologic changes that occur after major burn injury
2. Serum protein levels decrease, making agents that bind to albumin more pharmacologically active
3. Narcotic anesthesia amounts may be high because of developed tolerance
4. Amount of cardiac depression must be weighed if inhalation agents are used
5. Increased sensitivity to depolarizing neuromuscular blocking agents occurs and may result in hyperkalemic response
   a. Succinylcholine use contraindicated because of hyperkalemic response
6. Hyposensitivity to nondepolarizing neuromuscular blocking agents

B. Ventilatory needs
1. Intubation may be difficult because of burns of face and neck or limited oral mobility requiring use of fiberoptic bronchoscope
2. Hypermetabolic response results in increased oxygen consumption and carbon dioxide production
3. Chest wall compliance may be decreased if chest burns are present
4. Ventilation/perfusion mismatches may occur with pulmonary injuries
5. Patient may need increased minute ventilation because of hypermetabolic state and positive end-expiratory pressure (PEEP)
6. Monitor oxygen saturation and end-tidal carbon dioxide

C. Prevention of hypothermia
1. Room temperature maintained at 85° F
2. Use of warming blankets and warmed fluids
3. Temperature monitoring
4. Warmed inspired gases

D. Maintaining hemodynamic stability
1. May be prone to hypotension because of position changes as donor skin is obtained and burn wound prepared
2. Fluid loss through evaporation and bleeding
   a. Replacement with red blood cells and fresh frozen plasma
   b. Crystalloids to maintain adequate urine output without giving excess salt

E. Fluid resuscitation criteria
1. Calculated fluid requirements for first 24 to 48 hours after injury

2. Thermal injuries uncommonly taken to operating room during burn shock period (first 24 to 48 hours)
   a. Early excision after 24 hours to begin wound coverage to decrease metabolic rate and decrease wound infection
3. Calculated requirements (Parkland formula)
   a. 4 ml/kg/TBSA percent of injury
   b. One half of calculated requirements given over first 8 hours from time of injury
   c. One half of calculated requirements given over next 16 hours
   d. Fluids adjusted to maintain urinary output
      (1) Adult: 0.5 to 1 ml/kg/hr
      (2) Children: 1 to 2 ml/kg/hr
4. Fluids used
   a. Isotonic crystalloid
      (1) Normal saline
      (2) Lactated Ringer's
   b. Hypertonic saline may be used
      (1) Increases osmotic pull back to intravascular space
      (2) Decreases total fluid requirements and assists to minimize edema formation
   c. Colloids rarely used in first 12 hours after burn injury because of increased capillary permeability
5. Electrical injury fluid requirements
   a. More difficult to estimate fluid needs
   b. Injury greater internally than what is seen externally
   c. Calculate on the basis of Parkland formula
   d. Adjust fluids to maintain urinary output of 75 to 100 ml/hr in adults or 2 to 3 ml/kg/hr in children
   e. Add sodium bicarbonate to alkalinize urine, promoting myoglobin excretion
   f. Administer mannitol to increase urinary flow, promoting myoglobin excretion
6. Inadequate fluid resuscitation is primary cause of death in first 24 to 48 hours after injury

## POSTOPERATIVE CONCERNS FOR THE BURN PATIENT

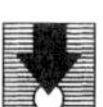

### NURSING DIAGNOSIS

Examples of related nursing diagnostic categories include:
- Alteration in tissue perfusion: peripheral
- Impaired gas exchange
- Pain
- Fluid volume deficit
- Hypothermia
- Potential for infection
- Body image disturbance
- Anxiety

**I. Airway and Ventilatory Needs**

A. Upper airway injuries
   1. Caused from heat injury to oronasopharynx and vocal cords
   2. Swelling usually peaks 48 hours after injury
   3. Edema may lead to obstruction
   4. Intubation performed early, often prophylactically

5. If patient is extubated postoperatively, observe for signs of obstruction (e.g., stridor, tachypnea, increased work of breathing, low $Sa_{O_2}$, low $Sv_{O_2}$)
6. Secure endotracheal tube
   a. Use ties in patients with face burns
   b. Tape will not adhere
   c. Avoid pressure on burned nose or ears
   d. Monitor ties for constriction as facial swelling increases

B. Lower airway injuries
1. Injuries below glottis are caused by chemical irritants released from smoke
2. Lower airway damage results in
   a. Increased airway irritability, laryngospasm, bronchospasm
   b. Bronchiolar edema and impaired airway flow
   c. Increased mucus production caused by chemical irritants
   d. Damage to epithelial lining of bronchial tree and alveolar cells
3. Management considerations
   a. Frequent assessment of respiratory function and airway patency
      (1) Respiratory effort
      (2) Chest wall expansion and symmetry
      (3) Monitor oxygenation with pulse oximeter and arterial blood gases
      (4) Monitor end-tidal $CO_2$
   b. Assess need for bronchodilator therapy
   c. Assess chest expansion
      (1) Constriction of nonexcised chest burns
      (2) Constriction of chest dressings
   d. Deep breathing and coughing to facilitate mucus mobilization
   e. Provide for oxygen and ventilatory needs
      (1) May need increased minute ventilation (rate or tidal volume or both) because of hypermetabolic state
      (2) Humidified oxygen
      (3) Prevent oxygen administration device from applying pressure if grafts have been placed on face or neck

## II. Circulatory Function

A. Blood and fluid loss may be significant

B. Monitor for signs of hypovolemia
1. Tachycardia
2. Decreased blood pressure and presence of pulsus paradoxsus
3. Delayed capillary refill
4. Monitor urinary output
   a. Maintain 30 to 50 ml/hr in adult
   b. Maintain 1 to 2 ml/kg/hr in children

C. Provide fluid replacement
1. Isotonic or hypertonic crystalloids
2. Colloids: red blood cells, fresh frozen plasma, albumin

D. Monitor circulatory function distal to burn
1. Distal to escharotomy sites every 15 to 30 minutes
2. Assess circulatory compromise caused by constricting dressings or splints
3. Assessment
   a. Pulses
   b. Capillary refill
   c. Movement and sensation
   d. Color

## III. Infection

A. Thorough hand washing and gloves are essential

B. Prevent cross contamination with other patients
C. Isolation precautions, including gowns, mask, and gloves, may be necessary in large burns
D. Aseptic wound technique
E. Frequent change of invasive catheters

## IV. Temperature Control

A. Assess body temperature every 30 minutes
B. Warm fluids and blood products before infusion
C. Use heat shields or warming blankets
D. Adjust room temperature to 75° to 85° F
E. Monitor for ST segment changes caused by myocardial ischemia

## V. Wound Care

A. Monitor graft and donor sites for bleeding
   1. Grafts will fail if blood collects beneath them
   2. Dressings usually not changed for first few days
B. Monitor status of sheet grafts that do not have dressing
   1. Assess for fluid and blood collection under graft
      a. Aspiration of fluid using syringe and small-gauge needle
      b. Remove fluid by "rolling" fluid to edges of graft with cotton tip applicator
   2. Avoid pressure or shearing
   3. Antimicrobial ointment may be applied to the edges and seams of graft
C. Maintain joint immobility if graft is over joint
D. Elevate grafted extremities to minimize edema and promote venous return

## VI. Pain Control

A. Pain is usually more severe at donor site than at grafted areas
B. May have high analgesic needs because of previous narcotic needs during wound care
C. Intravenous administration preferred over intramuscular in large burns because of poor absorption
D. Avoid aspirin-containing products

## VII. Emotional Support for Patients and Families

A. Patients and families must deal with change in physical appearance from first day after injury
B. Ongoing emotional support required
   1. Change in physical appearance
      a. Long-term results may be uncertain
      b. Must begin to adjust to fact that even with the best cosmetic results patients will never look the same again
   2. Possible changes in function if severe burns of extremities, hands, feet, face
C. Surgical procedure may be the first or one of many
   1. Expectations of each may differ
   2. May view regrafting as a setback because of graft failure or poor cosmetic result
D. Provide support appropriate to stage of adjustment that patient or family is experiencing
E. Use additional health care workers to assist in support (e.g., child life specialists, clergy, mental health practitioners, social worker)
F. Priorities of care: life, limbs, looks (in that order)

## VIII. Discharge Instructions for the Ambulatory Skin Graft Patient

A. Maintain dressing dry and intact
   1. Donor site dressing may exhibit some bloody drainage
   2. Avoid getting dressings wet

B. Keep grafted area immobile
   1. Avoid activities that would cause sheer
   2. Grafts over joint must remain immobile—may have splints in place
   3. Reinforce weight-bearing status or crutch walking for lower extremity grafts
   4. Elevate grafted extremity to limit edema
C. Pain management
   1. Reinforce that donor site may be more painful
   2. Instruct on use of prescribed analgesia
D. Notify physician for
   1. Temperature >38.5° C
   2. Numbness, paresthesia of grafted extremity
   3. Pain that is not controlled by analgesia
   4. Bleeding of graft or donor site
E. Reinforce follow-up instructions
   1. Dressing usually changed and graft evaluated 3 to 5 days after grafting

## BIBLIOGRAPHY


Abadir AR, Humayum SG (eds): *Anesthesia for Plastic and Reconstructive Surgery.* St. Louis, Mosby–Year Book, 1991.

Dinman S, Giovannone MK: The care and feeding of miscrovascular flaps: how nurses can help prevent flap loss. *Plast Surg Nurs* 14:154–164, 1994.

Fritsch DE, Yurko LC: Management of patients with burns. In Phipps WJ, Cassmeyer VL, Sands JK, Lehman MK (eds): *Medical-Surgical Nursing: Concepts and Clinical Practice.* St. Louis, Mosby, 1995.

Goodman T (ed): *Core Curriculum for Plastic and Reconstructive Surgical Nurses.* Pitman, NJ, Anthony J. Janetti, 1996.

Greenfield E, Jordan B: Advances in burn wound care. *Crit Care Nurs Clin North Am* 8:203–215, 1996.

Herndon DN: *Total Burn Care.* London, WB Saunders, 1996.

Johnson PC, Barker JH: Thrombosis and antithrombotic therapy in microvascular surgery. *Clin Plast Surg* 19:799–807, 1992.

Katex P: Reduction mammoplasty. *Plast Surg Nurs* 12(2):51–52, 60, 1992.

Khouri RK: Avoiding free flap failure. *Clin Plast Surg* 19:773–781, 1992.

Mangan MA: Current concepts in breast reconstruction. *Nurs Clin North Am* 29:763–776, 1994.

Miller RD (ed): *Anesthesia.* New York, Churchill Livingstone, 1994.

Netscher DT, Clamon J: Methods of reconstruction. *Nurs Clin North Am* 29:725–739, 1994.

Nguyen TT, Gilpin DA, Meyer NA, Herndon DN: Current treatment of severely burned patients. *Ann Surg* 223:14–25, 1996.

Rosenberg GJ, Gregory RO: Lasers in aesthetic surgery. *Clin Plast Surg* 23:29–48, 1996.

Ryan F, LaFourcade C: Skin care, chemical face peeling, and skin rejuvenation. *Plast Surg Nurs* 15:167–171, 1995.

Schmidling RE, Gordon SI, Davenport BB: Treating pressure ulcers with a myocutaneous flap. *Nursing* 22(7):86–89, 1992.

Spencer KW: Selection and preoperative preparation of plastic surgery patients. *Nurs Clin North Am* 29: 697–710, 1994.

Vasconez LO, Core GB, Oslin B: Endoscopy in plastic surgery. *Clin Plast Surg* 22:585–589, 1995.

Williams LA: Facial rejuvenation. *Nurs Clin North Am* 29:741–751.

Wirt SW, Algren CL, Arnold SL: Cleft lips and palates: A multidisciplinary approach. *Plast Surg Nurs* 12(4):140–145, 162, 1992.


## REVIEW QUESTIONS

**1. In evaluating a myocutaneous flap, which one of the following signs indicates circulatory compromise?**

A. The flap is warm to touch
B. The flap has bluish coloration
C. The flap has 2-second capillary refill
D. Venous and arterial sounds are heard by Doppler ultrasonography

**2. A 45-year-old woman is admitted after a reduction mammoplasty. Her care in the PACU includes:**

A. Monitoring for hematoma or swelling
B. Maintaining her arms in the abducted position
C. Promoting active use of her arms
D. Maintaining a light, loose dressing

**3. Which of the following is not true of the optimal anesthetic agent for the plastic surgery patient?**

A. Provides adequate analgesia
B. Promotes awakening free from coughing
C. Potentiates epinephrine
D. Provides a relatively bloodless surgical field

**4. A 25-year-old man has had a split-thickness skin graft to his right leg, extending from the thigh to the calf. In the PACU he complains of significant pain. Which of the following statements is correct?**

A. Early mobilization is important to promote blood flow, prevent contracture, and decrease pain
B. Pain medication may include narcotics and aspirin-containing nonnarcotics
C. Changes in metabolism in the burn patient result in decreased narcotic needs
D. The donor area will be more painful than the grafted area

**5. Which of the following statements indicates a positive body image and psychologic readiness for rhinoplasty?**

A. My husband really wants me to have this done.
B. I know I'll get the job after the surgery is completed.
C. I wanted to have this done before the dance next week.
D. I would like my nose to look like it did before it was broken.

**6. Anesthetic induction of deliberate hypotension during plastic surgery:**

A. Decreases blood loss at the surgical field
B. Is contraindicated for procedures of the face and neck
C. Is obtained through the use of narcotic anesthetics
D. Compromises organ perfusion

**7. Anesthetic administration is adjusted on the basis of metabolic changes in the major burn patient. Which of the following statements is true regarding anesthesia?**

A. Decreased amounts of narcotics are necessary
B. Hypokalemia results if depolarizing neuromuscular blocking agents are used
C. Increased amounts of protein-binding anesthetics are necessary if the patient is hypoproteinemic
D. Anesthetics are chosen that minimize cardiac depression

**8. Monitoring for hypovolemia is important in which of the following plastic surgery procedures?**

A. Lesion excision
B. Liposuction
C. Z-plasty
D. Blepharoplasty

**9. The appropriate patient positioning after plastic surgery is:**

A. Prone position after cleft lip repair
B. Supine, flat position after abdominoplasty
C. Side-lying position after otoplasty
D. Supine, head of the bed elevated to 45 degrees after rhinoplasty

**10. The operative report indicates a full-thickness burn has been tangentially excised and a mesh split-thickness sheet graft placed. Which of the following statements is true regarding the surgical procedure?**

A. Less bleeding occurs during tangential excision than fascial excision
B. The split-thickness skin graft is composed of the entire epidermis and dermis from the donor site
C. Hemostasis is necessary before the graft is placed
D. The mesh graft will have a better cosmetic result than a sheet graft

**ANSWERS:** 1. B, 2. A, 3. C, 4. D, 5. D, 6. A, 7. D, 8. B, 9. D, 10. C

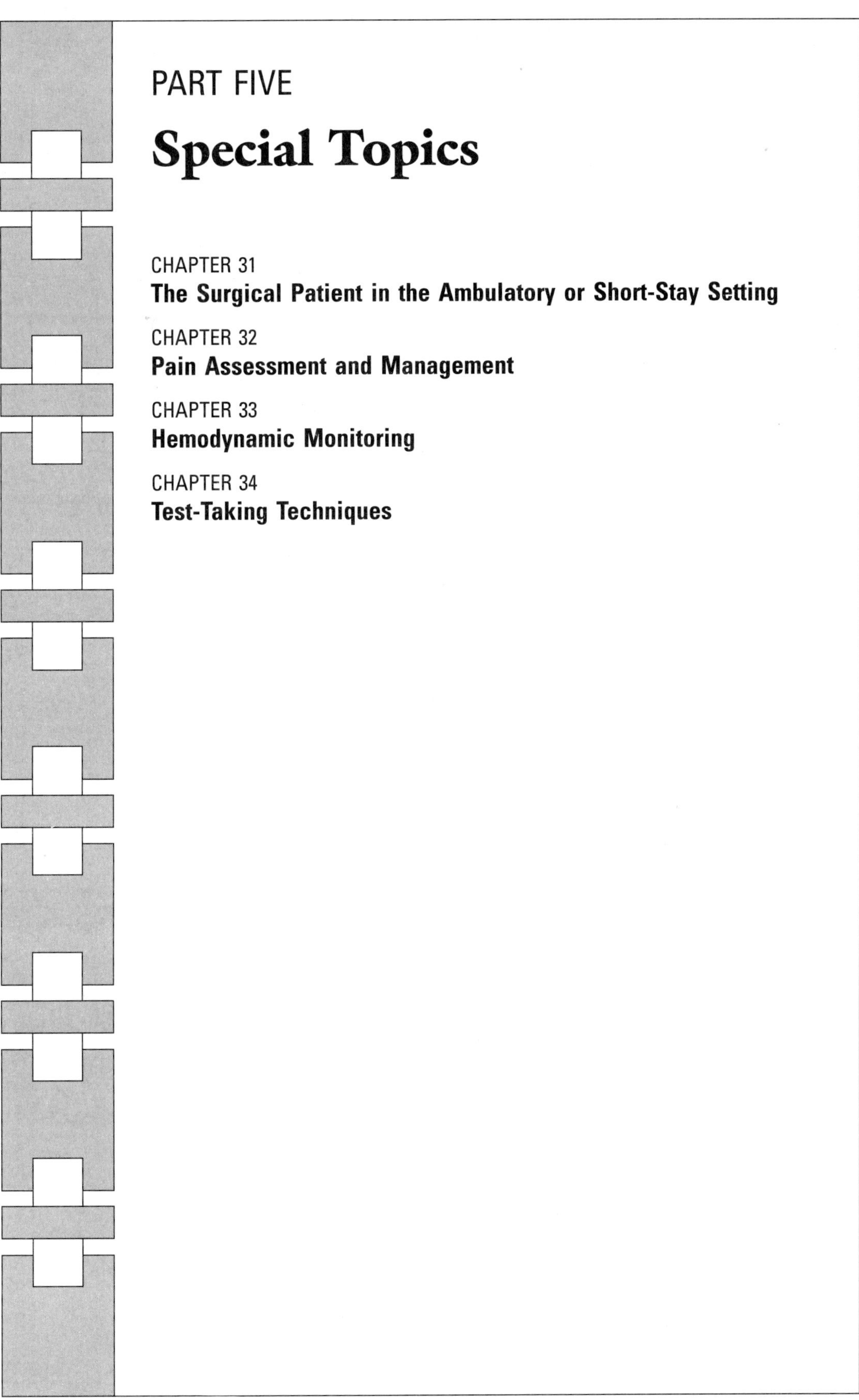

PART FIVE

# Special Topics

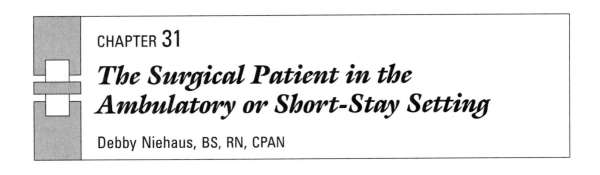

CHAPTER 31

# The Surgical Patient in the Ambulatory or Short-Stay Setting

Debby Niehaus, BS, RN, CPAN

## OBJECTIVES

**Study of the information represented by this outline will enable the learner to:**

1. Apply the nursing process to deliver safe, complete, and high-quality professional care to all perianesthesia patients in the ambulatory surgical setting.
2. Incorporate a perioperative nursing care approach with a problem- or goal-oriented plan to be implemented in preassessment, intraoperative, and postanesthesia care.
3. Monitor, intervene, and implement pain management with the ambulatory surgical patient.
4. Maintain appropriate communication with the family to minimize anxiety during the ambulatory surgical care.
5. Promote improved ability to cope with anxiety, evidenced by verbal understanding of perioperative events.

An increasing number of operative procedures that formerly would have required hospitalization are now being performed in an ambulatory surgical setting. The scope of ambulatory surgery has expanded beyond the previous confines of the hospital surgery suites to now include endoscopy, obstetrics, urology, emergency rooms, and special procedure units. An increasing number of outpatient surgical procedures are being done at hospital and privately owned, freestanding ambulatory surgery centers; at emergency care and medicenter facilities; and in physicians' offices. In the past 5 years outpatient procedures (ambulatory or short-stay in some areas of the country) have grown from 30% of all surgical cases scheduled to 70% of surgeries scheduled. Projections have been made that 85% of all surgical procedures will take place in an ambulatory or short-stay setting at the start of the next millenium.

Advances in medical technology and analgesia allow physicians to perform minimally invasive surgery with fewer serious side effects caused by postoperative pain and the effects of anesthesia. In this dynamic environment, traditional modes of providing surgical services must be modified to meet the demands of the consumers, physicians, changes in financial reimbursement, legal and professional standards, requirements of regulating bodies, and continuing educational needs.

The expanded role of the ambulatory care nurse demands knowledge, skill, creativity, autonomy, and flexibility to function efficiently in all phases of perianesthesia care. This chapter presents an overview of the ambulatory surgery environment and the key components to its success.

## THE AMBULATORY SURGERY ENVIRONMENT

**I. Changes**

A. Health care consumer

1. Educated, informed, involved in decision making
2. Expects comprehensive care in short time
   a. Competitive pricing, without increased risk

b. Quality
c. Pleasant, safe, caring environment
d. Convenience
e. Minimum time away from home, work, family, thus reducing alterations in activities of daily living and stress
f. Decrease risk of nosocomial infection (less than 5%)

B. Health care environment
1. Innovative, dynamic
2. Traditional ideas modified to meet consumer needs
a. Safe surgical care
b. State-of-the-art technologic support
c. Shortest possible time
d. Lowest possible cost and risk
e. Autonomous, attentive, knowledgeable staff
3. 60% to 70% of all surgical procedures now done in ambulatory or short-stay setting

C. Reimbursement structure
1. Dictates shorter length of stay for acute care, increase in ambulatory and short-stay care
2. Expansion in range of surgical procedures and acceptable candidates
a. Age no longer a barrier
b. Well-controlled systemic disease does not disqualify patient
3. Many operative procedures formerly requiring hospitalization now done in ambulatory setting
4. Cost of ambulatory setting: 40% to 50% less than same procedure with hospitalization
5. Up to 85% of all surgical procedures projected to be performed in ambulatory setting by 2000

## II. Challenges

A. Changes in nursing practice
1. Registered nurse (RN) challenged to be clinically efficient; deliver comprehensive, compassionate, quality care in abbreviated time frame
2. Change in primary focus from illness to wellness
3. Promotion of health and wellness before, during, and after surgical procedure
4. Perioperative nursing care needs unchanged, but time to meet needs has been sharply reduced
a. Emphasis on wellness, self-care after discharge
b. Objective: safe surgery, smooth recovery
5. Family inclusion in patient care

B. RN assumes major responsibility for ensuring
1. Appropriate, effective preassessment interview and preoperative screening
2. Preoperative assessment, evaluation
a. Physiologic and psychosocial assessment
b. Physical and psychosocial preparation
3. Patient and family education
4. Availability of support systems
5. Management of care in preoperative through postoperative phases
6. Discharge planning
7. Postdischarge follow-up

## III. Ambulatory Surgery Patient Selection Criteria

A. American Society of Anesthesiologists (ASA) physical status classifications
1. Physical status I
a. Healthy patient with no systemic disease
2. Physical status II
a. Mild systemic disease without functional limitations

b. Examples: chronic bronchitis, moderate obesity, diet-controlled diabetes mellitus, old myocardial infarction, and mild hypertension
3. Physical status III
    a. Severe systemic disease associated with definite functional limitations
    b. Examples: coronary artery disease with angina, insulin-dependent diabetes mellitus
4. Physical status IV not candidate for ambulatory surgery
    a. Severe systemic disease that is a constant threat to life
    b. Examples: organic heart disease with marked cardiac insufficiency, persisting angina, intractable dysrhythmia; advanced pulmonary, renal, hepatic, or endocrine insufficiency
5. Physical status V not candidate for ambulatory surgery
    a. Moribund patient who is not expected to survive without the operation
    b. Example: ruptured abdominal aneurysm with profound shock
6. Physical status VI not candidate for ambulatory surgery
    a. A declared brain-dead patient whose organs are being removed for donor purposes
7. Physical status E (emergency)
    a. Used to denote presumed poorer physical status of any patient in one of these categories who is operated on as an emergency

B. Physician and patient preference, usually elective procedure
C. Positive motivation
D. Good general health, assessed by physician and anesthesiologist
E. Systemic disease well controlled, low risk of hospital admission
F. Adequate or appropriate support systems
G. Insurance requirements
H. Extent of surgical procedure
I. Premature infant or expreemies who need postoperative apnea monitoring: not appropriate candidates
J. Age not disqualifier, assessed as an individual

## IV. Preoperative Preparation

A. Smooth, efficient system is essential
    1. Communicates trust, respect
    2. Sets stage for positive patient experience
    3. Compliance through understanding and organization
B. Planning allows every phase to move at a fast pace and efficiently without patients feeling rushed
C. Uncomplicated forms for collection of patient information facilitate complete documentation
    1. Health care team is provided with patient's history and medical, social, and emotional needs profile
D. Effective preoperative screening and evaluation are essential as more complex procedures are performed
    1. Special needs can be addressed
        a. Having an interpreter present from presurgical period to discharge
        b. Special positioning needed during surgery and after anesthesia phase because of preexisting physical condition
        c. Psychosocial and spiritual needs addressed
E. Preoperative or preadmission education is key to positive benefits and outcomes from surgical experience
    1. Instructs on preparation for surgery through accurate information to patient and family
    2. Provides information about physical and psychosocial outcomes expected with surgical experience
    3. Reduces patient anxiety and gives emotional support
    4. Prepares for self-care after discharge

5. Decreases potential for complications
6. Reduces number of cancellations because of noncompliance with preoperative instructions
7. Assesses current knowledge level
   a. Teaches on individual's level of understanding to promote positive outcomes
   b. Elderly, pediatric, visually or hearing impaired, mentally or physically handicapped persons have special needs

F. Active patient involvement in provision of care
   1. Attend preoperative educational session or tour facility
   2. Telephone or personal interview with ambulatory surgery nurse
      a. Patient can ask questions about surgery and instructions
      b. Opportunity to verbalize understanding of instructions and information exchanged
      c. Diminishes anxiety and stress and offers support in coping
      d. Begins planning for discharge
      e. Decreases and prevents postoperative complications
      f. Less need for postoperative analgesia
      g. Reduces length of stay at facility
      h. Improves patient satisfaction and postoperative compliance

G. Preoperative tours of facility may be helpful on individual or scheduled group basis for patient and family members
   1. Research shows tours are beneficial for pediatric patients in decreasing stress and fear on day of surgery

H. Slide presentation or video of 5 to 8 minutes may benefit
   1. Show at preadmission testing time or at facility tour
   2. Videos for patients and families to view at home can be useful
      a. Allows them to learn at their own pace and convenient

I. Teaching sessions are more productive when done before day of surgery because of higher level of stress and anxiety factors *(Refer to Chapter 6 for more details on patient education and learning strategies.)*

J. Success key: careful scheduling
   1. Accommodate and coordinate schedules of patients, anesthesiologists, and surgeons
   2. Personnel who understand perioperative process carry out scheduling
      a. Latex allergy or sensitive patients will be scheduled as the first case of the day and may be scheduled before the normal start time for the regular schedule
   3. Arrange necessary laboratory, electrocardiogram (ECG), x-ray work to be concurrent with anesthesia and nursing interviews; obtain history and physical examination for baseline data
   4. Eliminate or minimize waiting time; preoperative visit will help minimize this on day of surgery

K. Preadmission verbal and written instructions
   1. Information about NPO status before test or surgery
   2. Management of valuables: leave at home or with family
      a. May store valuables including jewelry, watches
      b. May need money for prescriptions on way home; have responsible party hold it
   3. Location of check-in and waiting room
   4. Expected arrival time on day of surgery; if pediatric patient, parent or caregiver to remain present at all times
   5. Responsible adult to drive patient home; if pediatric patient, recommend a second adult to care for child in transit
   6. What to do about medications
      a. Do not take medications the day of surgery unless instructed by anesthesiologist or surgeon and take only as directed
      b. Bring all prescription medications to the surgical facility on day of surgery

7. Appropriate clothing to wear: comfortable, loose fitting
8. Do not wear contact lenses, false eyelashes, wigs, and makeup
9. Arrange for child care for 24 hours after surgery because of drowsiness from anesthesia and pain medication (ideal)
10. Adult to stay with patient postoperatively
11. Home care instructions and restrictions
12. Ambulatory center telephone number with service hours listed
13. Available resources for meeting short- and long-term goals for care of patient
14. Map of area for family member to use in escorting patient to and from ambulatory center
15. Tours may be helpful to alleviate fear of the unknown for children before day of surgery
16. Preoperative instruction sheets given; emphasize teaching and provide information about taking or not taking usual medications
17. Preoperative anesthesia instruction and information sheet
18. Notification of center of any change in health status or problems that could delay or cancel surgery

L. Preoperative call on evening before surgery is valuable
   1. Communicates caring, individual importance
   2. Enhances assessment, patient education, patient compliance
   3. Reinforces patient's knowledge of procedure, need to arrive on time, and importance of instructions (i.e., NPO includes no gum, mints, chewing tobacco after midnight or time stated)
   4. Active listening fosters insight into patient's needs
   5. Capture information that would lead to cancellation, causing inconvenience to patient, family, staff, surgeon, anesthesia personnel, and loss of revenue for facility

## PREOPERATIVE ASSESSMENT

**I. Success Key: Communication Skills**

A. Effective communication enables nurse to
   1. Gain pertinent information
   2. Identify individual needs, resources required
      a. Physical, psychological, emotional
      b. Familial, spiritual, cultural, social
         (1) Spiritual or cultural needs as to wearing of medal or amulets during procedure discussed and compromise as to placement on the body if interferes with operative site
   3. Reduce anxiety; identify coping mechanisms
   4. Establish tone of wellness, self-care, and positive expectations
   5. Decrease likelihood of complications
   6. Verifies that informed consent has been given and signed
   7. Initiate care plan leading to safe and informed discharge
   8. Ensures the patient or responsible adult signs for receipt of preoperative instructions

B. Success key: assessment skills
   1. Assess physical, motor, sensory, or mental impairment
   2. Vital signs, including baseline $Sao_2$
   3. Astute nurse can uncover information, special needs, possible risk factors that may not have been previously noted and can share these with health care team
   4. Questions designed to elicit information
      a. Possible allergic reaction to drugs, environmental conditions, latex allergy/ sensitivity, or anesthesia
         (1) Latex-sensitive or allergic patients require strict policy and procedure guidelines

be followed in caring for the patient in preadmission and continues the day of surgery with a latex-free environment on admission, preoperative preparation, intraoperative, postoperative, and continued through discharge from the unit. *Latex allergy must be communicated to all care areas*

(2) A latex allergy cart complete with care guidelines, policy and procedure, supply and equipment resource manual, and all needed equipment and care supplies that are latex free to provide safe patient care from admission to discharge from the PACU

b. Nursing history and health history with note of current medical problems, chronic illness, or handicaps that may call for an alteration in usual care (i.e., asthma, systemic disease, familial tendencies) or need for
   (1) Diabetic Accucheck, pregnancy test
   (2) Nitro patch, asthma inhaler
   (3) Antinausea medication
   (4) Malignant hyperthermia precautions
   (5) Regional vs. general anesthesia
   (6) Steroid coverage
   (7) Latex allergy precautions (nonlatex supplies)
   (8) Special positioning
c. Nonverbal cues or casual statements may suggest need for further investigation
d. Drug use, physical or mental impairments or limitations, use of prostheses such as hearing aids
   (1) Current medications prescribed and any over-the-counter medications taken before admission
   (2) Many individuals do not consider over-the-counter medications significant
   (3) Recreational use of illegal drugs has increased
   (4) Alcohol, tobacco use could pose problems
e. Familial, cultural, spiritual considerations and individual coping mechanisms
   (1) Interpreter (support person) should be available if needed
   (2) Balance patient privacy with family-centered care
   (3) Previous response to illness, hospitalization, and surgery
   (4) In some cultures the decision for surgery is made by the head of the household or an elder, who are to be included in explanations about the surgery and its importance
f. Noncompliance with preoperative instructions
   (1) NPO, driving self, did not take prescribed medications, or took medication not ordered

5. Test results (laboratory, x-ray, ECG, pregnancy test) collected and abnormal values reported to anesthesiologist or surgeon

C. Success key: preoperative teaching
1. Assess understanding of procedure; confirm operative site
2. Reinforce patient's knowledge of procedure as explained by surgeon
3. Answer questions and continue to collect necessary data
   a. Health history, nursing history completed
   b. Goal setting, nursing care plan begun
   c. Written and verbal postoperative instructions given
      (1) Should be written for sixth grade reading level (see information on discharge, I,A,1, for list of instructions)
      (2) Provide copy of hospital discharge instructions and also available surgeon-specific written instructions
      (3) Inform patient and family that these instructions and teaching will be repeated and questions answered before discharge

      d. Patient and family education ongoing
      e. Communication to other members of care team
      f. Assessment of available home care
      g. Community support service needs
      h. Special programs for children, i.e., tours
      i. Question-and-answer time provided
      j. Paperwork completed and checked
   4. Misconceptions clarified at level of understanding
   5. Documentation of teaching: method of presentation and patient and family understanding noted on chart
   6. Learning enhanced with more than one approach (i.e., written, verbal, pictures, or through interpreter)

**II. Success Key: Special Attention**

A. Home health nurse assigned for postoperative home visit; if feasible, meet patient before surgery
   1. Home care, activity level discussed
   2. Individualized care plan formulated

B. Ancillary specialists (i.e., physical therapist and respiratory therapist) may need to meet with patient to address special postoperative care plan

C. Special attention given to support children undergoing surgery
   1. Play therapist may be employed to help child undergoing surgery
   2. Tours may be helpful in alleviating fear and stress
   3. Preoperative introduction to care team
   4. Special gifts, coloring books, or other programs to provide pleasant experience and personal touch
   5. Parents or guardian present until time for surgery
      a. May have parent accompany child to operating room
      b. Parents or guardian to remain in surgical facility

D. Special attention given to the known or suspected latex allergic or sensitive patient includes isolation from area where other patients are being readied with latex products (isolation room or recovery), bed covered so there is no direct contact with mattress, latex-free supply cart readily accessible before admission, allergy bracelet or signs clearly posted so traffic avoids area; communication of special attention conveyed to team
   1. No elasticized booties or bouffant caps; use paper surgeon caps for patient, nurses, doctors, and others caring for patient
   2. Latex-free BP cuffs (wrap patient arm or BP cuff with cotton stockinet and use regular cuff; protect arm from latex
   3. Use glass thermometer or latex-free probe covers if available
   4. Latex-free stethoscope tubing; or wrap regular stethoscope and monitor wires with nonlatex tape; use in all care areas
   5. Latex-free gloves and tourniquets to start IV, draw blood
   6. Oxygen cannula can be used; do not use masks because of elastic strap
   7. Jelco needles are latex free; use Durapore, Transpore or Microfoam tapes; Tegaderm *not* used because of latex adhesive paper
   8. IV bags if ports sealed and not used or glass IV bottles from pharmacy are used; latex-free tubing and stopcocks for IV access for medication or anesthesia with extension tubing added are used and found on latex-free cart
   9. Latex-free or glass syringes and needles are to be used
   10. Do not pierce rubber stopper on medicine vials; use single-use vials if possible
   11. Have emergency medications and latex-free supplies (i.e., AMBU bag) readily available

## III. Preoperative Medication

A. Preoperative medication administration ranges from none to a select few or to all ambulatory surgery patients
   1. May be taken by patient night before or preadmission as prescribed
      a. Patient directed by physician whether to take own insulin, antihypertensive, anticonvulsant, or steroid

B. Preoperative medications given before surgery
   1. Reduce anxiety, fear, and stress
   2. Lower incidence of nausea and vomiting
   3. Decrease discomfort and pain
   4. Reduce secretions and potential for aspiration and laryngospasm
   5. Prophylactic antibiotic to decrease chance of infection
      a. Follow hospital and recommended antibiotic protocols
      b. Monitor patient during antibiotic administration
   6. Preparation of surgical site (e.g., eyedrops)
   7. Management of diabetes, hypertension, seizures, or steroid replacement needs

C. Choice of preoperative medication depends on patient needs
   1. Level of anxiety
   2. Expectation of intraoperative and postoperative pain
   3. Desired outcomes or goals of anesthesiologist

D. Children may be given liquid medication preoperatively (i.e., a syrup that contains a tranquilizer, narcotic, and anticholinergic; or a tranquilizer mixed with syrup or juice

E. Preoperative medication may also be given intranasally, sublingually, intramuscularly, or intravenously

F. Monitor after any sedation narcotic; keep side rails up; tell patient what to expect, such as drowsiness or relaxation

G. Preoperative drugs often used in ambulatory setting (see Chapter 9 for additional information on these drugs)
   1. Narcotics: fentanyl (Sublimaze), morphine, alfentanil (Alfenta), meperidine (Demerol)
   2. Benzodiazepines: diazepam (Valium) oral or intravenously (IV), midazolam (Versed) IV, oral, or intramuscularly (IM)
   3. Antiemetics: droperidol (Inapsine), prochlorperazine (Compazine), ondansetron (Zofran)
   4. Histamine blockers: ranitidine (Zantac), cimetidine (Tagamet), and nizatidine (Axid)
   5. Gastrokinetic: metoclopramide (Reglan)
   6. Anticholinergics: atropine and glycopyrrolate (Robinul)

## IV. Goal Setting

A. Priorities established on the basis of
   1. Surgical procedure
   2. Medical and nursing diagnoses
   3. Type of anesthetic to be administered

**NURSING DIAGNOSIS**

Examples of related nursing diagnostic categories include

- Potential for airway obstruction
- Anxiety/ineffective coping patient or family
- Fear regarding anticipated pain or loss of control
- Potential knowledge deficit
- Impaired physical mobility
- Potential for grieving regarding altered body image
- Potential for injury
- Alteration in comfort/pain
- Alteration in comfort/nausea and vomiting
- Altered level of consciousness
- Alteration in parenting
- Alteration of body temperature
- Alteration in cardiovascular system
- Potential for infection
- Alteration in tissue perfusion
- Potential loss of self-control and privacy
- Potential for fluid deficit/excess
- Alteration in body elimination
- Potential for impaired verbal communication
- Potential for impaired sensory perception
- Potential or actual impairment of skin integrity

## PLANNING

**I. Standards of Perianesthesia Nursing Practice (1998)**

A. Published by the American Society of PeriAnesthesia Nurses (ASPAN); available through ASPAN's national office

B. Endorsed by American Society of Anesthesiologists

C. Set criteria by which quality of nursing care in all phases of perianesthesia care is judged

D. Guide professional nurse in providing for convenience without sacrificing quality in ambulatory or short-stay setting

E. Used to develop individualized nursing care plan

F. Provide guidelines for staffing phase I and phase II

G. Standards for PACU with recommended equipment needs, personnel management, educational guidelines, emergency care resources

**II. Success Key: Focus of Care Plan**

A. Uniqueness of each individual patient and standards of nursing practice

B. Facilitates continuity and quality care throughout perioperative process

**III. Goal Setting**

A. Bases for priorities

1. Standards of care, staff competencies
2. Surgical procedure
3. Type of anesthetic to be administered
4. Patient and family preferences; patient rights
5. Available resources

B. Strategies for achieving goals (nursing care plan) determined, documented, communicated to care team
   1. Effective communication is hallmark of quality care
      a. Enhances continuity and quality of care throughout
      b. Assists in meeting individual patient needs
      c. Reduces possible risks and liability
   2. Care plan may change if necessary as patient progresses through preoperative, intra-operative, and postoperative phases
      a. Input from all members of care team
      b. Gives direction for nursing care
   3. Plan includes nursing diagnosis, potential goals, and desired outcomes
   4. Plan contains goals that should be realistic, attainable, and focus on a positive patient outcome

## IMPLEMENTATION

**I. Postanesthesia Care, Phase I**
   A. Admission to PACU
   B. Ends with safe discharge to phase II
   C. Transfer to second stage of postanesthesia area, ends with discharge home

**II. Immediate Postanesthesia Care**
   A. PACU nurse assesses vital signs and airway patency, positions patient, applies oxygen, and ensures patient safety on admission; reporting should wait until accepting nurse has completed rapid initial assessment *unless* notified before admission of critical care need or to set up for care of latex-allergic patient
   B. Operating room (OR) circulating nurse reports events in OR that might provide insight for PACU nurse or influence nursing care (procedure, drains, special medications used during procedure [i.e., local anesthetics, antibiotics, and irrigations])
   C. Anesthesia personnel report
      1. Name and age
      2. Surgical procedure
      3. Range of vital signs, including $Sao_2$ baseline
      4. Anesthetic techniques and agents, including medications given and antagonists used, and any anesthetic complications
      5. Preoperative medications
      6. Estimated fluid and blood loss and any replacement
      7. Allergy medicine, environmental or latex (special note to isolate latex-allergic patients to provide safe care and to institute latex allergy precautions)
      8. Relevant preoperative physical and laboratory findings
      9. General health status of patient, including preoperative status and ASA classification
      10. Physical and mental impairments
      11. Any intraoperative complications, postoperative support required
      12. Information pertinent to postanesthesia care
   D. Initial assessment documentation
      1. Airway patency and respiratory function, including oxygen saturation ($Sao_2$) and, if available, end-tidal $CO_2$ ($P_{ETCO_2}$)
      2. Vital sign stability, including temperature
      3. Level of consciousness
      4. Condition of surgical site and dressing if present and note any drains or packing
      5. IV fluids, intake, and condition of IV site
      6. Urinary output
      7. Position and level of comfort

8. Sensory and motor control of areas affected by anesthetics
9. Numeric scoring system, such as Aldrete, can be used on admission and discharge to measure parameters of activity, respiration, circulation, consciousness, and color
   a. Note that revised Aldrete scale (1992) uses $Sao_2$ instead of color
10. Continue protective measures initiated preoperatively and intraoperatively using latex-free supplies and equipment noted preoperatively
    a. If elastic bandages used, must first cover extremity with a nonlatex covering to protect skin from contact

E. Nursing actions
1. Maintain patent airway: initiate chin hold, thrust, insert oral or nasal airway if needed to relieve obstruction
2. Suction endotracheal tube or oropharyngeal passages to clear excessive secretions
3. May place patient on side, if not contraindicated, especially if "full stomach" has been reported
   a. Preferred with children
   b. Maintained until conscious
4. Auscultate bilateral breath sounds with admission assessment and monitor respiratory status continually
5. Observe for hoarseness, croup, or stridor; if present, use cool mist oxygen, keep patient calm; consult an anesthesiologist immediately
6. Instruct awake patient in coughing (if not contraindicated by surgical procedure) or deep breathing exercises or both
7. Titrate oxygen per institution policy or anesthesia standing orders to maintain oxygen saturation greater than 90%; however, some patients are not at this level preoperatively and may not be at this level postoperatively; therefore consult anesthesia personnel for acceptable level of oxygen saturation
8. Assess respiratory effort, return of reflexes, muscle strength, measure of negative inspiratory force (NIF), and spontaneous tidal volume on patient with endotracheal tube; observe for any signs of pulmonary edema
9. Extubate patient when specified criteria have been met; place oxygen mask, face tent, mist mask, or nasal cannula; and assess ability to maintain $Sao_2$ above 90%
10. Oxygen should be continued on shivering patients to reduce chance of myocardial ischemia or other sequelae
11. Assess heart rate, rhythm, blood pressure on admission and according to policy during phase I stay or more often as dictated by problem identification and intervention; cardiac monitoring should be continuous in phase I
12. Monitor temperature on admission and discharge and more often if necessary to treat hypothermia or hyperthermia and to evaluate outcome of intervention
13. Elevate head of bed if no contraindications; keep side rails up for safety
14. Assess level of comfort, observe for splinting, and assess awake patient's verbal and nonverbal responses to pain
15. Request awake patient to rate level of pain (see Chapter 32)
16. Use alternative comfort methods (i.e., position change, warm blanket, and gentle touch) when appropriate
17. Titrate narcotic IV in small increments as indicated for pain control, IM injections of narcotic or nonsteroidal anti-inflammatory drugs, or oral medications, and evaluate effectiveness of these comfort measures
18. Observe for signs of nausea (e.g., excessive swallowing)
19. Administer antiemetic as ordered, and evaluate effectiveness
20. Evaluate fluid balance by assessing outputs, skin turgor, and blood pressure
21. Monitor as indicated for alteration in fluid volume, and titrate IV fluid rates as indicated
22. Observe IV site for signs of inflammation and infiltration
23. Observe patient for areas of tissue injury, redness, and skin breakdown; pad bony prominences; turn and change position to prevent tissue breakdown; check capillary

refill; and observe changes in temperature and warmth of all extremities and operative site

24. Acknowledge pain, anxiety, and fear and provide patient reassurance and comfort measures
    a. Assess verbal and nonverbal pain cues
25. Orient patient to time, place, and person with an explanation of events leading to PACU
26. Allow visitation by family member or companion when feasible
    a. Very important with pediatric or special need patients
27. Make provisions for interpreter or care giver of child or special-needs adult
28. Provide close observation of delayed awakening patient
29. Provide safe environment for staff and patients who may experience emergence delirium (padded side rails, soft restraints, pharmacologic intervention needs, staffing, and readily available assistance of anesthesia personnel)
30. Provide oral fluids or water and ice chips as allowed
31. Progression toward ambulation achieved by gradual elevation of patient's head and movement of extremities
    a. Include patient in plan as to progress toward moving to phase II and involve patient in care plan
32. Readiness for movement to phase II is individualized and may not be time based; includes physical recovery, emotional readiness, social considerations, and safety
33. Discharge to phase II care when criteria for institution have been met
    a. NOTE: Use of propofol and other short-acting anesthetic agents decreases time needed in phase I with a more alert patient able to be moved to phase II
    b. These patients have fewer side effects often seen with formerly used long-acting anesthetic agents

F. Postanesthesia care after regional and local anesthesia
1. Patients with spinal and epidural blocks need careful monitoring of vital signs, fluid intake and output, protection of extremities affected, and nurses skilled in recognizing central nervous system (CNS) complications
2. Observe and determine sensory level at which pinprick felt
    a. High spinal level can cause respiratory failure and may require assisted ventilation
3. Estimation of expected duration of effects
    a. Drug used
    b. Route of administration
    c. Addition of epinephrine (delays absorption of drug; prolongs block)
    d. Time given
4. Discharge made on the basis of hemodynamic stability and regression of sympathetic block
5. Observe for toxicity or allergic reactions to medication used in local infiltration, peripheral nerve blocks (brachial plexus, lumbar, etc.), or regional anesthesia (Bier blocks)
6. Mild symptoms can be prolonged numbness at injection site radiating to an extremity and adjoining tissue, redness, slight swelling at site, slight decrease in blood pressure
7. After a Bier block, observe for prolonged numbness of the extremity and any systemic release causing dizziness, tinnitus, drowsiness, or complaint of numbness of tongue or around lips
    a. More severe toxicity shown by cardiovascular and CNS bradycardia, AV block, decrease in cardiac output, hypotension, tremor, muscle twitching, convulsions, or regression to unconsciousness and leading to arrest
8. Pneumothorax should be suspected on any patient who has had a thoracic, neck, or shoulder block that results in shortness of breath, chest pain, and tachycardia
    a. Treat with supplemental oxygen, upright positioning, and pain medication; order x-ray film

G. Epidural and spinal anesthesia: specific considerations
  1. Hypotension caused by pooling of circulating blood volume in relaxed veins (sympathetic block), loss of volume during surgery, or bradycardia caused by blockade of cardioaccelerator fibers in high spinal anesthesia
     a. Must observe for pallor, disorientation, bradycardia
     b. Treat hypotension with vasopressor, atropine for bradycardia
  2. High spinal levels may need ventilatory support, emotional support, and careful observation; as level recedes, use of light sedation and supplemental oxygen will ease efforts
  3. Hydration with IV fluids helps to prevent postpuncture headaches; positioning with head elevated is acceptable; supine positioning in bed is not necessary unless spinal headache is already in progress
  4. Severe backache, reparalysis of legs, and/or progressive disorientation may mean an epidural hematoma, and action needs to be taken
  5. Patient with urinary retention caused by sympathetic block will need to have catheter inserted, and discharge may be prolonged
  6. Pruritus along with nausea and vomiting may result from narcotics used or histamine release; antiemetics and diphenhydramine (Benadryl) to treat; protect from complication of vomiting

H. Conditions before discharge after regional, epidural, or spinal anesthesia
  1. Patient can ambulate (providing could ambulate before surgery or is permitted postoperatively)
  2. Motor function has returned, and patient can void
  3. Level of block is receding
     a. Discharge criteria should state if it is acceptable to have patient go home with regional block in effect if no systemic involvement and a sling applied for safety to arm or crutches or wheelchair for leg safety
     b. Patient teaching must include need to protect extremity

I. Success key: postanesthesia nursing skills
  1. Broad base of knowledge
  2. Patients of all ages
  3. Many have serious systemic disease processes
  4. Able to revise plan of care to meet immediate needs

J. Understanding of anesthetic agents, drug interactions, reversal agents
  1. Particularly important in pain management
  2. Essential in maintaining respiratory competence

K. Complications
  1. Conditions tolerated as normal side effects of anesthesia in hospitalized patients are serious complications for ambulatory patients
     a. Nausea and vomiting
     b. Extended somnolence
     c. Pain
  2. Delayed recovery; may prevent discharge home or the need for continued care overnight or at an extended care unit

L. Success key: preparedness
  1. Emergencies
     a. Should not occur frequently in ambulatory setting; potential emergency ever present after anesthesia
     b. Must maintain emergency equipment, supplies, and staff skilled in their use
     c. Written policies and protocols
     d. Freestanding center must have predetermined plan and agreement with hospital for emergency admission of patients
  2. Hypoxemia may cause somnolence and confusion and lead to cardiac dysrhythmias
  3. Continuous assessment, evaluation, and intervention essential

4. Special supplies and equipment specific for pediatric patients are available to meet needs stated in competencies and Standards
5. Medication and equipment needed for malignant hyperthermia treatment should be assembled at one location, guidelines for treatment posted, and hotline number available
   a. See Chapter 17

M. Nursing care plan continues toward phase II goal of returning patient to a safe physiologic level, enabling discharge home
   1. Effective airway clearance
   2. Effective breathing pattern
   3. Adequate comfort level
   4. Tissue perfusion
   5. Temperature regulation
   6. Fluid volume balance
   7. Coping with physiologic response to surgery intervention
   8. Stability of vital signs
   9. Level of alertness, consciousness, and visual activity at baseline

## DOCUMENTATION

**I. Professional and Legal Responsibility**

A. Succinct recording of all pertinent patient care activities, attention to all needs, and legibility so that information is readily available, including
   1. Assessments
   2. Plans
   3. Interventions
   4. Evaluations
   5. Outcomes

B. Discharge documentation reflects patient's status with total assessment and patient readiness per discharge criteria

C. Discharge score recorded if numeric system used; scoring is an objective way to evaluate patient condition on multiple parameters from PACU admission to discharge

D. Note mode of transfer to phase II care and person accompanying patient, and report to receiving nurse

E. Predetermined discharge criteria approved by medical staff or anesthesia department provide for discharge to phase II
   1. If patient does not meet criteria, physician is notified, and observation is continued until later discharge or patient is admitted for additional recovery in observation unit
   2. In most facilities an anesthesiologist is in attendance or written discharge criteria are used by nurse for decision of when to discharge patient from PACU
   3. Deviation from accepted criteria requires physician's approval and notation in chart as to unmet criteria, nursing actions, and patient education
   4. Criteria for those patients ready to go to a recliner and then home are more stringent than those for patients being transferred to a 23-hour care unit or recovery care center
      a. Overnight observation and pain control at a 23-hour unit in the ambulatory surgery center or designated hospital unit after an outpatient procedure is a less costly environment than the acute care hospital setting and allows more complicated and extensive list of procedures to be done in a lower cost outpatient setting
      b. Recovery care centers provide low-cost alternative to hospitalization for patients having outpatient surgery who may need observation or care for 24 to 72 hours after surgery but not care in a more costly hospital setting
      c. Family members may stay with patient, and the center is staffed by registered nurses, usually at 5 : 1 ratio

d. Standards and guidelines apply to center accreditation
e. Home health care allows advanced procedures to be done in outpatient setting with recuperation in home

5. Patients going to phase II unit in a hospital setting to stay for multiple hours, recovery care center, or 23-hour unit for observation may be having some residual anesthesia or medication effect
   a. Need not be able to walk
   b. May need assistance with some activities of care
   c. May have nausea or pain requiring medications
   d. Need continued observation of nurses before ready for family or self-care
   e. Need for wound and dressing care assistance or management of drains or tubes

## II. Postanesthesia Care, Phase II

A. Begins with recovery from effects of anesthesia and evaluation of readiness to return home
   1. Phase II PACU nurses also may be caring for patients who have been to special procedure units and received sedation
   2. PACU nurses are assisting in care of patients receiving ambulatory acute and chronic pain management by anesthesiologist or physicians at ambulatory surgery centers

B. Report of patient status given to phase II care nurse
   1. Vital signs stable
   2. Physical and mental functions at preoperative level
   3. Success key: alert, insightful care
      a. Monitor vital signs and patient recovery status per institutional policy
      b. Watch for signs of impending complications not previously noted
         (1) Excessive bleeding or hematoma
         (2) Nausea and vomiting
         (3) Ineffective pain control
         (4) Loss of pulses to extremity; numbness; poor sensation; slow capillary refill; cool, pale skin color
         (5) Increasing somnolence, changes in sensorium
         (6) Allergic responses to medication, tape
   4. Dressings, perineal pads, and wound site (if no dressing present) are clean and dry, with no complications related to surgical procedure evident
   5. Peripheral pulses present, circulation and sensation to operated extremity intact
      a. May be discharged with residual numbness and lack of full movement resulting from use of local anesthetic or regional block per policy guidelines
      b. Sling or arm support device will be used for upper extremity still having effects of the block
      c. Postoperative sheet with neurovascular parameters should accompany any postoperative instructions
   6. Voiding if applicable
   7. Standing, walking without orthopnea, steady gait with minimal assistance when planning for discharge from phase II (not necessary for discharge to 23-hour unit)
      a. Crutch-walking instructions if indicated; written instructions or demonstration by nurse or physical therapist
      b. Return demonstration by patient of ability to use crutches appropriately or referral to physical therapist for gait training
      c. Determine appropriateness of crutch size
      d. For latex-allergic patients, cover axillary pads and handgrips with latex-free tape or apply cotton washcloths and secure with latex-free tape
   8. Instruction and patient demonstration of understanding and ability to manage other prostheses, braces, sling
   9. Patient can visit with family and friends and take light refreshments while resting (in lounge chair or wheelchair)

C. Criteria to determine readiness for discharge
   1. Vital signs stable and blood pressure within 20% of preoperative value
   2. Patient steady when upright and can ambulate (if able to preoperatively or permitted postoperatively) without dizziness
   3. Mental status and vision approaching preoperative status
   4. Nausea and vomiting controlled and oral fluids tolerated
      a. Be able to cough and swallow
      b. May not be required for all patients; clinical judgment
   5. Pain and discomfort reasonably controlled
   6. Operative site dry and dressing, if applied, intact
   7. Circulation not impaired by cast or dressing and motion and sensation at acceptable level
   8. Voiding after epidural and spinal anesthesia, hernia repair, pelvic procedures, urinary procedures, or in patients with history of retention
   9. Full motor, sensory, and sympathetic functions must return before patients receiving epidural or spinal anesthesia can be discharged
   10. Regional anesthesia still in effect to arm needs to be evaluated for adequate circulation and have sling or protection for numb extremity to avoid injury
   11. Need to be progressing toward assisted care and self-care

## EVALUATION AND DOCUMENTATION

**I. Professional and Legal Responsibility**

A. Hospital or facility written policy as to necessity for anesthesiologist to be present to discharge patients from PACU or statement in policy approved by anesthesia or medical staff that PACU nurse can discharge patient
   1. Phase II PACU nurse can discharge patients providing there is a written anesthesia or medical staff policy that allows nurse to discharge patient and patient meets policy criteria
   2. If patient does not meet criteria, PACU nurse needs to notify anesthesiologist or physician in charge of patient care to assess, evaluate, and give discharge order
   3. Anesthesiologist or physician may plan for additional observation in 23-hour unit, hospital setting, recovery care center, or home nursing care for patient unable to meet criteria to be discharged home under routine dismissal guidelines

B. All pertinent details of care, assessments, interventions, outcomes documented appropriately and legibly

C. Documentation of patient and family education and understanding acknowledged

D. Documentation of prescriptions for pain and antibiotics and printed information about medications given to responsible family member or companion

E. Documentation of providing physician and facility telephone numbers for emergencies or clarification of care after discharge

F. Documentation of discharge to care of responsible adult if patient has received anesthesia, medication, or sedation

## DISCHARGE

**I. Discharge Order by Surgeon or Anesthesiologist Per Policy**

A. Review of discharge instructions orally; patient and family have understanding verbalized and charted; copy of printed instructions (can include the following) given to patient and responsible adult as reinforcement of teaching
   1. A responsible person needs to drive you home; have someone stay with you today (if only local anesthesia given, may drive self)

2. Rest quietly and restrict activity for rest of day
3. Do not make important decisions, drink alcohol, drive a car, operate heavy machinery, cook, or handle dangerous household appliances and kitchen knives for 24 hours after anesthesia, IV sedation, or while taking pain medication
4. Do not take tranquilizers, sleeping pills, aspirin products, or over-the-counter medicine for next 24 hours, unless directed to
5. Check the operative site for signs of excessive bleeding, swelling, redness, or discoloration; notify your physician
6. Observe for signs of infection with dressing odor or temperature greater than 100° F; notify your physician immediately
7. Take prescription medication as directed by physician (take medicine with food to avoid stomach upset unless pharmacist or prescription container advises otherwise)
8. Start out on liquids and advance to soft diet; if nausea occurs, eat or drink nothing for 1 to 2 hours and then start back on fluid with progression to regular diet as tolerated
9. If nausea and vomiting persist, notify your physician
10. If unable to urinate, notify physician or emergency referral
11. Follow any other written or oral instructions from your physician and schedule your follow-up appointment as directed
12. Special instructions individualized as to procedure can be added to basic instructions given to all patients
    a. Application of ice, circulation check, elevation, sling, use of crutches and any prosthetic devices
    b. Dressing change, shower and bath restrictions
    c. Limits on stairs, lifting, sexual activity, return to work or school, and any prescribed exercise program
    d. Specialized instruction sheets or cards specific to individual surgeons

B. Patient meets discharge criteria and is assessed to be ready for discharge from phase II unit
C. Confirm availability of safe transport; competent individual to stay with patient at home (legal and professional responsibility) documented on discharge note
D. Provide for emergency after-hours care by giving telephone number of physician, facility, or emergency after-hours referral
E. Patient transported to car ambulatory or by wheelchair as per discharge policy
F. Discharge criteria and discharge instructions for pediatric patient should be adapted to the age and abilities of child
G. All documentation completed and charted legibly
H. Family and patient teaching important if latex allergy identified preoperatively or during this admission for care
   1. Patient and family made aware of need for medic alert tag for emergency situations and need to have auto-inject epinephrine kit and know how to use it
   2. Notify family doctor and other medical providers of allergy
   3. Parents need to notify school officials of the allergy and all doctors' offices that provide care so that precautions in providing care or in an emergency will be given
   4. *Communication* from preadmission, preoperatively, intraoperatively, and postoperatively through discharge is mandatory when caring for a latex-sensitive or allergic patient. Education of fellow health care providers, patients, families, and the general public of avoidance of latex products for noted and potential latex-allergic patients is needed
   5. Report any incident or adverse latex reaction or medical device to management and notification by administration to the Food and Drug Administration Reporting Program if applicable

## II. Follow-up Telephone Call Next Day Completes Care

A. Open-ended questions to elicit information from or about patient
B. Call should take place early the following day to give support, answer questions, evaluate any problems or complications that patient is experiencing; also, more likely to reach patient

C. Report of operative site and any bleeding or drainage
D. Pain management, medication, and comfort measures used
E. Nausea, vomiting, or dizziness
F. Fever, any signs of infection, circulation changes
G. Nutritional and elimination status
H. Any complications noted after discharge with need for treatment or follow-up should be reported to management, the surgeon, and if applicable the anesthesiologist and patient's family physician
I. Documentation includes call date, time, and name of caller, attempts to reach, and who provided information about patient
   1. All information received by caller on patient status
   2. Problem identification, complications, emergency room visits, or hospital admissions
   3. Resolution and follow-up with appropriate persons notified; assessment and evaluation to ensure problem does not recur
   4. Patient satisfaction with care or improvement suggestions
   5. Documentation will become part of medical record and be used in accreditation review for adherence to care plan
   6. Follow through of any problems or complaints may alleviate costly legal cases and promote goodwill
J. Outcomes of care and patient satisfaction can be monitored through follow-up telephone interview as an extension of aftercare to home and in addition can be source of information gathered for unit quality improvement program
   1. Outcomes measured by audits, indicators, and patient specifics that include follow-up telephone call
      a. See Chapter 2
   2. Other outcomes are in providing sense of caring and concern to patient and nurse feedback for job satisfaction
   3. Call is a personal touch and a great marketing tool in that word-of-mouth sharing to friends and family brings referrals
K. Questionnaires and opinion polls returned by patient and family as to care and satisfaction with facility, service, and staff also can become part of quality improvement program and be used for accreditation, documentation, and evaluation purposes

## BIBLIOGRAPHY

American Society of Post Anesthesia Nurses: *Ambulatory Post Anesthesia Nursing Outline: Content for Certification*. Richmond, Va, The Society, 1994.

American Society of PeriAnesthesia Nurses: *Standards of Perianesthesia Nursing Practice 1998*. Thorofare, NJ, The Society, 1998.

Bean M: Preparation for surgery in an ambulatory surgery unit. *J Post Anesth Nurs* 5(1):42–47, 1990.

Burden N: *Ambulatory Surgical Nursing*. Philadelphia, WB Saunders, 1993.

Burden N: Malignant hyperthermia in the ambulatory surgery setting. *J Post Anesth Nurs* 7(3):209, 1992.

Burden N: Telephone follow-up of ambulatory surgery patients following discharge is a nursing responsibility. *J Post Anesth Nurs* 7(4):256–261, 1992.

Caldwell LM: The influence of preference for information on preoperative stress and coping in surgical outpatients. *Appl Nurs Res* 4(4):177–183, 1991.

Callahan CR: Could pain management be the next big profit center? *Same Day Surgery* 16(11):161–164, 1992.

Carlson K: *Certification Review for Perianesthesia Nursing*. Philadelphia, W.B. Saunders, 1996.

Crawford FJ: Managing quality and reducing risks in ambulatory surgery. *Semin Periop Nurs* 1(3):153–166, 1992.

Documentation form serves as quality assurance tool for ASC. *Same Day Surgery* 14(5):64–67, 1990.

Eddy ME, Coslow BI: Preparation for ambulatory surgery: A patient education program. *J Post Anesth Nurs* 6(1):5–12, 1991.

Emmons M, McDonald S: *Exposing Latex Allergies*. Cincinnati, *The Cincinnati Enquirer*, Jan. 15, 1997.

Fallo PC: Developing a program to monitor patient satisfaction and outcome in the ambulatory surgery setting. *J Post Anesth Nurs* 6(3):176–180, 1991.

Federated Ambulatory Surgery Association: Expanding the scope of ambulatory surgery. *FASA Update* 10(2):9–14, 1993.

Figley E, Burden N: Preparing for the unexpected in the ambulatory surgery unit. *J Post Anesth Nurs* 6(2): 117–120, 1991.

Frost EAM: *Post Anesthesia Care Unit: Current Practice,* 2nd Ed. St Louis, CV Mosby, 1990.

Haines N: Same day surgery: Coordinating the education process. *AORN J* 55(2):573–578, 1992.

Heinen C, Paul M: "Operation information" for ambulatory surgical patients. *Nurs Management* (OR/ Ambulatory Surgery Edition) 23(8):64Q–64T, 1992.

Hill GJ: *Outpatient Surgery,* 3rd Ed. Philadelphia, WB Saunders, 1988.

Hill JM: Time saving formats for patient care planning in outpatient surgery units. *J Post Anesth Nurs* 6(3): 181–184, 1991.

Johnson and Johnson Medical Inc: Latex sensitivity: Its causes and implications to hospitals. 21130JH: 4–13, Jan. 31, 1995.

Lea SG, Phippen ML: Client education in the ambulatory surgery setting. *Semin Periop Nurs* 1(4):203–223, 1992.

Litwack K: *Post Anesthesia Care Nursing,* 2nd ed. St Louis, Mosby–Year Book, 1995.

Luckmann J (ed): *Saunders Manual of Nursing Care.* Philadelphia, W.B. Saunders, 1997.

Mamaril ME: Standard of care: Legal implications in the post anesthesia care unit. *J Post Anesth Nurs* 8(1): 13–20, 1993.

Noon B, Paul A: Ambulatory surgery: Integrating the preadmission program. *Nurs Management* (OR/ Ambulatory Surgery Edition) 23(7):112A, 112D, 112H, 1992.

Parnass SM: Problem management in the ambulatory surgery post anesthesia care unit. *Anesthesiol Clin North Am* 8(2):399–421, 1990.

Patient training, follow-up speed recovery. *Same Day Surgery* 15(1):1–4, 1991.

Petersen CA: Postoperative follow-up: Tracking compliance and complications. *Semin Periop Nurs* 1(4): 255–260, 1992.

Philip BK: Patients' assessment of ambulatory anesthesia and surgery. *J Clin Anesthesia* 4(5):355–358, 1992.

Phippen ML: Ambulatory surgery: Recovery to discharge. *Semin Periop Nurs* 1(4):249–254, 1992.

Poss C: Outpatient surgery documentation: Incorporating nursing diagnoses. *AORN J* 53(1):81, 83–86, 88–89, 1991.

Redmond M: The importance of good communication in effective patient-family teaching. *J Post Anesth Nurs* 8(2):109–112, 1993.

Redmond M: Latex allergy: Recognition and perioperative management. *J Post Anesth Nurs* 11(1):6–12, 1996.

Schiffer DH: Regional anesthesia: Considerations for the perioperative nurse. *Semin Periop Nurs* 2(1):23–32, 1993.

SDS units produce special risks for nursing liability. *Same Day Surgery* 16(3):55–57, 1992.

Shepherd S: Helping ambulatory surgery patients cope with emotions. *J Post Anesth Nurs* 5(2):103–105, 1990.

Stephenson ME: Discharge criteria in day surgery. *J Adv Nurs* 15(5):601–613, 1990.

Technique may reduce need for drugs, hasten recovery. *Same Day Surgery* 16(1):1–3, 1992.

Voeler-Lewis T, Andrea CM, Magee SS: Parent perceptions of pediatric ambulatory surgery: Using family feedback for program evaluation. *J Post Anesth Nurs* 7(2):106–114, 1992.

Yale E: Preoperative teaching strategy: Videotapes for home viewing. *AORN J* 57(4):901, 1993.

Young CM: The postoperative follow-up phone call: An essential part of the ambulatory surgery nurse's job. *J Post Anesth Nurs* 5(4):273–275, 1990.

## REVIEW QUESTIONS

**1. Which of the following patients is not an appropriate candidate for ambulatory surgery?**

A. Physical status (ASA class) I patient
B. Physical status (ASA class) II patient
C. Physical status (ASA class) III patient
D. Physical status (ASA class) IV patient

**2. Preoperative education is designed to do all of the following except:**

A. Reduce patient anxiety
B. Assess current knowledge level
C. Provide presurgical instructions
D. Completely eliminate day of surgery delays and cancellations

**3. In providing preoperative teaching about the use of prescription medications on the day of surgery, patients should be told:**
A. To take no medications on the day of surgery
B. To take all of their medications at bedtime the day before surgery
C. To only take medications given by injection or patch
D. To take medications only as directed by their anesthesiologist or surgeon

**4. Preoperative medications:**
A. Should routinely be administered to all ambulatory surgical patients
B. Are not used in ambulatory surgical patients because they delay discharge
C. Are indicated in consideration of the patient's need and the anesthesiologist's goal
D. Potentiate anesthetic agents and are therefore not widely used

**5. Phase I recovery is designed to:**
A. Provide immediate postanesthetic and postsurgical care
B. Be a place to begin family and patient teaching
C. Be used as a preoperative holding area for the pediatric ambulatory patient
D. Act as an overflow area if phase II is fully occupied

**6. In medicating an ambulatory surgical patient for pain:**
A. No IV or IM narcotics should be used because they will delay discharge
B. Only nonnarcotics should be used to prevent respiratory depression
C. Medications should be titrated if given IV and their effectiveness evaluated
D. Nonpharmacologic interventions should be tried only after pharmacologic intervention

**7. Before discharging a patient to home who has had a spinal anesthetic, the PACU nurse should verify that the patient:**
A. Has no headache or nausea and has received a minimum 1000 ml fluid bolus
B. Can void, can ambulate if age appropriate, and is normotensive
C. Has not developed a hematoma at injection site
D. Has received 25 mg of ephedrine IM to prevent orthostatic hypotension

**8. The three complications most likely to delay discharge of the ambulatory patient include:**
A. Local anesthetic toxicity, epidural hematoma, spinal headache
B. Nausea, pain, extended somnolence
C. Paresthesias, nerve damage, epistaxis
D. Orthostatic hypotension, inability to void, nausea

**9. Discharge criteria:**
A. May be used to guide patient transfer from phase I to phase II recovery
B. May be used to guide patient transfer from phase II to home
C. Must be approved by the medical staff or anesthesia department
D. All of the above

**10. Discharge home from phase II includes completing all except the following:**
A. Review discharge instructions, give the patient a copy, and document understanding
B. Confirm that responsible adult will take patient home
C. Provide information on how to contact the physician or surgery center should complications arise
D. Follow-up telephone call on only the patients who might get in trouble

**11. Precautions when caring for a latex allergic/sensitive patient include all except the following:**
   A. Provide isolated area for care preadmission through discharge to prevent contamination from airborne latex used on other patients
   B. Use stopcocks as entry to give IV drugs and anesthesia
   C. Secure IV with Tegaderm or paper tape
   D. Cover monitor wires and stethoscope tubing and O ring with an Durapore tape before caring for patient

**ANSWERS:** 1. D, 2. D, 3. D, 4. C, 5. A, 6. C, 7. B, 8. B, 9. D, 10. D, 11. C

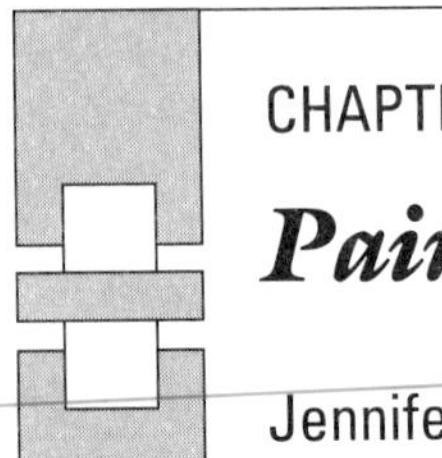

CHAPTER 32

# Pain Assessment and Management

Jennifer Ruth Consla, MSN, RN, CNS, CPAN
Cecil B. Drain, PhD, RN, CRNA, FAAN

## OBJECTIVES

**Study of the information represented by this outline will enable the learner to:**

1. Define pain, acute pain, and the three types of chronic pain.
2. Identify physiologic and psychologic effects of untreated pain.
3. Discuss causes of postoperative pain.
4. Compare and contrast four techniques of pain assessment.
5. Identify important principles of pediatric pain management.
6. Evaluate the pharmacologic interventions that can be used in the preoperative, phase I, or phase II PACU settings.
7. Compare and contrast the various routes of drug administration available in the phase I or phase II PACU.
8. Discuss the place of nonpharmacologic interventions for pain control in the phase I or phase II PACU.
9. State the importance of evaluating pain relief measures.

## I. Definition of Pain

A. Whatever the experiencing person says it is, existing whenever he or she says it does (McCaffery and Beebe, 1989)
   1. Emphasizes subjective nature of pain experience

B. Acute pain
   1. Brief duration
   2. Intensity subsides as healing takes place
   3. May range from mild to severe intensity
   4. Most pain in phase I or phase II PACU of this type

C. Chronic pain
   1. Lasts longer than 6 months
   2. Types
      a. Recurrent acute: has pain-free periods; examples: migraine headaches, sickle cell crisis
      b. Ongoing time-limited: has foreseeable end; example: cancer pain that ends with control of disease or death
      c. Chronic nonmalignant: not time-limited; no response to treatment
         (1) Not life-threatening
         (2) Persists beyond expected time despite treatment
         (3) Patients may present in phase I or phase II PACU for pain blocks; examples: low back pain; reflex sympathetic dystrophy (RSD)
            (a) RSD: syndrome of continuous limb pain, often burning in nature, usually occurring after an injury; variable sensory, motor, autonomic, and trophic changes

3. Patients with chronic pain may present in the phase I or phase II PACU for regional pain blocks, for epidural steroid injections, or following pain ablative surgery, i.e., rhizotomy or cordotomy

## II. Effects of Untreated Pain

A. Physiologic
  1. Decreases respiratory movement
     a. Abolishes normal sigh mechanism (yawn)
     b. Increases thoracic and abdominal splinting
     c. Ineffective cough mechanism
     d. Reduces lung compliance
     e. Reduces lung volumes
     f. Decreases ventilation/perfusion ratio ($\dot{V}/\dot{Q}$)
     g. Atelectasis in dependent lung zones
  2. Decreases mobility
     a. Increases risk of thromboembolism
  3. Exaggerates catecholamine response
     a. Increases systemic vascular resistance (SVR)
        (1) Increases risk of deep venous thrombosis
     b. Increases cardiac work
     c. Increases myocardial oxygen demand
  4. Increases potential for dysrhythmias and hypertension
     a. Increases risk for myocardial ischemia
  5. Delays return of bowel and gastric function

B. Psychologic
  1. Fear
  2. Helplessness
  3. Anxiety
  4. Anger
  5. Frustration

## III. Influences of Postoperative Pain

A. Site, nature, and duration of surgery
  1. Abdominal and intrathoracic procedures most painful

B. Physiologic and psychologic makeup of the patient
  1. Preexisting conditions
  2. Previous experience with pain

C. Preoperative pharmacologic and psychologic preparation
  1. Preemptive analgesia
     a. Prevention or reduction of pain before the operation
        (1) It is easier to prevent pain than to treat it once it has started
        (2) Early postoperative pain is a predictor to long-term pain
        (3) May reduce the incidence of chronic pain
     b. Attempts to block central sensitization to pain
     c. Reduction of noxious input to spinal cord during surgery can reduce immediate and long-term postoperative pain
     d. Local anesthetics, opioids, and NSAIDs are used alone or in combination as preemptive analgesics
     e. Analgesics can be administered locally, epidurally, intrathecally, or systemically
        (1) Preoperative medication should be given painlessly
  2. Preoperative teaching
     a. Describe pain assessment tool that will be used postoperatively
     b. Emphasize the importance of reporting pain
  3. Preoperative medication

D. Postoperative complications: unexpected events

E. Anesthetic management: before, during, and after surgery
F. Quality of postoperative care: phase I and phase II PACU nursing care

**IV. Assessment**

A. Agency for Health Care Policy and Research (Agency for Health Care Policy and Research, 1992) developed clinical practice guidelines for acute pain management
   1. Pain management guides for adults (publication No. 92-0019), pediatric (publication No. 92-0020), and families (publication No. 92-0021) are available free of charge by calling 1-800-358-9295
   2. Key principle of guidelines: The single, most reliable indicator of existence and intensity of pain, and any resultant distress, is the patient's self-report
      a. The patient is ultimate authority about his or her pain

B. Data collection drawn from variety of sources
   1. Patient: best source
   2. Family
   3. Culture
   4. Knowledge of surgical procedure
   5. Awareness of anesthetic agents and techniques used
   6. Anesthesiologist or anesthetist

C. Subjective reports
   1. Verbalizations by patient
   2. Not useful in preverbal or intubated patients

D. Physiologic signs
   1. Manifestations of sympathetic stimulation: tachycardia, hypertension, tachypnea, dilated pupils
   2. Should only be used in addition to subjective reports
   3. Not sensitive or specific to pain
      a. Signs of pain are also signs of hypoxemia

E. Behavioral indicators
   1. Crying, moaning, grimacing, guarding, repositioning, holding very still, restlessness in absence of hypoxemia
   2. Most reliable indicator in preverbal and nonverbal patients

F. Assessment tools
   1. Designed to quantify pain objectively
   2. Adjunct to self-report
   3. Useful in assessment, management, and evaluation of pain
   4. Ideal to instruct patient about scale preoperatively
   5. Should be available in languages suited to area or community
   6. Regardless of physiologic or behavioral signs, if patient rates pain as "severe" or as a "9," the pain is "severe" or a "9"
      a. Verbal rating scale: patient rates pain on scale of 0 to 10: 0 = no pain; 10 = worst possible pain
      b. Visual analog scale (VAS): patient determines intensity of pain

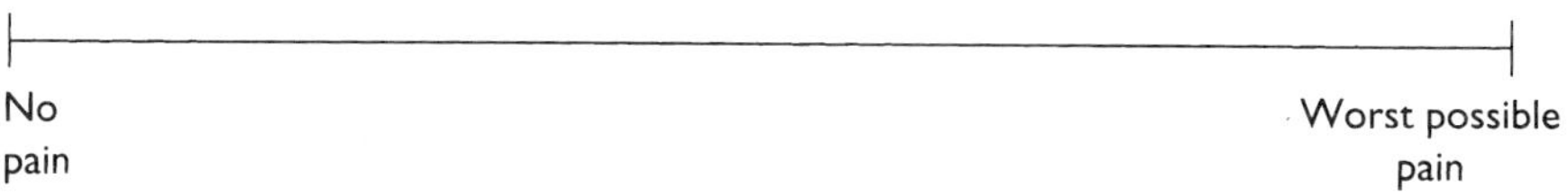


      c. Descriptive pain intensity scale: requires verbal ability

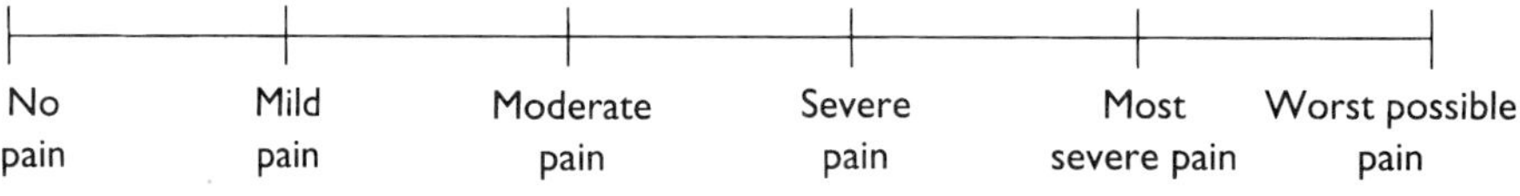

## V. Pediatric Pain Assessment

A. Influences on incidence and intensity
   1. Child's medical condition
   2. Type of surgery performed
   3. Type of anesthetic techniques and medications used
   4. Attitudes of health care providers toward pain management
      a. Children often undermedicated
      b. Fear that children cannot tolerate narcotics
      c. Despite ordered medications, frequently not given
      d. Myth that children do not feel pain: pain response confirmed even in neonates

B. Patients may be limited by development
   1. May be unable to communicate verbally
   2. Unable to understand time-limited nature of pain
   3. Unable to understand reasons for pain

C. Difficulties in assessment often lead to undertreatment or no treatment of pain

D. Self-report remains most reliable indicator of pain
   1. Behavioral indicators useful in preverbal children
      a. Lying still or sleeping does not indicate absence of pain
   2. Parents may be useful in interpreting behavior

E. Rating scales for children
   1. Faces rating scale for children 3 years of age or older
   2. Objective pain scale for children 6 months to 3 years
   3. CRIES scale for neonates through 6 months

**NURSING DIAGNOSIS**

Alteration in comfort: acute pain
1. Outcomes
   a. Patient reports pain is minimized, relieved, or controlled
   b. Patient verbalizes methods that provide relief
   c. Patient demonstrates relaxation skills as indicated for individual situation

Alteration in comfort: chronic pain
1. Outcomes
   a. See discussion of acute pain
   b. Patient is cooperating in pain management program

## VI. Pain Management

A. Patient has the right to best pain relief that may be safely provided

B. Pain management is a team effort between the patient, family, nurse, anesthesiologist or anesthetist, and surgeon

C. Pharmacologic and nonpharmacologic interventions

D. Patient must understand that it is acceptable to have pain, talk about pain, and to request medication
   1. Requiring pain medication will not cause addiction
      a. Addiction defined as psychologic dependence
   2. Request for pain medication is not a "bother" for the nurse
   3. Requiring pain medication does not make patient a "baby"

## VII. Pharmacologic Interventions

A. Nonsteroidal anti-inflammatory agents (NSAIDs)
   1. Indications: mild to moderate pain
   2. Mechanism of action: inhibit cyclooxygenase, an enzyme that catabolizes arachidonic

acid into prostaglandin; prostaglandins incite inflammatory response and activate nerve fibers that transmit pain
    a. All of the NSAIDs are analgesic, antipyretic, and antiinflammatory
3. Advantages of NSAIDs
    a. No respiratory depression
    b. Little physical tolerance
    c. No withdrawal
    d. Can be given orally
4. Disadvantages of NSAIDs
    a. Oral route not useful after anesthesia; only keterolac available parenterally
    b. Alteration in platelet aggregation
        (1) Increase risk of bleeding
        (2) Acetaminophen does not affect platelets
    c. Not indicated for management of severe pain
        (1) Limited use in immediate postoperative period
        (2) Can be combined with opioid to increase pain relief
5. Dosing information (Table 32–1)

B. Opioids
1. Indications: moderate to severe pain
    a. Should be given round the clock on day of surgery, not prn
2. Mechanism of action: bind to opiate receptors in brain and spinal cord
    a. $Mu_1$ ($\mu_1$) receptor: supraspinal analgesia and euphoria
    b. $Mu_2$ ($\mu_2$) receptor: respiratory depression and physical dependence
    c. Kappa ($\kappa$) receptor: spinal analgesia, sedation, nausea, vomiting, constipation (gastrointestinal effects)
    d. Delta ($\delta$) receptor: respiratory depression, physical dependence, nausea and vomiting, changes in affective behavior
    e. Sigma ($\sigma$) receptor: dysphoria, psychomimetic effects
3. Pure opioid agonists (Table 32–2): high affinity for $\mu$ receptors and less affinity (in descending order) for $\kappa$, $\delta$, and $\sigma$ receptors
    a. Produce analgesia, respiratory depression, gastrointestinal effects, physical dependence
        (1) Physical dependence unlikely (<1% chance) when opioid given for acute postsurgical pain, even if opioids given round the clock for 1 week
        (2) Physical dependence: occurrence of withdrawal symptoms when opioid suddenly stopped or an antagonist given
    b. Remifentanil (Ultiva) is a nonspecific esterase-metabolized pure opioid agonist
        (1) Rapid onset (<1 minute) and rapid offset (5 to 10 minutes) that does not have any accumulation regardless of dose or duration of infusion
        (2) Metabolized totally in 3 to 10 minutes: patients who received this drug intraoperatively will not have any analgesia from the drug in the phase I or phase II PACU
        (3) Should be administered *only* by an anesthesia practitioner
4. Mixed agonist-antagonists, such as pentazocine, nalbuphine, and butorphanol, have a high affinity for $\kappa$ and $\sigma$ receptors and moderate affinity for $\mu$ receptors
    a. Moderate analgesia, high sedation, high psychomimetic effects
5. Mixed agonist-antagonists, such as buprenorphine and dezocine, have high affinity at $\mu$ receptors with lower response than direct agonists
    a. Less analgesia than agonists
6. Advantages
    a. Control of moderate to severe pain
    b. Can be given orally, intramuscularly, intravenously, epidurally, intraspinally, or as patient-controlled analgesia
    c. Can be given IV and titrated to effect

**TABLE 32–1 Dosing Data for NSAIDs**

| DRUG | USUAL ADULT DOSE | USUAL PEDIATRIC DOSE* | COMMENTS |
|---|---|---|---|
| **Oral NSAIDs** | | | |
| Acetaminophen | 650–975 mg q4hr | 10–15 mg/kg q4hr | Acetaminophen lacks peripheral antiinflammatory activity of other NSAIDs |
| Aspirin | 650–975 mg q4hr | 10–15 mg/kg q4hr† | Standard against which other NSAIDs are compared; inhibits platelet aggregation; may cause postoperative bleeding |
| Choline magnesium trisalicylate (Trilisate) | 1000–1500 mg bid | 25 mg/kg bid | May have minimal antiplatelet activity; also available as oral liquid |
| Diflunisal (Dolobid) | 1000 mg initial dose followed by 500 mg q12h | | |
| Etodolac (Lodine) | 200–400 mg q6–8hr | | |
| Fenoprofen calcium (Nalfon) | 200 mg q4–6hr | | |
| Ibuprofen (Motrin, others) | 400 mg q4–6hr | 10 mg/kg q6–8hr | Available as several brand names and as generic; also available as oral suspension |
| Ketoprofen (Orudis) | 25–75 mg q6–8hr | | |
| Magnesium salicylate | 650 mg q4hr | | Many brands and generic forms available |
| Meclofenamate sodium (Meclomen) | 50 mg q4–6hr | | |
| Mefenamic acid (Ponstel) | 250 mg q6hr | | |
| Naproxen (Naprosyn) | 500 mg initial dose followed by 250 mg q6–8hr | 5 mg/kg q12hr | Also available as oral liquid |
| Naproxen sodium (Anaprox) | 550 mg initial dose followed by 275 mg q6–8hr | | |
| Salsalate (Disalcid, others) | 500 mg q4hr | | May have minimal antiplatelet activity |
| Sodium salicylate | 325–650 mg q3–4hr | | Available in generic form from several distributors |
| **Parenteral NSAID** | | | |
| Ketorolac tromethamine (Toradol) | 30 or 60 mg IM initial dose followed by 15 or 30 mg q6hr; oral dose following IM dosage: 10 mg q6–8hr | | Intramuscular dose not to exceed 5 days |

From the *Clinical Practice Guideline for Acute Pain Management: Operative or Medical Procedures and Trauma.* The complete guideline should be consulted. For more information or to receive copies of guideline materials, call 1-800-358-9295 or write AHCPR Clearinghouse, PO Box 8547, Silver Spring, MD 20907.

NOTE: Only the above NSAIDs have US Food and Drug Administration (FDA) approval for use as simple analgesics, but clinical experience has been gained with other drugs as well.

*Drug recommendations are limited to NSAIDs where pediatric dosing experience is available.

†Contraindicated in presence of fever or other evidence of viral illness.

**TABLE 32–2 Opioid Agonists**

Morphine
Codeine
Hydromorphone (Dilaudid)
Hydrocodone (in Lortab, Lorcet, Vicodin, others)
Levorphanol (Levo-Dromoran)
Meperidine (Demerol)
Methadone (Dolophine, others)
Oxycodone (Roxicodone, also in Percocet, Percodan, Tylox, others)
Oxymorphone (Numorphone)

   d. Rapid onset of action (except oral and intramuscular routes)
   e. Can be reversed with naloxone
7. Disadvantages
   a. Potentiated by general anesthetics and benzodiazepines
   b. Side effects of respiratory depression, sedation, gastrointestinal effects
   c. May cause hypotension
   d. Physical dependence with long-term use
   e. May develop tolerance to drug effects with prolonged use
      (1) May require increased doses of opioids to achieve same analgesic effect; tolerance does not equal addiction
8. Dosing information (Table 32–3)
   a. Table 32–3 also reflects equianalgesic doses of opioids
      (1) Allows for comparison of drug potency and selection of alternative drug therapy

C. Local anesthetics
   1. Indications: localized to systemic pain control
   2. Mechanism of action: interfere with nerve conduction, blocking transmission of pain (see Chapter 9)

**TABLE 32–3 Dosing Data for Opioids**

| DRUG | APPROXIMATE EQUIANALGESIC ORAL DOSE | APPROXIMATE EQUIANALGESIC PARENTERAL DOSE |
|---|---|---|
| **Opioid Agonist** | | |
| Morphine† | 30 mg q3–4hr (around-the-clock dosing)<br>60 mg q3–4hr (single dose or intermittent dosing) | 10 mg q3–4hr |
| Codeine‡ | 130 mg q3–4hr | 75 mg q3–4hr |
| Hydromorphone† (Dilaudid) | 7.5 mg q3–4hr | 1.5 mg q3–4hr |
| Hydrocodone (in Lorcet, Lortab, Vicodin, others) | 30 mg q3–4hr | Not available |
| Levorphanol (Levo-Dromoran) | 4 mg q6–8hr | 2 mg q6–8hr |
| Meperidine (Demerol) | 300 mg q2–3hr | 100 mg q3hr |
| Methadone (Dolophine, others) | 20 mg q6–8hr | 10 mg q6–8hr |
| Oxycodone (Roxicodone, also in Percocet, Percodan, Tylox, others) | 30 mg q3–4hr | Not available |
| Oxymorphone† (Numorphan) | Not available | 1 mg q3–4hr |
| **Opioid Agonist-Antagonist and Partial Agonist** | | |
| Buprenorphine (Buprenex) | Not available | 0.3–0.4 mg q6–8hr |
| Butorphanol (Stadol) | Not available | 2 mg q3–4hr |
| Nalbuphine (Nubain) | Not available | 10 mg q3–4hr |
| Pentazocine (Talwin, others) | 150 mg q3–4hr | 60 mg q3–4hr |

From the *Clinical Practice Guideline for Acute Pain Management: Operative or Medical Procedures and Trauma.* The complete guideline should be consulted. For more information or to receive copies of guideline materials, call 1-800-358-9295 or write AHCPR Clearinghouse, PO Box 8547, Silver Spring, MD 20907.

NOTE: Published tables vary in the suggested doses that are equianalgesic to morphine. Clinical response is the criterion that must be applied for each patient; titration to clinical response is necessary. Because cross tolerance among these drugs is not complete, it usually is necessary to use a lower than equianalgesic dose when changing drugs and to retitrate to response.

CAUTION: Recommended doses do not apply to patients with renal or hepatic insufficiency or other conditions affecting drug metabolism and kinetics.

*CAUTION: Doses listed for patients with body weight <50 kg cannot be used as initial starting doses in babies <6 months of age. Consult the *Clinical Practice Guideline for Acute Pain Management: Operative or Medical Procedures and Trauma* section on management of pain in neonates for recommendations.

3. Advantages
   a. Avoid side effects of opioids
      (1) But may be combined with opioids for epidural and spinal analgesia
   b. Administration by variety of techniques
      (1) Topical, infiltration, regional blockade
      (2) May last minutes to upward of 12 hours
      (3) Single dose or continuous infusion through catheter
4. Disadvantages
   a. Requires physician to administer or establish block or infusion
   b. Catheter placement usually requires hospitalization
   c. After local anesthetic wears off, patient often requires additional analgesia
   d. Require patient teaching if outpatient discharged to home with extremity block still in place
      (1) Protection of extremity
      (2) Circulatory status of extremity; capillary refill
      (3) Expected duration of block
      (4) Supplemental analgesia

| RECOMMENDED STARTING DOSE (ADULTS MORE THAN 50 kg BODY WEIGHT) | | RECOMMENDED STARTING DOSE (CHILDREN AND ADULTS LESS THAN 50 kg BODY WEIGHT)* | |
|---|---|---|---|
| **ORAL** | **PARENTERAL** | **ORAL** | **PARENTERAL** |
| 30 mg q3–4hr | 10 mg q3–4hr | 0.3 mg/kg q3–4hr | 0.1 mg/kg q3–4hr |
| 60 mg q3–4hr | 60 mg q2hr (intramuscular/ subcutaneous) | 1 mg/kg q3–4hr[§] | Not recommended |
| 6 mg q3–4hr | 1.5 mg q3–4hr | 0.06 mg/kg q3–4hr | 0.015 mg/kg q3–4hr |
| 10 mg q3–4hr | Not available | 0.2 mg/kg q3–4hr[§] | Not available |
| 4 mg q6–8hr | 2 mg q6–8hr | 0.04 mg/kg q6–8hr | 0.02 mg/kg q6–8hr |
| Not recommended | 100 mg q3hr | Not recommended | 0.75 mg/kg q2–3hr |
| 20 mg q6–8hr | 10 mg q6–8hr | 0.2 mg/kg q6–8hr | 0.1 mg/kg q6–8hr |
| 10 mg q3–4hr | Not available | 0.2 mg/kg q3–4hr[§] | Not available |
| Not available | 1 mg q3–4hr | Not recommended | Not recommended |
| Not available | 0.4 mg q6–8hr | Not available | 0.004 mg/kg q6–8hr |
| Not available | 2 mg q3–4hr | Not available | Not recommended |
| Not available | 10 mg q3–4hr | Not available | 0.1 mg/kg q3–4hr |
| 50 mg q4–6hr | Not recommended | Not recommended | Not recommended |

[†]For morphine, hydromorphone, and oxymorphone, rectal administration is an alternate route for patients unable to take oral medications, but equianalgesic doses may differ from oral and parenteral doses because of pharmacokinetic differences.

[‡]CAUTION: Codeine doses >65 mg often are not appropriate because of diminishing incremental analgesia with increasing doses but continually increasing constipation and other side effects.

[§]CAUTION: Doses of aspirin and acetaminophen in combination opioid/NSAID preparations must also be adjusted to the patient's body weight.

## VIII. Routes of Administration

A. Intravenous (IV)
   1. Rapid-onset, instant absorption
   2. Titrated to effect
   3. Most common method in phase I and phase II PACUs

B. Intramuscular (IM)
   1. Painful, frightening to children
   2. Delayed absorption, especially in vasoconstricted, hypotensive, hypothermic patients
   3. Unable to titrate
   4. Possibility of delayed respiratory depression
   5. Longer duration of action than IV administration

C. Oral (PO)
   1. Useful for outpatient being discharged to home
   2. May cause nausea and vomiting when given immediately after anesthesia
      a. Requires functioning gastrointestinal tract
   3. Unable to titrate
   4. Long duration
   5. Peak effect prolonged

D. Patient-controlled analgesia (PCA)
   1. Patient is best judge of pain; patient controls relief
   2. PO, IV, or epidural
   3. Requires specially designed, programmable infusion pump for IV or epidural administration
   4. Requires patient teaching (may be done preoperatively)
   5. Can be used with adults or children as young as age 5 years
      a. Only patient is to operate pump
      b. Parents are not to operate child's pump
   6. Physician to write dosing parameters

E. Epidural
   1. May be used for 1 to 4 days postoperatively
   2. Useful for orthopedic, thoracic, intraabdominal surgeries
   3. May be used for labor and delivery (obstetrics)
   4. Administered by infusion pump
   5. Common side effects include pruritus, urinary retention, nausea and vomiting, and respiratory depression
      a. Naloxone (Narcan) at bedside to treat respiratory depression
         (1) Pure narcotic antagonist
      b. Requires hourly assessment of respiratory status
         (1) Pulse oximetry useful adjunct in monitoring
      c. May require bladder catheterization
      d. Naloxone or diphenhydramine (Benadryl) to treat pruritus
      e. Standing orders facilitate problem management
      f. Nursing and patient education vital
   6. Requires approximately 2 hours to achieve therapeutic level of analgesia
      a. May require IV supplementation with opioids
   7. Numerous physiologic advantages
      a. Improves respiratory function
      b. Increases blood flow to extremities
      c. Decreases incidence of thromboembolism
      d. Blunts catecholamine release
      e. Decreases myocardial oxygen demand
      f. Stimulates gastrointestinal motility

8. ASPAN has developed a policy statement specific to the role of the registered nurse in management of analgesia by catheter techniques

## IX. Nonpharmacologic Interventions

A. Indications
   1. Patient request or preference
   2. Incomplete pain relief from pharmacologic intervention
   3. Intolerance of patient to pharmacologic intervention
   4. Patient instability prevents use of pharmacologic intervention
   5. Prolonged pain
   6. Designed to supplement, not substitute, pharmacologic intervention (Agency for Health Care Policy and Research, 1992)

B. Approaches
   1. Cognitive-behavioral
      a. Patient understands pain and takes active role in management
      b. Examples
         (1) Preparatory information
         (2) Relaxation
         (3) Imagery
         (4) Hypnosis
         (5) Biofeedback
         (6) Music therapy
      c. Some techniques require advanced education for nurses
      d. Goals
         (1) Change patient perception of pain
         (2) Alter pain behavior
         (3) Increase patient control over pain
   2. Physical therapeutic agents or modalities
      a. Examples
         (1) Application of heat or cold
         (2) Massage
         (3) Exercise
         (4) TENS (transcutaneous electronic nerve stimulation) therapy
         (5) Immobility
      b. Goals
         (1) Provide comfort
         (2) Correct physiologic dysfunction
         (3) Alter physiologic responses
         (4) Reduce fear associated with immobility

C. Implementation
   1. Nurse initiated: preparatory information, deep breathing, relaxation, application of warm blankets, touch
   2. Physician ordered: ice packs, TENS therapy, traction

## X. Evaluation of Pain Management

A. Process of control is ongoing

B. Must involve patient

C. Techniques of assessment used in evaluation

D. If effective, continue interventions and decrease as appropriate

E. If ineffective, reconsider options, medications, dosage, route, patient teaching
   1. Implement new ideas and reevaluate

F. Follow-up with outpatient
   1. Provide means for outpatient to seek help if pain unmanageable at home with prescribed intervention

## BIBLIOGRAPHY

Agency for Health Care Policy and Research, Public Health Service, U.S. Department of Health and Human Services, Acute Pain Management Guideline Panel: *Acute Pain Management: Operative or Medical Procedures and Trauma.* Clinical Practice Guideline (AHCPR pub no 92-0032). Rockville, Md, The Agency, Feb 1992.

American Society of PeriAnesthesia Nurses: *Standards of Perianesthesia Nursing Practice.* Thorofare, NJ, The Society, 1998.

Barash P, Cullen B, Stoelting R: *Clinical Anesthesia,* 3rd Ed. Philadelphia, Lippincott-Raven, 1997.

Hill K, Anderson C: Pediatric pain management: Clinical aspects for the nineties. *Semin Anesth* 16(2): 136–151, 1997.

Lubenow T, McCarthy R, Ivankovich A: Management of acute postoperative pain. *Clin Anesth Updates* 3(4):1–15, 1992.

McCaffery M, Beebe A: *Pain: Clinical Manual for Nursing Practice.* St Louis, CV Mosby, 1989.

Molloy A, Power I (eds): *Acute and Chronic Pain. Int Anesthesiol Clin* 35(2), 1997.

Orkin F: What do patients want? Preferences for immediate postoperative recovery. *Anesth Analg* 74:S225, 1992.

Souter, A, Fredman, B, White P: Controversies in the perioperative use of nonsteroidal anti-inflammatory drugs. *Anesth Analg* 79:1178–1190, 1994.

Stoelting R: *Pharmacology and Physiology in Anesthetic Practice,* 2nd Ed. Philadelphia, JB Lippincott, 1991.

Warfield C, Kahn C: Acute-pain management: Programs in U.S. hospitals and experiences and attitudes among U.S. adults. *Anesthesiology* 83:1090–1094, 1995.

Yaksh T: Physiology and pharmacology of the post-injury pain site. *Semin Anesth* 16(2):79–91, 1997.

## REVIEW QUESTIONS

**1. The most common type of pain experienced by the postsurgical patient is:**

A. Ongoing time-limited
B. Recurrent acute
C. Chronic nonmalignant
D. Acute

**2. How likely is it that psychologic dependence will occur as a result of treating pain with opioids around the clock for 1 week?**

A. <1%
B. 5%
C. 25%
D. >50%

**3. When a patient requests increasing amounts of an analgesic to control pain, this usually indicates:**

A. The patient is addicted
B. The patient is experiencing increased pain
C. The patient has developed tolerance to the drug
D. The patient is attempting to manipulate the health care system

**4. The potency of the pain relief measure selected for a patient should be determined on the basis of:**

A. The type of surgery performed
B. The opinion of the surgeon
C. The patient's reported pain intensity
D. Physiologic indicators of pain

**5. The best judge of the patient's pain intensity is the:**

A. Nurse
B. Patient
C. Patient's family
D. Anesthesiologist

**6. Analgesics for postoperative pain should initially be given:**
A. Around the clock on a fixed schedule
B. Only when the patient asks for medication
C. Only when the patient rates pain as a 5 or higher
D. Only when the nurse determines that the patient is in pain

**7. Which of the following equianalgesic doses is correct?**
A. Hydromorphone, 1.5 mg = morphine, 10 mg
B. Codeine, 50 mg = meperidine, 100 mg
C. Morphine, 2 mg = hydrocodone, 30 mg
D. Meperidine, 25 mg = morphine, 5 mg

**8. The recommended route of administration of opioid analgesics for patients with acute post-operative pain is:**
A. Intramuscular
B. Oral
C. Epidural
D. Intravenous

**9. Lisa Jones, 42-years-old, is admitted to the PACU after an abdominal hysterectomy. As her nurse, your assessment yields the following information: she is awake, alert, oriented, and pleasant. Her blood pressure is 110/70, heart rate 78, respiratory rate 14. She is requesting to see her husband. On a scale of 0 to 10, she rates her pain as a "9." She states an acceptable level of pain would be a "2." What is your assessment of Lisa's pain?**
A. 2
B. 4
C. 7
D. 9

**10. Although initial doses of a medication are based on a patient's body weight, which of the following statements is true about subsequent doses?**
A. Subsequent doses should be administered on a prn schedule
B. Subsequent doses should be based on the patient's response to the initial dose
C. Subsequent doses will be less than the initial dose because the intensity of the pain will decrease with time
D. Subsequent doses should continue to be based on the patient's weight

**11. Which of the following is the best indicator of pain relief?**
A. The patient is sleeping
B. The patient's vital signs are within the preoperative range
C. The patient states relief has been obtained
D. You have administered the highest allowed opioid dose

**12. In preverbal patients the best indicator of pain is/are:**
A. Physiologic signs
B. Behavioral indicators
C. The patient's care giver
D. The subjective report

**13. Which of the following statements about NSAIDs is true?**
A. NSAIDs have no place in the phase I or phase II PACU for acute pain management
B. NSAIDs can only be given orally and therefore can only be used for the patient in phase II recovery
C. NSAIDs can be combined with opioids to increase analgesia
D. NSAIDs are indicated for the management of severe pain

**14. Nonpharmacologic interventions for pain control are designed to:**
   A. Supplement pharmacologic interventions
   B. Replace pharmacologic interventions
   C. Treat pain when it is rated 5 or less
   D. Be used only in an acute care setting

**15. The ideal approach to pain management is:**
   A. The surgeon taking full responsibility for determining pain control measures
   B. The development of standing protocols to be applied to all patients
   C. The selection of one drug to be used for all patients in doses adjusted for weight
   D. A team approach involving the patient, nurse, surgeon, and anesthesiologist

**ANSWERS:** 1. D, 2. A, 3. C, 4. C, 5. B, 6. A, 7. A, 8. D, 9. D, 10. B, 11. C, 12. B, 13. C, 14. A, 15. D

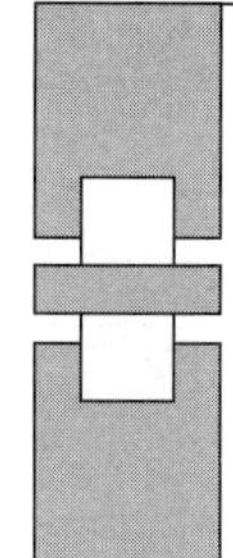

CHAPTER 33

# *Hemodynamic Monitoring*

D. George Dresden, MSN, RN, CCRN

## OBJECTIVES

**Study of the information represented by this outline will enable the learner to:**

1. Identify appropriate surgical patients for the use of intraoperative and postoperative hemodynamic pressure monitoring.
2. Describe cardiac physiology related to preload, afterload, and contractility.
3. Describe the normal pressure waveforms and values occurring in the right atrium (RA), pulmonary artery (PA), pulmonary artery occlusion (PAO) pressure and radial or femoral artery.
4. Describe the thermodilution technique for obtaining cardiac output (CO) measurement.
5. Describe the normal values derived from oximetric hemodynamic monitoring.
6. Give examples of nursing interventions and troubleshooting measures related to inaccurate pressure waveforms and/or values.

## I. Physiologic Variables Affecting Cardiovascular Function

A. Cardiac output (CO)
  1. Definition: amount of blood ejected by heart measured in liters per minute
    a. CO = Stroke volume (SV) × Heart rate (HR)
  2. Influences on CO
    a. Preload (right sided, left sided)
    b. Afterload
    c. Contractility
    d. Heart rate
    e. Atrioventricular synchrony

B. Right-sided preload = central venous pressure (CVP) or right atrial pressure
  1. Definition: filling volume of right ventricle, which stretches relaxed ventricular wall at end diastole (venous return to heart)
  2. Influences on right-sided preload
    a. Myocardial pumping
    b. Vascular tone
    c. Blood volume measured by central venous catheter or lumen port placed in superior vena cava
    d. Increased intrathoracic pressure (including positive end-expiratory pressure [PEEP])
    e. Tricuspid valve stenosis

C. Left-sided preload = left atrial pressure (LAP), pulmonary artery diastolic (PAD) pressure, pulmonary artery occlusion (wedge) pressure (PAOP)
  1. Influences on left-sided preload
    a. Compliance of left ventricle
    b. Myocardial pumping action
    c. Blood volume
  2. Optimal left-sided preload produces adequate CO without causing backflow
  3. Measured by pulmonary artery catheter or left atrial pressure catheter (LAP)

- D. Afterload
  1. Definition: resistance or impedance to blood ejection from either right or left ventricle
  2. Influences on right-sided afterload (also called pulmonary vascular resistance)
     a. Pulmonary hypertension
     b. Chronic obstructive pulmonary disease (COPD)
  3. Influences on left-sided afterload (also called systemic vascular resistance)
     a. Arteriolar constriction
     b. Hypertension
  4. Indirectly measured
- E. Contractility
  1. Definition: inherent capability to increase extent and force of muscle fiber shortening regardless of preload or afterload
  2. Indirectly measured through calculated right and left stroke work index
- F. Heart rate: variations alter stroke volume
- G. Atrioventricular synchrony
  1. Definition: coordinated contraction pattern between atria and ventricles
  2. Influences on atrioventricular synchrony
     a. Ischemia
     b. Infarction
     c. Conduction deficits
     d. Dysrhythmias
     e. Artificial pacemakers
  3. Loss of synchrony decreases CO, blood pressure, and stroke volume and increases LAP

**II. Direct Arterial Pressure Monitoring (Arterial Line)**

- A. Indications
  1. Cardiopulmonary bypass
  2. Potential intraoperative or postoperative wide variation in blood pressure
     a. Carotid endarterectomy
     b. Aortic aneurysm resection
     c. Craniotomies
  3. Strict blood pressure control mandated
  4. Multiple arterial blood gases or laboratory tests
  5. Titration of vasoactive medications
- B. Measurement
  1. Placement
     a. Radial artery (most frequent)
        (1) Allen test should be performed before insertion
     b. Femoral artery (site associated with greatest risk of infection)
     c. Brachial artery (uncommon)
  2. Arterial pressure waveform: two components (Fig. 33–1)
     a. Anacrotic limb: ejection of blood and systolic pressure
     b. Dicrotic limb: diastole
- C. Risks and complications
  1. Vascular compromise (e.g., thrombus, spasm)
  2. Disconnection: hemorrhage
  3. Accidental injection of drugs or air
  4. Infection
  5. Nerve damage
- D. Troubleshooting and nursing interventions (Fig. 33–2)

**III. CVP Monitoring**

- A. Indications
  1. Rapid infusion of fluid or blood
  2. Inability to cannulate peripheral veins

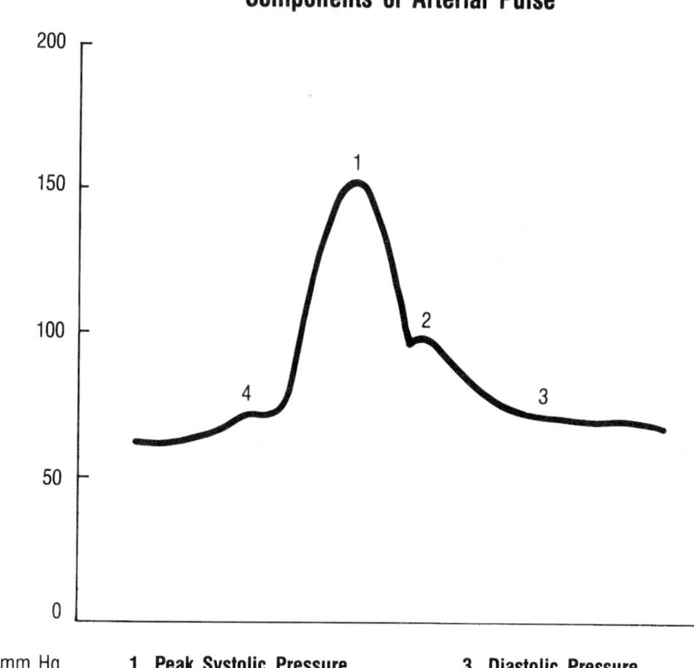


**FIGURE 33–1** Arterial pressure waveform. *1,* peak systolic pressure; *2,* dicrotic notch; *3,* diastolic pressure; *4,* anacrotic notch.

3. Administration of drugs that may cause peripheral sclerosis (i.e., potassium, epinephrine, chemotherapeutic agents, aminoglycosides)
4. Administration of hyperalimentation
5. Access site for temporary pacemakers
6. Assessment of fluid status

B. Measurement
1. Placement: catheter placed in major veins leading to superior vena cava (i.e., subclavian, internal jugular, femoral, or brachial vein or proximal lumen of a PA catheter)
2. Intermittent readings by means of water manometer (cm $H_2O$) (mm Hg × 1.36 = cm $H_2O$)
3. Continuous readings by means of pressure transducer (mm Hg)
4. Must be leveled for accurate reading at phlebostatic axis (Fig. 33–3)
    a. The transducer requires zeroing to atmospheric pressure only before insertion and at any time the tubing is disconnected or changed
5. Waveform (Fig. 33–4)
6. Readings (Table 33–1)
    a. RAP (right arterial pressure) = 2 to 6 mm Hg (through pulmonary artery catheter and is determinent of right ventricular end diastolic pressure [RVEDP])
    b. CVP (mean right atrial pressure) = 2 to 8 cm $H_2O$ (through CVP manometer)

C. See risks and complications of pulmonary artery catheters

D. Troubleshooting and nursing interventions (Fig. 33–5)

## IV. Pulmonary Artery Pressure (PAP) Monitoring (PA Catheter)

A. Indications
1. Existing preoperative medical conditions
    a. Cardiac disease
    b. Renal failure

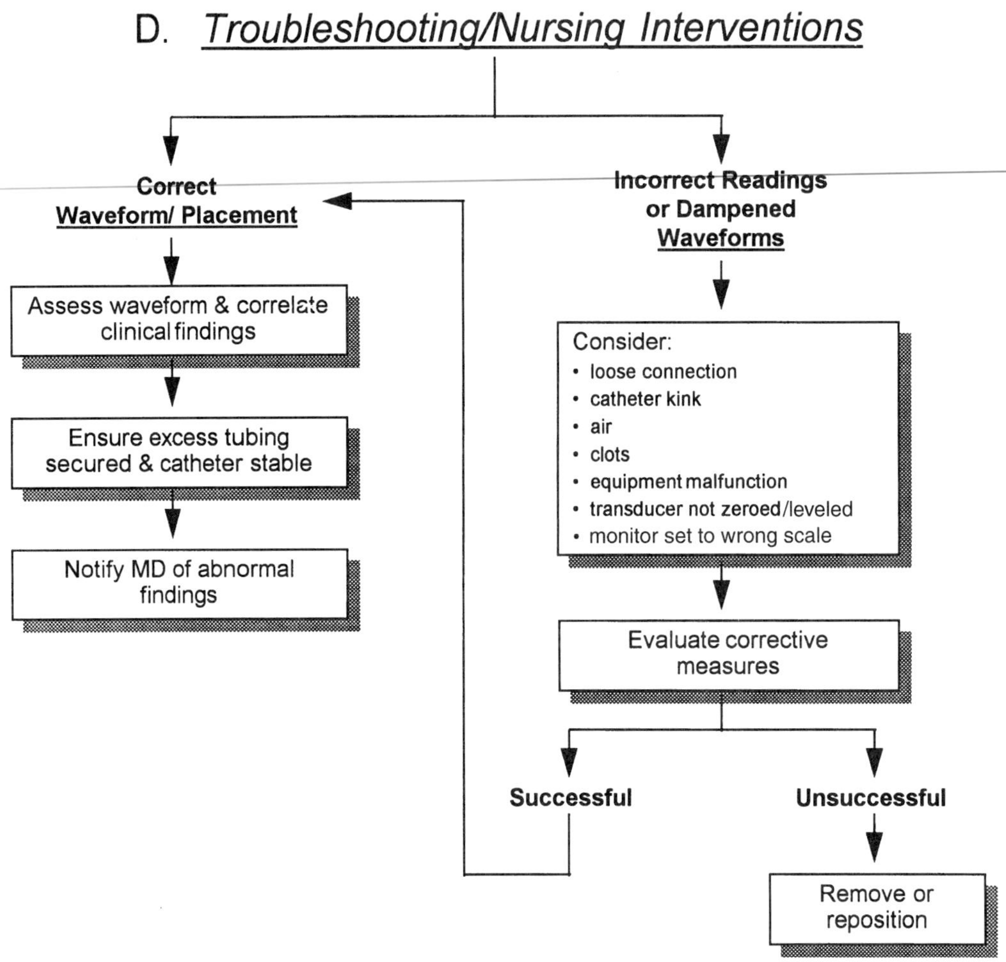

D. Troubleshooting/Nursing Interventions
Correct Waveform/ Placement
Assess waveform & correlate clinical findings
Ensure excess tubing secured & catheter stable
Notify MD of abnormal findings
Incorrect Readings or Dampened Waveforms
Consider:
• loose connection
• catheter kink
• air
• clots
• equipment malfunction
• transducer not zeroed/leveled
• monitor set to wrong scale
Evaluate corrective measures
Successful
Unsuccessful
Remove or reposition

**FIGURE 33–2** Flowchart of troubleshooting and nursing interventions in arterial pressure monitoring.

Fourth intercostal space
Midaxillary line
Phlebostatic axis

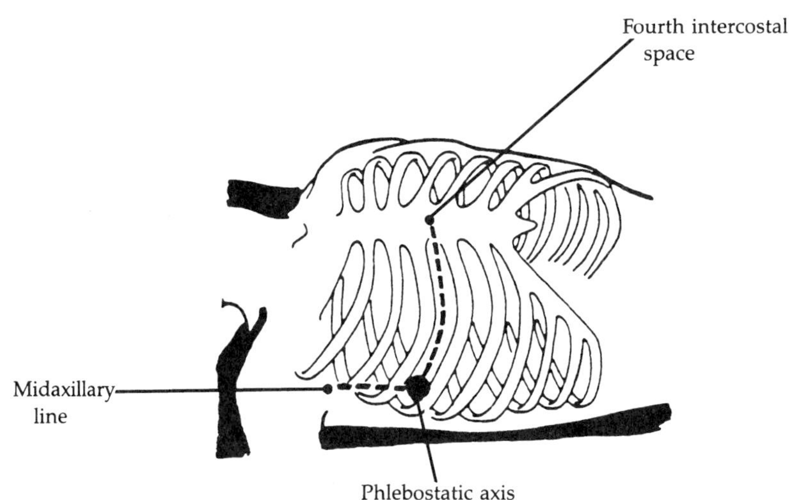

**FIGURE 33–3** Phlebostatic axis is an approximation of right atrium and is used for leveling air interface port of pressure monitoring system.

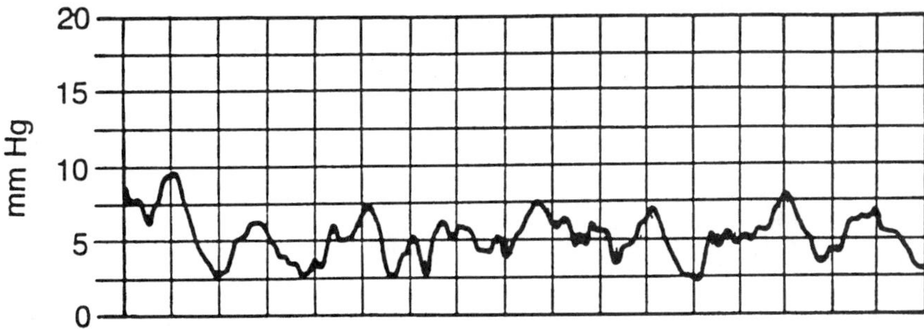


**FIGURE 33–4** Right arterial waveform.

c. Obesity
d. Gastrointestinal bleeding
e. Abdominal or head trauma
f. COPD

2. Thoracic or abdominal aortic aneurysms
3. Extensive intraabdominal resections
4. Prolonged orthopedic procedures
5. Use of mechanical assist devices
6. Titration of vasoactive drugs
7. Sepsis

B. Measurement

1. Placement: preferred sites are internal jugular, subclavian; may also be placed in brachial or femoral vein (rare)

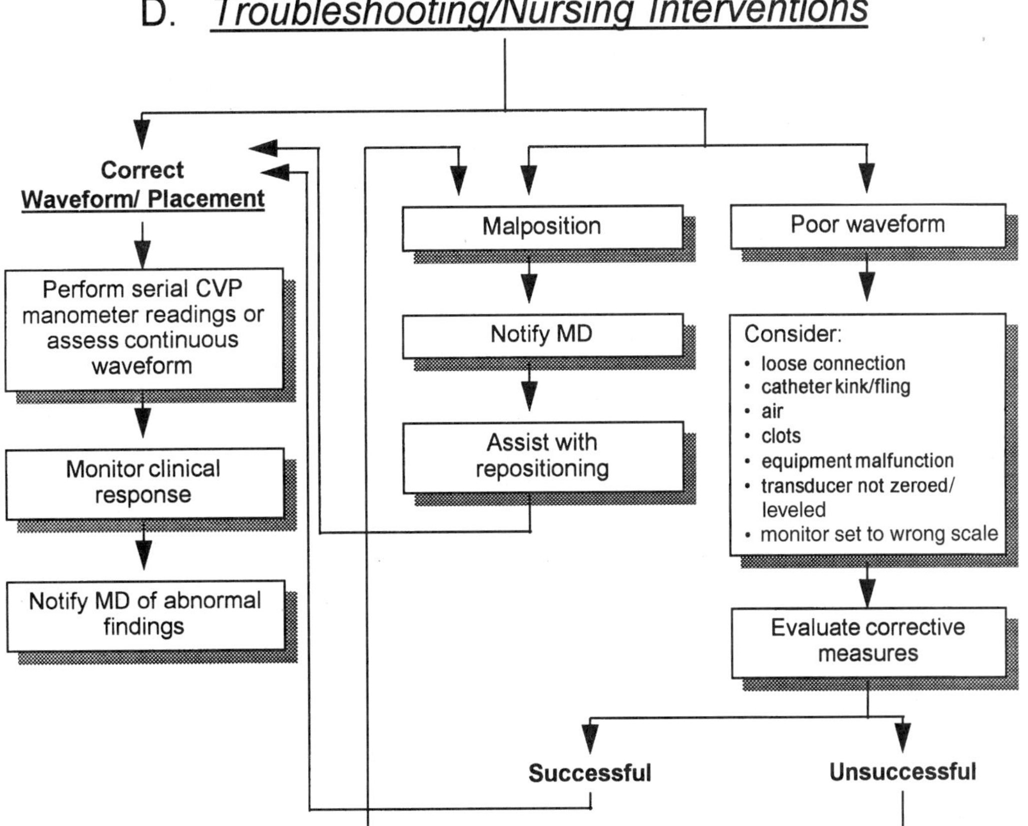


**FIGURE 33–5** Flowchart of troubleshooting and nursing interventions in central venous pressure monitoring.

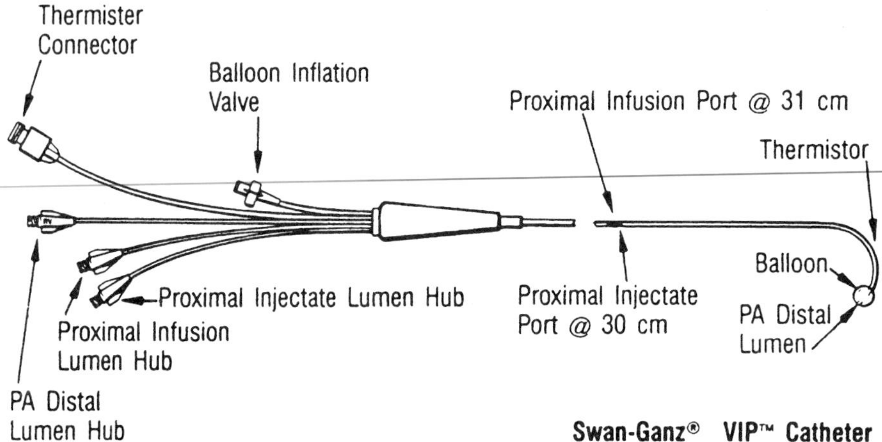


**FIGURE 33–6** Swan-Ganz VIP catheter. (Reprinted with permission of Baxter Healthcare Corporation, Edwards Critical-Care Division.)

2. Catheter: many types, including multiple infusion ports, transvenous pacer, and co-oximetric catheters (Fig. 33–6)
3. Air interface port must be leveled at phlebostatic axis (see Fig. 33–3) for accurate readings
4. Measure PAP and PAOP through distal port (see Fig. 33–6)
5. PAP
   a. Systolic: 20 to 30 mm Hg
   b. Diastolic: <10 to 20 mm Hg
   c. Mean PAP: <20 mm Hg (see Table 33–1)
   d. Reflects left- and right-sided heart pressures
   e. PA systolic pressure reflects right ventricular pressure
   f. Readings may be obtained in position of comfort for the patient, as long as this is performed consistently.
6. PAOP (PCWP): mean = 4 to 12 mm Hg (see Table 33–1)
   a. To obtain, must inflate balloon (see Fig. 33–6) with up to 1.5 ml of air for 7.5 Fr catheter (use syringe supplied with catheter or a 1 cc TB syringe), allowing syringe to passively refill
   b. Balloon must not be inflated for more than 15 seconds (risk of pulmonary artery infarction)

**TABLE 33–1 Hemodynamic Normal Values**

| PRESSURE | VALUE | RANGE |
|---|---|---|
| Right atrial pressure (RA) | Mean | 2–6 mm Hg |
| Central venous pressure (CVP) | Mean | 2–8 cm $H_2O$ |
| Right ventricular pressure (RV) | Systolic | 20–30 mm Hg |
| | Diastolic | <10 mm Hg |
| Pulmonary artery pressure (PAP) | Systolic | 20–30 mm Hg |
| | Diastolic | <10–20 mm Hg |
| | Mean | <20 mm Hg |
| Left arterial pressure (LAP) | Mean | 10 mm Hg |
| Pulmonary artery occlusion pressure (PAOP) or pulmonary capillary wedge pressure (PCWP) | Mean | 4–12 mm Hg |
| Left ventricular end diastolic pressure (LEVDP) | Mean | 4–12 mm Hg |
| Arterial pressure (MAP) | Mean | 70–100 mm Hg |

c. Reflects left atrial pressure and left ventricular end diastolic pressure (LVEDP)
d. PAOP should be within 2 to 5 mm Hg of PA diastolic pressure
e. Readings are obtained at end-expiration

7. Measurement variables
   a. PA diastolic pressure reflects LVEDP; therefore it is used as an indirect measure of LV function and diastolic filling
   b. PA diastolic pressure does not reflect LVEDP when heart rate >125 bpm or in cases of COPD, adult respiratory distress syndrome (ARDS), pulmonary emboli, or mitral stenosis
8. Waveforms (Fig. 33–7)

C. Significance of PAP and PAOP in surgical patients
   1. Elevated PAP (systolic) may be due to
      a. Pulmonary hypertension
      b. LV failure and mitral stenosis
      c. Constrictive pericarditis
      d. Cardiac tamponade
      e. Congestive heart failure
      f. Atrial or ventricular septal defects
   2. Elevated PAP (diastolic) may be due to
      a. LV failure
      b. Mitral stenosis
      c. Pulmonary hypertension
      d. Left-to-right shunts
   3. Elevated PAOP may be due to
      a. Constrictive pericarditis
      b. LV failure
      c. Mitral valve dysfunction
      d. Fluid overload
      e. Ischemia
   4. Decreased PAP and PAOP may be due to
      a. Hypotension
      b. Hypovolemia
      c. Vasodilating drugs causing decreased afterload

D. Risks and complications
   1. Carotid artery puncture with insertion (internal jugular approach)
   2. Infection
   3. Pulmonary artery rupture
   4. Thrombus or embolic event
   5. Air embolism
   6. Perforation of right ventricle

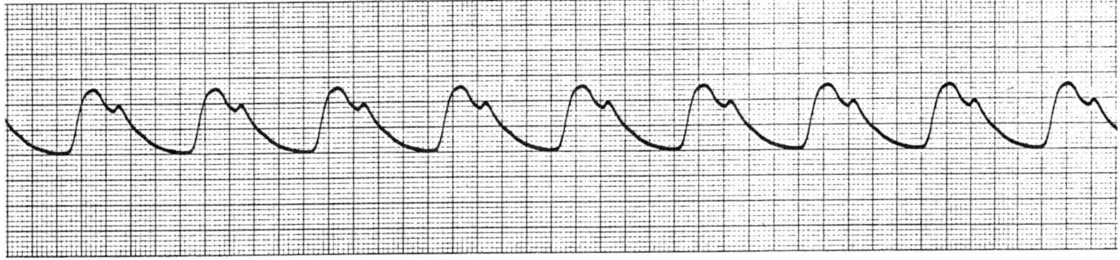

**FIGURE 33–7** PAP showing transition to PAOP (wedge) with balloon inflation.

7. Dysrhythmias
8. Pneumothorax resulting from insertion (subclavian approach)
9. Electrical microshocks
10. Catheter migration backward to right ventricle or forward to wedged (occlusion) position
11. Catheter knotting or kinking
12. Balloon rupture
13. Overwedging or failure to unwedge, resulting in pulmonary necrosis or infarction

E. Troubleshooting and nursing interventions (Fig. 33–8)

## V. Thermodilution Cardiac Output

A. Indications
1. Determination of hemodynamic calculations (Table 33–2)
2. Postoperative fluid management, balloon pump therapy, PEEP
3. Evaluation of effects of cardioactive drugs
4. Determination of myocardial ischemia
5. Evaluation for intraoperative myocardial infarction

B. Measurement
1. Types
   a. Invasive: thermodilution technique (Table 33–3)
   b. Noninvasive: continuous wave Doppler probe
   c. Thoracic electrical impedance
2. CO = 4–8 L/min (see Table 33–1)
3. Waveform (Fig. 33–9)

**TABLE 33–2 Hemodynamic Calculations**

| PRESSURE | FORMULA | VALUE |
|---|---|---|
| Mean arterial pressure (MAP) | Diastolic + ⅓ (Systolic – Diastolic) | 70–100 mm Hg |
| Cardiac output (CO) (L/min) | HR × SV | 4–8 L/min |
| Cardiac index (CI) (L/min/m$^2$) | CO/BSA | 2.7–4.2 L/min/m$^2$ |
| Stroke volume (SV) | CO/HR | 60–90 ml |
| Stroke index (SI) | SV/BSA or CI/HR | 40 ± 7 ml/beat/m$^2$ |
| Left ventricular stroke work index (LVSWI) | $\frac{1.36 \times (\text{MAP} - \text{PAOP}) \times \text{SI}}{100}$ | 45–60 g-m/beat/m$^2$ |
| Right ventricular stroke work index (RVSWI) | $\frac{1.36 \times (\text{MPAP} - \text{RAP}) \times \text{SI}}{100}$ | 7–12 g-m/beat/m$^2$ |
| Systemic vascular resistance (SVR) | $\frac{\text{MAP} - \text{RAP or CVP}}{\text{CO}} \times 80$ | 800–1200 dynes/sec/cm$^{-5}$ |
| | **or** | **or** |
| | $\frac{\text{MAP} - \text{RAP}}{\text{CO}}$ | 12–18 units |
| Pulmonary vascular resistance (PVR) | $\frac{\text{RAP} - \text{PAOP}}{\text{CO}} \times 80$ | 50—150 dynes/sec/cm$^{-5}$ |
| | **or** | **or** |
| | $\frac{\text{MAPA} - \text{PAOP}}{\text{CO}}$ | 0.5–1 unit |
| Ejection fraction (EF) | $\frac{\text{SV}}{\text{End diastolic volume}} \times 100$ | 60–75% (left ventricle) |
| Body surface area (BSA) | Use Dubois chart | 1.5–2 m$^2$ |

*MPAP,* Mean pulmonary artery pressure; *PAOP,* pulmonary artery occlusion pressure (wedge); *HR,* heart rate; *RAP,* right atrial pressure (CVP).

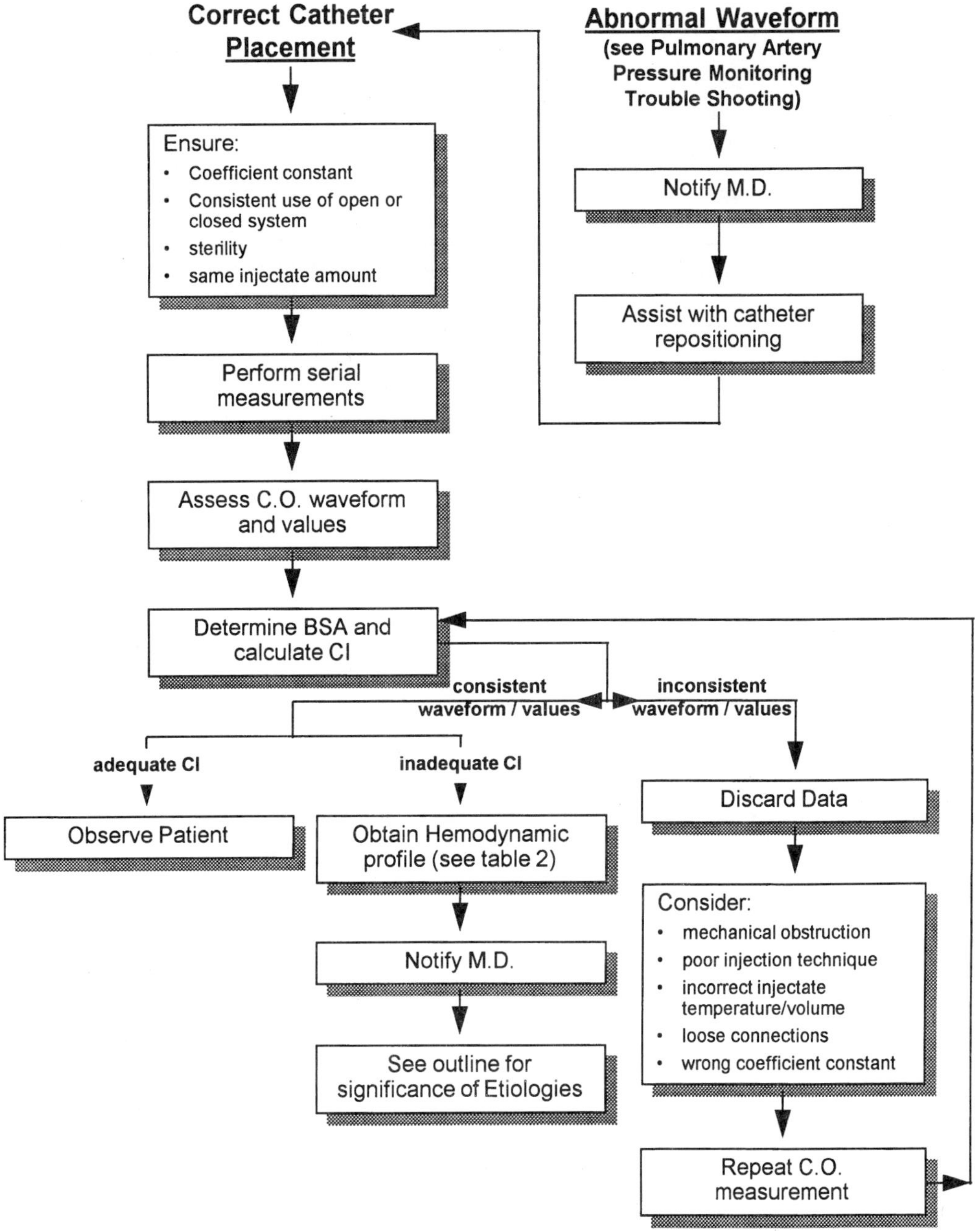


**FIGURE 33–8** Flowchart of troubleshooting and nursing interventions in pulmonary artery pressure monitoring.

4. Must be referenced to body surface area (BSA) through use of DuBois chart (considers height and weight) and is measured as cardiac index (CI): 2.7–4.2 L/min/m$^2$ (see Table 33–2); determines whether CO is adequate for a particular body size

C. Significance of CO in surgical patients
   1. Low CO (<4 L/min)
      a. Decreased myocardial contractility (e.g., cardiac tamponade, MI with LV failure)

**TABLE 33–3 Technique for Accurate Thermodilution Cardiac Output**

1. Use accurately measured injectate volume of 2.5, 5, or 10 ml (usually 10 ml normal saline for adults).
2. Room temperature (19°–24° C) injectate is used.
3. Use correct (K2) computation constant. This will vary with manufacturer, size of catheter, and injectate volume.
4. If medication is being administered through the proximal port, aspirate at least 10 ml before injection for CO and ensure straight shot (no 90-degree angle).
5. Inject rapidly and smoothly within 4 seconds; wait 60 seconds between injections.
6. A total of three to five injections should be obtained and averaged.
7. Perform each injection during the same time in the respiratory cycle (preferably end-expiration).
8. Visible inspection of CO curve is best to determine correct technique and accuracy (see Fig. 33–4).

b. Decreased PAOP
c. Vasoconstriction or increased systemic vascular resistance
d. Valvular heart disease (especially mitral)
e. Hypovolemia
f. Loss of vascular neural control (e.g., postoperative spinal anesthesia)
g. Dysrhythmias (especially significant tachycardias)
h. Drugs with negative inotropic effects
i. Metabolic disorders
j. Hypothermia
k. Constrictive pericarditis, restrictive cardiomyopathies

2. High CO (>8 L/min)
   a. Hypervolemia
   b. Vasodilatation or low systemic vascular resistance (sepsis)
   c. High metabolic rate (hyperthyroid states)

Troubleshooting and nursing interventions (Fig. 33–10)

**VI. Mixed Venous Oxygen Saturation ($S\bar{v}O_2$)**

A. $S\bar{v}O_2$ reflects extent of the body's $O_2$ demands being met by supply
B. $O_2$ supply depends on $PaO_2$ content and the efficiency of CO
C. Critically ill or postoperative patients have increased $O_2$ demands at the cellular level
D. If CO does not increase to compensate for increased $O_2$ demand, increased extraction of $O_2$ at the tissue level results in an $O_2$ imbalance
E. Normal $S\bar{v}O_2$ 60% to 80%
F. Increased $S\bar{v}O_2$ (80% to 95%) reflects decreased demand as a result of hypothermia or sepsis
G. Decreased $S\bar{v}O_2$ (<60%) reflects increased demand as a result of hypotension related to dysrhythmias, fever, pain, seizure, pump failure, hemorrhage, respiratory failure, hypoxia

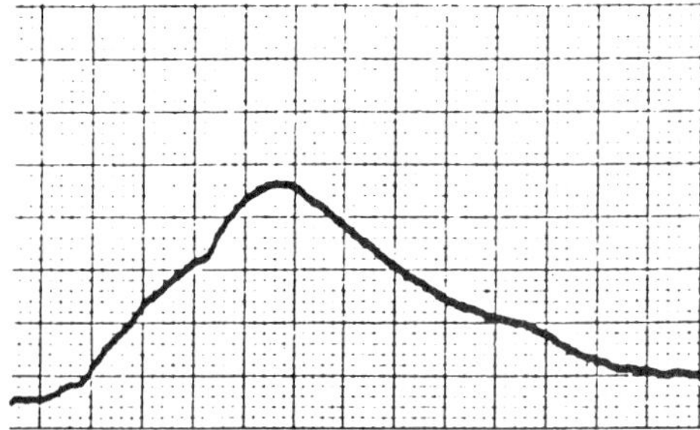
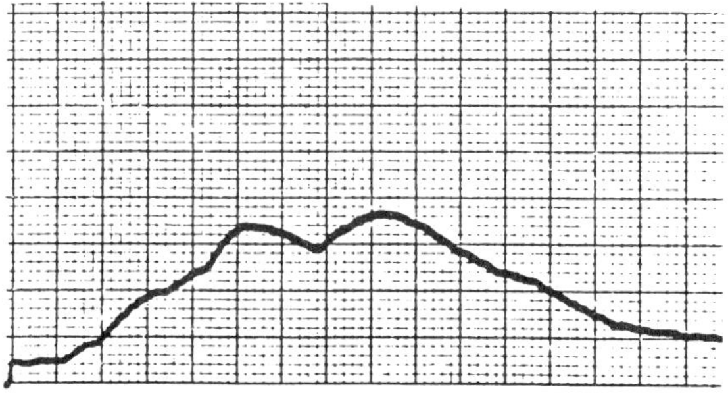

**FIGURE 33–9** **A,** Cardiac output waveform showing good technique. Note steady up slope, high amplitude curve with peak, and uniform descending down slope. **B,** Cardiac output waveform showing poor technique. Note nonsteady up slope, prolonged injection time, and varying curve heights.

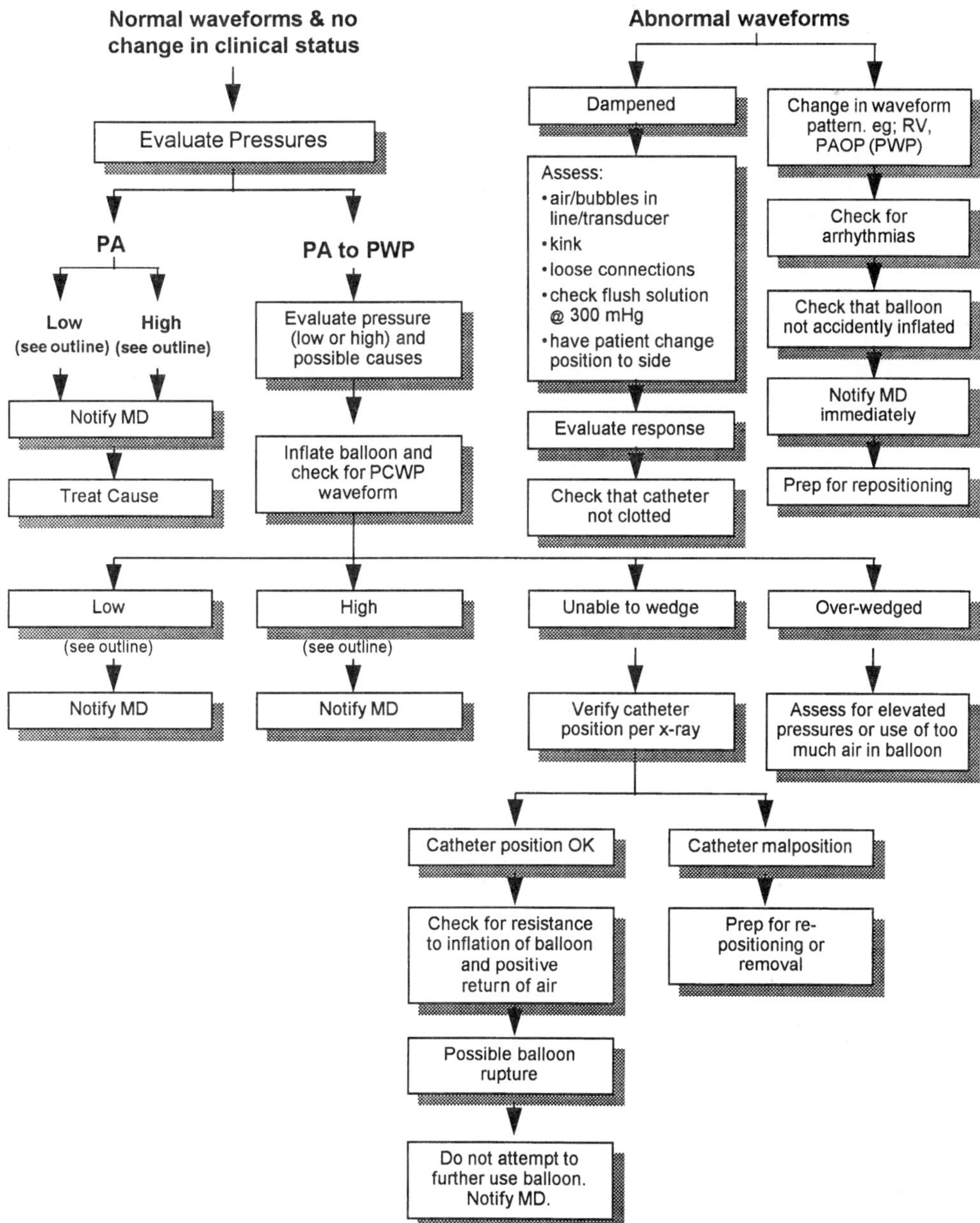


**FIGURE 33–10** Flowchart of troubleshooting and nursing interventions in thermodilution cardiac output.

## BIBLIOGRAPHY


Ahrens T, Taylor L: *Hemodynamic Waveform Analysis.* Philadelphia, WB Saunders, 1992.

Bedford RF: Invasive blood pressure monitoring. In Blitt C (ed): *Monitoring in Anesthesia and Critical Care Medicine* (2nd ed). New York, Churchill Livingstone, 1990.

Biga C, Bethel S: Hemodynamic monitoring in post anesthesia care units. *Crit Care Nurs Clin North Am* 3:83–94, 1991.

Blitt C: A philosophy of monitoring. In Blitt C (ed): *Monitoring in Anesthesia and Critical Care Medicine,* 2nd Ed. New York, Churchill Livingstone, 1990.

DeAngelis R: The cardiovascular system. In Alspach J, Williams S (eds): *Core Curriculum for Critical Care Nursing.* Philadelphia, WB Saunders, 1991.

Debrow M: Arterial pressure monitoring. In Williams S

(ed): *Decision Making in Critical Care Nursing.* Philadelphia, BC Decker, 1990.

Friesinger G, Williams S: Clinical competence in hemodynamic monitoring. *Circulation* 81:2036–2040, 1990.

Groom L, Frisch S, Elliott M: Reproducibility and accuracy of patient pulmonary artery pressure measurement in supine and lateral positions. *Heart Lung* 19:147–151, 1990.

Hines R, Barash P: Pulmonary artery catheterization. In Blitt C (ed): *Monitoring in Anesthesia and Critical Care Medicine,* 2nd Ed, New York, Churchill Livingstone, 1990.

Niehaus D: 1990's: Decade of awakening. *Breathline-ASPAN* 10:1, 1990.

Otto C: Central venous monitoring. In Blitt C (ed): *Monitoring in Anesthesia and Critical Care Medicine,* 2nd Ed. New York, Churchill Livingstone, 1990.

Saeger J, Palmer L: Issues of whether critically ill patients should be transferred directly from OR to ICU. *Breathline-ASPAN* 10:3, 1990.

Stiff JB: Monitoring modalities of the future. In Blitt C (ed): *Monitoring in Anesthesia and Critical Care Medicine,* 2nd Ed. New York, Churchill Livingstone, 1990.

Swan HJC, Ganz W: The Swan-Ganz catheter: Past and present. In Blitt C (ed): *Monitoring in Anesthesia and Critical Care Medicine,* 2nd Ed. New York, Churchill Livingstone, 1990.

## REVIEW QUESTIONS

**1. Preload is defined as:**
A. Arteriolar resistance to left ventricular emptying
B. Venous return to the heart
C. Vascular dilation
D. Stroke volume × Heart rate

**2. Preload is measured by:**
A. Systemic vascular resistance (SVR) and pulmonary vascular resistance (PVR)
B. Cardiac output (CO) and cardiac index (CI)
C. Central venous pressure (CVP) and right arterial pressure (RAP)
D. Central venous pressure (CVP) and pulmonary artery pressure (PAP)

**3. To prevent a pulmonary artery infarction, the balloon tip of a pulmonary artery catheter should be:**
A. Locked in a permanently inflated position
B. Filled only with normal saline
C. Filled with a maximum of 1.5 cc of air for no more than 15 seconds
D. Positioned in the right ventricle and advanced only as necessary

**4. To most accurately determine whether the heart is pumping blood adequately for a particular patient, which measurement should be obtained?**
A. Cardiac index
B. Body surface area
C. Contractility
D. Cardiac output

**5. A $S\bar{v}O_2$ measurement of 90% indicates**
A. Normal value
B. Hyperthermia
C. Sepsis
D. Hemorrhage

**6. The use of sodium nitroprusside will cause a reduction in:**
A. Right atrial pressure
B. Cardiac output
C. Contractility
D. Systemic vascular resistance

**7. The site associated with the greatest risk of infection after arterial line placement is the:**

A. Brachial artery
B. Radial artery
C. Carotid artery
D. Femoral artery

**8. A central venous pressure line may be placed in all of the following vessels except:**

A. Subclavian vein
B. External jugular vein
C. Internal jugular vein
D. Femoral vein

**9. CVP is an indicator of**

A. LVEDP
B. Afterload
C. PAOP
D. Preload

**10. Spinal anesthesia may produce all of the following except:**

A. A fall in central venous pressure
B. A fall in systemic vascular resistance
C. A fall in cardiac output
D. An increase in pulmonary artery occlusion pressure

**ANSWERS:** 1. B, 2. C, 3. C, 4. A, 5. C, 6. D, 7. D, 8. B, 9. D, 10. D

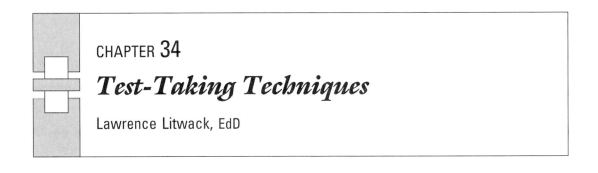

CHAPTER 34

# Test-Taking Techniques

Lawrence Litwack, EdD

## OBJECTIVES

**Study of the information represented in this outline will enable the learner to:**

1. Provide an understanding of the current purpose and structure of the CPAN (certification in perianesthesia nursing) and CAPA (certified ambulatory perianesthesia) examinations.
2. Provide specific test-taking cues to assist examinees preparing to take the CPAN or CAPA examination.
3. Provide examples of test items that illustrate the examinations' format.
4. Assist individuals preparing to take the CPAN and CAPA examinations.

**I. The Examination**

A. Purposes of certification
   1. Demonstration of concern for accountability to the general public for perianesthesia nursing practice
   2. Identification of professional nurses who have demonstrated professional achievement in providing care for patients during the perianesthesia period
   3. Enhancement of quality patient care
   4. Provision of personal satisfaction for the professional nurse
   5. Provision of employing agencies with a means of identifying professional achievement of an individual registered nurse (RN)

B. Background
   1. CPAN examination developed during 1985 and 1986 and first offered in November 1986; CAPA first offered November 1994
   2. Examinations developed by American Board of Perianesthesia Nursing Certification (ABPANC) under guidance of Professional Examination Service (PES), a professional firm that administers the examination
   3. Five-step process in examination development
      a. Role delineation and validation
         (1) Requires analysis or definition of content areas unique to specialty to be tested
         (2) Defines actual tasks, knowledge, and skills used by competent practitioner in performing job specific to an area of practice
         (3) Done by panel of currently practicing perianesthesia nurses representing different perianesthesia settings and major US geographic areas
         (4) Components
            (a) Domains: major areas in which perianesthesia nurse practices
            (b) Tasks: actions performed, recipients of actions, how and why actions are performed
            (c) Knowledge: specified body of information of a factual or procedural nature; includes knowledge of nursing diagnoses
            (d) Skill: proficient manual, verbal, or mental manipulation of data, people, or things; includes data interpretation

b. Validation study
   (1) Content validity: evidence demonstrating that individual examination questions accurately represent defined area of perianesthesia nursing practice
   (2) Done by ratings of each domain furnished by random sample of practicing perianesthesia nurses
c. Item (question writing)
   (1) Only questions ranked high in importance by ABPANC for competent, safe practice were accepted for test question bank
   (2) Items prepared by ABPANC and through mail solicitation from practitioners
d. Examination construction
   (1) ABPANC committee validates questions in each defined area of practice in accordance with the test specifications; direct care given heaviest weighting (degree of importance)

C. Examinations' revisions
   1. Examinations updated yearly by ABPANC
   2. Revisions based on review of need for update to keep up with changing practice in perianesthesia nursing

D. Eligibility
   1. Candidate must hold unrestricted RN licensure in the United States or any of its territories
   2. Candidate must have minimum of 1800 hours practice as RN within last 3 years in care, management, teaching, or research in any phase of perianesthesia care

E. Administration of examinations
   1. Given twice yearly in November and April
   2. Additional test sites possible with minimum of 10 registrants
   3. Special arrangements can be made for candidates with disabilities

F. Examinations' organization
   1. Examination: 200 multiple choice questions
   2. CAPA test blueprint
      a. Direct care (54%): 108 questions
      b. Education (24%): 48 questions
      c. Leadership (22%): 44 questions
   3. CPAN test blueprint
      a. Direct care (80%): 160 questions
      b. Leadership (20%): 40 questions
   4. Examination components of CAPA
      a. Domain I: Direct care
         (1) Collect and document pertinent patient data by interview, consultation, record review, and physical examination to assess the patient's health status and identify patient, family, and companion needs
         (2) Formulate a nursing diagnosis by analyzing collected data and collaborating with the patient, family or companion, and other health care providers to develop a plan of care for each patient
         (3) Develop a plan of care by identifying and prioritizing patient needs, especially as related to the impact of anesthesia, the procedure or surgical intervention, and discharge needs, by identifying available resources to anticipate and prevent potential complications and to establish goals for discharge readiness
         (4) Implement the plan of care by initiating appropriate nursing interventions to prevent complications and prepare the patient and family or companion for the patient's discharge readiness
         (5) Evaluate the results of nursing interventions by assessment of the patient's response to the implemented plan of care to determine the effectiveness of care or the need to modify it accordingly

(6) Provide for continuity of care by communicating the patient's health status and response to the plan of care with the patient, the patient's family or companion, and other health care providers, to facilitate optimum recovery

b. Domain II: Education
   (1) Collect and document pertinent learner characteristics by interview, consultation, record review, and physical examination to assess educational needs of the patient and family or companion
   (2) Formulate a nursing diagnosis by analyzing collected data and by collaborating with the patient, family or companion, and other healthcare providers to develop a teaching plan for each patient and family or companion
   (3) Develop a teaching plan by identifying and prioritizing patient needs to individualize patient and family or companion education
   (4) Provide education to the patient and the patient's family or companion to prepare the patient both physically and emotionally for the potential impact of anesthesia, the procedure or surgical intervention, and the plan of care to assist the patient and family or companion in recognizing and accepting their joint responsibility for the patient's well-being
   (5) Provide education to the patient and the patient's family or companion to prepare the patient both physically and emotionally for the consequences of anesthesia, the procedure or surgical intervention, and the plan of care to assist the patient and family or companion in recognizing and accepting their joint responsibilities for the patient's predischarge and postdischarge care
   (6) Evaluate the results of the teaching provided by assessing the comprehension of the information by the patient and family or companion to determine the effectiveness of the teaching or the need to modify it accordingly

c. Domain III: Leadership
   (1) Participate in the development, implementation, and evaluation of standards and projected outcomes of patient care by utilizing available resources to promote the highest quality of patient care
   (2) Use available resources within the organization framework to provide for an environment conducive to the highest quality of patient care
   (3) Maintain competence by seeking and sharing information pertinent to ambulatory surgery nursing to promote the highest quality of patient care

5. Examination components of CPAN
   a. Domain I: Direct care
      (1) Collect and communicate pertinent patient data (including but not limited to consultation, record review, and physical examination) to assess the patient's health status and identify patient problems
      (2) Formulate and communicate a nursing diagnosis by analyzing collected data and by collaborating, when appropriate, with the health-care team and the patient's family/significant others to develop a plan of care for each patient
      (3) Develop and communicate a plan of care by identifying and prioritizing patient needs and by identifying available resources to establish short- and long-term goals
      (4) Implement and communicate the plan of care by initiating appropriate nursing interventions to assist the patient's return to optimal health status
      (5) Evaluate and communicate the results of nursing interventions by ongoing patient assessment and the application of total quality management principles or research protocols to ensure the quality of patient care
   b. Domain II: Leadership
      (1) Contribute to the development, implementation, and evaluation of patient care standards and outcomes by research and total quality management (TQM) to ensure consistent quality care

(2) Collaborate in the management of the patient care environment by utilizing available resources to ensure consistent quality care
(3) Promote sharing of knowledge by use of available resources to advance the practice of perianesthesia nursing

6. Role delineation of expected knowledge
    a. Information sources and retrieval mechanisms
    b. Normal diagnostic values
    c. Anatomy, physiology, and pathophysiology of body systems
    d. Surgical and procedural interventions; anesthesia techniques
    e. Pharmacology and drug interactions (know generics)
    f. Medical terminology
    g. Documentation techniques and requirements
    h. Risk factors
    i. Physical, psychosocial, and cognitive assessment
    j. Perioperative or periprocedural process
    k. Nursing diagnosis, terminology, and process
    l. Scope of nursing practice
    m. Appropriate interventions; available resources
    n. Discharge planning
    o. Potential complications
    p. Psychological support
    q. Diagnostic and therapeutic technology
    r. Acceptable deviations from normal
    s. Prevailing nurse practice act and standards of nursing practice
    t. Organization governance
    u. Patient's bill of rights
    v. Ethical guidelines of professional practice
    w. Licensure and credentialing requirements; regulatory agencies and their guidelines
    x. Teaching, research, and evaluation methods
    y. Quality assurance and risk management
    z. Change theory
7. Role delineation of expected skills
    a. Interviewing
    b. Verbal and written communication
    c. Assessment
    d. Data interpretation
    e. Critical thinking
    f. Setting priorities
    g. Clinical and technologic nursing
    h. Evaluation
    i. Networking
    j. Written policy and procedures
    k. Management

G. Examination format
    1. 4 hours
    2. 200 multiple-choice questions with four choices for each question

H. Determining readiness to take examination
    1. Obtain application from Professional Examination Service, 475 Riverside Drive, New York, NY 10115-0089
    2. Read application carefully for requirements and deadlines
    3. Meet eligibility requirements
    4. Register to take test; requests for CPAN and CAPA certification application should be

made at least 6 months before examination date because of examination registration deadlines, which are 7 to 9 weeks before test date

5. Use practice guide to diagnose areas needing study
6. Consider taking review course or workshop
7. Use review text and materials
   a. Do not rely solely on any *one* source to study
   b. Use multiple sources, including *Journal of Perianesthesia Nursing*, perianesthesia and ambulatory surgical nursing texts, physiology texts, current *ASPAN Standards of Perianesthesia Nursing Practice*

I. After examination
   1. Report of results usually takes 5 weeks
   2. Passing information (CPAN and CAPA)
      a. Pass rate averages approximately 75%
   3. Examination may be retaken if necessary; no limit on number of times
   4. Nurses who successfully pass the examination are able to use the title CPAN or CAPA during 3-year certification period

## II. Multiple-Choice Examinations

A. Format
   1. Multiple-choice question consists of two parts
      a. The stem: usually in form of question or incomplete statement
      b. The responses: several alternatives that are possible answers to question or conclusions for incomplete statement in stem
   2. Types of items
      a. One best answer type
         (1) Consists of stem that is either question or incomplete statement
         (2) Stem followed by four choices, one of which is correct answer
         (3) Select best or most appropriate choice; example:

            *The most common cause of postoperative hypoxemia is:*
            A. Aspiration
            B. Pneumothorax
            C. Atelectasis
            D. Pulmonary edema

            Answer: C

      b. One best answer: negative stem type
         (1) Requires switch from positive to negative thinking
         (2) Stem will include words *except, not,* or *least*
         (3) Consists of stem that is question or incomplete statement
         (4) Stem followed by four choices, one of which is wrong, most inappropriate, or least likely; example:

            *Infants aged 3 to 24 months who are separated from their mothers and a secure environment for a long period are least likely to show:*
            A. Apathy and withdrawal
            B. Compulsive interest in food
            C. Inability to give and receive attention
            D. Retardation in skeletal growth

            Answer: B

      c. One best answer: case history type
         (1) Consists of brief description of patient or problem situation followed by two or more questions related to patient or problem

(2) Case history may include any or all of the following types of information
   (a) Patient history
   (b) Signs and symptoms
   (c) Laboratory findings
   (d) Diagnosis
   (e) Treatment
(3) Example (questions 1–3):

A 14-year-old girl is admitted to the postanesthesia care unit (PACU) after a posterior spinal fusion for scoliosis. Her only medical history is juvenile-onset diabetes. Anesthesia was general, and the operating room course was unremarkable. One hour after admission she is still unresponsive to verbal and tactile stimuli.

1. *Possible causes of the delayed awakening may include all of the following except:*
   A. Prolonged drug effects
   B. Hypothermia
   C. Her young age
   D. Hypoglycemia

   Answer: C

2. *When a diabetic patient undergoes surgery, the most important goal of care is:*
   A. Prevention of hyperglycemia
   B. Administration of insulin preoperatively
   C. Monitoring of blood glucose levels
   D. Prevention of hypoglycemia

   Answer: D

3. *Priorities of care for this patient include:*
   A. Neurologic and respiratory assessment
   B. Cardiovascular and metabolic assessment
   C. Orthopedic and neurologic assessment
   D. Orthopedic and respiratory assessment

   Answer: A

B. Test-taking techniques
   1. Read directions carefully
   2. Review answer sheet; complete requested information carefully and accurately
   3. Be careful to record each answer beside correct number on answer sheet
   4. Because there is no penalty for guessing, answer every question
   5. Allow approximately 1 minute per question; if stuck, leave blank for the moment and go on to the next one
      a. *If skipping an item, make sure to skip a space on answer sheet so that correct answer is placed with correct number*
   6. Look at stem to see what the emphasis is; which answer emphasizes same thing?
   7. Identify key words or phrases in both stem and answers; circling key words or phrases on test booklet will help to focus your attention
   8. Can write on test booklet; do not make any stray marks on answer sheet
   9. Read all choices, even if you think first or second choice is correct
   10. Evaluate each choice as true or false
      a. One best answer type
         (1) As you read stem, underline or circle words or phrases that seem important

(2) As you read alternatives, circle or underline words or phrases that are repeated in two or more alternatives; this will help to focus
(3) Read each alternative and make your best judgment as to whether you believe it is true or false
(4) Select one true, best, or most appropriate answer; example:

*The benzodiazepine with the longest half-life is:*
(F) A. Midazolam
(T) B. Diazepam
(F) C. Lorazepam
(F) D. Flumazenil

Answer: B

b. One best answer: negative stem type
(1) Circle or underline negative word in stem
(2) Omit negative word; read each alternative and make your best judgment as to whether you believe it is true or false
(3) Select one false or least appropriate answer; example:

*Risk factors for pulmonary embolism include all of the following except:*
(T) A. Immobility
(T) B. Malignancy
(F) C. Anticoagulation
(T) D. Obesity

Answer: C

11. Do not read into a question information or interpretations that are not there; take question as it is
12. If two answers overlap or mean the same, both are probably incorrect if there is only one correct alternative
13. Your first response is usually best; do not change it unless you have a logical, definite reason for doing so
14. Concentrate on basic principles; examination is given nationally so that questions will not be specific to your state or clinical facility
15. Look for key indicators (all, none, always, good, bad, except, should, first, must, only, never, usually, most often, no, is not, some, sometimes, chief, one, greatest, least, few, seldom, many, frequent)
    a. Absolute statements (all, none, always, never, good, bad, is, is not, only) are usually false or incorrect
    b. Generalizations are usually only partially true
    c. Relative statements are more likely to be true
    d. Qualifiers (most, some, usually, sometimes) are more likely to be true
    e. The broader the statement, the greater the likelihood it is untrue
16. If one answer is much longer or shorter than all others, it is more likely to be correct answer
17. If one answer has more parts, it is more likely to be correct
18. Select answer that is reasonable or attainable under ordinary circumstances
19. If asked for immediate or prioritized action, base selection on professionally identified priorities
20. Answers that are exceptions to the general rule or that are controversial are likely to be false
21. Do not look for pattern to answers; correct answers are usually arranged randomly

C. General guidelines
1. It is sensible to review before taking test; concentrate on major areas and general

principles; examination covers a large body of knowledge; planning and calculation of study hours should be done well in advance
2. Evaluate areas reflected on the examination that you do not do on a day-to-day basis, and brush up on the areas with which you are least familiar
3. It is useless to attempt to cram the night before test
4. It is better to relax, do something different the night before test, and get a good night's sleep
5. Eat a good breakfast that morning
6. Allow sufficient time to get to examination; call in advance for directions if necessary; be on time; be prepared (lots of no. 2 pencils, eraser, admission card, photo identification); dress comfortably—bring a sweater or dress in layers to allow for warm or cool room
7. Arrive with positive attitude; avoid participating in last minute, self-defeating, worry-focused conversations with fellow test takers; even if you do not pass, it will be a valuable learning experience

## BIBLIOGRAPHY


American Board of PeriAnesthesia Nursing Certification: *Certification Handbook & Application.* New York, Professional Examination Service, 1998.

American Society of PeriAnesthesia Nurses, *Standards of Perianesthesia Nursing Practice.* Thorofare, NJ, The Society, 1995.

Corsico, RJ: Developing a valid certification program. *J Post Anesth Nurs* 3(6):379–382, 1988.

Litwack, L, Linc L, Bower D: *Evaluation in Nursing: Principles and Practice.* New York, National League for Nursing, 1985.

Mullen CA: Strategies for Success: Preparing for the Certification Examination, *J Peri Anesth Nurs* 11(5):324–329, 1996.

Nugent PM, Vitale BA: *Test Success: Test-Taking Techniques for Beginning Nursing Students,* 2nd Ed. Philadelphia, FA Davis, 1997.

Role Delineation Validation Study for the Ambulatory Surgery Nurse Certification Program. *American Board of PeriAnesthesia Nursing Certification.* New York, Professional Examination Service, 1997.

Sides MB, Korchek N: *Nurse's Guide to Successful Test-Taking* (pp 29–76). Philadelphia, Lippincott, 1994.


For additional information, contact:

ABPANC
475 Riverside Ave, 7th Floor
New York, NY 10715-0089
(800) 622-7262
FAX (212) 367-4256

## REVIEW QUESTIONS

**1. Which one of the following is not a purpose of certification?**

A. To demonstrate concern for accountability for safe practice
B. To provide advanced credentialing for nurses
C. To enhance quality patient care
D. To provide employers with a means of identifying professional achievement of RNs

**2. The process of examination development includes all of the following steps except:**

A. Role delineation
B. Item writing
C. Passing point determination
D. Selection of examiners

**3. Which of the following is not a domain of practice addressed on the CAPA examination?**

A. Direct care
B. Education
C. Research
D. Leadership

**4. The eligibility requirements for the CPAN and CAPA examination include all of the following except:**

A. At least 10 years' experience as an RN in direct care
B. Must be licensed RN in the United States or its territories
C. Must have at least 1800 hours of practice in perianesthesia nursing within last 3 years
D. Practice may be in care, management, teaching, and/or research

**ANSWERS:** 1. B, 2. D, 3. C, 4. A

# *Index*

Note: Page numbers in *italics* refer to illustrations; page numbers followed by t refer to tables.

## C

**I**

## J



## K



## L

**O**

## Q



## R

## U